Symptoms and Neuropathological Mechanisms of Psychiatric Disorders

Symptoms and Neuropathological Mechanisms of Psychiatric Disorders

Editor: Harvey Wilson

hayle medical

New York

Hayle Medical,
750 Third Avenue, 9th Floor,
New York, NY 10017, USA

Visit us on the World Wide Web at:
www.haylemedical.com

ISBN 978-1-64647-587-2 (Hardback)

Cataloging-in-Publication Data

Symptoms and neuropathological mechanisms of psychiatric disorders / edited by Harvey Wilson.
p. cm.
Includes bibliographical references and index.
ISBN 978-1-64647-587-2
1. Psychology, Pathological. 2. Psychiatry. 3. Mental illness. 4. Neuropsychology. 5. Neuropsychiatry. I. Wilson, Harvey.
RC435 .S96 2023
616.89--dc23

Contents

Preface

Psychiatric disorder refers to a behavioral or mental pattern, which causes significant distress or impairment of personal functioning. These features can be remitting, persistent and relapsing or may happen as single episodes. Some of the prominent symptoms of psychiatric disorders are excessive fear and worry, poor concentration, feelings of excessive guilt or low self-worth, and alternating depressive episodes with periods of manic symptoms. The area of medicine which studies the nervous system tissues in order to diagnose diseases is known as neuropathology. Organic brain diseases and degenerative diseases exhibit clear morphological and neurohistological abnormalities, and can be efficiently studied within the domain of neuropathology. However, psychiatric illnesses generally do not manifest homogenous brain pathology, and research is ongoing in studying the neuropathological mechanisms of psychiatric disorders. This book presents the symptoms and neuropathological mechanisms of psychiatric disorders. It presents researches and studies performed by experts across the globe. The extensive content of this book provides the readers with a thorough understanding of the subject.

This book is the end result of constructive efforts and intensive research done by experts in this field. The aim of this book is to enlighten the readers with recent information in this area of research. The information provided in this profound book would serve as a valuable reference to students and researchers in this field.

At the end, I would like to thank all the authors for devoting their precious time and providing their valuable contribution to this book. I would also like to express my gratitude to my fellow colleagues who encouraged me throughout the process.

Editor

1

Altered Regional Cerebral Blood Flow of Right Cerebellum Posterior Lobe in Asthmatic Patients with or without Depressive Symptoms

*Yuqun Zhang [1,2], Yuan Yang [3], Ze Wang [4], Rongrong Bian [1,2], Wenhao Jiang [1,2], Yingying Yin [1,2], Yingying Yue [1,2], Zhenghua Hou [1,2] and Yonggui Yuan [1,2]**

[1] Department of Psychosomatics and Psychiatry, ZhongDa Hospital, School of Medicine, Southeast University, Nanjing, China, [2] Institute of Psychosomatics, School of Medicine, Southeast University, Nanjing, China, [3] Department of Respiration, ZhongDa Hospital, Southeast University, Nanjing, China, [4] Center for Cognition and Brain Disorders and the Affiliated Hospital, Hangzhou Normal University, Hangzhou, China

***Correspondence:**
Yonggui Yuan
yygylh2000@sina.com

Background: Asthma is a chronic disease appeared to be associated with depression. But the underpinnings of depression in asthma remain unknown. In order to understand the neural mechanisms of depression in asthma, we used cerebral blood flow (CBF) to probe the difference between depressed asthmatic (DA) and non-depressed asthmatic (NDA) patients.

Methods: Eighteen DA patients, 24 NDA patients and 57 healthy controls (HC) received pulsed arterial spin labeling (pASL) scan for measuring CBF, resting-state functional magnetic resonance imaging (rs-fMRI) scan, severity of depression and asthma control assessment, respectively.

Results: Compared to NDA, DA patients showed increased regional CBF (rCBF) in the right cerebellum posterior lobe. Compared to HC, DA, and NDA patients all showed significantly decreased rCBF in the right cerebellum posterior lobe.

Conclusions: We showed the first evidence of altered rCBF in the right cerebellum posterior lobe in asthma using pASL, which appeared to be involved in the neuropathology in asthma.

Clinical Trial Registration: An investigation of therapeutic mechanism in asthmatic patients: based on the results of Group Cognitive Behavioral Therapy (Registration number: ChiCTR-COC-15007442) (http://www.chictr.org.cn/usercenter.aspx).

Keywords: depression, asthma, cerebral blood flow, pulsed arterial spin labeling, cerebellum

INTRODUCTION

Asthma was a chronic inflammatory condition that swelled and narrowed the airways, leading to dyspnea, coughing, and tightening of the chest. To et al. (1) showed the global prevalence rates of doctor-diagnosed asthma, clinical/treated asthma and wheezing in adults were 4.3, 4.5, and 8.6% respectively, and varied by as much as 21-fold amongst the 70 countries. Ding et al. (2) assessed the population of asthma in urban China with data from 2010 to 2013 in China National Health and Wellness Survey and reported that the prevalence of asthma was 30.73%. Several epidemiology studies consistently documented that depression was prevalent in patients with asthma, and was associated with uncontrolled asthma and poor quality of life (3–5).

Over the past decades, functional magnetic response imaging (fMRI) proved itself a useful technique to detect and quantitate sites of activation in the brain and to map circuits that might be associated with or involved in the underpinnings of emotion in asthma. Rosenkranz et al. (6–8) explored the neural circuitry underlying the interaction between emotion and asthma symptoms used task fMRI, the findings consistently indicated that neurophenotypes of asthma might be identified by neural activity of brain circuits previously implicated in emotion regulation, especially the insula and anterior cingulate cortex (ACC). In addition, dyspnea shared emotion-related brain network also has been suggested, including the insula, ACC, amygdala and medial thalamus (9). On the basis of previous studies, Busse (10) summarized minutely how was the central nervous system involved in allergic airway response in asthma and how this related to stress. This review emphasized the important role of emotion-related neural networks in asthma attack and maintenance processing. Subsequently, neural circuits turned to be a critical joint linked asthma and emotion. However, previous research predominantly focused on the neurobiological mechanisms of fear and anxiety in asthma, a better understanding of the biological pathogenesis of depression was required.

Increasing evidence revealed abnormal glucose metabolism and cerebral blood flow (CBF) of certain brain regions in depressed patients, such as hippocampus (11), right prefrontal and (12, 13) and striatal regions (12). In patients with chronic obstructive pulmonary disease (COPD), Yildiz et al. (14) reported increased CBF at rest because cerebral autoregulation-mediated vasodilatation to overcome COPD exacerbation induced hypoxia. Enhanced CBF appeared when healthy subjects experiencing hypoxia and hypercapnia (15), which might be explained by the tendency of upregulating $PaCO_2$, a potent cerebral vasodilator (16). Considering abnormal ventilation of asthmatic patients, the aberrant $PaCO_2$ level might also exist in certain brain regions. Unfortunately, studies exploring CBF in depressed asthmatic (DA) patients were not found, although the abnormalities were identified in both depression (11) and asthmatic (17) patients separately. Here, we adopted a method of arterial spin labeling (ASL) perfusion magnetic resonance imaging (MRI) which is a technique for quantifying regional brain perfusion and requiring no radioactive source or contrast agent (18), to investigate the regional CBF (rCBF) in asthmatic patients. ASL perfusion MRI renders the interpretation of quantitative measurements of the rCBF, a physiological parameter, easier than the assessment of the blood-oxygen-level-dependent (BOLD) effect at resting state (13, 19). Pulsed ASL (pASL) uses a short radio frequency pulse to invert the blood water spins in a very short time and provides signal-to-noise ratio as well as increased physiological noise (20).

To the current study's best knowledge, the pattern of rCBF changes in DA patients has not been characterized by pASL studies. So, a data-driven analysis was chosen to study the data according to the complexity and multidimensional causes of DA together with variability between individuals. We identified regions of interest (ROI) with abnormal rCBF between DA and non-depressed asthmatic (NDA), healthy controls (HC) groups. ROIs were then used as seeds to find out the rCBF alterations in DA patients and provided evidence for exploring the mechanism of depression in asthma.

MATERIALS AND METHODS

Participants and Evaluations

According to the scores of 17 items Hamilton depression rating scale (HDRS-17), asthmatic patients were divided into DA (HDRS-17 $\geq$ 7) and NDA (HDRS-17 $<$ 7) group. As shown in **Figure 1** (a flow diagram) and **Table 1** (listing demographic data), 18 DA patients (mean age was 53.61 years, 9 males and 9 females), 24 NDA patients (mean age was 50.58 years, 9 males and 15 females) and 57 HC (mean age was 45.63 years, 23 males and 34 females) participated in this study after attrition and data cleaning. HDRS-17 was used to assess the depression of all participants. The asthma control test (ACT) is a self-rating scale and used to measure asthma control level in asthmatic patients. This study was carried out in accordance with the recommendations of the ethics committee of Zhongda Hospital with written informed consent from all subjects. All subjects gave written informed consent in accordance with the Declaration of Helsinki. The protocol was approved by the ethics committee of Zhongda Hospital, Southeast University.

Inclusion/Exclusion Criteria

Participants who met the following criteria entered asthma group: (1) met the diagnostic criteria of bronchial asthma and during non-acute attacks; (2) 18 years old or above; (3) right handedness; (4) education to junior high school or above; (5) there is no electronic and metal equipment in body (such as cardiac pacemaker, defibrillator, stent, et al.); (6) participants sign the informed consent form. Inclusion criteria of HC: HDRS-17 $<$ 7 and the above item (2) $\sim$ (6) in the inclusion criteria of asthmatic patients.

Participants with one of following items were excluded: (1) other serious disease of the respiratory system; (2) history of other mental disorders, alcohol, and drug dependence; (3) organic brain disorders and cardio, hepar, kidney abnormality; (5) women during pregnancy or lactation.

Brain Image Acquisition

Imaging was performed on a 3-Tesla Siemens Magnetom Symphony scanner using a homogeneous birdcage head coil. Subjects laid supine with the head snugly fixed by a belt and foam pads to minimize head motion. High-resolution 3-dimensional T1-weighted scans were performed using the Siemens product magnetization prepared rapid gradient echo (MPRAGE) sequence [repetition time (TR) = 1,900 ms, echo time (TE) = 2.48 ms; flip angle (FA) = 9°; acquisition matrix = 256 × 256; field of view (FOV) = 250 × 250 mm^2; thickness = 1.0 mm, gap = 0; time = 4 min 18 s]. ASL perfusion MRI was performed using the Siemens product pASL PICORE

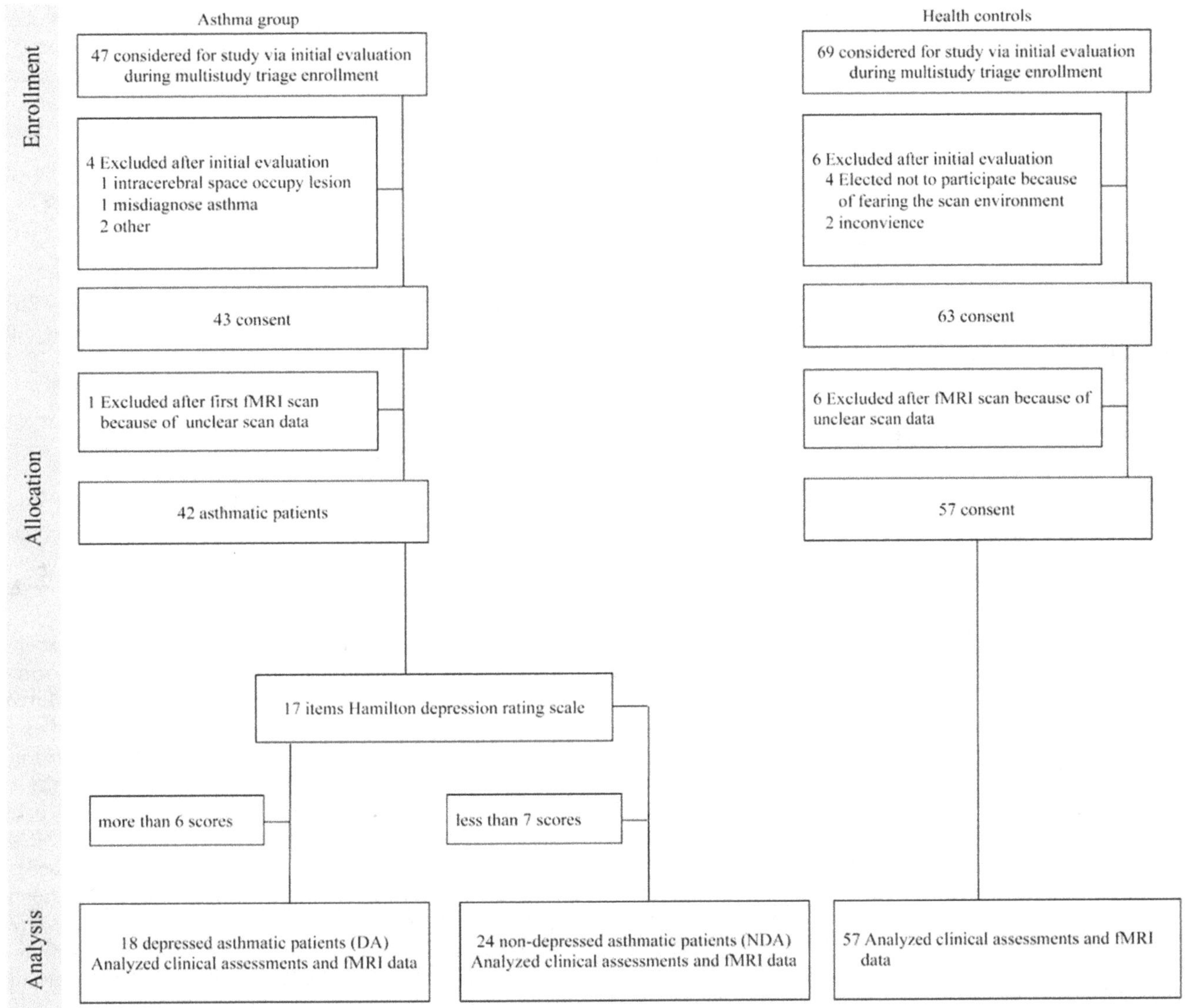

FIGURE 1 | Flow diagram. fMRI indicated functional magnetic resonance imaging.

Q2T sequence (TR = 4,000 ms, TE = 12 ms; TI1 = 600 ms, TI2 = 1,600 ms; FA = 90°; maxtrix = 64 × 64; FOV = 220 × 220 mm^2; 27 axial slices; thickness = 4 mm; gap = 1 mm, total scan time = 7 min 14 s).

Preprocessing Protocol

All the image data were reconstructed and inspected by two experienced radiologists. T1 images were manually checked for quality controls. pASL data were processed using SPM12 (http://www.fil.ion.ucl.ac.uk/spm) and ASLtbx (21). To avoid the spurious motion artifacts due to the systematic labeling and non-labeling in ASL, motion corrections were performed using the amended motion correction algorithm implemented in ASLtbx (21, 22). The raw ASL images were then high pass filtered to keep the higher half frequency band. The pASL images were then co-registered to the T1 images and spatially smoothed with a 6 mm full-width-half-maximum (FWHM) kernel, followed by pairwise control/label image subtraction and CBF quantification. After rejecting the outlier CBF volumes using the prior-guided adaptive outlier cleaning algorithm, mean CBF map was created from the remaining CBF volumes and were registered into the MNI space using the transformation obtained through the structural image.

Statistical Analysis

Predictive Analytic Software (PASW) Statistics 18 package was employed (IBM Corporation, Armonk, NY, USA) to complete the analyses. Age, education, and HDRS-17 scores were performed by one-way analysis of variance (ANOVA). Gender was compared by means of the Chi-square test. Duration of illness and ACT scores were analyzed by independent sample t-test. $P < 0.05$ were considered to indicate statistical significance.

CBF comparisons were processed with REST software (23). Statistical tests across groups were performed using a voxel-based, one-way analysis of covariance (ANCOVA), with age, gender and education level as covariates, followed by *post-hoc* two-sample t-tests. AlphaSim correction based on Monte Carlo simulation algorithm was used to correct for multiple comparisons [single voxel P value = 0.025, FWHM = 6 mm, with 61 × 73 × 61 mm^3 gray matter mask, which yielded a corrected threshold of $P < 0.025$, cluster size > 2025 mm^3/75 voxels (http://afni.nimh.nih.gov/pub/dist/doc/manual/AlphaSim.pdf)]. The *post-hoc* two-sample t-tests were conducted within a mask showing significant differences obtained from the ANCOVA analysis, with AlphaSim corrections (single voxel P-value = 0.025, FWHM = 6 mm, which yielded a corrected threshold of $P < 0.025$, cluster size > 162 mm^3/6 voxels).

Brain regions were selected as ROI only when they were exhibiting significant differences both between the DA and NDA groups and between DA and HC groups. Mean CBF values were extracted within each of these ROIs, then Pearson correlation coefficients were computed between the extracted CBF values within these ROIs and the clinical assessments of DA patients by PASW 18.0, and the significance level was set at $P < 0.05$ (two-tailed).

RESULTS

Demographic and Clinical Data

Table 1 showed the demographic and clinical variables. No significant differences in participants' gender, education, and durations of asthma were found between groups. The age of DA was significantly elder than HC ($P < 0.05$). It would be a covariate in the following statistical analysis of CBF. There was a significant difference in HDRS-17 scores among the three groups ($P < 0.001$). And the ACT scores were significantly different between DA and NDA group ($P < 0.01$).

Group Differences of CBF

As displayed in **Table 2** and **Figure 2**, the DA patients showed increased rCBF in the right cerebellum posterior lobe (CPL) compared than in NDA patients. In addition, DA patients exhibited lower rCBF in the right CPL compared with HC. Significantly decreased CBF value was also observed in the right CPL in the NDA group relative to HC.

Correlations Between CBF Values and Clinical Assessments

The present study used partial correlation analysis to explore the relationships between mean CBF values in the right CPL and two scales (HDRS-17 and ACT). It revealed that no significant correlations were found between CBF values and HDRS-17, ACT scores respectively either in DA or NDA group.

DISCUSSIONS

To our knowledge, this study at the first time used pASL method to explore the relationship between altered rCBF and depression in asthmatic patients. DA patients exhibited increased CBF values in the right CPL compared with NDA patients, and reversed result compared with HC.

Stoodley and Schmahmann (24) highlighted the widely functions of cerebellum, which included sensorimotor control, language, spatial, and executive functions. Moreover, positron emission tomography (PET) and fMRI studies have demonstrated that cerebellar activation was also involved in the emotional processing paradigms (24, 25), especially the right CPL (26, 27). It further supported our finding that DA patients showed increased rCBF in the right CPL compared with NDA. In patients with late-onset depression, the excessive cerebellar FC with medial prefrontal lobe displayed significant correlation with depression symptoms (28). Su et al. (29) summarized the cerebral metabolism of depression patients based on PET, suggesting that altered metabolism in cerebellum is likely to play a key role in

TABLE 1 | Demographics and clinical characteristics of participants.

	DA (n = 18)	NDA (n = 24)	HC (n = 57)	*P-value*
Age (years)	53.61 ± 9.08*	50.58 ± 10.57	45.63 ± 14.70	0.05[a]
Gender (male/female)	9/9	9/15	23/34	0.723[b]
Education (years)	11.89 ± 2.56	11.75 ± 2.64	12.42 ± 3.60	0.643[a]
Duration of asthma (years)	22.86 ± 20.19	21.41 ± 19.27	–	0.815[c]
HDRS-17 scores	11.06 ± 4.40**††	2.21 ± 1.47#	0.89 ± 1.35	<0.001[a]
ACT scores	15.00 ± 4.38	19.58 ± 4.31	–	0.002[c]

Data are expressed as mean ± standard deviation. [a]One-way ANOVA; [b]Chi-square test; [c]Independent-sample t-test.

*DA vs. HC, *P < 0.05, **P < 0.001; DA vs. NDA, ††P<0.001; NDA vs. HC, #P<0.05. DA, depressed asthma; NDA, non-depressed asthma; HC, healthy controls; HDRS-17, 17 items Hamilton Depression Rating Scale; ACT, asthma control test.*

TABLE 2 | Regions showing significant differences in rCBF between groups.

Peak area	Side	MNI coordinates X	Y	Z	Voxels	Peak t-value
ANCOVA						
Cerebellum posterior lobe	R	21	−51	−48	90	6.5089
DA-NDA						
Cerebellum posterior lobe	R	18	−51	−45	20	3.5013
DA-HC						
Cerebellum posterior lobe	R	42	−48	−51	12	−3.6889
NDA-HC						
Cerebellum posterior lobe	R	21	−51	−48	78	−3.4643

ANCOVA, threshold was set at P < 0.025 (AlphaSim-corrected, cluster size > 2,025 mm^3 voxels); Two-sample t-test, threshold was also set at P < 0.025 (AlphaSim-corrected, cluster size > 162 mm^3 voxels). X, Y, Z, coordinates of primary peak locations in the MNI space. rCBF, regional cerebral blood flow; MNI, Montreal Neurological Institute space; BA, Brodmann area; R, right; ANCOVA, analysis of covariance; DA, depressed asthma; NDA, non-depressed asthma; HC, healthy controls.

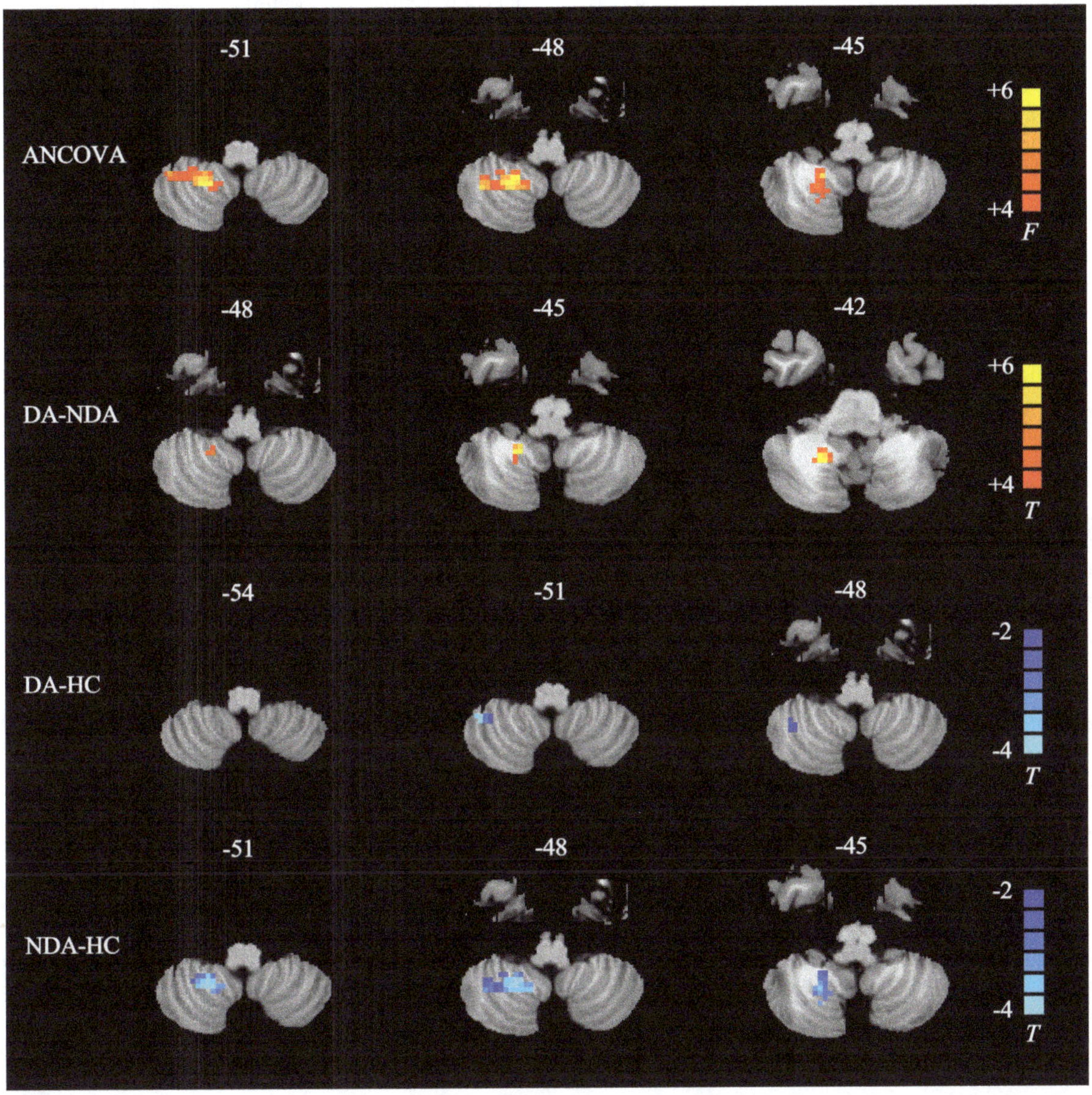

FIGURE 2 | Statistical maps showing rCBF differences in different brain regions between DA, NDA, and HC groups. ANCOVA, significantly increased in rCBF among DA, NDA and HC groups ($P < 0.025$, AlphaSim corrected); Higher rCBF was in the right cerebellum posterior lobe; the red color bar indicates the *F*-value from ANCOVA among three groups. DA-NDA, significantly increased in rCBF of DA patients compared with NDA patients ($P < 0.025$, AlphaSim corrected); the DA patients showed higher CBF in the right cerebellum posterior lobe; the red color bar indicates the t value from independent sample *t*-test between DA and NDA groups. DA-HC, significantly decreased in rCBF of DA patients compared with HC ($P < 0.025$, AlphaSim corrected); the DA patients showed lower rCBF in the right cerebellum posterior lobe; the blue color bar indicates the t value from independent sample *t*-test between DA and HC groups. NDA-HC, significantly decreased in rCBF of NDA patients compared with HC patients ($P < 0.025$, AlphaSim corrected); the NDA patients showed lower rCBF in the right cerebellum posterior lobe; the blue color bar indicates the t value from independent sample *t*-test between NDA and HC groups. ANCOVA, analysis of covariance; DA, depressed asthma; NDA, non-depressed asthma; HC, healthy controls.

the pathophysiology of depression. Several metabolism-related investigations suggested that the MDD patients exhibited enhanced metabolism in the right CPL (29–31). The previous study also reported decreased CBF in the cerebellum in patients with depression disorder (32), however the similar finding was not found in DA patients. Thus, the increased rCBF in the right CPL might be associated with the depression in asthmatic patients. However, in the current study, DA and NDA patients displayed decreased rCBF in the right CPL compared with HCs. We deduced that it might be influenced by other factors such as cognitive function (24).

Stoodley et al. (24, 33–36) made a series of studies to explore the function of human cerebellum through neuroimaging. Their findings demonstrated that the posterior lobe was also involved in higher-level tasks, including language and verbal working memory, spatial tasks, executive function besides emotional processing, especially the region of lobule VI which was reported in our study. For asthmatic patients, they followed doctors' recommendations less frequently, subsequently led to a vicious circle (37). However, underlying this were serious cognitive dysfunctions which contributed to difficulties in understanding given advice and putting it into practice (37, 38). In contrast, Ray et al. (39) reported that poor asthma control and airway obstruction were not associated with poor performance on various measures of cognitive function in older adults with asthma. Although limited research presented inconsistent results, cognitive dysfunction existed in asthmatic patients was consistent approbation. Unfortunately, we did not explore the relationship between asthma and cognitive function in the current study, research focusing on the related issues needed to be investigated in the future.

Evidence of aberrant activities in ACC and insula were often discovered whatever in emotion disorders or asthma (7–9, 40, 41). von Leupoldt et al. (9, 40, 42) explored a series studies of dyspnea in asthmatic patients and healthy participants used task fMRI. Their findings suggested that emotion-related brain regions including ACC and insula showed abnormal BOLD signal while experiencing dyspnea from mild to severe. However, both regions did not exhibit dysfunctions used the method of pASL in the current study. We detected that methodological differences (task vs. resting state and BOLD vs. pASL) would be the main possible reasons for the lack of ACC and insula dysfunctions in our study.

Significantly correlations between CBF values of the right CPL and HDRS-17 scores were not found whatever in DA or NDA group in the current study. A regional cerebral metabolism study suggested that different depressive symptom clusters might have different neural structures in unipolar depression, and depression symptom clusters predominantly correlated with the cerebral metabolism in right insula, temporal cortex, and ACC (43). CPL was a critical node possessed various functions (24), the insignificant correlation between the CBF values and HDRS-17 scores might be influenced by other confused factors (e.g., aberrant ventilation, cognitive function). It suggested that the altered rCBF in the right CPL might independent of depression severity and asthma control.

There are some limitations to our study. First, since the current study mainly focused on the differences of rCBF between asthmatic patients with and without depression, we adopted only HDRS-17 and ACT for the evaluation of depressive- and asthma control- level in participants. More cognitive-related tests were required to adequately describe patients cognitive profile, and to confirmed the speculations that the abnormal rCBF in right CPL might reflect impaired cognitive function in asthmatic patients. Second, our study involved a relatively small sample, and the number of the subjects in the three groups did not match perfectly. To control for the effects of the differences in age among the three groups, this variable was considered as covariates and regressed out in the statistical analysis.

In summary, this was the first study to explore the potential mechanism of depression in asthma using pASL. The findings demonstrated that the increased rCBF in the right CPL would be involved in the neuropathology of depression in asthma.

AUTHOR CONTRIBUTIONS

YZ took responsibility for the content of the manuscript; YZ and ZW were responsibility for the data and analysis; YZ, YYang and RB were charge for patient recruitment; WJ, YYin, YYue, ZH provided language help for this study; YYuan was responsibility for experimental design.

ACKNOWLEDGMENTS

This work was supported by National Natural Science Foundation of China (grant number 81771480, YYuan) and the Fundamental Research Funds for the Central Universities (Southeast University, grant number 2242016K41053).

REFERENCES

1. To T, Stanojevic S, Moores G, Gershon AS, Bateman ED, Cruz AA, et al. Global asthma prevalence in adults: findings from the cross-sectional world health survey. *BMC Public Health* (2012) **12**:204. doi: 10.1186/1471-2458-12-204
2. Ding B, DiBonaventura M, Karlsson N, Ling X. Asthma-chronic obstructive pulmonary disease overlap syndrome in the urban Chinese population: prevalence and disease burden using the 2010, 2012, and 2013 China National Health and Wellness Surveys. *Int J Chron Obstruct Pulmon Dis.* (2016) **11**:1139–50. doi: 10.2147/COPD.S103873
3. Liu S, Wu R, Li L, Liu L, Li G, Zhang X, et al. The prevalence of anxiety and depression in Chinese asthma patients. *PLoS ONE* (2014) **9**:e103014. doi: 10.1371/journal.pone.0103014
4. Lu Y, Ho R, Lim TK, Kuan WS, Goh DY, Mahadevan M, et al. Psychiatric comorbidities in Asian adolescent asthma patients and the contributions of neuroticism and perceived stress. *J Adolesc Health* (2014) **55**:267–75. doi: 10.1016/j.jadohealth.2014.01.007
5. Ciprandi G, Schiavetti I, Rindone E, Ricciardolo FL. The impact of anxiety and depression on outpatients with asthma. *Ann Allergy Asthma Immunol.* (2015) **115**:408–14. doi: 10.1016/j.anai.2015.08.007
6. Rosenkranz MA, Busse WW, Johnstone T, Swenson CA, Crisafi GM, Jackson MM, et al. Neural circuitry underlying the interaction between emotion and asthma symptom exacerbation. *Proc Natl Acad Sci USA.* (2005) **102**:13319–24. doi: 10.1073/pnas.0504365102
7. Rosenkranz MA, Busse WW, Sheridan JF, Crisafi GM, Davidson RJ. Are there neurophenotypes for asthma? *Functional brain imaging of the interaction between emotion and inflammation in asthma. PLoS ONE* (2012) **7**:e40921. doi: 10.1371/journal.pone.0040921
8. Rosenkranz MA, Davidson RJ. Affective neural circuitry and mind-body influences in asthma. *Neuroimage* (2009) **47**:972–80. doi: 10.1016/j.neuroimage.2009.05.042
9. von Leupoldt A, Sommer T, Kegat S, Baumann HJ, Klose H, Dahme B, et al. Dyspnea and pain share emotion-related brain network. *Neuroimage* (2009) **48**:200–6. doi: 10.1016/j.neuroimage.2009.06.015
10. Busse WW. The brain and asthma: what are the linkages? *Chem Immunol Allergy* (2012) **98**:14–31. doi: 10.1159/000336495
11. Suzuki H, Matsumoto Y, Ota H, Sugimura K, Takahashi J, Ito K, et al. Hippocampal blood flow abnormality associated with depressive symptoms and cognitive impairment in patients with chronic heart failure. *Circ J* (2016) **80**:1773–80. doi: 10.1253/circj.CJ-16-0367

12. Cantisani A, Koenig T, Stegmayer K, Federspiel A, Horn H, Müller TJ, et al. EEG marker of inhibitory brain activity correlates with resting-state cerebral blood flow in the reward system in major depression. *Eur Arch Psychiatry Clin Neurosci.* (2015) **266**:755–64. doi: 10.1007/s00406-015-0652-7
13. Kaichi Y, Okada G, Takamura M, Toki S, Akiyama Y, Higaki T, et al. Changes in the regional cerebral blood flow detected by arterial spin labeling after 6-week escitalopram treatment for major depressive disorder. *J Affect Disord.* (2016) **194**:135–43. doi: 10.1016/j.jad.2015.12.062
14. Yildiz S, Kaya I, Cece H, Gencer M, Ziylan Z, Yalcin F, et al. Impact of COPD exacerbation on cerebral blood flow. *Clin Imaging* (2012) **36**:185–90. doi: 10.1016/j.clinimag.2011.08.021
15. Curran-Everett D, Zhang Y, Jones RH, Jones MD Jr. Hypoxia, hypercapnia, and hypertension: their effects on pulsatile cerebral blood flow. *J Appl Physiol.* (1995). **79**:870–8. doi: 10.1152/jappl.1995.79.3.870
16. Ogoh S, Ainslie PN. Cerebral blood flow during exercise: mechanisms of regulation. *J Appl Physiol.* (2009) **107**:1370–80. doi: 10.1152/japplphysiol.00573.2009
17. Bowton DL, Stump DA, Anderson R. Effect of chronic theophylline therapy on brain blood flow and function in adult asthmatics. *Am J Respir Crit Care Med.* (1994) **150**:1002–5. doi: 10.1164/ajrccm.150.4.7921428
18. Detre JA, Alsop DC. Perfusion magnetic resonance imaging with continuous arterial spin labeling: methods and clinical applications in the central nervous system. *Eur J Radiol.* (1999) **30**:115–24. doi: 10.1016/S0720-048X(99)00050-9
19. Zhu S, Fang Z, Hu S, Wang Z, Rao H. Resting state brain function analysis using concurrent BOLD in ASL perfusion fMRI. *PLoS ONE* (2013) **8**:e65884. doi: 10.1371/journal.pone.0065884
20. Wang Z. Characterizing early Alzheimer's disease and disease progression using hippocampal volume and arterial spin labeling perfusion MRI. *J Alzheimers Dis.* (2014) **42**(Suppl. 4):S495–502. doi: 10.3233/JAD-141419
21. Wang Z, Aguirre GK, Rao H, Wang J, Fernández-Seara MA, Childress AR, et al. Empirical optimization of ASL data analysis using an ASL data processing toolbox: ASLtbx. *Magn Reson Imaging* (2008) **26**:261–9. doi: 10.1016/j.mri.2007.07.003
22. Wang Z. Improving cerebral blood flow quantification for arterial spin labeled perfusion MRI by removing residual motion artifacts and global signal fluctuations. *Magn Reson Imaging* (2012) **30**:1409–15. doi: 10.1016/j.mri.2012.05.004
23. Song XW, Dong ZY, Long XY, Li SF, Zuo XN, Zhu CZ, et al. REST: a toolkit for resting-state functional magnetic resonance imaging data processing. *PLoS ONE* (2011) **6**:e25031. doi: 10.1371/journal.pone.0025031
24. Stoodley CJ, Schmahmann JD. Functional topography in the human cerebellum: a meta-analysis of neuroimaging studies. *Neuroimage* (2009) **44**:489–501. doi: 10.1016/j.neuroimage.2008.08.039
25. Van Overwalle F, Baetens K, Mariën P, Vandekerckhove M. Social cognition and the cerebellum: a meta-analysis of over 350 fMRI studies. *Neuroimage* (2014) **86**:554–72. doi: 10.1016/j.neuroimage.2013.09.033
26. Paradiso S, Robinson RG, Boles Ponto LL, Watkins GL, Hichwa RD. Regional cerebral blood flow changes during visually induced subjective sadness in healthy elderly persons. *J Neuropsychiatry Clin Neurosci.* (2003) **15**:35–44. doi: 10.1176/jnp.15.1.35
27. Wildgruber D, Riecker A, Hertrich I, Erb M, Grodd W, Ethofer T, et al. Identification of emotional intonation evaluated by fMRI. *Neuroimage* (2005) **24**:1233–41. doi: 10.1016/j.neuroimage.2004.10.034
28. Yin Y, Hou Z, Wang X, Sui Y, Yuan Y. Association between altered resting-state cortico-cerebellar functional connectivity networks and mood/cognition dysfunction in late-onset depression. *J Neural Transm.* (2015) **122**:887–96. doi: 10.1007/s00702-014-1347-3
29. Su L, Cai Y, Xu Y, Dutt A, Shi S, Bramon E. Cerebral metabolism in major depressive disorder: a voxel-based meta-analysis of positron emission tomography studies. *BMC Psychiatry* (2014) **14**:321. doi: 10.1186/s12888-014-0321-9
30. Hwang JP, Lee TW, Tsai SJ, Chen TJ, Yang CH, Lirng JF, et al. Cortical and subcortical abnormalities in late-onset depression with history of suicide attempts investigated with MRI and voxel-based morphometry. *J Geriatr Psychiatry Neurol.* (2010) **23**:171–84. doi: 10.1177/0891988710363713
31. Fujimoto T, Takeuchi K, Matsumoto T, Fujita S, Honda K, Higashi Y, et al. Metabolic changes in the brain of patients with late-onset major depression. *Psychiatry Res.* (2008) **164**:48–57. doi: 10.1016/j.pscychresns.2007.03.010
32. Liao W, Wang Z, Zhang X, Shu H, Wang Z, Liu D, et al. Cerebral blood flow changes in remitted early- and late-onset depression patients. *Oncotarget* (2017) **8**:76214–22. doi: 10.18632/oncotarget.19185
33. Stoodley CJ, Schmahmann JD. Evidence for topographic organization in the cerebellum of motor control versus cognitive and affective processing. *Cortex* (2010) **46**:831–44. doi: 10.1016/j.cortex.2009.11.008
34. Stoodley CJ. The cerebellum and cognition: evidence from functional imaging studies. *Cerebellum* (2012) **11**:352–65. doi: 10.1007/s12311-011-0260-7
35. Stoodley CJ, Valera EM, Schmahmann JD. An fMRI study of intra-individual functional topography in the human cerebellum. *Behav Neurol.* (2010) **23**:65–79. doi: 10.1155/2010/840942
36. Stoodley CJ, Valera EM, Schmahmann JD. Functional topography of the cerebellum for motor and cognitive tasks: an fMRI study. *Neuroimage* (2012) **59**:1560–70. doi: 10.1016/j.neuroimage.2011.08.065
37. Bratek A, Zawada K, Beil-Gawełczyk J, Beil S, Sozanska E, Krysta K, et al. Depressiveness, symptoms of anxiety and cognitive dysfunctions in patients with asthma and chronic obstructive pulmonary disease (COPD): possible associations with inflammation markers: a pilot study. *J Neural Transm.* (2015) **122**(Suppl. 1):S83–91. doi: 10.1007/s00702-014-1171-9
38. O'Conor R, Wolf MS, Smith SG, Martynenko M, Vicencio DP, Sano M, et al. Health literacy, cognitive function, proper use, and adherence to inhaled asthma controller medications among older adults with asthma. *Chest* (2015) **147**:1307–15. doi: 10.1378/chest.14-0914
39. Ray M, Sano M, Wisnivesky JP, Wolf MS, Federman AD. Asthma control and cognitive function in a cohort of elderly adults. *J Am Geriatr Soc.* (2015) **63**:684–91. doi: 10.1111/jgs.13350
40. von Leupoldt A, Sommer T, Kegat S, Eippert F, Baumann HJ, Klose H, et al. Down-regulation of insular cortex responses to dyspnea and pain in asthma. *Am J Respir Crit Care Med.* (2009) **180**:232–8. doi: 10.1164/rccm.200902-0300OC
41. Herigstad M, Hayen A, Wiech K, Pattinson KT. Dyspnoea and the brain. *Respir Med.* (2011) **105**:809–17. doi: 10.1016/j.rmed.2010.12.022
42. von Leupoldt A, Brassen S, Baumann HJ, Klose H, Buchel C. Structural brain changes related to disease duration in patients with asthma. *PLoS ONE* (2011) **6**:e23739. doi: 10.1371/journal.pone.0023739
43. Dunn RT, Kimbrell TA, Ketter TA, Frye MA, Willis MW, Luckenbaugh DA, et al. Principal components of the Beck Depression Inventory and regional cerebral metabolism in unipolar and bipolar depression. *Biol Psychiatry* (2002) **51**:387–99. doi: 10.1016/S0006-3223(01)01244-6

2

Bidirectional Causal Connectivity in the Cortico-Limbic-Cerebellar Circuit Related to Structural Alterations in First-Episode, Drug-Naive Somatization Disorder

Ranran Li[1]*, Feng Liu*[2]*, Qinji Su*[3]*, Zhikun Zhang*[3]*, Jin Zhao*[1]*, Ying Wang*[1]*, Renrong Wu*[1]*, Jingping Zhao*[1*] *and Wenbin Guo*[1*]

[1] *Department of Psychiatry, Second Xiangya Hospital of Central South University, Changsha, China,* [2] *Department of Radiology, Tianjin Medical University General Hospital, Tianjin, China,* [3] *Mental Health Center of the First Affiliated Hospital, Guangxi Medical University, Nanning, China*

Correspondence:
Jingping Zhao
zhaojingping@csu.edu.cn
Wenbin Guo
guowenbin76@csu.edu.cn

Background: Anatomical and functional deficits in the cortico-limbic-cerebellar circuit are involved in the neurobiology of somatization disorder (SD). The present study was performed to examine causal connectivity of the cortico-limbic-cerebellar circuit related to structural deficits in first-episode, drug-naive patients with SD at rest.

Methods: A total of 25 first-episode, drug-naive patients with SD and 28 healthy controls underwent structural and resting-state functional magnetic resonance imaging. Voxel-based morphometry and Granger causality analysis (GCA) were used to analyze the data.

Results: Results showed that patients with SD exhibited decreased gray matter volume (GMV) in the right cerebellum Crus I, and increased GMV in the left anterior cingulate cortex (ACC), right middle frontal gyrus (MFG), and left angular gyrus. Causal connectivity of the cortico-limbic-cerebellar circuit was partly affected by structural alterations in the patients. Patients with SD showed bidirectional cortico-limbic connectivity abnormalities and bidirectional cortico-cerebellar and limbic-cerebellar connectivity abnormalities. The mean GMV of the right MFG was negatively correlated with the scores of the somatization subscale of the symptom checklist-90 and persistent error response of the Wisconsin Card Sorting Test (WCST) in the patients. A negative correlation was observed between increased driving connectivity from the right MFG to the right fusiform gyrus/cerebellum IV, V and the scores of the Eysenck Personality Questionnaire extraversion subscale. The mean GMV of the left ACC was negatively correlated with the WCST number of errors and persistent error response. Negative correlation was found between the causal effect from the left ACC to the right middle temporal gyrus and the scores of WCST number of categories achieved.

Conclusions: Our findings show the partial effects of structural alterations on the cortico-limbic-cerebellar circuit in first-episode, drug-naive patients with SD. Correlations are observed between anatomical alterations or causal effects and clinical variables in patients with SD, and bear clinical significance. The present study emphasizes the importance of the cortico-limbic-cerebellar circuit in the neurobiology of SD.

Keywords: somatization disorder, resting-state functional magnetic resonance imaging, voxel-based morphometry, cortico-limbic-cerebellar, gray matter volume, granger causality analysis

INTRODUCTION

Somatization disorder (SD) is characterized by a history of various unexplained physical symptoms in many organ systems. This disorder begins before age of 30 and occurs for many years, leading to repeated treatment seeking or significant impairment in social/occupational function (1). Lifetime prevalence of SD varies from 0.2 to 2% in women and less than 0.2% in men (2). In the Diagnostic and Statistical Manual of Mental Disorders-IV (DSM-IV), SD is characterized by multiple, recurring, affecting many organ systems, with at least four pain symptoms, two gastrointestinal symptoms, one sexual symptom and one pseudoneurological symptom. Each of the symptoms cannot be explained by a general medical condition, or in factitious disorder or malingering (3). The occurrence of somatization symptoms is commonly assessed by self-report questionnaires. A large amount of questionnaires are available to assess self-report somatization symptoms (4), such as the screen for Somatoform Symptoms (5), Physical Health Questionnaire-15 (6), and somatization subscale of the symptom checklist-90 (SCL-90) (7). Among these questionnaires, the SCL-90 and Physical Health Questionnaire-15 were deemed as the suitable scales for assessing somatization symptoms.

Although evidence suggests that dissociation amnesia, childhood emotional/physical abuse, and unsupportive family environment are associated with SD (8), its neurobiology remains unclear. The functional neuroimaging methods allow us to investigate neural changes in patients with SD (9–14). For instance, Garcia-Campayo et al. (14) reported that patients with SD exhibited hypoperfusion in the frontal, cerebellar, and temporoparietal brain areas under single-photon-emission computed tomography (SPECT). Moreover, increased glutamatergic activity in the posterior cingulate cortex (PCC) was observed in patients with SD by magnetic resonance spectroscopy techniques (9). By contrast, regional cerebral hypometabolism in the right precentral gyrus, caudate nuclei, and left putamen was found in patients with SD by using positron emission tomography techniques (15). Recently, abnormal activities in the anterior ventral precuneus, PCC, and anteromedial thalamus were correlated with the somatization severity of SD (16). Patients with SD showed increased regional activity in the bilateral superior medial prefrontal cortex (MPFC) and decreased regional activity in the left precuneus (12). The same researchers also found a positive correlation between increased activity in the bilateral superior MPFC and the scores of SCL-90 (12), and an increase in the right inferior temporal gyrus functional connectivity (FC) in patients with SD (13). Moreover, a variety of literatures reported correlations between abnormal FC or neural activity within brain areas of the default-mode network (DMN) and somatization severity or personality (10, 11, 17, 18). Impaired brain activity has been shown in patients with SD under an emotional empathy task by using functional magnetic resonance imaging (fMRI) (19), such as reduced activity in the bilateral parahippocampal gyrus, left amygdala, and left superior temporal gyrus, suggesting that these brain regions are responsible for emotional regulation and emotional memory.

Limited structural imaging studies have shown that patients with SD exhibit anatomical alterations, including reduced pituitary and amygdala volume and increased caudate nucleus volume (20–22). By contrast, no significant white matter differences were found between patients with SD and healthy controls by using diffusion tensor imaging at the corrected level (23). However, the same study showed that patients with SD had significantly decreased fractional anisotropy values in the right cingulate cortex and right inferior fronto-occipital fasciculus compared with controls at the uncorrected level in the same study (23), and the fractional anisotropy values of the two brain regions are correlated with the severity of somatization symptoms.

Furthermore, cerebellar alterations were observed in patients with SD, such as increased cerebellar-DMN FC (10) and decreased regional homogeneity in the left cerebellum (24). In addition, a recent study found that patients with persistent somatoform pain disorder showed increased FC between the sensorimotor network and cerebellar network (25). In a study comparing empathic deficits in patients with somatoform disorder using fMRI during an empathy task, de Greck et al. (19) observed lower activity in several brain regions, such as the bilateral parahippocampal gyrus, left amygdala, left superior temporal gyrus, left postcentral gyrus, bilateral cerebellum, and left posterior insula.

The aforementioned studies revealed that the cortico-limbic-cerebellar circuit may play a crucial role in the neurobiology of the SD. However, several methodological drawbacks should be taken into consideration when interpreting these findings. First, some studies have used structural MRI for data analysis without combining with fMRI to analyze neural activity or FC in patients with SD, thus preventing the understanding of the relationship between anatomical and functional alterations. Second, most studies have adopted regions of interest (ROI) or independent component analysis (ICA). The reported results might be affected by the selection of ROIs or uncertainty of ICA signal separation. Importantly, the altered information flow of the cortico-limbic-cerebellar circuit remains unclear based on prior studies.

In the present study, we used voxel-based morphometry (VBM) to examine whole-brain GMV differences in patients with SD, and brain areas with abnormal GMV were selected as seeds. Then, Granger causality analysis (GCA) was employed to examine abnormal causal connectivity of the seeds with other voxels of the entire brain. The GCA method is based on the predictive value of the current time series Y from the past value of time series X for reasoning that the causal influence from X causes Y (26). The Granger effect was assessed by a signed regression coefficient β (27, 28). Here, we aimed to determine the anatomical deficits and causal connectivity related to anatomical deficits in a group of first-episode, drug-naive patients with SD. Based on the abovementioned researches, we hypothesized that patients with SD would show anatomical deficits of the cortico-limbic-cerebellar circuit, and causal effects would decrease with the anatomical deficits (see **Figure 1**). We also examined the correlations between the abnormal GMV or causal connectivity, and clinical variables (i.e., symptom severity and cognitive function) in the patients.

MATERIALS AND METHODS

Participants

A total of 56 right-handed subjects were recruited for this study, including 26 first-episode, drug-naive patients with SD and 30 healthy controls. Diagnosis of SD was determined through a consensus of two experienced clinical psychiatrists by using the Structural Clinical Interview of the Diagnostic and Statistical Manual of Mental Disorders-IV (SCID), Patient's Edition (29). Healthy controls were recruited from the community and were screened to exclude lifetime psychiatric illness by the non-patient edition of the SCID. Moreover, healthy controls with a history of psychiatric illness in first-degree relatives were also excluded. Exclusion criteria for all subjects included severe medical or neurological diseases, substance abuse or loss of consciousness history, mental retardation, contraindications for MRI scanning, and other psychiatric disorders, such as schizophrenia, bipolar disorder, anxiety disorders, and personality disorders. As depressive symptoms were common in patients with SD, patients with comorbidity of depression were not excluded. However, the presence of depressive symptoms should occur after the onset of somatization symptoms. Six patients with SD presented comorbidity with major depressive disorder in the current study. In addition, none of the healthy controls had a personal history of psychiatric or severe physical disease and craniocerebral operations.

All subjects were evaluated through the following tests by two experienced psychiatrists (ZZ and WG): symptom severity of somatization, depression, and anxiety were assessed by the somatization subscale of SCL-90 (7), Hamilton Rating Scale for Depression (HAMD, 17 items) (30), and Hamilton Anxiety Scale (HAMA) (31); Eysenck Personality Questionnaire (EPQ) (32) was used to assess personality dimensions; and cognitive function was assessed by the Wisconsin Card Sorting Test (WCST) (33) and Wechsler Adult Intelligence Scale (WAIS): digit symbol coding (34).

This study was carried out in accordance with the recommendations of the local ethics committee of the First Affiliated Hospital of Guangxi Medical University. All subjects gave a written informed consent in accordance with the Declaration of Helsinki.

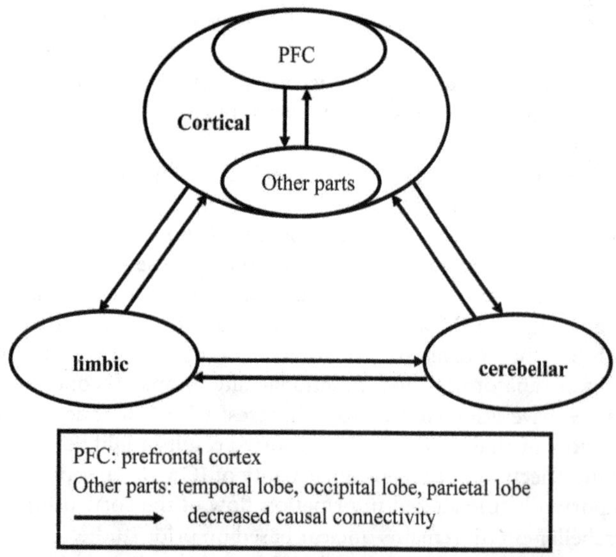

FIGURE 1 | Hypothesized model in first-episode, drug-naive somatization disorder: overall reduced causal connectivities in the cortico-limbic-cerebellar circuit.

MRI Acquisition and Functional Data Preprocessing

Whole-brain imaging was acquired on a 3.0 T Siemens scanner. Functional data were preprocessed with the software DPABI in Matlab (35). Details of MRI acquisition and functional data preprocessing are provided in the Supplementary Files.

Anatomical Analyses

Each image was manually checked for gross anatomical abnormalities and image artifacts. The images were processed with the VBM8 toolbox (http://dbm.neuro.uni-jena.de/vbm) and SPM8 (http://www.fil.ion.ucl.ac.uk/spm). First, the images were normalized to the same template using a 12 parameter affine transformation. Afterward, each participant's images were segmented to identify tissue-signal intensities, combined with prior knowledge of probability maps. The images were then spatially normalized to the template space and resampled to $1.5 \times 1.5 \times 1.5\,mm^3$. To eliminate non-brain tissue voxels from dural venous sinuses, skull, scalp, and diplopic space, an automated brain extraction procedure was used. Finally, the optimally normalized segmented images were modulated, and the obtained images were smoothed with an 8 mm full-width half-maximum Gaussian kernel.

Two-sample t-tests were conducted to determine GMV differences between patients with SD and healthy controls. Age was used as a covariate to minimize the potential effects of this variable. For multiple comparisons, the significance threshold was set at $p < 0.05$ for multiple comparisons corrected by the Gaussian Random Field (GRF) theory (voxel significance: $p < 0.001$, cluster significance: $p < 0.05$).

GCA Processing

Four brain regions, the right cerebellum Crus I, right middle frontal gyrus (MFG), left anterior cingulate cortex (ACC), and left angular gyrus (AG), with abnormal GMV were selected as seeds. The peak voxel of each seed was selected as a 6 mm-radius spherical seed for GCA processing. Voxel-wise coefficient GCA was performed by using the REST software (36). Granger causality was conducted by vector autoregressive models to explore whether the past variable of a time series could predict the current variable of another time series correctly. A signed regression coefficient β was used to estimate the Granger effect (27, 28). Positive/negative β may indicate an excitatory/inhibitory effect or positive/negative feedback (37). There were two analyses for each seed: seed-to-whole-brain and whole-brain-to-seed analyses. The former was conducted to estimate the driving effect from the seed to other brain regions of the whole brain, including excitatory and inhibitory effects. The latter was used to estimate the feedback effect from other brain regions of the whole brain to the seed, including positive and negative feedback. Two sample *t*-tests were used to compare the causal effects between patients and controls. The framewise displacement (FD) values were computed for all subjects. Age and the mean FD values were used as covariates in the group comparisons to minimize the potential effects of these variables. The significance threshold was set at $p < 0.05$ (GRF corrected).

Correlation Analyses

To identify the correlations between abnormal GMV or causal effect and symptoms in patients with SD, partial correlation analyses were conducted after controlling for the HAMD and HAMA scores to rule out the potential effects of depression and anxiety. The statistical threshold was set at $p < 0.05$ (Bonferroni corrected).

TABLE 1 | Characteristics of the participants.

Variables	Patients (n = 25)	Controls (n = 28)	p-value
Age (years)	41.00 ± 10.76	38.71 ± 9.59	0.42[b]
Sex (male/female)	4/21	6/22	0.73[a]
Years of education (years)	7.72 ± 4.39	7.82 ± 2.59	0.92[b]
FD (mm)	0.08 ± 0.03	0.10 ± 0.05	0.02[b]
Illness duration (months)	59.12 ± 62.22		
Somatization subscale of SCL-90	28.48 ± 10.37	14.32 ± 3.44	<0.001[b]
HAMD	18.84 ± 7.31	2.60 ± 1.83	<0.001[b]
HAMA	22.96 ± 10.95	0.53 ± 0.99	<0.001[b]
Digit symbol-coding of WAIS	8.28 ± 2.87	9.64 ± 2.15	0.06[b]
EPQ			
Extraversion	46.84 ± 11.02	49.75 ± 9.65	0.31[b]
Psychoticism	50.52 ± 9.01	45.00 ± 8.54	0.03[b]
Neuroticism	57.36 ± 9.18	46.78 ± 10.24	<0.001[b]
Lie	49.44 ± 12.31	47.96 ± 11.01	0.65[b]
WCST			
Number of categories achieved	3.52 ± 1.76	3.89 ± 1.66	0.43[b]
Number of errors	22.84 ± 9.12	24.71 ± 8.91	0.45[b]
WCST-Pre	20.04 ± 9.48	22.82 ± 8.72	0.27[b]

[a] The p-value for sex distribution was obtained by a chi-square test.
[b] The p-values were obtained by two sample t-tests.
FD, Framewise displacement; HAMD, Hamilton depression scale; HAMA, Hamilton anxiety scale; SCL-90, Symptom Checklist-90; EPQ, Eysenck Personality Questionnaire; WAIS, Wechsler Adult Intelligence Scale; WCST-Pre, persistent error response of Wisconsin Card Sorting Test.

RESULTS

Demographics and Clinical Characteristics of Participants

The data of one patient and two controls were eliminated due to excessive head motion. As shown in **Table 1**, no significant differences were found between patients and controls in regard to age, sex ratio, education level, digit symbol coding of WAIS, EPQ extraversion and EPQ lie scores, and WCST scores. Relative to healthy controls, patients with SD showed significantly higher scores in the SCL-90 somatization subscale, HAMD, HAMA, and EPQ psychoticism and neuroticism scales. Furthermore, the controls exhibited higher FD values than those of the patients.

Anatomical Abnormalities Between Groups

Relative to the controls, patients with SD showed significantly reduced GMV in the right cerebellum Crus I and significantly increased GMV in the left ACC, right MFG, and left AG (**Table 2** and **Figure 2**). These four brain regions were selected as seeds for further GCA analyses.

Voxel-Wise GCA: Seed-To-Whole-Brain Analysis

As shown in **Table 3** and **Figure 3** (**Supplementary Figure S1**), the patients exhibited excitatory effect from the left ACC to the left cerebellum Crus II, bilateral MFG/superior frontal gyrus, and right middle temporal gyrus (MTG) relative to the controls. In addition, the patients showed excitatory effect from the right MFG to the right fusiform gyrus/cerebellum vermis IV, V, left lingual gyrus/cerebellum vermis VI, cerebellum vermis IX, left inferior temporal gyrus, and bilateral middle cingulate cortex. Moreover, the patients exhibited inhibitory effect from the right cerebellum Crus I to the left middle occipital gyrus/inferior occipital gyrus/cerebellum VI, left superior MPFC, and left superior MPFC/ACC, from the left ACC to the left supplementary motor area.

Voxel-Wise GCA: Whole-Brain-To-Seed Analysis

Patients with SD showed positive feedback from the left MFG to the right cerebellum Crus I and from the left superior temporal gyrus, bilateral PCC/precuneus, right inferior frontal gyrus, right precentral gyrus/postcentral gyrus, and right postcentral gyrus to the left AG compared with healthy controls. By contrast, causal effects from the left cerebellum Crus II, right MTG, and right superior frontal gyrus to the left ACC, as well as from the left cerebellum Crus I and II, cerebellum IV, V, bilateral lingual gyrus/cerebellum vermis VI, and right superior parietal lobule to the right MFG decreased in the patients (**Table 3**, **Figure 4** and **Supplementary Figure S2**).

TABLE 2 | Regions with abnormal gray matter volume in the patients.

Cluster location	Peak (MNI)			Number of voxels	*T*-value
	x	*y*	*z*		
Right Cerebellum Crus I	36	−75	−28.5	27	−3.4839
Left Anterior Cingulate Cortex	−12	18	27	35	4.7333
Right Middle Frontal Gyrus	51	15	30	24	3.9673
Left Angular Gyrus	−39	−63	33	25	4.3977

MNI, Montreal Neurological Institute.

Correlations Between Anatomical Alterations or Causal Effects and Clinical Variables in Patients With SD

As shown in **Figure 5**, the mean GMV of the right MFG was negatively correlated with the scores of the somatization subscale of SCL-90 ($r = -0.46$, $p = 0.027$) and persistent error response of WCST ($r = -0.415$. $p = 0.049$) in the patients. Significantly negative correlations were observed between the causal effect from the right MFG to the bilateral middle cingulate cortex and scores of WCST number of categories achieved ($r = -0.649$, $p = 0.001$) and between the causal effect from the right MFG to the right fusiform gyrus/cerebellum IV and V and the EPQ extraversion scores ($r = -0.422$, $p = 0.045$). Moreover, the mean GMV of the left ACC was positively associated with the scores of WCST number of categories achieved ($r = 0.467$, $p = 0.025$) and negatively associated with the WCST number of errors and persistent error response ($r = -0.589$, $p = 0.003$; $r = -0.627$, $p = 0.001$). Significantly negative correlation was observed between the causal effect from the left ACC to the right MTG and the scores of WCST number of categories achieved ($r = -0.472$, $p = 0.023$), and a positive correlation was found between the causal effect from the right MTG to the left ACC and scores of WCST number of categories achieved ($r = 0.487$, $p = 0.019$).

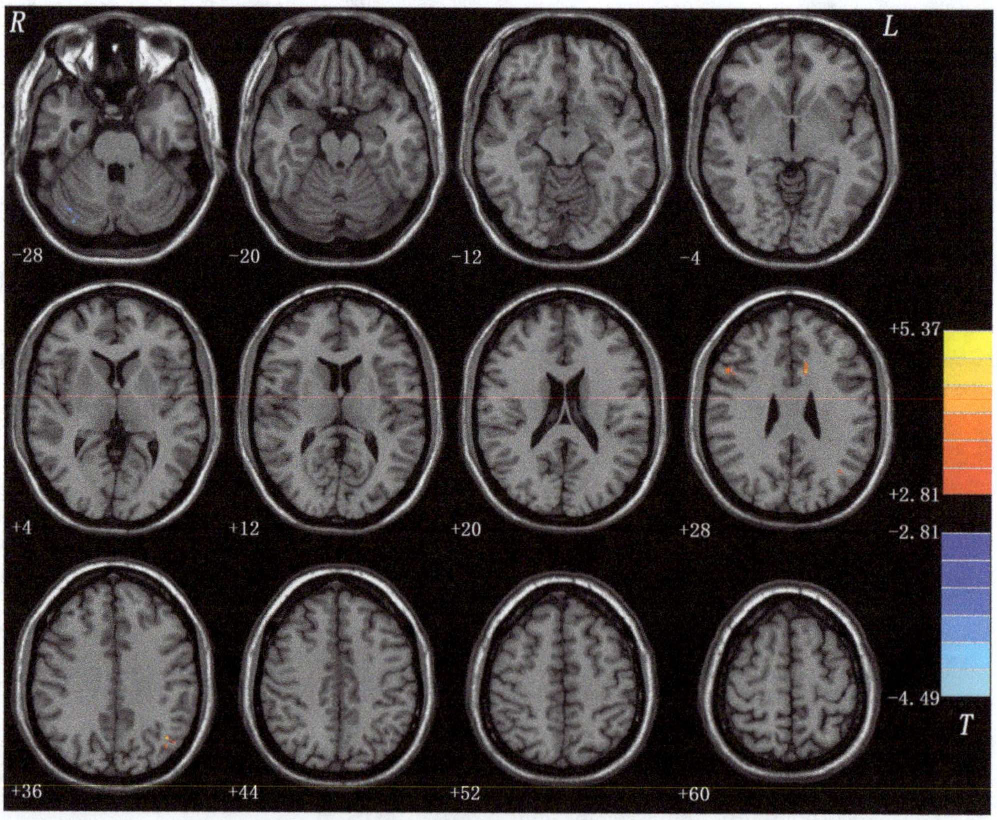

FIGURE 2 | Regions with abnormal gray matter volume in the patients.

TABLE 3 | Regions with abnormal causal effect with the seeds in the patients.

Cluster location	Peak (MNI)			Number of voxels	*T*-value[a]
	x	*y*	*z*		
SEED-TO-WHOLE-BRAIN EFFECT					
Seed: Right cerebellum crus I					
Left Middle Occipital Gyrus/Inferior Occipital Gyrus/Cerebellum VI	−45	−78	−6	235	−3.9323
Left Superior MPFC/ACC	−6	51	27	412	−4.3354
Left Superior MPFC	−9	39	51	63	−5.2241
Right Superior Temporal Gyrus	39	−39	12	34	4.1831
Seed: Left ACC					
Left Cerebellum Crus II	−45	−60	−45	49	3.9294
Left Middle Frontal Gyrus/Superior Frontal Gyrus	−30	45	9	59	3.8802
Right Middle Frontal Gyrus/Superior Frontal Gyrus	24	60	12	93	4.5407
Right Middle Temporal Gyrus	42	−66	15	42	4.1405
Left Supplementary Motor Area	−9	−12	57	51	−3.5602
Seed: Right middle frontal gyrus					
Left Inferior Temporal Gyrus	−42	9	−39	33	3.7493
Cerebellum Vermis IX	3	−51	−36	32	3.6072
Right Fusiform Gyrus/Cerebellum IV, V	21	−36	−18	120	4.2073
Left Lingual Gyrus/Cerebellum Vermis VI	−12	−39	−6	248	4.8860
Bilateral Middle Cingulate Cortex	−3	−3	33	35	3.8098
Seed: Left angular gyrus					
None					
WHOLE-BRAIN-TO-SEED EFFECT					
Seed: Right cerebellum crus I					
Left Middle Frontal Gyrus	−36	33	36	48	3.9856
Seed: Left ACC					
Left Cerebellum Crus II	−42	−63	−36	67	−4.0615
Right Middle Temporal Gyrus	39	−66	18	46	−4.1778
Right Superior Frontal Gyrus	24	63	12	38	−4.5013
Seed: Right middle frontal gyrus					
Left Cerebellum Crus I, II	−42	−51	−42	171	−4.225
Bilateral Lingual Gyrus/Cerebellum Vermis VI	3	−78	−24	337	−4.4932
Cerebellum IV, V	−6	−39	−9	48	−4.2817
Right Superior Parietal Lobule	24	−72	51	93	−4.2222
Seed: Left angular gyrus					
Left Superior Temporal Gyrus	−54	−12	6	78	4.3236
Right Inferior Frontal Gyrus	63	12	6	34	5.2976
Bilateral PCC/Precuneus	0	−15	48	174	3.6941
Right Precentral Gyrus/Postcentral Gyrus	54	−12	42	57	3.5997
Right Postcentral Gyrus	42	−33	54	37	3.9333

(Continued)

TABLE 3 | Continued

[a]*A positive/negative T value represents an increased/decreased causal effect; MNI, Montreal Neurological Institute; MPFC, Medial Prefrontal cortex; ACC, Anterior Cingulate Cortex; PCC, Posterior Cingulate Cortex.*

DISCUSSION

The current findings reveal that the causal connectivity of the cortico-limbic-cerebellar circuit is partly affected by structural alterations in patients with SD. The primary results include bidirectional cortico-limbic connectivity abnormalities, bidirectional cortico-cerebellar connectivity abnormalities, bidirectional limbic-cerebellar connectivity abnormalities, and bidirectional causal effects among the cortical regions (**Figures 3, 4**). Moreover, correlations between anatomical alterations or causal effects and clinical variables are observed in patients with SD, and bear clinical significance.

Gray matter deficits in the bilateral amygdala or pituitary have been reported in patients with SD by using manual volumetric analysis (20, 21). Inconsistent with these studies, the present study demonstrates that patients with SD showed increased GMV in several cortical areas, including the right MFG, left ACC, and left AG. Several factors merit consideration in interpreting the increased GMV seen in our study. First, the magnetic resonance field strength may have contributed to such increases. Previously, Atmaca et al. (20) and Yildirim et al. (21) utilized a 1.5 T magnetic resonance scanner. In the current study, we used a 3.0 T scanner, which had higher signal-to-noise ratio, better image quality, and higher resolution than the 1.5 T scanner. Second, all patients were females in the previous studies, whereas there were four male patients in our study. Sex differences in GMV may account for the inconsistency (38). Importantly, Atmaca et al. and Yildirim et al. recruited chronic and medicated patients, whereas we recruited first-episode and drug-naive patients. Therefore, the patients in our study may present with early-stage neuronal pathology at the onset of somatization symptoms.

The MFG is involved in working memory, executive functions, attention, and language skills (39–42). Increased GMV in the right MFG has not been reported in patients with SD, but increased FC in the left MFG in patients with SD has been found (43). Furthermore, negative associations were found between the GMV of the right MFG and somatization subscale of SCL-90 and persistent error response of WCST in patients with SD in this study, indicating that patients with a smaller right MFG volume experienced more severe somatic symptoms and impaired executive function. Moreover, a negative correlation was observed between the increased driving connectivity from the right MFG to the bilateral middle

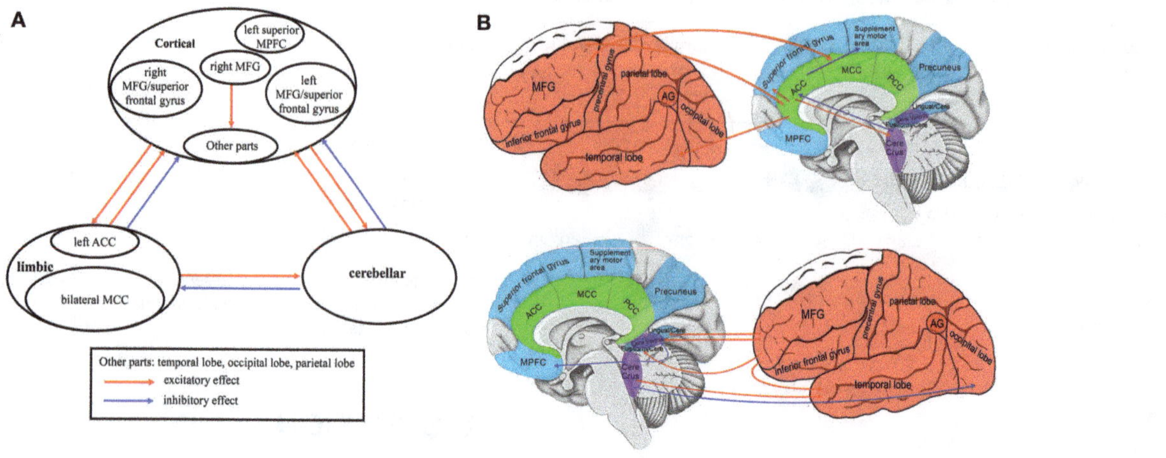

FIGURE 3 | Integrated model of voxel-wise Granger causality analyses in first-episode, drug-naive somatization disorder (Seed-to-Whole-Brain Analyses): affected causal connectivities in the cortico-limbic-cerebellar circuit **(A)**. Brain regions and circuitry implicated in first-episode, drug naive somatization disorder (Seed-to-Whole-Brain Analyses) **(B)**. MFG, Middle Frontal gyrus; MPFC, Medial Prefrontal Cortex; ACC, Anterior Cingulate Cortex; MCC, Middle Cingulate Cortex; PCC, Posterior Cingulate Cortex; AG, Angular Gyrus; Cere Crus, Cerebellum Crus; Cere Vermis, Cerebellum Vermis; Lingual/Cere, Lingual Gyrus/Cerebellum Vermis; Fusiform/Cere, Fusiform Gyrus/Cerebellum. Lateral cortical regions are shown in red, medial cortical regions in blue, subcortical regions in green, and cerebellum regions in purple. The functional pathways in **(A,B)** are indicated with red arrows (excitatory effect) and blue arrows (inhibitory effect).

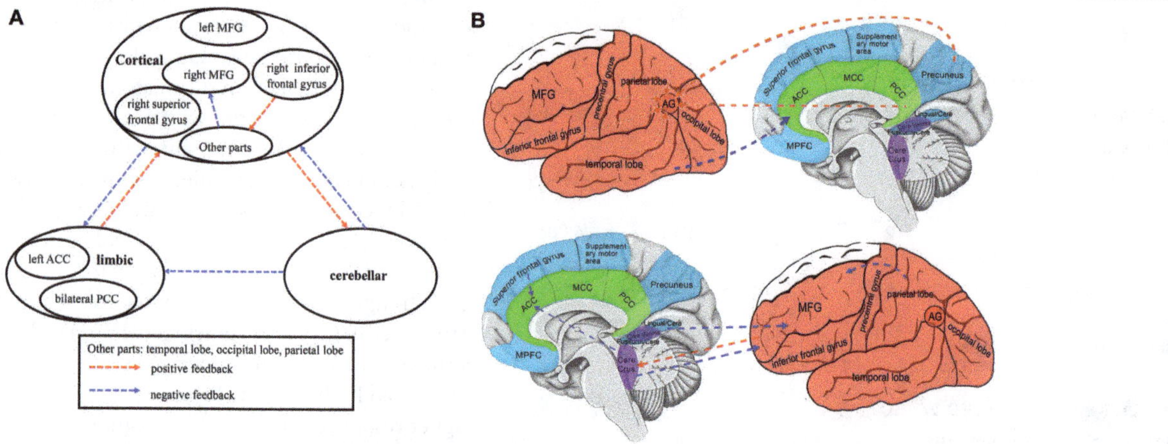

FIGURE 4 | Integrated model of voxel-wise Granger causality analyses in first-episode, drug-naive somatization disorder (Whole-Brain-to-Seed Analyses): affected causal connectivities in the cortico-limbic-cerebellar circuit **(A)**. Brain regions and circuitry implicated in first-episode, drug naive somatization disorder (Whole-Brain-to-Seed Analyses) **(B)**. MFG, Middle Frontal gyrus; MPFC, Medial Prefrontal Cortex; ACC, Anterior Cingulate Cortex; MCC, Middle Cingulate Cortex; PCC, Posterior Cingulate Cortex; AG, Angular Gyrus; Cere Crus, Cerebellum Crus; Cere Vermis, Cerebellum Vermis; Lingual/Cere, Lingual Gyrus/Cerebellum Vermis; Fusiform/Cere, Fusiform Gyrus/Cerebellum. Lateral cortical regions are shown in red, medial cortical regions in blue, subcortical regions in green, and cerebellum regions in purple. The functional pathways in **(A,B)** are indicated with red dotted arrows (positive feedback) and blue dotted arrows (negative feedback).

cingulate cortex and number of categories achieved on the WCST scores in patients, suggesting that patients with increased cortico-limbic connectivity would show prominent dysfunction in executive function. A negative correlation was also found between the EPQ extraversion scores and increased driving effect from the right MFG to the right fusiform gyrus/cerebellum IV, V in the patients, demonstrating that patients with a low EPQ extraversion (introversion) score reflect increased cortico-cerebellar connectivity. Patients who were introverts tend to be reserved, show solitary in behavior, and seek internal stimuli. Due to personality traits concentrating on internal stimuli, introverts may be more concerned about their own internal physical discomfort and be inclined to have a high risk of experiencing SD. Increased connectivity in the lobule IX-left superior MPFC with a negative correlation with the EPQ extraversion scores has been reported in patients with SD (10). In line with these findings, the present study emphasizes the importance of the cortico-limbic-cerebellar circuit in the neurophysiological mechanism of SD.

The ACC plays an important role in cognitive, emotional regulation, social evaluation, and awareness (44–47).

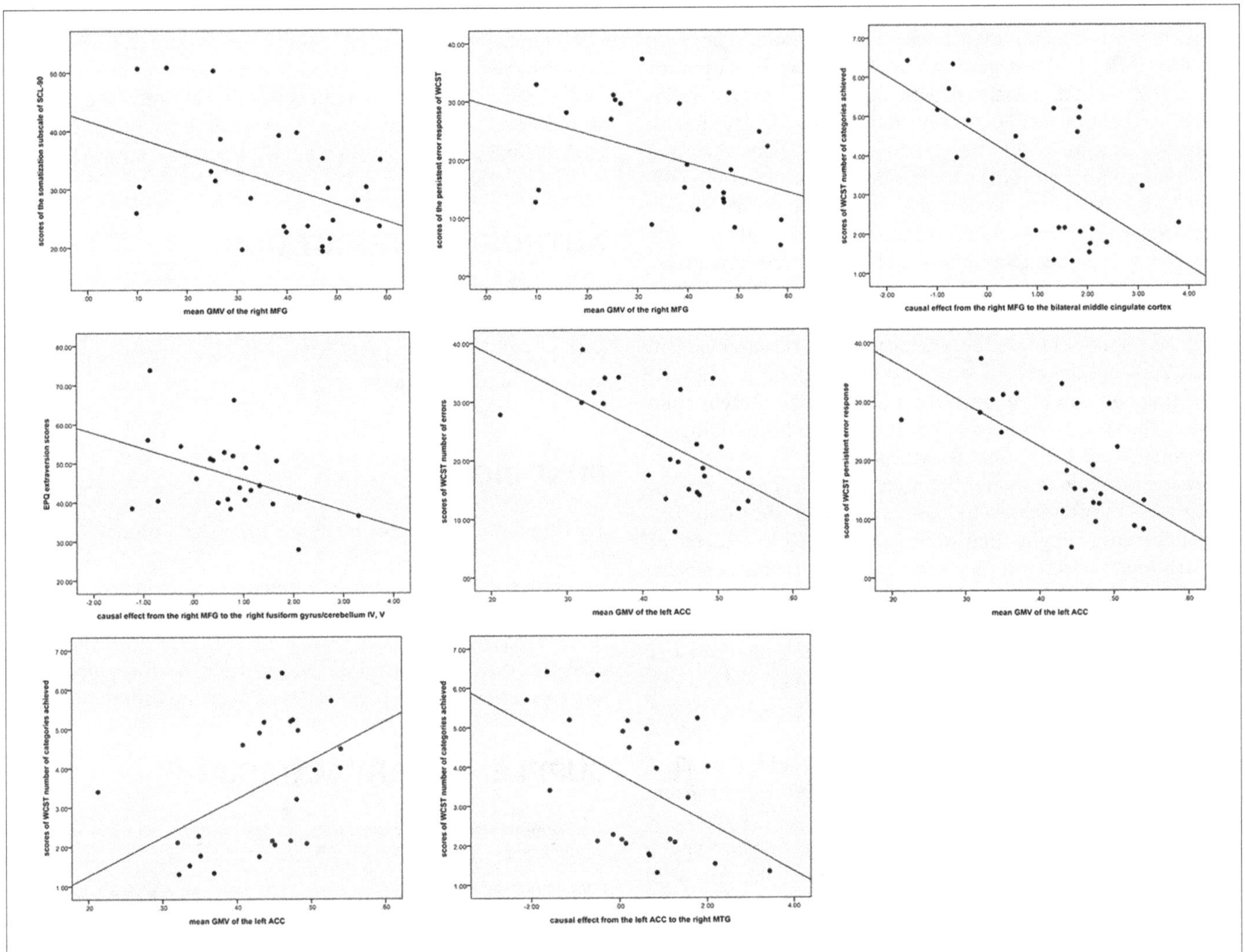

FIGURE 5 | Correlations between abnormal GMV or causal effects and clinical variables in patients with somatization disorder. GMV, gray matter volume; ACC, anterior cingulate cortex; WCST, Wisconsin Card Sorting Test; WCST-Pre, persistent error response of WCST; MFG, middle frontal gyrus; MTG, middle temporal gyrus.

Intriguingly, anatomical alterations of the left ACC and increased connectivity of ACC are correlated with cognitive function. First, the mean GMV of the left ACC negatively correlates with the WCST number of errors and persistent error response scores, and positively correlates with the WCST number of categories achieved scores. These correlations suggest that patients with a smaller GMV of the left ACC may display more serious cognitive impairment, such as dysfunction abstract reasoning and problem solving. ACC plays a crucial role in cognition and emotional regulation, especially in the monitoring of conflict processing (48). Our findings are in line with the results that ACC has a strong connectivity with areas involved in cognition and sensorimotor processing (49). Second, a negative correlation was observed between increased driving effect from the left ACC to the right MTG and scores of WCST number of categories achieved, corresponding to the positive correlation between decreased feedback from the right MTG to the left ACC and scores of WCST number of categories achieved. The MTG, located between the superior temporal and inferior temporal gyri, is involved in cognitive processes, such as semantic memory processing and multimodal sensory integration (50). Taken together, these findings suggest that the left ACC and increased driving effect from the left ACC to the right MTG might be an important anatomical substrate of cognitive deficits in patients with SD.

The AG plays an important role in semantic processing, language, number processing, memory retrieval, attention, reasoning, and social cognition (51, 52). A recent study suggests that patients with SD were associated with lower voxel-mirrored homotopic connectivity in the AG/supramarginal gyrus (11). Therefore, our finding of increased GVM in the AG may provide an understanding of the pathophysiology of SD.

Converging evidence suggests that the cerebellum is involved in sensorimotor control, cognitive function, and emotional control (53–56). Previous SPECT study in patients with SD found hypoperfusion in cerebellum region in four out of eleven patients with SD (14). Decreased cerebellar activity has also been found in patients with somatoform disorder during emotional empathy by using fMRI (19), suggesting that there may be important clinical significance associated with disorder-related alteration in the cerebellum. MPFC, a key node in the DMN, has an extensive connection with the affective limbic regions, including the hippocampus, amygdala, and hypothalamus. Additionally, MPFC and ACC are important parts of cortical midline structures, which play a crucial role in emotional regulation, self-referential processing, and sensory and higher-order processing. Cortical midline structures play a mediating effect in self-referential processing between sensory (sensory cortex) and advanced cognitive processing (lateral cortex). Considering many studies showing the involvement of the cerebellum in cognitive processing and emotional regulation (56–58), the present study suggests that the cerebellum is involved in the neurobiology of SD through a cerebellar-frontal connectivity.

Several limitations should be taken into consideration when interpreting the present results. First, the current study is a cross-sectional study. Longitudinal studies are needed to understand the treatment effects on the altered cortico-limbic-cerebellar circuit in SD. Second, patients with SD showed a high rate of comorbidity with depression in our study, which could have affected our findings. However, to exclude the potential effects of depression and anxiety, the HAMD and HAMA scores were used as covariates in the correlation analyses. Hence, comorbidity with depression and anxiety may have limited effects on our results. Finally, the sample size was relatively small. A large sample size is needed to confirm or refute the current results.

Despite these limitations, this study is the first to explore the causal connectivity affected by structural alterations in patients with SD at rest. These findings demonstrate the partial effects of structural alteration on the cortico-limbic-cerebellar circuit in first-episode, drug-naive patients with SD. Correlations are observed between anatomical alterations or causal effects and clinical variables in patients with SD, and bear clinical significance. The present study emphasizes the importance of the cortico-limbic-cerebellar circuit in the neurobiology of SD.

AUTHOR CONTRIBUTIONS

RL, FL, QS, ZZ, JZ, YW, RW, JZ, and WG: acquired the data, designed the study, contributed to data analysis, interpretation of data and wrote the article. All authors reviewed and gave final approval of publication.

FUNDING

This study was supported by grants from the National Key R&D Program of China (2016YFC1307100 and 2016YFC1306900) and the National Natural Science Foundation of China (Grant Nos. 81571310, 81630033, 81771447, 81622018, and 81471363). The funders had no role in the study design, data collection, data analysis, data interpretation, and writing of the report. The corresponding authors had full access to all the data in the study.

SUPPLEMENTARY MATERIAL

Supplementary Figure S1 | Voxel-wise Granger causality analyses in patients with somatization disorder: Seed-to-Whole-Brain Analyses.

Supplementary Figure S2 | Voxel-wise Granger causality analyses in patients with somatization disorder: Whole-Brain-to-Seed Analyses.

REFERENCES

1. Mai, F. Somatization disorder: a practical review. *Can J Psychiatry* (2004) **49**:652–62. doi: 10.1177/070674370404901002
2. Escobar JI, Burnam MA, Karno M, Forsythe A, Golding JM. Somatization in the community. *Arch Gen Psychiatry* (1987) **44**:713–8. doi: 10.1001/archpsyc.1987.01800200039006
3. van Dessel NC, van der Wouden JC, Dekker J, van der Horst HE. Clinical value of DSM IV and DSM 5 criteria for diagnosing the most prevalent somatoform disorders in patients with medically unexplained physical symptoms (MUPS). *J Psychosom Res.* (2016) **82**:4–10. doi: 10.1016/j.jpsychores.2016.01.004
4. Zijlema WL, Stolk RP, Lowe B, Rief W, White PD, Rosmalen JG. How to assess common somatic symptoms in large-scale studies: a systematic review of questionnaires. *J Psychosom Res.* (2013) **74**:459–68. doi: 10.1016/j.jpsychores.2013.03.093
5. Rief W, Hiller W, Fichter MM. Somatoform symptoms in depressive and panic syndromes. *Int J Behav Med.* (1995) **2**:51–65. doi: 10.1207/s15327558ijbm0201_5
6. Kroenke K, Spitzer RL, Williams JB. The PHQ-15: validity of a new measure for evaluating the severity of somatic symptoms. *Psychosom Med.* (2002) **64**:258–66. doi: 10.1097/00006842-200203000-00008
7. Derogatis LR, Rickels K, Rock AF. The SCL-90 and the MMPI: a step in the validation of a new self-report scale. *Br J Psychiatry* (1976) **128**:280–9. doi: 10.1192/bjp.128.3.280
8. Brown RJ, Schrag A, Trimble MR. Dissociation, childhood interpersonal trauma, and family functioning in patients with somatization disorder. *Am J Psychiatry* (2005) **162**:899–905. doi: 10.1176/appi.ajp.162.5.899
9. Fayed N, Andres E, Rojas G, Moreno S, Serrano-Blanco A, Roca M, et al. Brain dysfunction in fibromyalgia and somatization disorder using proton magnetic resonance spectroscopy: a controlled study. *Acta Psychiatr Scand.* (2012) **126**:115–25. doi: 10.1111/j.1600-0447.2011.01820.x
10. Wang H, Guo W, Liu F, Chen J, Wu R, Zhang Z, et al. Clinical significance of increased cerebellar default-mode network connectivity in resting-state patients with drug-naive somatization disorder. *Medicine* (2016) **95**:e4043. doi: 10.1097/MD.0000000000004043
11. Su Q, Yao D, Jiang M, Liu F, Long L, Dai Y, et al. Decreased interhemispheric functional connectivity in insula and angular gyrus/supramarginal gyrus: significant findings in first-episode, drug-naive somatization disorder. *Psychiatry Res.* (2016) **248**:48–54. doi: 10.1016/j.pscychresns.2016.01.008
12. Su Q, Yao D, Jiang M, Liu F, Jiang J, Xu C, et al. Dissociation of regional activity in default mode network in medication-naive, first-episode somatization disorder. *PLoS ONE* (2014) **9**:e99273. doi: 10.1371/journal.pone.0099273
13. Su Q, Yao D, Jiang M, Liu F, Jiang J, Xu, C, et al. Increased functional connectivity strength of right inferior temporal gyrus in first-episode, drug-naive somatization disorder. *Aust N Z J Psychiatry* (2015) **49**:74–81. doi: 10.1177/0004867414553949

14. Garcia-Campayo J, Sanz-Carrillo C, Baringo T, Ceballos C. SPECT scan in somatization disorder patients: an exploratory study of eleven cases. *Aust N Z J Psychiatry* (2001) **35**:359–63. doi: 10.1046/j.1440-1614.2001.00909.x
15. Hakala M, Karlsson H, Ruotsalainen U, Koponen S, Bergman J, Stenman H, et al. Severe somatization in women is associated with altered cerebral glucose metabolism. *Psychol Med.* (2002) **32**:1379–85. doi: 10.1017/S0033291702006578
16. Lemche E, Giampietro VP, Brammer MJ, Surguladze SA, Williams SC, Phillips, ML. Somatization severity associated with postero-medial complex structures. *Sci Rep.* (2013) **3**:1032. doi: 10.1038/srep01032
17. Song Y, Su Q, Jiang M, Liu F, Yao D, Dai Y, et al. Abnormal regional homogeneity and its correlations with personality in first-episode, treatment-naive somatization disorder. *Int J Psychophysiol.* (2015) **97**:108–12. doi: 10.1016/j.ijpsycho.2015.05.012
18. Wei S, Su Q, Jiang, M, Liu F, Yao D, Dai Y, et al. Abnormal default-mode network homogeneity and its correlations with personality in drug-naive somatization disorder at rest. *J Affect Disord.* (2016) **193**:81–8. doi: 10.1016/j.jad.2015.12.052
19. de Greck M, Scheidt L, Bolter AF, Frommer J, Ulrich C, Stockum E, et al. Altered brain activity during emotional empathy in somatoform disorder. *Hum Brain Mapp.* (2012) **33**:2666–85. doi: 10.1002/hbm.21392
20. Atmaca M, Sirlier B, Yildirim H, Kayali A. Hippocampus and amygdalar volumes in patients with somatization disorder. *Prog Neuropsychopharmacol Biol Psychiatry* (2011) **35**:1699–703. doi: 10.1016/j.pnpbp.2011.05.016
21. Yildirim H, Atmaca M, Sirlier B, Kayali A. Pituitary volumes are reduced in patients with somatization disorder. *Psychiatry Investig.* (2012) **9**:278–82. doi: 10.4306/pi.2012.9.3.278
22. Hakala M, Karlsson H, Kurki T, Aalto S, Koponen S, Vahlberg T, et al. Volumes of the caudate nuclei in women with somatization disorder and healthy women. *Psychiatry Res.* (2004) **131**:71–8. doi: 10.1016/j.pscychresns.2004.03.001
23. Zhang J, Jiang M, Yao D, Dai Y, Long L, Yu M, et al. Alterations in white matter integrity in first-episode, treatment-naive patients with somatization disorder. *Neurosci Lett.* (2015) **599**:102–8. doi: 10.1016/j.neulet.2015.05.037
24. Li Q, Xiao Y, Li Y, Li L, Lu N, Xu Z, et al. Altered regional brain function in the treatment-naive patients with somatic symptom disorder: a resting-state fMRI study. *Brain Behav.* (2016) **6**:e00521. doi: 10.1002/brb3.521
25. Zhao Z, Huang T, Tang C, Ni K, Pan X, Yan C, et al. Altered resting-state intra- and inter- network functional connectivity in patients with persistent somatoform pain disorder. *PLoS ONE* (2017) **12**:e0176494. doi: 10.1371/journal.pone.0176494
26. Demirci O, Stevens MC, Andreasen NC, Michael A, Liu J, White T, et al. Investigation of relationships between fMRI brain networks in the spectral domain using ICA and Granger causality reveals distinct differences between schizophrenia patients and healthy controls. *Neuroimage* (2009) **46**:419–31. doi: 10.1016/j.neuroimage.2009.02.014
27. Hamilton JP, Chen G, Thomason ME, Schwartz ME, Gotlib IH. Investigating neural primacy in Major Depressive Disorder: multivariate Granger causality analysis of resting-state fMRI time-series data. *Mol Psychiatry* (2011) **16**:763–72. doi: 10.1038/mp.2010.46
28. Guye M, Regis J, Tamura M, Wendling F, McGonigal A, Chauvel P, et al. The role of corticothalamic coupling in human temporal lobe epilepsy. *Brain* (2006) **129**(Pt 7):1917–28. doi: 10.1093/brain/awl151
29. Wade T, Glasofer DR, Brown AJ, Riegel M. Structured Clinical Interview for DSM-IV (SCID). In: Wade T, editor. *Structured Clinical Interview for DSM-IV (SCID)* (2015). p. 1–4.
30. Hamilton M. A rating scale for depression. *J Neurol Neurosurg Psychiatry* (1960) **23**:56–62. doi: 10.1136/jnnp.23.1.56
31. Hamilton M. The assessment of anxiety states by rating. *Br J Med Psychol.* (1959) **32**:50–5. doi: 10.1111/j.2044-8341.1959.tb00467.x
32. Eysenck SB, Eysenck HJ. The questionnaire measurement of psychoticism. *Psychol Med.* (1972) **2**:50–5. doi: 10.1017/S0033291700045608
33. Greve KW, Stickle TR, Love JM, Bianchini KJ, Stanford MS. Latent structure of the wisconsin card sorting test: a confirmatory factor analytic study. *Arch Clin Neuropsychol.* (2005) **20**:355–64. doi: 10.1016/j.acn.2004.09.004
34. Wechsler, D. *Wechsler Adult Intelligence Scale.* 3rd edn. San Antonio, TX: The Psychological Corporation (1997).
35. Yan CG, Wang XD, Zuo XN, Zang, YF. DPABI: Data Processing &; Analysis for (Resting-State) Brain Imaging. *Neuroinformatics* (2016) **14**:339–51. doi: 10.1007/s12021-016-9299-4
36. Song XW, Dong ZY, Long XY, Li SF, Zuo XN, Zhu CZ, et al. REST: a toolkit for resting-state functional magnetic resonance imaging data processing. *PLoS ONE* (2011) **6**:e25031. doi: 10.1371/journal.pone.0025031
37. Guo W, Liu F, Liu J, Yu L, Zhang J, Zhang Z, et al. Abnormal causal connectivity by structural deficits in first-episode, drug-naive schizophrenia at rest. *Schizophr Bull.* (2015) **41**:57–65. doi: 10.1093/schbul/sbu126
38. Kennedy KM, Erickson KI, Rodrigue KM, Voss MW, Colcombe SJ, Kramer AF, et al. Age-related differences in regional brain volumes: a comparison of optimized voxel-based morphometry to manual volumetry. *Neurobiol Aging* (2009) **30**:1657–76. doi: 10.1016/j.neurobiolaging.2007.12.020
39. Japee S, Holiday K, Satyshur MD, Mukai I, Ungerleider LG. A role of right middle frontal gyrus in reorienting of attention: a case study. *Front Syst Neurosci.* (2015) **9**:23. doi: 10.3389/fnsys.2015.00023
40. Liu CL, Hue CW, Chen CC, Chuang KH, Liang KC, Wang YH, et al. Dissociated roles of the middle frontal gyri in the processing of Chinese characters. *Neuroreport* (2006) **17**:1397–401. doi: 10.1097/01.wnr.0000233090.00463.35
41. Miller EK, Cohen JD. An integrative theory of prefrontal cortex function. *Annu Rev Neurosci.* (2001) **24**:167–202. doi: 10.1146/annurev.neuro.24.1.167
42. Belger A, Puce A, Krystal JH, Gore JC, Goldman-Rakic P, McCarthy G. Dissociation of mnemonic and perceptual processes during spatial and nonspatial working memory using fMRI. *Hum Brain Mapp.* (1998) **6**:14–32. doi: 10.1002/(SICI)1097-0193(1998)6:1<14::AID-HBM2>3.0.CO;2-O
43. Guo W, Liu F, Chen J, Wu R, Li L, Zhang Z, et al. Anatomical distance affects cortical-subcortical connectivity in first-episode, drug-naive somatization disorder. *J Affect Disord.* (2017) **217**:153–8. doi: 10.1016/j.jad.2017.04.008
44. Caetano SC, Kaur S, Brambilla P, Nicoletti M, Hatch JP, Sassi RB, et al. Smaller cingulate volumes in unipolar depressed patients. *Biol Psychiatry* (2006) **59**:702–6. doi: 10.1016/j.biopsych.2005.10.011
45. Giuliani NR, Drabant EM, Gross JJ. Anterior cingulate cortex volume and emotion regulation: is bigger better? *Biol Psychol.* (2011) **86**:379–82. doi: 10.1016/j.biopsycho.2010.11.010
46. Lane RD, Reiman EM, Axelrod B, Yun LS, Holmes A, Schwartz GE. Neural correlates of levels of emotional awareness. Evidence of an interaction between emotion and attention in the anterior cingulate cortex. *J Cognitive Neurosci.* (1998) **10**:525–35. doi: 10.1162/089892998562924
47. Dedovic K, Slavich GM, Muscatell KA, Irwin MR, Eisenberger NI. Dorsal anterior cingulate cortex responses to repeated social evaluative feedback in young women with and without a history of depression. *Front Behav Neurosci.* (2016) **10**:64. doi: 10.3389/fnbeh.2016.00064
48. Bush G, Luu P, Posner MI. Cognitive and emotional influences in anterior cingulate cortex. *Trends Cogn Sci.* (2000) **4**:215–22. doi: 10.1016/S1364-6613(00)01483-2
49. Stevens FL, Hurley RA, Taber KH. Anterior cingulate cortex: unique role in cognition and emotion. *J Neuropsychiatry Clin Neurosci.* (2011) **23**:121–5. doi: 10.1176/jnp.23.2.jnp121
50. Cabeza R, Nyberg L. Imaging cognition II: an empirical review of 275 PET and fMRI studies. *J Cognitive Neurosci.* (2000) **12**:1–47. doi: 10.1162/08989290051137585
51. Seghier ML. The angular gyrus: multiple functions and multiple subdivisions. *Neuroscientist* (2013) **19**:43–61. doi: 10.1177/1073858412440596
52. Binder JR, Frost JA, Hammeke TA, Cox RW, Rao SM, Prieto T. Human brain language areas identified by functional magnetic resonance imaging. *J Neurosci.* (1997) **17**:353–62. doi: 10.1523/JNEUROSCI.17-01-00353.1997
53. Schmahmann JD, Caplan D. Cognition, emotion and the cerebellum. *Brain* (2006) **129**(Pt 2):290–2. doi: 10.1093/brain/awh729
54. Glickstein M, Doron K. Cerebellum: connections and functions. *Cerebellum* (2008) **7**:589–94. doi: 10.1007/s12311-008-0074-4

55. Doron KW, Funk CM, Glickstein M. Fronto-cerebellar circuits and eye movement control: a diffusion imaging tractography study of human cortico-pontine projections. *Brain Res.* (2010) **1307**:63–71. doi: 10.1016/j.brainres.2009.10.029
56. Strata P. The emotional cerebellum. *Cerebellum* (2015) **14**:570–7. doi: 10.1007/s12311-015-0649-9
57. Schmahmann JD. The role of the cerebellum in cognition and emotion: personal reflections since 1982 on the dysmetria of thought hypothesis, and its historical evolution from theory to therapy. *Neuropsychol Rev.* (2010) **20**:236–60. doi: 10.1007/s11065-010-9142-x
58. Sacchetti B, Scelfo B, Strata P. Cerebellum and emotional behavior. *Neuroscience* (2009) **162**:756–62. doi: 10.1016/j.neuroscience.2009.01.064

3

Aberrant Neural Activity in Patients with Bipolar Depressive Disorder Distinguishing to the Unipolar Depressive Disorder: A Resting-State Functional Magnetic Resonance Imaging Study

Meihui Qiu[1†], *Huifeng Zhang*[1†], *David Mellor*[2], *Jun Shi*[3], *Chuangxin Wu*[1], *Yueqi Huang*[1], *Jianye Zhang*[4], *Ting Shen*[5*] and *Daihui Peng*[1*]

[1] Division of Mood Disorders, Shanghai Mental Health Center, Shanghai Jiao Tong University School of Medicine, Shanghai, China, [2] School of Psychology, Faculty of Health, Deakin University, Melbourne, VIC, Australia, [3] Institute of Biomedical Engineering, School of Communication and Information Engineering, Shanghai University, Shanghai,China, [4] Department of Medical Imaging, Shanghai Mental Health Center, Shanghai Jiao Tong University School of Medicine, Shanghai, China, [5] Department of Psychiatry, Shanghai Mental Health Center, Shanghai Jiao Tong University School of Medicine, Shanghai, China

***Correspondence:**
Ting Shen
shen.t@126.com
Daihui Peng
pdhsh@126.com

†Joint first authors.

This study aims to explore the intrinsic patterns of spontaneous activity of bipolar depression (BD) patients by analyzing the fractional amplitude of low frequency fluctuation (fALFF) that help differentiate BD from unipolar depressive disorder(UD). Twenty eight patients with BD, 47 patients with UD and 29 healthy controls were enrolled to receive the resting-state functional magnetic resonance imaging (rs-fMRI) scans. The group differences of fALFF values were calculated among three groups. In addition, the correlations between the clinical variables and mfALFF values were estimated. The brain regions with activation discrepancies among three groups are located in precuneus, the left middle temporal gyrus (MTG) and left inferior parietal lobe (IPL) and lingual gyrus. Compared with HC group, BD group shows decreased fALFF in precuneus, the left IPL and increased fALFF in lingual gyrus remarkably; UD group shows significantly decreased fALFF in precuneus, the left MTG and the left IPL. On the contrast of patients with UD, patients with BD have significantly increased fALFF value in the left precuneus, the left MGT and lingual gyrus. Furthermore, a negative correlation is found between the mfALFF values in precuneus and the scores of cognitive impairment factor in the UD group. The similar pattern of intrinsic activity in PCC suggests depressive state-dependent change. The aberrant patterns of intrinsic activity in precuneus, the IPL and lingual gyrus might be provide quantitative nodes that help to conduct further study for better distinguishing between BD and UD.

Keywords: bipolar disorder, unipolar depressive disorder, fractional amplitude of low frequency fluctuation, resting-state, functional magnetic resonance imaging

INTRODUCTION

Bipolar disorder, characterized by abnormal mood, cognitive dysfunctions, changes of behaviors, and disturbed circadian rhythms, ranks the twelfth burdens of all diseases in terms of disability-adjusted of Life Years (1). The precise diagnosis and efficient treatment have generally been limited by the fact that the dynamic process of bipolar disorder is dominated by depression or elevated mood (mania or hypomania). The hypomania is even more difficult to recognized in its earlier onset (2). More importantly, most individuals with bipolar disorder (58–71%) have depressive onset polarity, which usually show some overlapping clinical manifestations with the UD, such as depressed mood, retardation of thinking, and cognitive impairment. A latest meta-analysis for prospective transition from UD to bipolar disorder, reported that almost a quarter of individuals with UD transitioned to bipolar disorder after more than 12 years follow-up (3). Furthermore, the misdiagnosis of bipolar disorder would result in the delay of treatment, exerting a heavy economic burden on patients' families and the society (4, 5). Hence, it is imperative to find appropriate methods to distinguish bipolar disorder patients from individuals with UD, which could help to minimize the impact of mixed diagnoses in early therapeutic intervention.

Unfortunately, the current diagnostic schema for bipolar disorder, which is still based on descriptive psychopathology rather than clearly elucidating the neuropathophysiology, has failed to identify BD precisely (6). The current advances in multi-modal neuroimaging studies of bipolar disorder have effectively found the alterations in both brain structure and function, including gray matter morphology (7, 8), white matter integrity (9), and local/global network connectivity (10, 11), which could provide reliable neurobiological markers for bipolar disorder. Importantly, considerable neuroimaging studies have suggested that compared with UD patients, individuals with BD had significantly abnormal patterns of subcortical and cortical activity (12–14). Therefore, considering intrinsic neural characteristics without task-specific neural function, resting-state functional magnetic resonance (rs-fMRI) can provide useful biomarkers (3, 15, 16), which investigate the basic activity of brain during awake and resting state based on the blood oxygenation level dependent (BOLD) signal (17). However, only few studies based on rs-fMRI data directly compared BD with UD. Liu et al revealed that significant alteration of connectivity models of default mode network (DMN) were found in bipolar depressive disorder compared with unipolar depression using the pLiNGAM algorithm (18). Two additional studies (19, 20) showed abnormal values of regional homogeneity (ReHo) in BD group compared with UD group. These functional neuroimaging studies estimated functional integrity of neural circuitries relevant to neuropathophysiological processes in bipolar disorder, which have provided us with holistic information of patterns within brain networks from the perspective of functional integration, by measuring regional activity, using blood-oxygen level dependent (BOLD) signal change, and functional connectivity, using techniques examining the extent of coupling of time series of activity between neural regions of interest. However, most of previous studies used seed-voxel analysis to explore the regional brain activity (21). Studies of the intrinsic functional dynamics based on global brain voxels between BD and UD groups are insufficient.

For these reasons, it's important to explore the intrinsic spontaneous brain activity measured by resting-state fMRI (RS-fMRI) in samples of depression (22), Individual differences in spontaneous brain activity may reflect distinct experiences and learning histories (23). Considering the widespread region features of BOLD-fMRI signal, Zou et al. firstly applied the fast Fourier Transform technique to process the low frequency (0.01-0.08 Hz) signal of the whole brain voxels (24). The low frequency signals were further standardized by full frequency amplitude (0–0.25 Hz), which were defined as the fractional amplitude of low-frequency fluctuations (fALFF) (24). The fALFF might reflect the features of spontaneous neural activity, which is related to the rate of regional glucose metabolism and reflecting regional brain activity abnormalities at baseline (25, 26), avoid the influences of physiological noise, and provide the information about the brain impairment (24). The fALFF has been applied to directly reveal the spontaneous activity of each brain region and to precisely demonstrate that the significant alteration of cortical intrinsic activity is existed in many psychiatric disorders, such as schizophrenia, UD and obsessive-compulsive disorder (27–29). Although some neuroimaging studies by fALFF analysis showed the alterations of spontaneous activities of cortical-limbic circuits in patients with UD (30, 31), no studies found the similar changes in patients with BD. Furthermore, the abnormality of spontaneous neuronal activity in patients with UD and BD has not been totally elucidated. Evidences obtained from existing studies using the fALFF approach are insufficient and inconsistent.

There were insufficient studies to evaluate the alterations of global regions in characteristics of spontaneous neural activity between patients with BD and patients with UD by fALFF value. Accordingly, in the present study, we aimed to investigate the abnormal regions in BD and UD by analyzing fALFF. We hypothesized that individuals with BD, compared to UD and HCs, would exhibit aberrant intrinsic activity by fALFF value based on rs-fMRI data, extrapolating a potential clue to distinguish patients with BD from population with depression.

MATERIALS AND METHODS

Participants

Twenty-eight patients with BD, 47 patients with UD were enrolled from out-patient departments in Shanghai Mental Health Center. Twenty-nine healthy volunteers were recruited from society by advertisement as well. Diagnosis of BD and UD were based on the Structured Clinical Interviews for Diagnostic and Statistical Manual fourth edition (DSM-IV), the 24-item Hamilton rating scale for depression (HAMD) >20 (32), and the Young Mania Rating Scale (YMRS) <7 (33). Exclusion criteria for all participants included meeting any other diagnosis criteria of current or past Axis I and Axis II psychiatric disorders of DSM-IV, current alcohol/substance dependence ,or abuse (within 6 months of study), positive urinary toxicology screening at baseline, serious neurological or medical disorders, positive pregnancy test or lactation, a history of head trauma, and general contraindications to MRI, a history of electroconvulsive therapy. All participants were right-handed Han Chinese with more than 9 years of schooling. The study was approved by the Investigational Review Board (IRB00002733-Shanghai mental health center, China), and written informed consent was obtained from all subjects before inclusion in the study.

Image Acquisition

Brain imaging data were acquired using magnetic resonance scanning (Siemens 3.0T). High-resolution T1 images were acquired by the gradient recalled echo (GRE) sequence as the following parameters: repetition time (TR) = 2,300 ms, echo time (TE) = 2.96 ms, field of view (Fov) = 24 × 24 cm^2, slice thickness = 1.0 mm, 192 slices, gap = 0.0 mm, voxel = 1.0 × 1.0 × 1.0 mm^3, matrix = 240 × 256, scanning time = 9 min 14 s. Resting-state images were collected by echo planar imaging (EPI) sequence as the following parameters: TR/TE = 2,000/30 ms, Fov = 220 *220 mm, slice thickness = 4.0 mm, 33 slices, gap = 0.6 mm, voxel = 3.4 × 3.4 × 4.0 mm^3, 200 bolds with GRAPPA on. For each participant, the rs-fMRI scanning lasted for 6 min and 46 s. During the scanning, the participants were kept awake with eyes closed, body still, and their respiration regular.

Functional Imaging Data Preprocessing

All images were processed by Data Processing Assistant for Resting-State fMRI (DPARSF) based on Statistical Parametric Mapping (SPM8) (http://www.fil.ion.ucl.ac.uk/spm) and the toolbox for Data Processing & Analysis of Brain Imaging (DPABI, http://rfmri.org/DPABI). For each participant's data, the first 10 time points and the data with excessive head motion (shift >2.5 mm, degree of rotation >2.5°) were discarded to ensure the steady state. After realignment using a 6 degrees-of-freedom linear transformation without re-sampling, we co-registered the individual structural images (T1-weighted MPRAGE) to the mean functional image. Then the structural images were segmented into gray matter, white matter, and cerebrospinal fluid. Based on the Diffeomorphic Anatomical Registration Through Exponentiated Lie algebra (DARTEL) tool, these segmented images was used to compute transformation parameters that coregistered individual native space to Montreal Neurological Institute (MNI). The nuisance covariates, as the Friston 24-parameter model, were to regress out from the realigned data, including the six head motion parameters, the first time derivations, signals of the global brain, cerebrospinal fluid and white matter. The remaining images were standardized by MNI system and re-sampled to 3*3*3 mm^3 voxels, and operated spatial smooth adopting 8 mm full width at half maximum (FWHM) so as to enhance the image signal-to-noise ratio. After preprocessing, 3 participants from UD group, 3 from BD group and 2 from HC group were respectively excluded with the standard of head motion.

fALFF Analysis

The fALFF was computed with Resting-State fMRI Data Analysis Toolkit (REST) (http://www.restfmri.net). After undergoing a band-pass filter (0.01–0.08 Hz) (34) and linear-trend removing, we calculated the power spectrum by transforming the time series of each voxel with a fast Fourier transform (FFT). A ratio of the low-frequency amplitude averaged (0.01–0.08 Hz) to the power spectrum of the entire frequency range (0–0.25 Hz) was computed at each voxel to obtain the fALFF (24). For standardization, the fALFF value was further divided by the global mean fALFF value within a group-based gray matter (GM) mask that was generated by the mean GM map (threshold = 0.15) of all subjects, and the mean fALFF (mfALFF) was obtained.

Statistical Analysis

Demographic and clinical data were analyzed using SPSS, version 19.0 (SPSS, Inc., Chicago). The differences of voxel-based fALFF among BD group, UD group, and HC groups were analyzed by the REST using one-way analysis of variance (ANOVA), with age, gender and education level as covariates. Significant differences were set at the threshold of voxel-wise $P < 0.001$ (uncorrected), with a cluster size >10 voxels. The mean fALFF values of brain regions with significant differences were extracted for further *post-hoc* analysis among three groups. Statistical significance for *post-hoc* analysis was set at $P < 0.01$. Then, we performed the Pearson correlation analyses between the mean fALFF values of the brain regions showing significant group differences and the clinical characteristic variant (e.g., total HAMD and HAMA scores). Notably, the scale of HAMD was broken into seven factors based on its Chinese version: anxiety/somatization, change of weight, cognitive dysfunction, atypical circadian rhythm, retardation, sleep disorder, and desperation (35). The threshold for statistical significance was set at $P < 0.05$.

RESULTS

Demographics and Clinical Characteristics

The demographic and clinical data of 28 participants with BD (14 male/14 female, aged 19–45 years, mean ± SD: 31.79 ± 12.83), 47 participants with UD (20 male/27 female, aged 21–51 years, mean ± SD: 38.11±13.16), and 27 healthy controls (17 male/10 female, aged 21–43 years, mean ± SD: 33.72±9.77) were respectively shown in the **Table 1**. There were no statistical differences in both age and gender among three groups.

Differences of mfALFF Values Among Groups

The significant differences of mfALFF values as the result of ANOVA among UD, BD, and healthy control groups were shown in **Figure 1**. The anatomical location of brain regions and intensity of activity were described in **Table 2**. The brain regions with significant differences were located in precuneus, the left MTG, the left IPL, and lingual gyrus.

By a *post-hoc* test, BD group showed a significant increase of mfALFF value in lingual gyrus ($p = 0.000$), but significant decrease of mfALFF value in precuneus ($p = 0.000$), and the left

TABLE 1 | Clinical characteristics of participants among groups.

Characteristics		I ($n = 28$)	II ($n = 47$)	III ($n = 27$)	$Z/F/c^2$	*P*
Age (Year)		31.79 ± 12.83	38.11 ± 13.16	33.72 ± 9.77	2.63	0.08
Onset Age (Year)		22.39 ± 8.82	33.98 ± 12.87	/	−3.82	<0.001
Gender	M	14	20	17	3.46	0.15
	F	14	27	10		
Education level (Year)		13.32 ± 3.37	11.26 ± 2.86	13.59 ± 3.30	6.43	<0.001
Scores of HAMD		31.04 ± 7.92	30.06 ± 7.45	/	−0.53	0.59
Scores of HAMA		13.86 ± 6.01	15.39 ± 6.01	/	1.07	0.29
Attack Frequency		4.64 ± 2.91	1.85 ± 1.72	/	−5.10	<0.001
Illness Course (Month)		109.79 ± 126.93	55.66 ± 98.20	/	−3.81	<0.001
Psychotropic medications, n		23	25			
Antidepressants, n		6	25			
Lithium, n		7	0			
Antiepileptic, n		15	2			
Anxiolytics, n		4	5			
Antipsychotics, n		12	2			
Medication-free		5	22			

I, bipolar depression group; II, unipolar depression disorder group; III, healthy control group. Chi-square test, gender; ANOVA, age, education level; T-test, scores of HAMD, scores of HAMA, onset age, attack frequency, illness course.

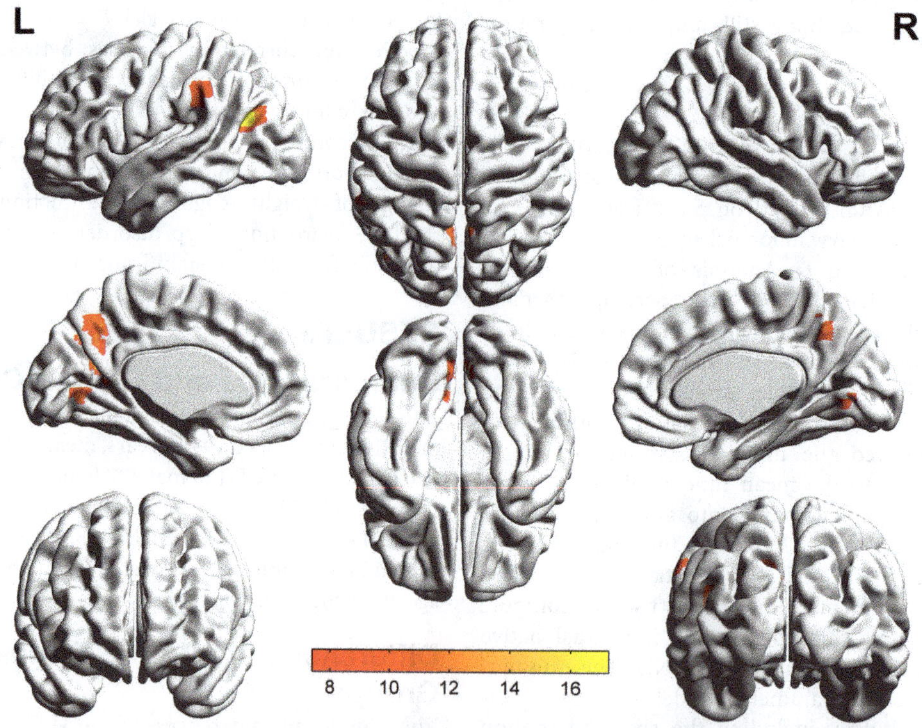

FIGURE 1 | Statistical maps showing ANOVA results of mfALFF value among patients with UD, BD, and HCs. The different regions mainly including precuneus, the left MTG, the left IPL, and lingual gyrus. Threshold was set at voxel-wise $P < 0.001$ (uncorrected), with a cluster size >10 voxels. The resulting images are overlaid on the MNI1152 template. The color bars represent the range of *F*-value.

IPL ($p = 0.000$) vs. healthy control group. Relative to the control group, a significant decreased mfALFF values were observed in the left precuneus ($p = 0.001$), precuneus ($p = 0.000$), the left MTG ($p = 0.000$), and the left IPL ($p = 0.000$) in UD group. Remarkable increased of mfALFF values in the left precuneus ($p = 0.000$), the left MTG ($p = 0.000$), and lingual gyrus

($p = 0.004$) were observed in BD group in contrast to UD group. Details are shown in **Table 3** and **Figure 2**.

Correlation Analysis With the Clinical Characteristics

We found a negative correlation between the cognitive disorder (factor 3 of HAMD) and the mfALFF value of precuneus in UD group, as shown in **Figure 3**. There were not any other significant relationships between the different fALFF values in the left PCC, the left IPL and lingual gyrus with clinical variants such as onset age, illness course, scores of HAMD, and scores of HAMA as well.

DISCUSSION

In the current study, we examined the fALFF changes in patients with BD and UD compared with healthy controls by using resting-state fMRI. The results revealed that fALFF values noticeably varied in precuneus, the left MTG, the left IPL, and lingual gyrus among BD, UD, and HC group. These altered values mainly occurred in DMN (excluding lingual gyrus) in the UD patients. The results also showed that the score of thought disorder factor in patients with UD was negatively correlated with the fALFF values in the precuneus. However, we noticed the altered neural activity of lingual gyrus, precuneus and the left IPL in patients with BD in comparison with HC group. Meanwhile, BD patients showed significantly increased fALFF values in the left precuneus, the left MGT and lingual gyrus relative to UD patients.

TABLE 2 | Brain regions with significant differences of mfALFF values in ANCOVA among UD, BD, and HC groups.

Brain regions	L/R	Cluster size (voxels)	BA	MNI Coordinate (mm)			F
				x	y	z	
Precuneus	L	40	7	−18	−57	21	16.62
				−12	−63	36	16.37
	/	15	7	0	−57	45	14.11
MTG	L	15	39	−39	−66	21	16.60
IPL	L	11	40	−57	−36	33	10.50
Lingual gyrus	/	11	18	0	−69	0	11.77

ANCOVA, analysis of covariance; BA, brodmann area; MNI, Montreal Neurological Institute; HC, healthy control; L, Left; R, Right.

This research indicated that the decreased intrinsic activity located in part of DMN including precuneus, the left MGT and left IPL in patients with UD relative to HCs. The DMN is composed of cerebral regions which are activated when the brain is wakefully rest, but are deactivated during the goal-oriented tasks (36). DMN is thought to be related to cognitive function of self-awareness, episodic memory, salience, and interactive modulation (37, 38). Previous neuroimaging studies have highlighted the involvement of DMN in the pathophysiology of UD by index of functional connectivity, effective connectivity, Reho, and fALFF (39). Among these different analysis methods, the fALFF analysis allows us to directly detect regional signal changes of spontaneous activity at rest (24). Our results also highlighted the importance of fALFF analysis in reflecting intrinsic neural activity within specific regions inside of the DMN.

In present study, subjects with UD showed decreased spontaneous neural activity of the left MTG compared to both subjects with BD and HC participants. As a part of DMN, the lateral temporal regions are considered to process sentence comprehension and language (40–42), especial the retrieval of lexical-syntactic information from memory (43). Our results were in line with previous findings. For example, Guo et al found decreased ALFF values in the left MTG (44). Meanwhile, decreased fALFF values in the left MTG was observed in first-episode, treatment-naïve patients with major depressive disorder (30, 45). Evidences from task-fMRI studies also supported the abnormality of the MTG in UD patients, as patients exhibited decreased activation in the left MTG during sad facial expression recognition (46). On the other hand, one study found that, compared to UD patients, BD patients showed decreased activation in the MTGduring emotional processing task (47). Thus, the finding of MTG in this study might be part of neural underpinning for the different clinical characteristics in depressive state between UD and BD patients.

Precuneus, serving as a core hub of the DMN, may be related to self-referential processing and mental representations (48). Similar to previous studies (19, 45, 49), our study reported decreased fALFF value of precuneus in UD patient and BD patients. We also found that there existed a drastic negative

TABLE 3 | Brain regions with significant differences of mfALFF values inter-groups.

Brain regions	BD	UD	HC	P-value		
				UD vs. BD	UD vs. N	BD vs. N
L_Precuneus	1.370 ± 0.124	1.243 ± 0.090	1.336 ± 0.104	0.000*	0.001*	0.666
Precuneus	1.023 ± 0.063	1.034 ± 0.078	1.165 ± 0.106	1.000	0.000*	0.000*
L_MTG	1.170 ± 0.121	1.052 ± 0.081	1.182 ± 0.088	0.000*	0.000*	1.000
L_IPL	1.068 ± 0.088	1.083 ± 0.079	1.187 ± 0.081	1.000	0.000*	0.000*
Lingual gyrus	1.167 ± 0.137	1.075 ± 0.112	1.010 ± 0.106	0.004*	0.066	0.000*

**Means $p < 0.01$.*

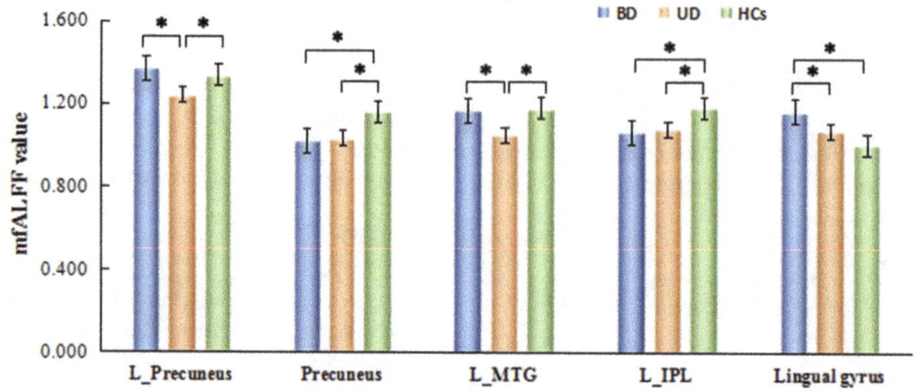

FIGURE 2 | Brain regions with significant differences of mfALFF values inter-groups. *Means $p < 0.001$.

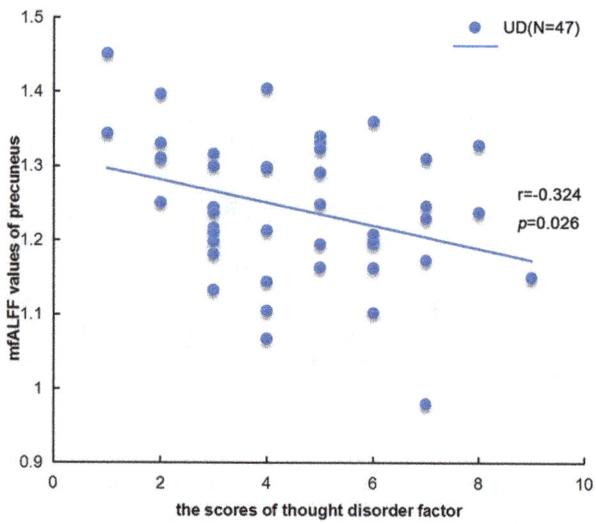

FIGURE 3 | Correlation analysis between mfALFF values of precuneus in UD group and thought disorder factor (factor 3 of HAMD). $n = 47$, $p < 0.05$.

correlation between the fALFF values of precuneus and the score of cognitive disorder. A meta-analysis reported the decreased brain activity in posterior precuneus in first-episode, drug-naïve UD patients (50), while Zhu et al. found that the decreased functional connectivity between precuneus and other regions of posterior medial cortex was negatively correlated with the overgeneral autobiographical memory (AM) (51). Furthermore, undergoing the sad mood induction, patients with chronic UD showed the decreased functional connectivity between precuneus and PCC (52). In our study, we found that the fALFF values of precuneus in BD group were significantly higher than UD group. Meanwhile, structural differences in precuneus have been found in comparisons between BD and UD patients (53). Young et al. also reported the decreased activity of precuneus in BD patients relative to UD patients during specific AM of negative memories (54). Therefore, it might be suggested that the abnormal spontaneous neural activity in precuneus may play an important role in AM (54), and maybe provide further evidence for distinguishing the differentiation of affective disorders.

The UD and BD group also showed decreased fALFF value in IPL compared to HC groups. Previous studies have found that IPL plays a critical role in emotional regulation, self-referential processing and response inhibition (55), while IPL is also observed to be related with monetary rewards (56). Several previous studies found the functional changes of IPL in patients with UD (30, 56–58). Guo et al. found that UD patients had decreased functional connectivity between the left cerebral lobule and the left IPL compared to healthy controls (57), which maybe related with the deficits of cognitive control in patients with UD (58). Our study also found decreased fALFF value in IPL of the patients with BD compared to HC. Previous studies (53, 59) indicated the alterations in cerebral blood flow or gray matter volume of IPL in BD might be related to the prominent deficits in response inhibition. Therefore, the further studies about IPL among the patients of UD and BD should be carried out in terms of the cognitive control function, which may present the similar symptom in depressive state.

Lingual gyrus was another region with significantly increased fALFF values in BD group, compared with both UD group and HC group. Lingual gyrus, as the key region of visual cognitive network, helps process the facial recognition and emotion recognition (60). Lingual gyrus also plays an important role in the integration of visual information and introspective stimuli. Xu et al. firstly found the decreased value of fALFF in lingual gyrus in patients with BD (61). The altered function of lingual gyrus in BD patients have been found to be associated with the deficits of visual sensory processing (62) and episodic memory (63). Taken together, our result indicates that the decrease of fALFF values in lingual gyrus might be the sensible index reflecting the visual cognitive dysfunction in BD.

The main limitation of the present study is uncontrolled effects of medication, especially that medication load was higher for individuals with BD than for those with UD, which might lead to type II errors (64), although our findings are similar to previous studies. Secondly, patients with BD in our study showed earlier age of onset, more depressive episodes and longer illness course relative to UD patients. These atypical characteristics of depressive episode are regarded as risk factors for bipolar disorder (65). Thirdly, the relatively small sample size would be a limitation for the interpreting of our potential findings. Although the sample size in our study is comparable to many previously published studies, larger-sized sample should hypothetically yield more representative results (66). However, one previous study also argued that the inter-subject correlation (ISC) statistics with 20 subjects had converged close to a large sample ISC statistics with 130 subjects averagely (67). Finally, our study failed to replicate the results in the other independent sample due to the limited sample size. Considering all the above mentioned, further work, combining clinical phenotype, and adopting longitudinal methods, is required to replicate our findings and to provide more conclusive evidences.

CONCLUSION

In summary, patients with BD showed distinctive pattern of intrinsic activity in the lingual gyrus compared to UD patients and HCs, suggesting potential different pathophysiological mechanisms of BD. The similar fALFF changes located in the precuneus and the left IPL between BD and UD patients might be associated with the coexisted symptoms in depressive state. Furthermore, the significant aberrant spontaneous neural activity in left MTG and the left precuneus may provide potential neural underpinning to distinguish BD from UD. Therefore, aberrant brain intrinsic activity may highlight new perspectives on investigating neuroimaging-based biomarkers in future studies of BD vs. UD.

AUTHOR CONTRIBUTIONS

MQ, DP, and TS conceived and designed the experiments. MQ, DP, TS, JZ, HZ, and YH performed the experiments. MQ, DP, JS, and CW analyzed the data. MQ, DM, HZ, DP, and TS wrote the paper.

ACKNOWLEDGMENTS

This study was funded by the National Natural Science Foundation of China (81571327), the Guiding Medical Project of Science and Technology Commission of Shanghai Municipality (16411965300) and the Project of Science Committee of Health Department of Shanghai Municipal Government (201640003).

REFERENCES

1. Mathers C, Fat D M, Boersma JT. World Health Organization. *The Global Burden of Disease: 2004 Update* (2008).
2. Etain B, Lajnef M, Bellivier F, Mathieu F, Raust A, Cochet B, et al. Clinical expression of bipolar disorder type I as a function of age and polarity at onset: convergent findings in samples from France and the United States. J *Clin Psychiatry* (2012) **73**:e561–6. doi: 10.4088/JCP.10m06504
3. Ratheesh A, Davey C, Hetrick S, Alvarez-Jimenez M, Voutier C, Bechdolf A, et al. (2017). A systematic review and meta-analysis of prospective transition from major depression to bipolar disorder. *Acta Psychiatr Scand.* **135**:273–84. doi: 10.1111/acps.12686
4. Goodwin G M. Bipolar depression and treatment with antidepressants. *Br J Psychiatry* (2012) **200**:5–6. doi: 10.1192/bjp.bp.111.095349
5. Rosa A R, Reinares M, Michalak E E, Bonnin C M, Sole B, Franco C, et al. Functional impairment and disability across mood states in bipolar disorder. *Value Health* (2010) **13**:984–8. doi: 10.1111/j.1524-4733.2010.00768.x
6. Gitlin M. Treatment-resistant bipolar disorder. *Mol Psychiatry* (2006) **11**:227–40. doi: 10.1038/sj.mp.4001793
7. Fears SC, Schür R, Sjouwerman R, Service SK, Araya C, Araya X, et al. Brain structure-function associations in multi-generational families genetically enriched for bipolar disorder. *Brain* (2015) **138**:2087–102. doi: 10.1093/brain/awv106
8. Wise T, Radua J, Nortje G, Cleare A J, Young A H, Arnone D. Voxel-based meta-analytical evidence of structural disconnectivity in major depression and bipolar disorder. *Biol Psychiatry* (2016) **79**:293–302. doi: 10.1016/j.biopsych.2015.03.004
9. Martino M, Magioncalda P, Saiote C, Conio B, Escelsior A, Rocchi G, et al. Abnormal functional-structural cingulum connectivity in mania: combined functional magnetic resonance imaging-diffusion tensor imaging investigation in different phases of bipolar disorder. *Acta Psychiatr Scandinav.* (2016) **134**:339–49. doi: 10.1111/acps.12596
10. Stoddard J, Gotts S J, Brotman M A, Lever S, Hsu D, Zarate C, et al. Aberrant intrinsic functional connectivity within and between corticostriatal and temporal-parietal networks in adults and youth with bipolar disorder. *Psychol Med.* (2016) **46**:1509–22. doi: 10.1017/S0033291716000143
11. Cardoso de Almeida JR, Phillips ML. Distinguishing between unipolar depression and bipolar depression: current and future clinical and neuroimaging perspectives. *Biol Psychiatry* (2013) 73:111–8. doi: 10.1016/j.biopsych.2012.06.010
12. Satterthwaite TD, Kable JW, Vandekar L, Katchmar N, Bassett DS, Baldassano CF, et al. Common and dissociable dysfunction of the reward system in bipolar and unipolar depression. *Neuropsychopharmacology* (2015) **40**:2258–68. doi: 10.1038/npp.2015.75
13. Rive MM, Mocking RJT, Koeter MWJ, Van Wingen G, De Wit SJ, Van Den Heuvel OA, et al. State-Dependent differences in emotion regulation between unmedicated bipolar disorder and major depressive disorder. *JAMA Psychiatry* (2015). **72**:687. doi: 10.1001/jamapsychiatry.2015.0161
14. Li M, Das T, Deng W, Wang Q, Li Y, Zhao L, et al. Clinical utility of a short resting-state MRI scan in differentiating bipolar from unipolar depression. *Acta Psychiatr Scand.* (2017) **136**:288–299. doi: 10.1111/acps.12752
15. Raichle ME. Two views of brain function. *Trends Cogn Sci.* (2010) **14**:180–90. doi: 10.1016/j.tics.2010.01.008
16. Peterson A, Thome J, Frewen P, Lanius R A. Resting-state neuroimaging studies: a new way of identifying differences and similarities among the anxiety disorders? *Can J Psychiatry* (2014) **59**:294–300. doi: 10.1177/070674371405900602
17. Ogawa S, Tank D W, Menon R, Ellermann J M, Kim S G, Merkle H, et al. Intrinsic signal changes accompanying sensory stimulation: functional brain mapping with magnetic resonance imaging. *Proc Natl Acad Sci USA.* (1992). **89**:5951–5.
18. Liu Y, Wu X, Zhang J, Guo X, Long Z, Yao L. Altered effective connectivity model in the default mode network between bipolar and unipolar depression based on resting-state fMRI. *J Affect Disord.* (2015) **182**:8–17. doi: 10.1016/j.jad.2015.04.009
19. Liang MJ, Zhou Q, Yang KR, Yang XL, Fang J, Chen WL, et al. Identify changes of brain regional homogeneity in bipolar disorder and

unipolar depression using resting-state FMRI. *PLoS ONE* (2013) **8**:e79999. doi: 10.1371/journal.pone.0079999
20. Liu CH, Ma X, Wu X, Zhang Y, Zhou FC, Li F, et al. Regional homogeneity of resting-state brain abnormalities in bipolar and unipolar depression. *Prog Neuropsychopharmacol Biol Psychiatry* (2013) **41**:52–9. doi: 10.1016/j.pnpbp.2012.11.010
21. Chen JE, Glover GH. Functional magnetic resonance imaging methods. *Neuropsychol Rev.* (2015) **25**:289–313. doi: 10.1007/s11065-015-9294-9
22. Fox M D, Raichle ME. Spontaneous fluctuations in brain activity observed with functional magnetic resonance imaging. *Nat Rev Neurosci.* (2007) **8**:700–11. doi: 10.1038/nrn2201
23. Wei L, Duan X, Zheng C, Wang S, Gao Q, Zhang Z, et al. Specific frequency bands of amplitude low-frequency oscillation encodes personality. *Hum Brain Mapp.* (2014). **35**:331–9. doi: 10.1002/hbm.22176
24. Zou QH, Zhu CZ, Yang Y, Zuo XN, Long XY, Cao QJ, et al. An improved approach to detection of amplitude of low-frequency fluctuation (ALFF) for resting-state fMRI: fractional ALFF. *J Neurosci Methods* (2008) **172**:137–41. doi: 10.1016/j.jneumeth.2008.04.012
25. Nugent AC, Martinez A, D'Alfonso A, Zarate CA, Theodore WH. The relationship between glucose metabolism, resting-state fMRI BOLD signal, and GABAA-binding potential: a preliminary study in healthy subjects and those with temporal lobe epilepsy. *J Cereb Blood Flow Metab.* (2015) **35**:583–91. doi: 10.1038/jcbfm.2014.228
26. Margulies DS, Bottger J, Long X, Lv Y, Kelly C, Schafer A, et al. Resting developments: a review of fMRI post-processing methodologies for spontaneous brain activity. *Magma* (2010) **23**:289–307. doi: 10.1007/s10334-010-0228-5
27. Guo Wb, Liu F, Xue ZM, Xu XJ, Wu RR, Ma CQ, et al. Alterations of the amplitude of low-frequency fluctuations in treatment-resistant and treatment-response depression: a resting-state fMRI study. *Progr Neuro Psychopharmacol Biol Psychiatry* (2012) **37**:153–60. doi: 10.1016/j.pnpbp.2012.01.011
28. Guo W, Song Y, Liu F, Zhang Z, Zhang J, Yu M, et al. Dissociation of functional and anatomical brain abnormalities in unaffected siblings of schizophrenia patients. *Clin Neurophysiol.* (2015) **126**:927–32. doi: 10.1016/j.clinph.2014.08.016
29. Cheng Y, Xu J, Nie B, Luo C, Yang T, Li H, et al. Abnormal resting-state activities and functional connectivities of the anterior and the posterior cortexes in medication-naive patients with obsessive-compulsive disorder. *PLoS ONE* (2013) **8**:e67478. doi: 10.1371/journal.pone.0067478
30. Wang L, Dai W, Su Y, Wang G, Tan Y, Jin Z, et al. Amplitude of low-frequency oscillations in first-episode, treatment-naive patients with major depressive disorder: a resting-state functional MRI study. *PLoS ONE* (2012) **7**:e48658. doi: 10.1371/journal.pone.0048658
31. Liu F, Guo W, Liu L, Long Z, Ma C, Xue Z, et al. Abnormal amplitude low-frequency oscillations in medication-naive, first-episode patients with major depressive disorder: a resting-state fMRI study. *J Affect Disord.* (2013) **146**:401–6. doi: 10.1016/j.jad.2012.10.001
32. Hamilton M. Development of a rating scale for primary depressive illness. *Br J Soc Clin Psychol.* (1967) **6**:278–96.
33. Young RC, Biggs JT, Ziegler VE, Meyer DA. A rating scale for mania: reliability, validity and sensitivity. *Br J Psychiatry* (1978) **133**:429–35.
34. Biswal B, Zerrin Yetkin F, Haughton VM, Hyde JS. Functional connectivity in the motor cortex of resting human brain using echo-planar mri. *Magne Reson Med.* (1995) **34**:537–41.
35. Zhang M. *Handbook of Rating Scales in Psychiatry.* Hunan: Hunan Science and Technology Press. (1998) 121–26.
36. Raichle ME, MacLeod AM, Snyder AZ, Powers WJ, Gusnard DA, Shulman GL. A default mode of brain function. *Proc Natl Acad Sci USA.* (2001) **98**:676–82. doi: 10.1073/pnas.98.2.676
37. Uddin LQ. Salience processing and insular cortical function and dysfunction. *Nat Rev Neurosci.* (2015) **16**:55–61. doi: 10.1038/nrn3857
38. Weissman-Fogel I, Moayedi M, Taylor K S, Pope G, Davis KD. Cognitive and default-mode resting state networks: do male and female brains "rest" differently? *Hum Brain Mapp.* (2010) **31**: 1713–26. doi: 10.1002/hbm.20968
39. Whitfield-Gabrieli S, Ford JM. Default mode network activity and connectivity in psychopathology. *Annu Rev Clin Psychol.* (2012) **8**:49–76. doi: 10.1146/annurev-clinpsy-032511-143049
40. Friederici AD. Pathways to language: fiber tracts in the human brain. *Trends Cogn Sci.* (2009) **13**:175–81. doi: 10.1016/j.tics.2009.01.001
41. Saur D, Kreher BW, Schnell S, Kummerer D, Kellmeyer P, Vry MS, et al. Ventral and dorsal pathways for language. *Proc Natl Acad Sci USA.* (2008) **105**:18035–40. doi: 10.1073/pnas.0805234105
42. Xu J, Wang J, Fan L, Li H, Zhang W, Hu Q, et al. Tractography-based parcellation of the human middle temporal gyrus. *Sci Rep.* (2015) **5**:18883. doi: 10.1038/srep18883
43. Snijders TM, Vosse T, Kempen G, Van Berkum JJ, Petersson KM, Hagoort P. Retrieval and unification of syntactic structure in sentence comprehension: an FMRI study using word-category ambiguity. *Cereb Cortex* (2009) 19:1493–503. doi: 10.1093/cercor/bhn187
44. Guo W, Liu F, Yu M, Zhang J, Zhang Z, Liu J, et al. Functional and anatomical brain deficits in drug-naive major depressive disorder. *Prog Neuropsychopharmacol Biol Psychiatry* (2014) **54**:1–6. doi: 10.1016/j.pnpbp.2014.05.008
45. Shen T, Qiu M, Li C, Zhang J, Wu Z, Wang B, et al. Altered spontaneous neural activity in first-episode, unmedicated patients with major depressive disorder. *Neuroreport* (2014) **25**:1302–7. doi: 10.1097/wnr.0000000000000263
46. Jiang W, Yin Z, Pang Y, Wu F, Kong L, Xu K. Brain functional changes in facial expression recognition in patients with major depressive disorder before and after antidepressant treatment: a functional magnetic resonance imaging study. *Neural Regen Res.* (2012) **7**:1151–7. doi: 10.3969/j.issn.1673-5374.2012.15.005
47. Cerullo MA, Eliassen JC, Smith CT, Fleck DE, Nelson EB, Strawn JR, et al. Bipolar I disorder and major depressive disorder show similar brain activation during depression. *Bipolar Disord.* (2014) **16**:703–12. doi: 10.1111/bdi.12225
48. Cavanna AE, Trimble MR. The precuneus: a review of its functional anatomy and behavioural correlates. *Brain* (2006) **129**(Pt 3):564–83. doi: 10.1093/brain/awl004
49. Liu F, Hu M, Wang S, Guo W, Zhao J, Li J, et al. Abnormal regional spontaneous neural activity in first-episode, treatment-naive patients with late-life depression: a resting-state fMRI study. *Prog Neuropsychopharmacol Biol Psychiatry* (2012) **39**:326–31. doi: 10.1016/j.pnpbp.2012.07.004
50. Zhong X, Pu W, Yao S. Functional alterations of fronto-limbic circuit and default mode network systems in first-episode, drug-naive patients with major depressive disorder: a meta-analysis of resting-state fMRI data. *J Affect Disord.* (2016) **206**:280–6. doi: 10.1016/j.jad.2016.09.005
51. Zhu X, Wang X, Xiao J, Liao J, Zhong M, Wang W, et al. Evidence of a dissociation pattern in resting-state default mode network connectivity in first-episode, treatment-naive major depression patients. *Biological Psychiatry* (2012) **71**:611–7. doi: 10.1016/j.biopsych.2011.10.035
52. Renner F, Siep N, Arntz A, van de Ven V, Peeters F P, Quaedflieg C W, et al. Negative mood-induction modulates default mode network resting-state functional connectivity in chronic depression. *J Affect Disord.* (2017) **208**:590–6. doi: 10.1016/j.jad.2016.10.022
53. Fung G, Deng Y, Zhao Q, Li Z, Qu M, Li K, et al. Distinguishing bipolar and major depressive disorders by brain structural morphometry: a pilot study. *BMC Psychiatry* (2015) **15**:298. doi: 10.1186/s12888-015-0685-5
54. Young KD, Bodurka J, Drevets WC. Differential neural correlates of autobiographical memory recall in bipolar and unipolar depression. *Bipolar Disord.* (2016) **18**:571–82. doi: 10.1111/bdi.12441
55. Tao H, Guo S, Ge T, Kendrick KM, Xue Z, Liu Z, et al. Depression uncouples brain hate circuit. *Mol Psychiatry* (2013) **18**:101–11. doi: 10.1038/mp.2011.127
56. Zhang WN, Chang SH, Guo LY, Zhang KL, Wang J. The neural correlates of reward-related processing in major depressive disorder: a meta-analysis of functional magnetic resonance imaging studies. *J Affect Disord.* (2013) **151**:531–9. doi: 10.1016/j.jad.2013.06.039
57. Guo W, Liu F, Liu J, Yu L, Zhang Z, Zhang J, et al. Is there a cerebellar compensatory effort in first-episode, treatment-naive major depressive disorder at rest? *Prog Neuropsychopharmacol Biol Psychiatry* (2013) **46**:13–8. doi: 10.1016/j.pnpbp.2013.06.009
58. Stange JP, Bessette KL, Jenkins LM, Peters AT, Feldhaus C, Crane NA, et al. Attenuated intrinsic connectivity within cognitive control network among individuals with remitted depression: temporal stability and association with negative cognitive styles. *Hum Brain Mapp.* (2017) **38**:2939–54. doi: 10.1002/hbm.23564

59. Dev SI, McKenna BS, Sutherland AN, Shin DD, Liu TT, Wierenga CE, et al. Increased cerebral blood flow associated with better response inhibition in bipolar disorder. *J Int Neuropsychol Soc.* (2015) **21**:105–15. doi: 10.1017/s135561771400112x
60. Wang Y, Zhong S, Jia Y, Zhou Z, Wang B, Pan J, et al. Interhemispheric resting state functional connectivity abnormalities in unipolar depression and bipolar depression. *Bipolar Disord.* (2015) **17**:486–95. doi: 10.1111/bdi.12315
61. Xu J, Rees G, Yin X, Song C, Han Y, Ge H, et al. Spontaneous neuronal activity predicts intersubject variations in executive control of attention. *Neuroscience* (2014) **263**:181–92. doi: 10.1016/j.neuroscience.2014.01.020
62. Phan KL, Wager T, Taylor SF, Liberzon I. Functional neuroanatomy of emotion: a meta-analysis of emotion activation studies in PET and fMRI. *Neuroimage* (2002) **16**:331–48. doi: 10.1006/nimg.2002.1087
63. Oertel-Knochel V, Reuter J, Reinke B, Marbach K, Feddern R, Alves G, et al. Association between age of disease-onset, cognitive performance and cortical thickness in bipolar disorders. *J Affect Disord.* (2014) **174C**:627–35. doi: 10.1016/j.jad.2014.10.060
64. Hafeman DM, Chang KD, Garrett AS, Sanders EM, Phillips ML. Effects of medication on neuroimaging findings in bipolar disorder: an updated review. *Bipolar Disord.* (2012) **14**:375–410. doi: 10.1111/j.1399-5618.2012.01023.x
65. Diler RS, Goldstein TR. Characteristics of depression among offspring at high and low familial risk of bipolar disorder. *Bipolar Disord.* (2017) **19**:344–52. doi: 10.1111/bdi.12508
66. Chen X, Lu B, Yan CG. Reproducibility of R-fMRI metrics on the impact of different strategies for multiple comparison correction and sample sizes. *Hum Brain Mapp.* (2018) **39**:300–18. doi: 10.1002/hbm.23843
67. Pajula J, Tohka J. How many is enough? Effect of sample size in inter-subject correlation analysis of fMRI. *Comput Intell Neurosci.* (2016) **2016**:2094601. doi: 10.1155/2016/2094601.

4

The Impact of Whole Brain Global Functional Connectivity Density Following MECT in Major Depression: A Follow-Up Study

Xiao Li[1], Huaqing Meng[1], Yixiao Fu[1], Lian Du[1], Haitang Qiu[1], Tian Qiu[1], Qibin Chen[2], Zhiwei Zhang[3] and Qinghua Luo[1]**

[1] Department of Psychiatry, The First Affiliated Hospital of Chongqing Medical University, Chongqing, China, [2] Department of Anesthesiology, The First Affiliated Hospital of Chongqing Medical University, Chongqing, China, [3] Department of Radiology, The First Affiliated Hospital of Chongqing Medical University, Chongqing, China

***Correspondence:**
Zhiwei Zhang
zhangzhiwei@hospital.cqmu.edu.cn
Qinghua Luo
luoqinghua@hospital.cqmu.edu.cn

To explore the alteration of global functional connectivity density (gFCD) in depressive patients after modified electroconvulsive therapy (MECT) and analyze the relationship between gFCD and clinical outcome. Thirty-seven subjects were evaluated based on the diagnostic criteria of the International Classification of Diseases-10 (ICD-10), consisting of a depressive group (24 patients after follow-ups) and a healthy control group with 13 normal individuals. All participants received Hamilton Depression Scale (HAMD) scores and resting-state functional magnetic resonance imaging scans. The gFCD significantly increased in the posterior-middle insula, the supra-marginal gyrus and the dorsal medial prefrontal cortex (dmPFC) before MECT treatment compared to healthy controlled patients. The gFCD statistically expanded in the perigenual anterior cingulate cortex (pgACC), the orbitofrontal cortex bilaterally and the left-supra-marginal gyrus after MECT, and it decreased notably in the posterior insula. The gFCD in the pgACC and the right orbital frontal cortex of depressive group before MECT showed a positive correlation with HAMD scores with treatment. Conforming to the impact of gFCD in depressive patients after MECT, the aforementioned brain region may become an indicator of MECT effect.

Keywords: depression, electroconvulsive therapy, brain, functional connectivity, fMRI methods

INTRODUCTION

Major depressive disorder (MDD) is one of the most common mental disorders; however, limited therapeutic options are available, creating an enormous individual and societal burden. An estimated 30% of patients with MDD still suffer from functional impairment and antidepressant drugs are only partially effective (1). Modified Electroconvulsive therapy (MECT) is known as a useful treatment for MDD and works by eliciting controlled, transient seizures in both acute and maintenance sessions (2). Several meta-analyses have confirmed the antidepressant effectiveness of MECT for depression (3–5).

However, not all patients respond to MECT. Approximately only 50% of patients experience remission when receiving right-unilateral MECT with optimal parameters, and the specific neural mechanism of action still remains unclear. Until now, the modulatory effect of MECT on brain functional connectivity density (FCD) has only been reported in a few studies. Some found the dorsal-lateral prefrontal cortex (DLPFC) was crucial for achieving a therapeutic response by MECT (6–8). Previous studies have shown symptom recovery in some regions, such as the amygdala or the subgenual anterior cingulated cortex (sgACC) (9, 10). Cano et al. (11) found that substantial intra-limbic functional connectivity (FC) decreases predicted a later increase in limbic–prefrontal FC, which could predict clinical improvement at the end of a course of ECT.

As a voxel-wise, data-driven method, functional connectivity density mapping (FCDM) is widely used to test the density distribution of whole-brain resting-state FC (12–14), such as resting-state global functional connectivity density (rs-gFCD). Rs-gFCD is been referred to as the level of centrality (15) or intrinsic connectivity contrast (16). For some neuropsychiatric disorders, rs-gFCD was suggested to be a biomarker (15, 17, 18). Increased FCDs shows the elevated number and strength of FC may indicate its important role for understanding the mechanism in these brain areas. Kandilarova et al. (19) found, according to spectral dynamic causal modeling, that significantly reduced strength of the connection from the MFG (i.e., dorsolateral prefrontal cortex) to the anterior insula was shown in patients, and a strong connection was found between the anterior insula and the amygdala. This research may be used to predict treatment response.

Neuroimaging research of ECT has particularly assessed brain function before and after treatment (20–22), but have not tried to characterize functional changes occurring at various treatment phases. These measurements may have important clinical utility as an outcome predictor (23) and may help to reveal the mechanism of antidepressant treatments.

In this study, we hypothesized that a complex interaction between MECT-induced gFCD changes and clinical improvement will emerge in patients with MDD. Therefore, to demonstrate this relationship, we assessed a group of patients with MDD and compared them to healthy controls. We used functional magnetic resonance imaging to examine developments in global functional connectivity density and assessed alterations in Hamilton depression scale (HAMD) scores during MECT. We measured gFCD in the depressive group before MECT and in the healthy controls, and after 8 courses of MECT, we tested gFCD in the depressive group again. The specific objectives of the study were as follows: [1] to assess changes in specific regions throughout the course of ECT and [2] to expose the relationship between ECT-induced gFCD changes and clinical response.

MATERIALS AND METHODS

Participants

Twenty-four patients and 13 demographically similar healthy control subjects received informed consent forms for participation in the research, which was approved by the First Affiliated Hospital of Chongqing Medical University. All the methods followed relevant regulations. Diagnostic assessment and response were assessed by experienced psychiatrists in depression and relevant scales. All the patients would take a clinical assessment before ECT including routine blood testing, chest X-rays, and brain CT scans (11). They were all experiencing MDD as defined by the ICD-10 and were screened using the Hamilton Depression Scale (pre-ECT 31.3 $\pm$ 8.6; post-ECT8.58 $\pm$ 5.62; healthy-control 2.21 $\pm$ 1.25). Subjects were excluded if they: (i) had a neurological or serious physical condition or any history of alcohol or drug abuse, or any other somatic diseases, or morphological anomalies of the brain, (ii) had any surgically-placed electronic or metal materials that might interfere with fMRI assessment, (iii) slept while scanning and/or (iv) had head motion exceeding 3 mm in translation or 3 degrees in rotation. The Local Medical Ethics Committee of the First Affiliated Hospital of Chongqing Medical University reviewed and confirmed the study protocol. Written informed consent was obtained from all subjects.

Electroconvulsive Therapy

The patients underwent modified bi-frontotemporal ECT which was conducted using a Thymatron (TM) DGx (Somatics LLC, Lake Bluff, IL, USA), which is the brief-pulse, constant-current apparatus at the psychiatry department of the First Affiliated Hospital of Chongqing Medical University (24). The first three courses of ECT took place on continued days and the left courses of ECT were performed every 2 days, and it would have a break on weekends. After eight courses, ECT was continued if depressive symptoms had not changed sufficiently, as determined by a clinician, with a maximum of 12 courses of ECT. The initial dosage was confirmed based on age, weight and sex. Anesthesia was induced with succinylcholine (0.5–1 mg/kg) and diprivan (1.5–2 mg/kg).

MRI Data Acquisition

A 3.0 Tesla MRI system (GE Signa) was used to obtain imaging data in the First Affiliated Hospital of Chongqing Medical University. Patients were asked to close their eyes peacefully and to keep their heads stable throughout MRI process and keep awake. After the MRI scan, they would be asked whether they had fallen asleep during the process (24). Resting-state fMRI images were collected using the following EPI sequence: repetition time: 2000 ms; echo time: 30 ms; flip angle: 90°; field of view: 240 $\times$ 240 mm^2; matrix: 64 $\times$ 64; slice thickness: 5 mm; and number of slices: 33 axial slices. Two hundred volumes were obtained, resulting in a 400s scan time, then 3D T1-weighted anatomical images were collected (repetition time: 8.35 ms; flip angle: 12°; echo time: 3.27 ms; field of view: 240 $\times$ 240 mm^2; matrix: 256 $\times$ 256; slice thickness: 1 mm; and the number of sagittal slices is 156) (25).

Pre-processing and Quality Control

Data Processing & Analysis of Brain Imaging (DPABI) was used to assess resting-state data (26). The first 10 volumes of the functional images were abandoned to account for signal equilibrium (27). Slice timing and head motion correction were conducted in sequence for the remaining time points. The covariates, including head motion, white matter signal and cerebrospinal fluid signal, were regressed out from the time series of every voxel. Here, the Friston 24-parameter model was used to regress out head motion effects. To decrease effects of high-frequency noise and low-frequency drift, a 0.01–0.1 Hz band-pass filter was used. The registered images were spatially normalized to the Montreal Neurological Institute (MNI) template. The images were resampled to 3-mm cubic voxels. To smooth the normalized images, a 6-mm full width at half maximum Gaussian kernel was used. Additionally, the scrubbing procedure was employed, excluding any volume with a frame-wise dependent value exceeding 0.5, with the two subsequent volumes and one preceding volume. Finally, normalization quality was monitored by checking the normalization images subject by subject (28).

Functional Connectivity Density

We used the DPARSF toolbox to calculate the functional connectivity density (FCD) of each voxel. High FCDs indicates increased strength and number of the respective FC, showing its significance in the brain. Between all the brain voxels, Pearson's correlation coefficients were calculated, so that the whole-brain functional connectivity matrix for each subject could be constructed. The degree centrality maps were computed using 0.3 (we also used 0.4 as the threshold for determining edges and found the results was similar) as the threshold for determining edges (12). Thus, the whole-brain maps were obtained by computing the number of voxels where the connections with other voxels in the BOLD time series exceeded the threshold in a whole-brain weighted graph.

Statistical Analysis

First, the two-sample *T*-Test was selected to test the group differences in gFCD between pre-ECT MDD patients and the control group in a voxel-wise manner by using a general linear model with age, gender, and the motion (Mean FD) as nuisance covariates. A correction for multiple comparisons was performed using $p < 0.05$ with family-wise error (FWE), which is correct at the voxel level. Second, to investigate the therapeutic effect of ECT, the paired sample *T*-test was also used to test the differences between MDD before treatment and after treatment using ECT in a voxel-wise manner. Because the results may be easily impacted by noise, a conservative statistical threshold was specified at cluster level $p < 0.05$, which is correct with an underlying voxel level of $p < 0.001$(AlphaSim corrected) using DPABI (26) software. Additionally, one-way ANOVA was performed to test the difference in the ROI regions based on previous paired sample t results (pre-treatment vs. post-treatment) among the healthy controls, pre-treatment MDD and post-treatment MDD.

The statistical analysis of one-way ANOVA was implemented by SPSS 20 (IBM SPSS Statistics for Windows, Version 20.0, IBM Corp, Armonk, NY, USA). To characterize the relationship between HAMD scores and pre-/post- treatment, we computed Pearson's correlation analysis. Each group was compared with others by using a Bonferroni *post hoc* test with $p < 0.05$.

RESULTS

Demographic Data and Psychological Measurements

The psychological measurements and demographic data are listed in **Table 1**. In comparison with the healthy controls and post-treatment depressive subjects, the pre-treatment depressive subjects had more serious depressive symptoms according to HAMD scores. One-way ANOVA analyses indicated that the scores on the HAMD were remarkably different among the three groups ($F = 232.4, p < 0.001$). A pairwise comparison found that post-treatment periods were characterized by significantly lower depressive symptoms than pre-treatment intervals ($F = -22.8$, $p < 0.001$), yet subjects in the post-treatment stage still experienced markedly higher depressive symptoms compared to healthy control subjects ($F = 6.4$, $p < 0.001$). The depressive group and the healthy controls did not differ considerably with age ($t = -0.55$, p = 0.59) or sex ($t = -0.81, p = 0.43$). Compared with the healthy controls, the depressive patients had more years of education ($t = -3.7$, $p < 0.001$). The individual scores from the HAMD of all participants are shown along with the mean in **Table 1**, excluding 6 patients who refused further treatment because of symptom recovery at an early stage.

Significant Differences Between Pre-treatment Periods and Healthy Controls in Global Functional Connectivity Density (gFCD)

In contrast with the healthy controls, the depressive patients in the pre-treatment phase exhibited a significantly increased gFCD in the posterior-middle insula, supra-marginal gyrus, and dorsal medial prefrontal cortex (all $p < 0.05$ with family wise error corrected, **Figure 1**). No regions showed decreased gFCD under the same statistical threshold.

TABLE 1 | The demographic data and psychological measurements of the healthy controls, pre-treatment and post-treatment depressive subjects.

Characteristic	Pre-treatment	Post-treatment	Control	Value	P
Age, mean (SD), y	32.5 (11.7)	/	33.3 (10.4)	$t = -0.55$	$p = 0.59$
Sex (male/female)	10/14	10/14	5/9	$t = -0.79$	$p = 0.43$
*Education years, mean (SD), y	11.1 (2.86)	/	15.1 (3.47)	$t = -3.9$	$p < 0.001$
Body Weight, mean (SD), Kg	54.1	N/A	57.2	$t = -1.46$	$p = 0.15$
HAMD, mean (SD)	31.3 (8.6)	8.58 (5.62)	2.21 (1.25)	$F = 164$	$p < 0.001$
Head Motion (FD), mean (SD)	0.089 (0.03)	0.113 (0.09)	0.104 (0.03)	$F = 1.54$	$p = 0.23$

*Results are $P < 0.05$.

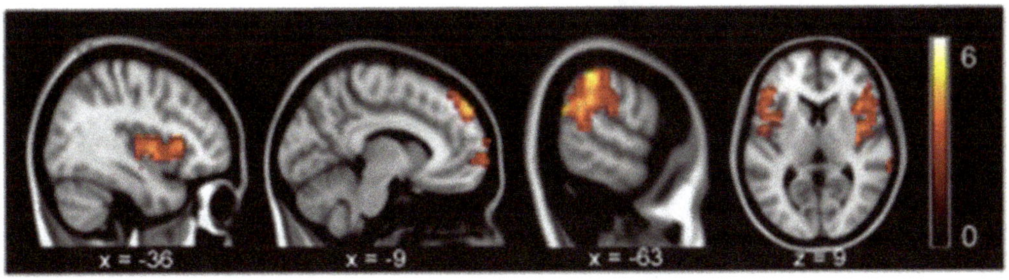

FIGURE 1 | gFCD in pre-treatment revealed significant increases in the posterior-middle insula, supramarginal gyrus, and dorsal medial prefrontal cortex compared to the controls ($p < 0.05$, FEW).

Significant Differences Between Pre-treatment and Post-treatment Stages in Global Functional Connectivity Density (gFCD)

Compared to the depressive patients in the pre-treatment period, the post-treatment depressive patients exhibited an obviously increased gFCD in the perigenual anterior cingulate cortex (pgACC), orbitofrontal cortex bilaterally and the left-supra-marginal gyrus. Moreover, depressive patients in the post-treatment stage exhibited decreased gFCD in the posterior insula compared to the pre-treatment phase (AlphaSim corrected $p < 0.001$ under voxel level uncorrected and cluster level under $p < 0.05$ familywise error corrected, **Figure 2**; **Table 2**).

The results from the correlation analyses revealed that the gFCD activity in the pgACC ($r = 0.46$, $p = 0.024$) and right orbital frontal cortex ($r = 0.5$, $p = 0.013$) in the pre-treatment interval had a significant correlation with the post-treatment period HAMD scores (see **Figure 3**). However, there was no correlation between the gFCD pre-MECT and HAMD scores pre-MECT ($p > 0.05$). There was also no noticeable correlation between post-treatment gFCD and HAMD scores. The changes of gFCD and the differences of HAMD scores also had no significant correlation. These results indicated that the gFCD activity present in pre-treatment may predict the post-treatment outcome.

DISCUSSION

In the present study, we assessed the gFCD changes in patients with MDD before and after MECT. The results demonstrated that, compared to the healthy controls, there was increased gFCD in the posterior-middle insula, supra-marginal gyrus, and dorsal medial prefrontal cortex of pre-ECT MDD patients.

The post-treatment results exhibited significantly increased gFCD in the perigenual anterior cingulate cortex (pgACC), orbitofrontal cortex bilaterally and the left-supra-marginal gyrus. These upshots were associated with decreased HAMD scores, and statistical analysis demonstrated that such connectivity changes were related to clinical outcome.

Orbitofrontal Cortex

The orbitofrontal cortex (OFC) is important in complex human behaviors. OFC cortico-striatal circuits are consistently involved in many mental disorders, such as depression. Structurally, the OFC reveals remarkable decreased volumes in medication-naïve MDD patients compared to MDD patients who take medications (29). Additionally, Webb et al. (30) found higher depressive symptoms were related to reduce gray matter volume in the left rACC (extending into the OFC). Likewise, significant decreases have been observed not only in OFC gray matter, but also in the ventral striatum and amygdala in MDD patients (30, 31). Furthermore, the changes may last through the whole life. According to a previous study, no significant differences were observed in total gray matter volume of OFC, or in total OFC volume between MDD children and healthy controls (32). Interestingly, Rajkowska et al. (33) obtained post-mortem samples from elderly depressed patients that showed that the density of pyramidal neurons in the OFC was particularly low, which shows more severe neuronal pathology changes in older MDD patients than in younger patients. Studies show that, compared with control subjects, significant hyperactivity is observed in the mOFC and VMPFC for MDD patients (34–40). At the same time, some research shows that, for medication-naïve MDD patients, the resting cerebral blood flow (rCBF) of the OFC was upregulated, while after taking antidepressants, reduced metabolism was observed in these regions (41). Thus, there is a positive correlation with MDD patients. Nevertheless, the correlation between symptom severity and rCBF of these areas remains somewhat of a mystery. This research suggests that activation of these areas can be a complemental reaction for decreasing negative emotional action. Specifically, some results revealed an inverse correlation between decreased functional connectivity within the medial division of the orbitofrontal circuit and the severity of symptoms, which matches our conclusions (42).

Insula

Some large trials demonstrated that pre-treatment regional insula activity could prognosticate the specific treatment that would be efficacious at the individual patient level. Dunlop et al. (43) found preliminary evidence that a putative right anterior insula metabolism biomarker could predict treatment outcomes,

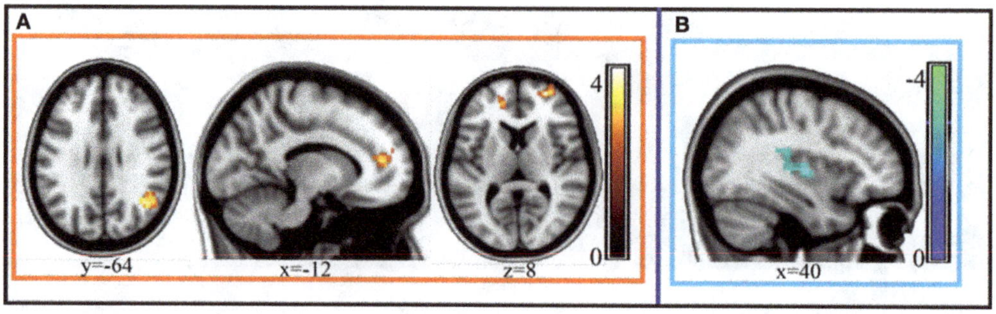

FIGURE 2 | gFCD of the depressive group statistically increased in the perigenual anterior cingulate cortex (pgACC), orbitofrontal cortex bilaterally and the left-supramarginal gyrus after MECT ($p < 0.05$, FEW). **(A)** Statistical increased gFCD in these regions post treatment. **(B)** Statistical decreased gFCD in these regions post treatment.

TABLE 2 | Significant difference between different groups in global functional connectivity density (gFCD).

Brain regions	MNI coordinates			Voxel size	Peak T value
	x	*y*	*z*		
PRETREATMENT vs. CONTROL					
Increased gFCD					
Middle insula (left)	−36	6	3	234	4.93
Posterior middle insula (right)	39	−3	3	310	4.87
Supramarginal gyrus (left)	−63	−51	30	296	5.68
Dorsal medial prefrontal cortex(DMPFC) (left)	−9	54	42	154	5.42
Decreased gFCD					
No					
POST-TREATMENT vs. PRETREATMENT					
Increased gFCD					
Perigenual anterior cingulate cortex (pgACC) (left)	−12	45	12	231	4.16
Right supramarginal gyrus (right)	54	−63	33	470	4.78
Orbitofrontal cortex (left)	−24	57	3	217	3.97
Decreased gFCD					
[a]Right insula (right)	36	−15	6	110	−4.03

[a]*Results are $P < 0.05$, corrected for multiple comparisons at a cluster level with AlphaSim, with an underlying voxel level of $P < 0.001$, uncorrected under whole brain analyses.*

even in children (43). Belden et al. (44) found there was some kind of correlation between structural abnormalities of anterior insula volume and the neurobiology of depression from early childhood. Consequently, the function and structure of insula are significant for presaging the clinical outcomes of depression. Some previous studies indicated that low functional connectivity density in the insula leads to better clinical outcomes in MDD, but there is no research to reveal upregulated connectivity in ACC/VMPFC, PCC/pC, dACC and insula within RSNs that are correlated with MDD pathology. Regression results showed that areas related to clinical response overlapped mostly with areas that exhibited abnormal connectivity. ACC/VMPFC, dACC and the left insula are the hub areas of the default mode network (DMN) and SN. These areas displayed prominent performance (highest sensitivity = 100% and highest specificity = 82%) in distinguishing therapeutic effect (45). Some recent researches specified that, in contrast with MDD patients who not attempted suicide, those who have attempted suicide showed hyper-activity resting-state functional connectivity (RSFC) of the left amygdala with the right insula (46). Our corollary showed increased gFCD in the insula before treatment, which matches previous studies.

Dorsal Medial Prefrontal Cortex

Chaotic network connectivity is observed in MDD core networks, which include DMN, of which the dorsal medial prefrontal cortex (dmPFC) is one part. Both pharmaceutical treatments and electroconvulsive therapy and repetitive transcranial magnetic stimulation can work in DMN. One previous study showed that, after using rTMS just in the dmPFC region, the symptoms became better (47). Previous studies have demonstrated abnormal changes in resting-state functional connectivity strength in several brain regions and brain networks (48–50); research has further shown that resting-state functional connectivity density is mainly located in the medial prefrontal cortex, posterior cingulated cortex,

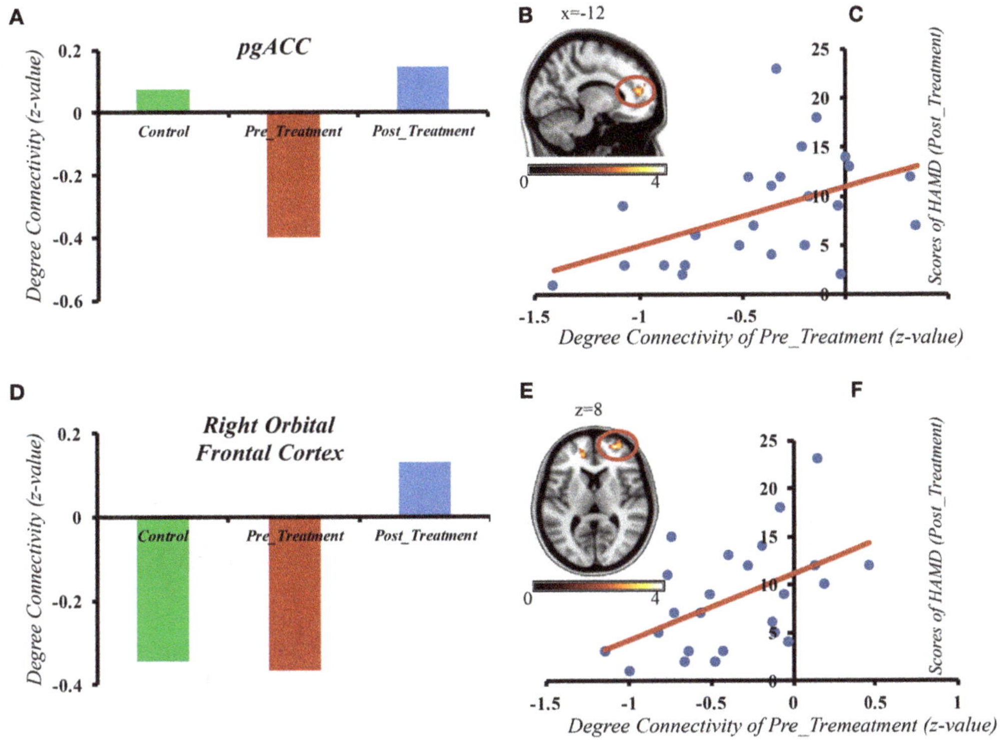

FIGURE 3 | The gFCD in the pgACC and right orbital frontal cortex of depressive patients before MECT shows a positive correlation with HAMD scores after treatment. **(A)** gFCD in pgACC in three different groups. **(B)** gFCD in pgACC. **(C)** The gFCD in the pgACC of depressive patients pre MECT shows a positive correlation with HAMD scores post treatment. **(D)** gFCD in Right Orbital Frontal Cortex in three different groups. **(E)** gFCD in Right Orbital Frontal Cortex. **(F)** The gFCD in the Right Orbital Frontal Cortex of depressive patients pre MECT shows a positive correlation with HAMD scores post treatment.

precuneus and occipital lobe. MDD patients show lower medial prefrontal cortex volumes. Research on a non-clinical sample found that, in the dorsal medial prefrontal cortex, male subjects with higher levels of depressive qualities seem to have lower volumes of gray matter (51). Even in a subclinical sample, the dorsal medial prefrontal cortex was shown to be a potentially significant biomarker for treatment outcomes in depression. In our study, we found increased gFCD in dmPFC in depressive patients. These outcomes match some previous research, such as how—compared with healthy control group—increased within-network connectivity was observed in the dmPFC of MDD patients (52), and another study showed increased resting-state FC between the medial prefrontal cortex and other DMN structures in patients who suffered from major depressive episodes (53). So, we predict increased gFCD exists not only in dmPFC its own, but also dmPFC with other brain regions.

Perigenual Anterior Cingulate Cortex (pgACC)

Previous studies indicated that abnormal structure of the anterior cingulate cortex (ACC) is also frequently linked with major depression disorder (54–56). Dysfunction in networks including the ACC and caudate nucleus has been demonstrated to underlie many core symptoms of MDD such as anhedonia, decreased energy and intellectual disability (7). In addition, Wu et al. (57) found a remarkble reduction of functional connectivity strength (FCS) in sgACC in MDD patients. Taken together, this research supports a neurotrophic model of MDD and antidepressant effects, showing that ECT may cause functional alterations within prefrontal and limbic areas.

Furthermore, we also found that gFCD in the pgACC and the right orbital frontal cortex of depressive patients before ECT had a positive correlation with HAMD scores after treatment. Previous research has shown that the alteration of limbic and prefrontal networks is continuous during symptom remission. Early antidepressant effects can be observed at the limbic level, and the following effects can be observed in the PFC (6, 11, 58). Cano et al. (11) found that early, substantial decreased intralimbic FC significantly exhibited a subsequent increase in limbic-prefrontal FC, which meant better clinical outcomes could come from an ECT session. The gFCD in the pgACC and the right orbital frontal cortex of depressive patients before MECT showed a positive correlation with HAMD scores after treatment, which suggests that functional disturbances in MDD may be associated with compensatory activity enhancement in some regions. In severe depression, the compensatory enhancement is more obvious. Our results may provide evidence for finding a new predictor of treatment outcome.

In the present study, our research focuses on describing treatment outcomes with gFCD and MECT. However, previous studies have shown that regardless of function or structure, the regional insula, ACC, OFC, supra-marginal gyrus, and dorsal medial prefrontal cortex may be important biomarkers for treatment outcomes of depression. Some studies have shown decreased gFCD in the left occipital lobe of depressive patients while our study found that the gFCD in the pgACC and right orbital frontal cortex of depressive patients before MECT demonstrated a positive correlation with HAMD scores after treatment, suggesting that the level of gFCD in the pgACC and right orbital frontal cortex may also be core indicators of treatment outcome.

This study has some limitations. These include the small number of patients; replication with a larger sample is warranted and the healthy control sample was also small. We did not add a subgroup analysis and there were no other psychopathological or neurocognitive assessments in our research, and we did not follow the healthy controls; therefore, further research is needed.

CONCLUSION

We found abnormal gFCD in the posterior-middle insula, supra-marginal gyrus, and dorsal medial prefrontal cortex in depressive patients after MECT. MECT influenced brain gFCD in depressive patients by increasing gFCD in the perigenual anterior cingulate cortex (pgACC), orbitofrontal cortex bilaterally and the left-supra-marginal gyrus while decreasing gFCD in the posterior insula after 8 courses of MECT. The gFCD in the pgACC and right orbital frontal cortex of depressive patients before MECT revealed a positive correlation with treatment outcome, demonstrating that the above brain region may be a strong indicator of MECT effect.

AUTHOR CONTRIBUTIONS

XL contributed to data collection and wrote the paper. HM, YF, LD, HQ, TQ, and QC helped revise the paper. ZZ and QL designed the experiment and revised the paper.

FUNDING

The National Science and Technologic of China (2015BAI13B02).

ACKNOWLEDGMENTS

This work was supported by a grant from the National Science and Technology Program of China (2015BAI13B02), the Foundation of the First Affiliated Hospital of Chongqing Medical University (PYJJ2017-27), the Pre-research Natural Science Foundation of Chongqing Medical University (NSFYY201607) and the Medical research project of the Chongqing Health and Family Planning Commission (2017MSXM024).

REFERENCES

1. Rush AJ, Trivedi MH, Wisniewski SR, Nierenberg AA, Stewart JW, Warden D, et al. Acute and longer-term outcomes in depressed outpatients requiring one or several treatment steps: a STAR D report. *Am J Psychiatry.* (2006) 163:1905–7. doi: 10.1176/ajp.2006.163.11.1905
2. Fink M, Taylor MA. Electroconvulsive therapy: evidence and challenges. *J Am Med Assoc.* (2007) 298:330–2. doi: 10.1001/jama.298.3.330
3. The UK ECT Review Group. Efficacy and safety of electroconvulsive therapy in depressive disorders: a systematic review and meta-analysis. *Lancet.* (2003) 361:799–8. doi: 10.1016/S0140-6736(03)12705-5
4. Pagnin D, de Queiroz V, Pini S, Cassano GB. Efficacy of ECT in depression: a meta-analytic review. *J ECT.* (2004) 20:13–20. doi: 10.1097/00124509-200403000-00004
5. Weiner R, Lisanby SH, Husain MM, Morales OG, Maixner DF, Hall SE, et al. Electroconvulsive therapy device classification: response to FDA advisory panel hearing and recommendations. *J Clin Psychiatry.* (2013) 74:38–42. doi: 10.4088/JCP.12cs08260
6. Mayberg HS. Modulating dysfunctional limbic-cortical circuits in depression: towards development of brain-based algorithms for diagnosis and optimized treatment. *Br Med Bull.* (2003) 65:193–207. doi: 10.1093/bmb/65.1.193
7. Price JL, Drevets WC. Neurocircuitry of mood disorders. *Neuropsychopharmacology* (2010) 35:192–216. doi: 10.1038/npp.2009.104
8. Lu Q, Li H, Luo G, Wang Y, Tang H, Han L, et al. Impaired prefrontalamygdala effective connectivity is responsible for the dysfunction of emotion process in major depressive disorder: a dynamic causal modeling study on MEG. *Neurosci Lett.* (2012) 523:125–30. doi: 10.1016/j.neulet.2012.06.058
9. Seminowicz DA, Mayberg HS, McIntosh AR, Goldapple K, Kennedy S, Segal Z, et al. Limbic-frontal circuitry in major depression: a path modeling metanalysis. *Neuroimage.* (2004) 22:409–18. doi: 10.1016/j.neuroimage.2004.01.015
10. Anand A, Li Y, Wang Y, Wu J, Gao S, Bukhari L, et al. Antidepressant effect on connectivity of the mood-regulating circuit: an fMRI study. *Neuropsychopharmacology.* (2005) 30:1334–44. doi: 10.1038/sj.npp.1300725
11. Cano M, Cardoner N, Urretavizcaya M, Martínez-Zalacaín I, Goldberg X, Via E, et al. Modulation of limbic and prefrontal connectivity by electroconvulsive therapy in treatment-resistant depression: a preliminary study. *Brain stimuli.* (2016) 9:65–71. doi: 10.1016/j.brs.2015.08.016
12. Tomasi D, Volkow ND. Functional connectivity density mapping. *Proc Natl Acad Sci USA.* (2010) 107:9885–90. doi: 10.1073/pnas.1001414107
13. Tomasi D, Volkow ND. Association between functional connectivity hubs and brain networks. *Cereb Cortex.* (2011) 21:2003–13. doi: 10.1093/cercor/bhq268
14. Tomasi D, Volkow ND. Functional connectivity hubs in the human brain. *Neuroimage.* (2011) 57:908–17. doi: 10.1016/j.neuroimage.2011.05.024
15. Buckner RL, Sepulcre J, Talukdar T, Krienen FM, Liu H, Hedden T, et al. et al. Cortical hubs revealed by intrinsic functional connectivity: mapping, assessment of stability, and relation to Alzheimer's disease. *J Neurosci.* (2009) 29:1860–73. doi: 10.1523/JNEUROSCI.5062-08.2009
16. Martuzzi R, Ramani R, Qiu M, Shen X, Papademetris X, Constable RT. A whole-brain voxel based measure of intrinsic connectivity contrast reveals local changes in tissue connectivity with anesthetic without a priori assumptions on thresholds or regions of interest. *Neuroimage.* (2011) 58:1044–50. doi: 10.1016/j.neuroimage.2011.06.075
17. Tomasi D, Shokri-Kojori E, Volkow ND. High-resolution functional connectivity density: hub locations, sensitivity, specificity, reproducibility, and reliability. *Cereb Cortex.* (2015) 26:3249–59. doi: 10.1093/cercor/bhv171
18. Zhuo C, Zhu J, Wang C, Qu H, Ma X, Qin W. Different spatial patterns of brain atrophy and global functional connectivity impairments in major depressive disorder. *Brain Imaging Behav.* (2017) 11:1678–89. doi: 10.1007/s11682-016-9645-z
19. Kandilarova S, Stoyanov D, Kostianev S, Specht K. Altered resting state effective connectivity of anterior insula in depression. *Front. Psychiatry.* (2018) 9:83. doi: 10.3389/fpsyt.2018.00083

20. Beall EB, Malone DA, Dale RM, Muzina DJ, Koenig KA, Bhattacharrya PK, et al. Effects of electroconvulsive therapy on brain functional activation and connectivity in depression. *J ECT.* (2012) 28:234–41. doi: 10.1097/YCT.0b013e31825ebcc7
21. Perrin JS, Merz S, Bennett DM, Currie J, Steele DJ, Reid IC, et al. Electroconvulsive therapy reduces frontal cortical connectivity in severe depressive disorder. *Proc Natl Acad Sci USA.* (2012) 109:1464–8. doi: 10.1073/pnas.1117206109
22. Abbott CC, Lemke NT, Gopal S, Thoma RJ, Bustillo J, Calhoun VD, et al. Electroconvulsive therapy response in major depressive disorder: a pilot functional network connectivity resting state fMRI investigation. *Front Psychiatry.* (2013) 4:10. doi: 10.3389/fpsyt.2013.00010
23. Papakostas GI, Fava M. Predictors, moderators, and mediators (correlates) of treatment outcome in major depressive disorder. *Dialog Clin Neurosci.* (2008) 10:439–51. Available online at: https://www.ncbi.nlm.nih.gov/pmc/articles/PMC3181892/
24. Du L, Qiu H, Liu H, Zhao W, Tang Y, Fu Y, et al. Changes in Problem-Solving Capacity and Association With Spontaneous Brain Activity After a Single Electroconvulsive Treatment in Major Depressive Disorder. *J ECT.* (2016) 32:49–54. doi: 10.1097/YCT.0000000000000269
25. Du L, Liu H, Du W, Chao F, Zhang L, Wang K, et al. Stimulated left DLPFC-nucleus accumbens functional connectivity predicts the anti-depression and anti-anxiety effects of rTMS for depression. *Transl Psychiatry.* (2018) 7:3. doi: 10.1038/s41398-017-0005-6
26. Yan CG, Wang XD, Zuo XN, Zang YF. DPABI: Data Processing & Analysis for (Resting-State) Brain Imaging. *Neuroinformatics.* (2016) 14:339–51. doi: 10.1007/s12021-016-9299-4
27. Tian X, Wei D, Du X, Wang K, Yang J, Liu W, et al. Assessment of trait anxiety and prediction of changes in state anxiety using functional brain imaging: a test-retest study. *Neuroimage.* (2016) 133:408–16. doi: 10.1016/j.neuroimage.2016.03.024
28. Liu W, Liu H, Wei D, Sun J, Yang J, Meng J, et al. Abnormal degree centrality of functional hubs associated with negative coping in older Chineseadults who lost their only child. *Biol Psychol.* (2015) 112:46–55. doi: 10.1016/j.biopsycho.2015.09.005
29. Bora E, Harrison BJ, Davey CG, Yücel M, Pantelis C. Meta-analysis of volumetric abnormalities in cortico-striatal-pallidal-thalamic circuits in major depressive disorder. *Psychol Med.* (2012) 42:671–81 . doi: 10.1017/S0033291711001668
30. Webb CA, Weber M, Mundy EA, Killgore WD. Reduced gray matter volume in the anterior cingulate, orbitofrontal cortex and thalamus as a function of mild depressive symptoms: a voxel-based morphometric analysis. *Psychol Med.* (2014) 44:2833–43. doi: 10.1017/S0033291714000348
31. Koolschijn PC, van Haren NE, Lensvelt-Mulders GJ, Hulshoff Pol HE, Kahn RS. Brain volume abnormalities in major depressive disorder: a meta-analysis of magnetic resonance imaging studies. *Hum Brain Mapp.* (2009) 30:3719–35 . doi: 10.1002/hbm.20801
32. Chen HH, Rosenberg DR, MacMaster FP, Easter PC, Caetano SC, Nicoletti M, et al. Orbitofrontal cortex volumes in medication naïve children with major depressive disorder: a magnetic resonance imaging study. *J Child Adolesc Psychopharmacol.* (2008) 18:551–6. doi: 10.1089/cap.2007.053
33. Rajkowska G, Miguel-Hidalgo JJ, Dubey P, Stockmeier CA, Krishnan KR. Prominent reduction in pyramidal neurons density in the orbitofrontal cortex of elderly depressed patients. *Biol Psychiatry.* (2005) 58:297–306. doi: 10.1016/j.biopsych.2005.04.013
34. Baxter LR, Schwartz JM, Phelps ME, Mazziotta JC, Guze BH, Selin CE, et al. Reduction of prefrontal cortex glucose metabolism common to three types of depression. *Arch Gen Psychiatry.* (1989) 46:243–50. doi: 10.1001/archpsyc.1989.01810030049007
35. Drevets WC, Videen TO, Price JL, Preskorn SH, Carmichael ST, Raichle ME. A functional anatomical study of unipolar depression. *J Neurosci.* (1991) 12:3628–41. doi: 10.1523/JNEUROSCI.12-09-03628.1992
36. Biver F, Goldman S, Delvenne V, Luxen A, De Maertelaer V, Hubain P, et al. Frontal and parietal metabolic disturbances in unipolar depression. *Biol Psychiatry.* (1994) 36:381–8. doi: 10.1016/0006-3223(94)91213-0
37. Galynker II, Cai J, Ongseng F, Finestone H, Dutta E, Serseni D. Hypofrontality and negative symptoms in major depressive disorder. *J Nucl Med.* (1998) 39:608–12.
38. Mayberg HS, Lozano AM, Voon V, McNeely HE, Seminowicz D, Hamani C, et al. Deep brain stimulation for treatment-resistant depression. *Neuron.* (2005) 45:651–60. doi: 10.1016/j.neuron.2005.02.014
39. Nofzinger EA, Buysse DJ, Germain A, Price JC, Meltzer CC, Miewald JM, et al. Alterations in regional cerebral glucose metabolism across waking and non-rapid eye movement sleep in depression. *Arch Gen Psychiatry.* (2005) 62:387–96. doi: 10.1001/archpsyc.62.4.387
40. Greicius MD, Flores BH, Menon V, Glover GH, Solvason HB, Kenna H, et al. et al. Resting-state functional connectivity in major depression: abnormally increased contributions from subgenual cingulate cortex and thalamus. *Biol Psychiatry.* (2007) 62:429–37. doi: 10.1016/j.biopsych.2006.09.020
41. Drevets WC, Price JL, Simpson JR, Todd RD, Reich T, Vannier M, et al. Subgenual prefrontal cortex abnormalities in mood disorders. *Nature.* (1997) 386:824–7. doi: 10.1038/386824a0
42. Cheng W, Rolls ET, Qiu J, Liu W, Tang Y, Huang CC, et al. Medial reward and lateral non-reward orbitofrontal cortex circuits change in opposite directions in depression. *Brain* (2016) 139:3296–309. doi: 10.1093/brain/aww255
43. Dunlop BW, Kelley ME, McGrath CL, Craighead WE, Mayberg HS. Preliminary findings supporting insula metabolic activity as a predictor of outcome to psychotherapy and medication treatments for depression. *J Neuropsychiatry Clin Neurosci.* (2015) 27:237–9. doi: 10.1176/appi.neuropsych.14030048
44. Belden AC, Barch DM, Oakberg TJ, April LM, Harms MP, Botteron KN, et al. Anterior insula volume and guilt: neurobehavioral markers of recurrence after early childhood major depressive disorder. *JAMA Psychiatry.* (2015) 72:40–8. doi: 10.1001/jamapsychiatry.2014.1604
45. Ge R, Blumberger DM, Downar J, Daskalakis ZJ, Dipinto AA, Tham JCW, et al. Abnormal functional connectivity within resting-state networks is related to rTMS-based therapy effects of treatment resistant depression: a pilot study. *J Affect Disord.* (2017) 218:75–81. doi: 10.1016/j.jad.2017.04.060
46. Kang SG, Na KS, Choi JW, Kim JH, Son YD, Lee YJ. Resting-state functional connectivity of the amygdala in suicide attempters with major depressive disorder. *Prog Neuropsychopharmacol Biol Psychiatry.* (2017) 77:222–7. doi: 10.1016/j.pnpbp.2017.04.029
47. Dunlop K, Gaprielian P, Blumberger D, Daskalakis ZJ, Kennedy SH, Giacobbe P et al. MRI-guided dmPFC-rTMS as a treatment for treatment-resistant major depressive disorder. *J Vis Exp.* (2015) 11:53129. doi: 10.3791/53129
48. Cordes D, Haughton V, Carew JD, Arfanakis K, Maravilla K. Hierarchical clustering to measure connectivity in fMRI resting-state data. *Magn Reson Imaging.* (2002) 20:305–17. doi: 10.1016/S0730-725X(02)00503-9
49. Mezer A, Yovel Y, Pasternak O, Gorfine T, Assaf Y. Cluster analysis of resting-state fMRI time series. *Neuroimage.* (2009) 45:1117–25. doi: 10.1016/j.neuroimage.2008.12.015
50. Zhuo C, Zhu J, Qin W, Qu H, Ma X, Tian H, et al. Functional connectivity density alterations in schizophrenia. *Front Behav Neurosci.* (2014) 8:404. doi: 10.3389/fnbeh.2014.00404
51. Carlson JM, Depetro E, Maxwell J, Harmon-Jones E, Hajcak G. Gender moderates the association between dorsal medial prefrontal cortex volume and depressive symptoms in a subclinical sample. *Psychiatry Res.* (2015) 233:285–8. doi: 10.1016/j.pscychresns.2015.06.005
52. Zhu X, Zhu Q, Shen H, Liao W, Yuan F. Rumination and default mode network subsystems connectivity in first-episode, drug-naive young patients with major depressive disorder. *Sci Rep.* (2017) 7:43105. doi: 10.1038/srep43105
53. Zhang B, Li S, Zhuo C, Li M, Safron A, Genz A, et al. Altered task-specific deactivation in the default mode network depends on valence in patients with major depressive disorder. *J Affect Disord.* (2017) 207:377–83. doi: 10.1016/j.jad.2016.08.042
54. Lorenzetti V, Allen NB, Fornito A, Yücel M. Structural brain abnormalities in major depressive disorder: a selective review of recent MRI studies. *J Affect Disord.* (2009) 117:1–17. doi: 10.1016/j.jad.2008.11.021
55. Rogers MA, Kasai K, Koji M, Fukuda R, Iwanami A, Nakagome K, et al. Executive and prefrontal dysfunction in unipolar depression: a review of neuropsychological and imaging evidence. *Neurosci Res.* (2004) 50:1–11. doi: 10.1016/j.neures.2004.05.003

56. Drevets WC, Price JL, Furey ML. Brain structural and functional abnormalities in mood disorders: implications for neurocircuitry models of depression. *Brain Struct Funct.* (2008) 213:93–118. doi: 10.1007/s00429-008-0189-x
57. Wu H, Sun H, Xu J, Wu Y, Wang C, Xiao J, et al. Changed hub and corresponding functional connectivity of subgenual anterior cingulate cortex in major depressive disorder. *Front Neuroanat.* (2016) 10:120. doi: 10.3389/fnana.2016.00120
58. DeRubeis RJ, Siegle GJ, Hollon SD. Cognitive therapy vs. medications for depression: treatment outcomes and neural mechanisms. *Nat Rev Neurosci.* (2008) 9:788–96. doi: 10.1038/nrn2345

5

Reduced White Matter Integrity with Cognitive Impairments in End Stage Renal Disease

Yi Yin[1,2†]*, Meng Li*[2†]*, Chao Li*[1]*, Xiaofen Ma*[2]*, Jianhao Yan*[2]*, Tianyue Wang*[2]*, Shishun Fu*[1,2]*, Kelei Hua*[1,2]*, Yunfan Wu*[1,2]*, Wenfeng Zhan*[2] *and Guihua Jiang*[1,2*]

[1] *Guangdong Second Provincial General Hospital, Third School of Clinical Medicine, Southern Medical University, Guangzhou, China,* [2] *Department of Medical Imaging, Guangdong Second Provincial General Hospital, Guangzhou, China*

Correspondence:
Guihua Jiang
GH.jiang2002@163.com

† *These authors have contributed equally to this work.*

Background: End-stage renal disease (ESRD) is a serious public health problem, which can often lead to multiorgan dysfunction, such as cerebrovascular disease and cognitive damage. It is essential to understand cognitive impairment in patients with ESRD to develop better ESRD treatment and prevent further cognitive impairment. Cognitive impairment is believed to be related to structural abnormalities in the brain.

Purpose: To investigate white matter microstructural abnormalities in patients with ESRD using TBSS analysis of DTI and to explore the possible mechanisms underlying the impaired cognitive function.

Materials and Methods: A TBSS analysis of DTI data was to investigate the microstructural changes in their WM over the whole brain. We chose the white matter tracts or regions with significantly reduced FA as the regions of interest (ROIs), Pearson's correlations were performed between clinical indicators (Mini-Mental State Examination (MMSE), digit span task scores, serum creatinine, blood urea nitrogen and hemodialysis duration) and the mean FA value of the ROIs in the ESRD patients.

Results: Lower FA and higher MD, AD and RD values were observed in widespread and symmetrical WM in ESRD patients than healthy controls (HCs), Pearson correlation analysis revealed a significantly positive correlation between the Mini-Mental State Examination (MMSE) scores and FA values in the right corona radiata and left anterior thalamic radiation (ATR) and demonstrated a significantly negative correlation between FA values and the serum creatinine and blood urea nitrogen in the ATR ($P < 0.01$) in addition, digit span task scores positively correlate with the FA value in the left anterior rather than in the corona radiata. No cluster survived when we adopted the False Discovery Rate (FDR) correction to multiple comparisons.

Conclusion: Our study indicate widespread impairment of the white matter in ESRD patients. Damage to the thalamic radiation and corona radiata may affect cognitive function in ESRD patients, the reduced integrity of ATR may tend to affect the working memory while the damage to the corona radiata may involve the executive function impaired in ESRD patients. The accumulation of serum creatinine and blood urea nitrogen may contribute to the WM impairment.

Keywords: end-stage renal disease, tract-based spatial statistics, white matter, cognitive function, serum creatinine, blood urea nitrogen

INTRODUCTION

End-stage renal disease (ESRD) is a serious public health problem [1, 2]. It occurs when glomerular filtration (GFR) falls below 15/mL/min/1.73 m^2. In China, approximately 270,000 patients with ESRD must accept dialysis or renal transplantation therapy to sustain their lives, and both these treatments are extremely costly [3, 4]. ESRD can often lead to multiorgan dysfunction, such as cerebrovascular disease and cognitive damage [5]. Increasingly, attention has focused on cognitive damage because approximately 90% of ESRD patients exhibit impairment of cognitive function [6], which may profoundly affect the quality of their lives. Understanding cognitive impairment in patients with ESRD is important because it can be used to plan ESRD treatment and so prevent further cognitive impairment in the early stage.

In previous studies, participants with aggravated chronic kidney disease (CKD) (eGFR < 30) were more likely to have significant cognitive impairment, such as naming and attention [3, 7, 8, 14]. Abnormal brain functional connectivity was also observed in ESRD patients with resting-state functional MRI (r-fMRI) [9]. For example, an r-fMRI study found that ESRD patients exhibited significantly decreased functional connectivity with the posterior cingulate cortex (PCC) in the left middle temporal gyrus, the right anterior cingulate gyrus, and the bilateral medial superior frontal gyrus, which suggested a spatially specific disruption of functional connectivity of the default mode network (DMN) [10]. In addition to this fMRI study, there were also some structural abnormalities reported in ESRD patients, and some diffusion tensor imaging (DTI) studies detected changes in the WM in ESRD patients using several analytical methods, including region of interest (ROI) [9], voxel-based analysis (VBA) [11], and diffusion tensor tractographies (DTTs) [12], these studies found some microstructural abnormalities in ESRD patients, for example, the VBA study concluded that voxelwise DTI analysis is helpful in the detection of white matter alterations caused by hemodialysis. DTTs and r-fMRI detected structural and functional alterations in the DMN in the brain after renal transplantation in patients with ESRD [12]. This study showed the DMN may be damaged in the ESRD patients. However, this study was limited by its arbitrary choice of fibers for use with DTTs, which did not facilitate comprehensive assessment of microstructural changes in the WM. Although these studies showed WM microstructural changes in patients with ESRD, both the ROI and the DTTs methods are known to have low reproducibility due to the lack of a clear and consistent standard, and the results are dependent on the location and size of the ROI selected by the researcher. These smoothing and alignments are not accurate enough for VBA, which may affect the results. Tract-based spatial statistics (TBSS) is a recently developed DTI analytical method that require smoothness or a hypothesis [13–15], which renders it non-susceptible to the disadvantages of the conventional ROI or VBA-method [16]. To the best of our knowledge, a few studies have reported some white matter (WM) abnormalities using TBSS methods, for example, Kong et al. [14] found diffuse interstitial brain edema and moderate WM integrity disruption occurring in ESRD patients, which correlated with cognitive dysfunction, and serum urea levels might be a risk factor for these WM changes. Zhang et al. [13] found structural damages to radiation and associative fiber tracts may account for the cognitive deficits especially in executive function in ESRD patients. As we know, besides executive function, cognitive function involving working memory, and we found the working memory impaired in some ERSD patients in the neuropsychological tests. Recently, a study [18] indicated anterior thalamic radiation (ATR) abnormalities have a possible link with cognitive abnormalities (e.g., working memory) in schizophrenia. However, similar findings were not reported in patients with ESRD. The working memory may also impaired in ERSD patients, and the reduced integrity of ATR may related to the impaired working memory. The study has used TBSS methods to assess the structural abnormalities of the WM in ESRD patients.

The purpose of this study was to investigate microstructural changes in the white matter over the whole brain in ESRD patients using TBSS. Correlation analysis was performed between ESRD-related WM microstructural alterations and biochemical variables, digit span test scores and MMSE scores to detect the mechanism underlying cognitive impairment in ESRD patients.

MATERIALS AND METHODS

Subjects

This study was approved by the Research Ethics Review Board of the Institute of Mental Health at the Guangdong Second Provincial General Hospital, and written informed consent was obtained from each participant. The inclusion criteria of our study for the ESRD patients were as follows: (a) confirmed ESRD diagnosis according to the K/DOQI classification of CKD; (b) age between 20 to 60 years, female or male; (c) no history of kidney transplant or acute renal failure (ARF); (d) undergoing regular hemodialysis 3 times weekly at hospital and (e) right handedness. Exclusion criteria included a history of traumatic brain injury, psychiatric disease, or ischemic disease including acute ischemic cerebrovascular disease. Forty ESRD patients were recruited from July 2013 to June 2015. Among 40 patients, 4 with severe mental disorders or infarcts were excluded from the study, and one patient was excluded because of movement artifacts and poor image quality.

Finally, 35 ESRD patients (38.3 $\pm$ 10.9 years; 30 males) were enrolled in the present study. The duration of dialysis and renal disease were recorded from the patients' case histories. Here, 40 age-and sex-matched healthy controls (HCs) (41.6 $\pm$ 11.2 years; 33 males) were recruited in Guangzhou.

Assessment of Neurocognition

All participants underwent MMSE, digit span test and multiple biochemical tests before MR data acquisition. The digit span test is used to measure digital storage capabilities in working memory. Subjects can see or hear a series of numbers, and are responsible for correctly recalling the sequence of numbers. The sequence of numbers tested in each trial is longer. The criterion for digit span test score is the longest number of consecutive numbers that can be accurately remembered. The biochemical tests included Scr and BUN. The MMSE tests were performed by trained psychometricians.

Image Acquisition

MR Imaging was performed by using a 1.5T MR system (Achieva Nova-Dual; Philips) at the Department of Medical Imaging, Guangdong Second Provincial General Hospital with an eight-channel head coil. To exclude subjects with visible brain abnormalities, conventional imaging was performed using an axial T1-weighted image and T2-fluid attenuated inversion recovery (T2-FLAIR) image. DTI was performed with 32 diffusion gradient directions ($b = 800$ s/mm^2 along 32 non-collinear directions) plus a reference image (i.e., $b = 0$) using a single shot spin echo planar sequence. The parameters were as follows: TR = 10,793 ms, TE = 62 ms, field of view = 230 × 230 mm^2, matrix = 128 × 128, slice thickness = 2 mm, no slice gap, voxel size = 2 × 2 × 2 mm^3.

Data Processing

All DTI images were processed using the PANDA toolbox (Version1.3.1, released 2016) based on the FSL [17]. Analysis of DTI parameters (MD, AD, and RD) was performed using TBSS implemented in FSL automatically. First, FA maps were calculated for all subjects from the DTI data after eddy-current-induced distortions and correct for head motion. Then, the FA data were spatially normalized into 1 × 1 × 1 mm^3 Montreal Neurological Institute (MNI) 152 Space. Next, the mean FA (FA threshold > 0.2) image was created and thinned to create a mean FA skeleton. Finally, each subject's aligned FA data were projected onto this skeleton. MD, AD, and RD maps were also mapped onto the template using projection vectors from each individual's FA-to-skeleton transformation, and similarly conducted like FA images. After voxel-wise group comparisons, the skeletal regions showing significant differences were labeled using the JHU White-Matter Tractography Atlas in FSL.

The demographic, biochemical, and clinical characteristics were analyzed using the Statistical Package for the Social Sciences (SPSS) version 19.0 (SPSS Inc., Chicago, IL, US) and Student's t-tests were performed to compare the differences between the patients and the HCs with respect to age, education, and cognitive results. Gender differences were assessed using the Pearson Chi-Square test. The level of statistical significance was set at 0.05 (two tailed). Differences in diffusion indices between the ESRD group and HCs were assessed using voxel-wise two sample t-tests by FSL. Nonparametric permutation tests were conducted based on 5,000 random permutations. The clusters with a Threshold-Free Cluster Enhancement (TFCE) uncorrected P-value of less than 0.05 were reported, then we adopted the False Discovery Rate (FDR) correction to multiple comparisons.

Outlining Region-of-Interest

We chose the white matter tracts or regions with significantly reduced FA as the regions of interest (ROIs), and then abstract the mean FA value of each ROIs, were delineated on FA images using Analyze AVW™ (Mayo Foundation, Rochester, Minnesota). b0 images are displayed with the FA image to help guide ROI delineation. ROIs were outlined by manually tracing the FA image and the position was confirmed on the b0 image. The same operator, who was unaware of the diagnostic team, tracked all ROIs. Mean FA value was computed to generate the total mean FA value for each ROIs.

TABLE 1 | Demographic and clinical characteristics of ESRD patients and healthy controls.

Variable	ESRD (n = 35)	HCs (n = 40)	P-value
Age (years)	38.3 ± 10.9	41.6 ± 11.2	0.117[a]
Gender (M/F)	30/5	33/7	> 0.999[b]
Level of education (years)	11.3 ± 2.8	11.5 ± 2.5	0.153
Duration of dialysis (m)	16.3 ± 5.8	–	–
Duration of disease (m)	83.25 ± 33.65	–	–
Serum calcium (mmol/L)	2.5 ± 0.4	2.2 ± 0.3	0.513[b]
Serum creatinine (μmol/L)	826.3 ± 432.4	155 ± 228.6	< 0.001[b]
Blood urea nitrogen (mmol/L)	18.3 ± 8.5	5.3 ± 1.6	< 0.001[b]
MMSE score	25.69 ± 3.43	28.69 ± 5.13	0.006[b]
Digit span test score	7.3 ± 1.3	9.6 ± 1.6	0.009[b]

Values are represented as mean ± standard deviation. ESRD, end-stage renal disease; HCs, healthy controls. MMSE, Mini-Mental State Examination.
[a] P-value was obtained by chi-square test.
[b] P-value was obtained by two-side two-sample t-test.

Correlation Analysis

Pearson correlation analysis was performed between the mean FA value of each above significant clusters and the MMSE, digit span test, serum creatinine, serum urea levels, and duration of dialysis and disease respectively, we adopted the False Discovery Rate (FDR) correction to multiple comparisons.

RESULTS

Demographic Information and Behavioral Tests

The demographic, biochemical, and clinical characteristics for all the participants are shown in **Table 1**. There were no significant differences with respect to age, gender, or level of education between the ESRD patients and the healthy controls patients showed lower MMSE scores and digit span test score than healthy controls ($P = 0.006$) ($P = 0.009$).

TBSS

ESRD patients showed lower FA than HCs, mainly in bilateral corona radiata, bilateral ATR, bilateral inferior fronto-occipital fasciculus, the body and genu of the corpus callosum, bilateral superior longitudinal fasciculus (SLF), WM in the frontal lobe, and right inferior longitudinal fasciculus (**Table 2**; **Figure 1**). Specifically, widespread and symmetrical abnormal WM with increased MD, AD, and RD was observed in deep brain regions in ESRD patients, including corpus callosum, bilateral corticospinal tract, SLF, ATR, cingulate gyrus, superior temporal gyrus, and inferior prefrontal cortex (**Figure 2**). Unfortunately, we found no cluster survived when adopted the False Discovery Rate (FDR) correction to multiple comparisons.

TABLE 2 | White matter tracts or regions with significantly reduced FA in patients and in healthy controls.

Regions within the Brain	Side	MNI Coordinates (mm) (*x, y, z*)	Cluster Voxels
Corona radiata	L	(−18, 40, 3)	2108
	R	(20, 42, 0)	2682
Anterior thalamic radiation	L	(−28, −69, 25)	1356
	R	(29, −65, 23)	1102
Inferiofronto-occipital fasciculus	L	(−35, −65, 2)	763
	R	(39, −36, 1)	473
Body of corpus callosum	N/A	(−11, 5, 33)	513
Genu of corpus callosum	N/A	(−13, 31, 13)	352
Superior longitudinal fasciculus	L	(−44, −10, 25)	231
	R	(43, −6, 26)	132
Inferior longitudinal fasciculus	R	(34, −65, −1)	84

R indicates right, L, left, N/A, not applicable, MNI, Montreal Neurological Institute. All $P < 0.05$, uncorrected.

Correlation Analysis

Pearson correlation analysis revealed that the digit span test scores was positively correlate with the FA value in the left ATR ($r = 0.810$, $p < 0.01$, uncorrected) (**Figure 2**). And also revealed a significantly positive correlation between the MMSE score and FA values in the right corona radiata ($r = 0.632$, $P < 0.01$, uncorrected) and the left ATR ($r = 0.658$, $P < 0.01$, uncorrected) (**Figure 3**), and we found a significantly negative correlation between FA value and the serum creatinine in the right ATR ($r = -0.706$, $P < 0.01$, uncorrected) (**Figure 4**) and a significantly negative correlation between FA value and the blood urea nitrogen in the left ATR ($r = -0.704$, $P < 0.01$, uncorrected) (**Figure 5**) and the right corona radiata ($r = -0.701$, $P < 0.01$, uncorrected). We found no cluster survived when we adopted the False Discovery Rate (FDR) correction to multiple comparisons. There was no significant correlation between the MMSE scores and other non-FA indices and also show no significant correlation between FA value and sex, serum creatinine, serum urea levels, and duration of dialysis and disease (all $P > 0.05$).

DISCUSSION

We used TBSS to explore the integrity of WM in ESRD patients and to further examine the relationship between WM microstructure, MMSE scores, and biochemical indicators. ESRD patients showed decreased FA and increased MD, AD, and RD, mainly in the bilateral corona radiata and ATR, and the body and genu of the corpus callosum. Several structural abnormalities, such as the FA value in the left ATR, are negatively associated with the level of serum creatinine and blood urea nitrogen and positively associated with MMSE and digit span test scores.

The ESRD patients showed reduced FA in the ATR. Previous studies showed that the ATR is associated with memory encoding [18, 19]. In one study that performed on rats, working memory was found to be impaired after the thalamic radiation became damaged, so the thalamic radiation appears to be necessary to maintain the performance of working memory [20]. In another study [21], researchers found that the thalamic radiation is disproportionally larger and more complex in humans than in other mammals, adjusting for body size, which may contribute to humans' special cognitive abilities, such as working memory and language. This supports the hypothesis that reduced integrity of the ATR may affect the cognitive function of ESRD patients. The MMSE scores and digit span test scores were found to be positively correlated with FA values in the left ATR in ESRD patients. The performance of the digital span test is closely related to the working memory ability, and improving the language memory ability can help master the new language. Zhang et al. [13] indicated damages to the white matter may affect executive function in the ESRD patients, but didn't report that the working memory was impaired. Our results indicated the working memory was also impaired in ESRD patients. One possible explanation for the impaired working memory in ESRD patients is that the anterior thalamic nuclei process afferent information from the hippocampus, which is involved in cognitive functions such as working memory, and they project mainly toward the anterior cingulate cortex. Reduced integrity of the ATR may disrupt this process, and the ATR is thought to consist of default mode network (DMN) [22–24]. DMN is thought to be involved in the core processes of human cognition, including the integration of cognitive and emotional processing, mind wandering, and monitoring of the surrounding environment [24–27]. Harciarek et al. found that the DMN recovered shortly after renal transplantation in ESRD patients [28]. In this way, the reduced integrity of the ATR in our study suggested that the working memory is impaired in ESRD patients.

We also found decreased FA values in the corona radiata, which was consistent with previous studies. For example, one study performed using the VBA-method showed that the FA value of the bilateral corona radiata was decreased in ESRD patients [11]. Another study suggested that structural damages to the corona radiata may disrupt neural transmission and affect the central executive network [29]. The decreased FA value in the corona radiata suggests it may affect the executive function in ESRD patients. The corona radiata is an important group of nerves because of its role in the relationship between regions in the brain. It contains afferent nerves that send messages of sensory input from the body to the brain, and the efferent nerves send motor control function messages from the brain to the body [30]. This means that the corona radiata carries messages to and from the body, and the reduced microstructure integrity observed in the corona radiata in this study indicate the impaired function of sensory input function and motor control in ESRD patients.

In addition, ESRD patients showed decreased FA and increased MD, AD, and RD, mainly consistent with the white matter regions that FA reduced. MD, AD, and RD reflect the overall or direction-specific capability of tissue water diffusion. These indices usually increase when WM undergoes demyelination, axon loss, or some other process. This suggested that decreased FA may be caused by both increased AD and

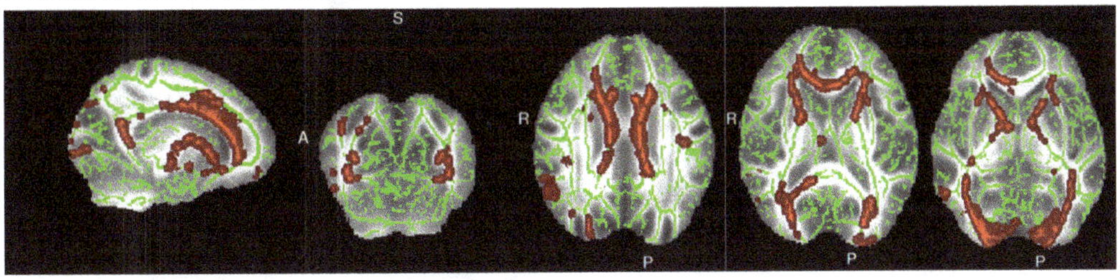

FIGURE 1 | Inter-group differences for FA in ESRD patients and healthy controls.

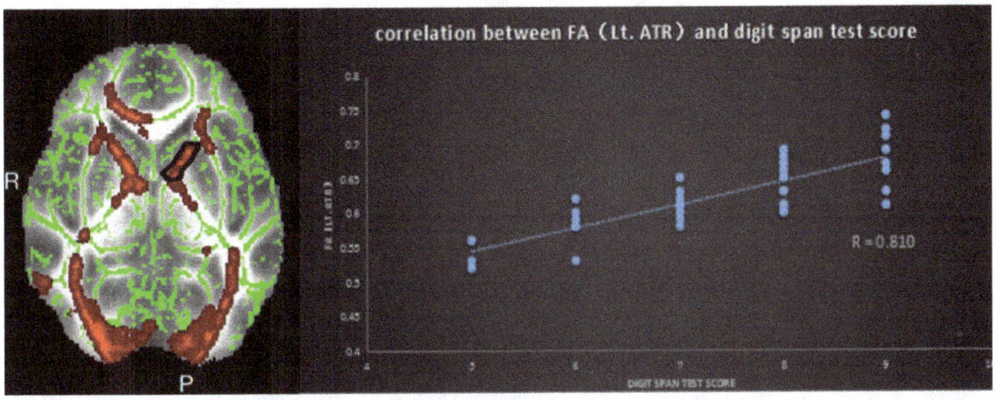

FIGURE 2 | Relationship between mean FA and digit span test scores in ESRD; region-of-interest maps **(Left side)** are displayed with the corresponding graphs **(Right side)**. Significant positive correlation between FA values for the left anterior thalamic radiation with MMSE scores. Lt.ATR indicates left anterior thalamic radiation.

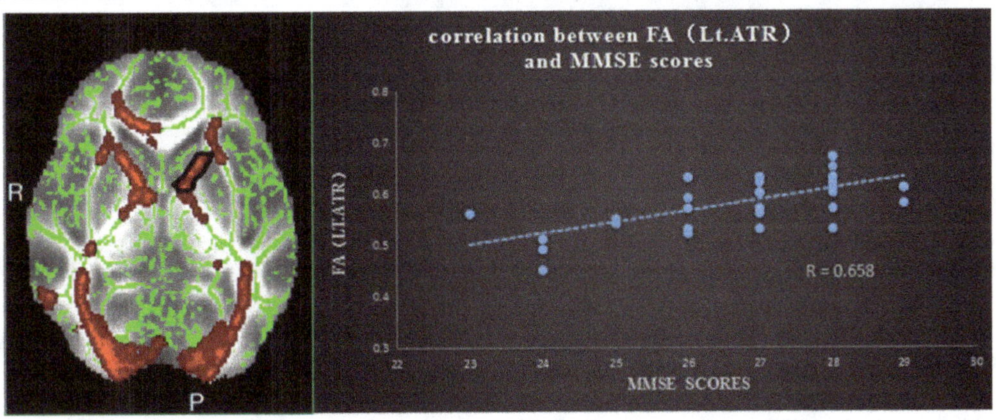

FIGURE 3 | Relationship between mean FA and MMSE scores in ESRD; region-of-interest maps **(Left side)** are displayed with the corresponding graphs **(Right side)**. Significant positive correlation between FA values for the left anterior thalamic radiation with MMSE scores. Lt.ATR indicates left anterior thalamic radiation.

increased RD, indicating that both demyelination and axonal injury may lead to the WM impairment in ESRD patients, which is partially consistent with previous DTI studies [8, 31]. Using DTI, Zhang et al. showed significant increases in RD values but no significant changes in AD values [13]. Another study, which used VBA, showed both increased RD and AD values in some WM regions [11], but the results showed no consistent relationship to abnormal brain structure in patients with ESRD. Hsieh found that the FA value in patients with ESRD was significantly reduced compared to the control group in the whole brain region by using manual region-of-interest analysis [32]. The FA value generally reduce in the elderly and long-term hemodialysis patients. This may be related to degeneration of axons and demyelination of white matter. The decrease of FA and the increase of MD may attributed to macroscopic tissue damage and the destruction of the microstructural integrity

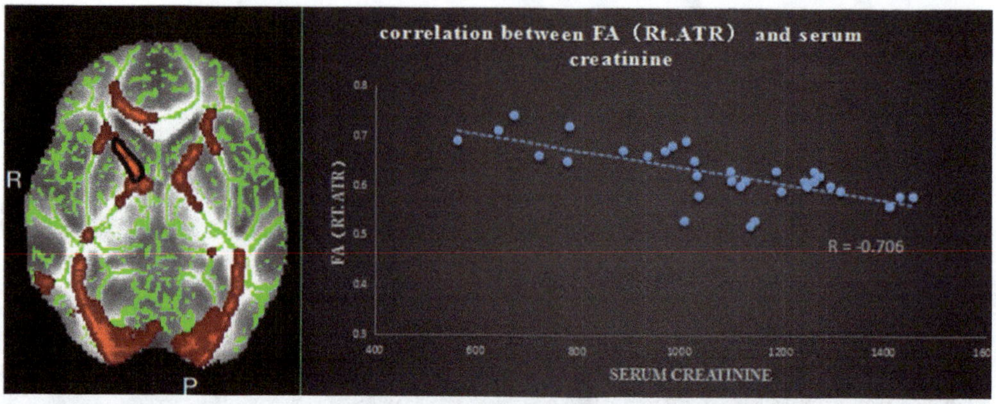

FIGURE 4 | Relationship between mean FA and the serum creatinine in ESRD; region-of-interest maps **(Left side)** are displayed with the corresponding graphs **(Right side)**. Significant negative correlation between FA values for the right anterior thalamic radiation with the serum creatinine. Rt.ATR indicates right anterior thalamic radiation.

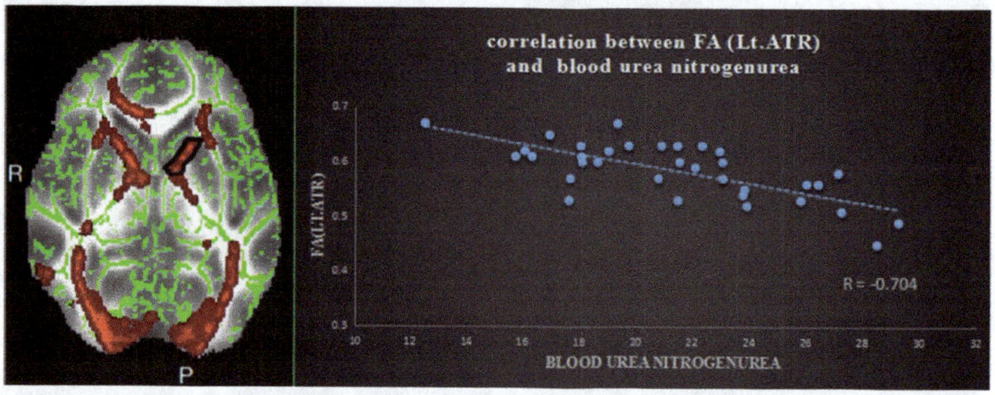

FIGURE 5 | Relationship between mean FA and blood urea nitrogen in ESRD; region-of-interest maps **(Left side)** are displayed with the corresponding graphs **(Right side)**. Significant negative correlation between FA values for the left anterior thalamic radiation with blood urea nitrogen in ESRD. Lt.ATR indicates left anterior thalamic radiation.

caused by interstitial edema. Moreover, they found the positive correlation between MD and RD values and duration of dialysis suggests that dialysis may be a factor in white matter demyelination. Long-term dialysis leads to interstitial edema and demyelination leading to pons of axons. They believe that dialysis has a broad impact on the white matter structure of patients with ESRD. Interstitial edema of patients with ESRD in dialysis may explain cognitive impairment in patients with ESRD [14]. However, our study didn't found any relationship between dialysis duration and FA, MD, AD, and RD value. One possible reason could be that the sample difference, which may affect the result. The other possible reason could be the heterogeneity of subjects due to the lack of more rigorous subject recruitment. A further study with a larger sample of subjects is needed to address this issue in the future. In addition, there is reason to believe that, in addition to dialysis may lead to brain cognitive impairment, patients with ESRD itself can also damage the brain structure and thus affect cognitive function due to renal failure caused the accumulation of toxic substances.

Finally, this study shows the positive correlation of serum creatinine and blood urea nitrogen with the reduced FA in the bilateral ATR. One previous study [29] suggested that serum creatinine and blood urea nitrogen may cause reduced WM integrity. One possible explanation for this is that renal function damage may lead to accumulation of metabolic agents, and these neural toxicities could lead to the demyelination and axonal injury [33]. Some studies [6, 34] have shown that serum creatinine and blood urea nitrogen are associated with cognitive dysfunction in patients with ESRD, and neuropsychologic performance has been shown to improve after renal transplantation. In a recent resting-state fMRI study, Bai et al. [31] reported similar findings in patients with ESRD and observed that metabolic agents were associated with altered functional connectivity in patients with ESRD. Our results indicate that serum creatinine and blood urea nitrogen may contribute to the cognitive impairment. It is essential to take steps to control the level of serum creatinine and blood urea nitrogen to prevent further impairment of cognitive function in ESRD patients.

The present work has several limitations that must be considered. First, the MRI scanning parameters were suboptimal (e.g., 1.5-T scanner) for the current dataset. Second, we only observed patients at the end stage of choric kidney disease because chronic kidney disease can be classified into 5 stages, and it progresses to ESRD when the glomerular filtration rate (GFR) falls below 15 ml/1.73 m^2, more studies should be performed in the future to explore cognitive impairment in CKD before the end stage because this cognitive impairment is mild and may reverse if detected and treated promptly. Finally, we found no cluster survived if we adopted the False Discovery Rate (FDR) correction to multiple comparisons. One possible reason could be that the sample size was not large enough in our study (35 patients), which may affect the statistical power, the other possible reason could be the heterogeneity of subjects due to the lack of more rigorous subject recruitment. A further study with a larger sample of subjects is needed to address this issue in the future.

In conclusion, the results of our study indicate the reduced integrity of the corona radiata and ATR may be related to cognitive function in ESRD patients. the impaired cognitive function involve not only in executive function but also involving the working memory. In addition, from a pathological perspective, this study indicates that the accumulation of metabolic agents such as serum creatinine and blood urea nitrogen may contribute to cognitive impairment in ESRD patients. These findings may facilitate understanding of the relationship between WM microstructural abnormalities and physiological alterations in ESRD. Although the pathophysiology is complicated, and there may be many factors that affect this WM impairment, this study provides an effective approach for exploring WM abnormalities in ESRD patients.

AUTHOR CONTRIBUTIONS

GJ: Designed experiments; XM, JY, and TW: Carried out experiments; CL: Analyzed experimental results; KH, SF, and YW: Analyzed sequencing data and developed analysis tools. WZ: Assisted with collecting data; YY and ML: Wrote the manuscript.

ACKNOWLEDGMENTS

This work was supported by grants from the National Natural Science Foundation of China (No.81471639, 81771807,81701111), the Natural Science Foundation of Guangdong (Grant Number:2015A030313723, 2016A020215125, 2017A020215077) and the science foundation of Guangdong Second Provincial General Hospital (YQ2015-011).

REFERENCES

1. Jahanian H, Ni WW, Christen T, Moseley ME, Kurella Tamura M, Zaharchuk G. Spontaneous BOLD signal fluctuations in young healthy subjects and elderly patients with chronic kidney disease. *PLoS ONE* (2014) **9**:e92539. doi: 10.1371/journal.pone.0092539
2. Siddiqi L, Hoogduin H, Visser F, Leiner T, Mali WP, Blankestijn PJ. Inhibition of the renin-angiotensin system affects kidney tissue oxygenation evaluated by magnetic resonance imaging in patients with chronic kidney disease. *J Clin Hyperten.* (2014) **16**:214–8. doi: 10.1111/jch.12263
3. Kurella Tamura M, Yaffe K, Hsu CY, Yang J, Sozio S, Fischer M, et al. Cognitive Impairment and Progression of CKD. *Am J Kidney Dis.* (2016) **68**:77–83. doi: 10.1053/j.ajkd.2016.01.026
4. Prasad PV, Thacker J, Li LP, Haque M, Li W, Koenigs H, et al. Multi-parametric evaluation of chronic kidney disease by MRI: a preliminary cross-sectional study. *PLoS ONE* (2015) **10**:e0139661. doi: 10.1371/journal.pone.0139661
5. Inoue T, Kozawa E, Okada H, Inukai K, Watanabe S, Kikuta T, et al. Noninvasive evaluation of kidney hypoxia and fibrosis using magnetic resonance imaging. *J Am Soc Nephrol.* (2011) **22**:1429–34. doi: 10.1681/ASN.2010111143
6. Gupta A, Lepping RJ, Yu AS, Perea RD, Honea RA, Johnson DK, et al. Cognitive function and white matter changes associated with renal transplantation. *Am J Nephrol.* (2016) **43**:50–7. doi: 10.1159/000444334
7. Li S, Ma X, Huang R, Li M, Tian J, Wen H, et al. Abnormal degree centrality in neurologically asymptomatic patients with end-stage renal disease: a resting-state fMRI study. *Clin Neurophysiol.* (2016). **127**:602–9. doi: 10.1016/j.clinph.2015.06.022
8. Inoue T, Kozawa E Ishikawa M, Okada H. [Assessment of chronic kidney disease using functional MRI]. *Nihon Jinzo Gakkai Shi.* (2015) **57**:1225–32.
9. Chen HJ, Zhang LJ, Lu GM. Multimodality MRI findings in patients with end-stage renal disease. *BioMed Res Int.* (2015) **2015**:697402. doi: 10.1155/2015/697402
10. Ma X, Tian J, Wu Z, Zong X, Dong, J. Zhan W, et al. Spatial disassociation of disrupted functional connectivity for the default mode network in patients with end-stage renal disease. *PLoS ONE* (2016) **11**:e0161392. doi: 10.1371/journal.pone.0161392
11. Chou MC, Hsieh TJ, Lin YL, Hsieh YT, Li WZ, Chang JM, et al. Widespread white matter alterations in patients with end-stage renal disease: a voxelwise diffusion tensor imaging study. *Am J Neuroradiol.* (2013) **34**:1945–51. doi: 10.3174/ajnr.A3511
12. Zhang LJ, Wen J, Liang X, Qi R, Schoepf UJ, Wichmann JL, et al. Brain default mode network changes after renal transplantation: a diffusion-tensor imaging and resting-state functional MR imaging study. *Radiology* (2016) **278**:485–95. doi: 10.1148/radiol.2015150004
13. Zhang R, Liu K, Yang L, Zhou T, Qian S, Li B, et al. Reduced white matter integrity and cognitive deficits in maintenance hemodialysis ESRD patients: a diffusion-tensor study. *Eur Radiol.* (2015) **25**:661–8. doi: 10.1007/s00330-014-3466-5
14. Kong X, Wen JQ, Qi RF, Luo S, Zhong JH, Chen HJ, et al. Diffuse Interstitial brain edema in patients with end-stage renal disease undergoing hemodialysis. *Medicine* (2014) **93**:e313. doi: 10.1097/MD.0000000000000313
15. Wang WJ, Pui MH, Guo Y, Wang LQ, Wang HJ, Liu M. 3T magnetic resonance diffusion tensor imaging in chronic kidney disease. *Abdom Imaging* (2014) **39**:770–5. doi: 10.1007/s00261-014-0116-y
16. Liu Z, Xu Y, Zhang J, Zhen J, Wang R, Caiet S, et al. Chronic kidney disease: pathological and functional assessment with diffusion tensor imaging at 3T MR. *Eur Radiol.* (2015) **25**:652–60. doi: 10.1007/s00330-014-3461-x
17. Smith S.M, Jenkinson M, Johansen-Berg H, Rueckert D, Nichols TE, Mackay CE, et al. Tract-based spatial statistics: voxelwise analysis of multi-subject diffusion data. *Neuroimage* (2006) **31**:1487–505. doi: 10.1016/j.neuroimage.2006.02.024
18. Mamah D, Conturo TE, Harms MP, Akbudak E, Wang L, McMichael AR, et al. Anterior thalamic radiation integrity in schizophrenia: a diffusion-tensor imaging study. *Psychiatry Res.* (2010) **183**:144–50. doi: 10.1016/j.pscychresns.2010.04.013
19. Watanabe Y, Funahashi S. Thalamic mediodorsal nucleus and working memory. *Neurosci Biobehav Rev.* (2012) **36**:134–42. doi: 10.1016/j.neubiorev.2011.05.003

20. Newman LA, Burk, JA. Effects of excitotoxic thalamic intralaminar nuclei lesions on attention and working memory. *Behav Brain Res.* (2005) **162**:264–71. doi: 10.1016/j.bbr.2005.03.018
21. Rodriguez A, Whitson J, Granger R. Derivation and analysis of basic computational operations of thalamocortical circuits. *J Cogn Neurosci.* (2004) **16**:856–77. doi: 10.1162/089892904970690
22. van den Heuvel MP, Hulshoff PH. Exploring the brain network: a review on resting-state fMRI functional connectivity. *Eur Neuropsychopharmacol.* (2010) **20**:519–34. doi: 10.1016/j.euroneuro.2010.03.008
23. Ye Q, Su F, Shu H, Gong L, Xie CM, Zhou H, et al. Shared effects of the clusterin gene on the default mode network among individuals at risk for Alzheimer's disease. *CNS Neurosci Ther.* (2017) **23**:395–404. doi: 10.1111/cns.12682
24. Wang Y, Tang W, Fan X, Zhang J, Geng D, Jiang K, et al. Resting-state functional connectivity changes within the default mode network and the salience network after antipsychotic treatment in early-phase schizophrenia. *Neuropsychiatr Dis Treat.* (2017). **13**:397–406. doi: 10.2147/NDT.S123598
25. Ni L, Wen J, Zhang LJ, Zhu T, Qi R, Xu Q, et al. Aberrant default-mode functional connectivity in patients with end-stage renal disease: a resting-state functional MR imaging study. *Radiology* (2014) **271**:543–52. doi: 10.1148/radiol.13130816
26. Zhu X, Zhu Q, Shen H, Liao W, Yuan F, et al, Rumination and default mode network subsystems connectivity in first-episode, drug-naive young patients with major depressive disorder. *Sci Rep.* (2017) **7**:43105. doi: 10.1038/srep43105
27. Greicius MD, Krasnow B, Reiss AL, Menon V, et al. Functional connectivity in the resting brain: a network analysis of the default mode hypothesis. *Proc Natl Acad Sci USA.* (2003) **100**:253–8. doi: 10.1073/pnas.0135058100
28. Harciarek M, Biedunkiewicz B, Lichodziejewska-Niemierko M, Debska-Slizien A, Rutkowski B, et al. Continuous cognitive improvement 1 year following successful kidney transplant. *Kidney Int.* (2011) **79**:1353–60. doi: 10.1038/ki.2011.40
29. Kim HS, Park JW, Bai DS, Jeong JY, Hong JH, Son SM, et al. Diffusion tensor imaging findings in neurologically asymptomatic patients with end stage renal disease. *NeuroRehabilitation* (2011) **29**:111–6. doi: 10.3233/NRE-2011-0684
30. Vemuri P, Knopman DS, Jack Jr CR, Lundt ES, Weigand SD, Zuk SM, et al, Association of kidney function biomarkers with brain mri findings: the BRINK study. *J Alzheimer's Dis.* (2016) **55**:1069–82. doi: 10.3233/JAD-160834
31. Bai Z, Ma X, Tian J, Dong J, He J, Zhan W, et al. Brain microstructural abnormalities are related to physiological alterations in end-stage renal disease. *PLoS ONE* (2016) **11**:e0155902. doi: 10.1371/journal.pone.0155902
32. Hsieh TJ, Chang J-M, Chuang H-Y, Ko C-H, Hsieh M-L, Liu G-C, et al. End-stage renal disease: *in vivo* diffusion-tensor imaging of silent white matter damage. *Radiology* (2009) **252**:518–25. doi: 10.1148/radiol.2523080484
33. Mogi M, Horiuchi M. Clinical interaction between brain and kidney in small vessel disease. *Cardiol Res Pract.* (2011) **2011**:306189. doi: 10.4061/2011/306189
34. Yamada K, Shinmoto H, Oshio K, Ito S, Kumagai H, Kaji T, et al. Diffusion-weighted MR imaging for the assessment of renal function: analysis using statistical models based on truncated gaussian and gamma distributions. *Magn Reson Med Sci.* (2016) **15**:237–45. doi: 10.2463/mrms.mp.2015-0067

6

Altered Structural Covariance Among the Dorsolateral Prefrontal Cortex and Amygdala in Treatment-Naïve Patients with Major Depressive Disorder

*Zhiwei Zuo[1], Shuhua Ran[1], Yao Wang[1], Chang Li[1], Qi Han[1], Qianying Tang[2], Wei Qu[2] and Haitao Li[1]**

[1] Department of Radiology, Affiliated Southwest Hospital, Army Medical University, Chongqing, China, [2] Department of Psychology, Affiliated Southwest Hospital, Army Medical University, Chongqing, China

***Correspondence:**
Haitao Li
liihait@163.com

Background: Impairments in cognitive and emotional processing are a characteristic of major depressive disorder (MDD), and the dorsolateral prefrontal cortex (DLPFC) and amygdala are involved in these processes. However, the structural covariance between these two areas in patients with MDD has not been examined. Whether anatomical patterns are further damaged or compensated in untreated multiple-episode MDD compared to those in first-episode MDD is unclear.

Methods: Structural magnetic resonance imaging was performed in 35 treatment-naïve, currently depressed patients with MDD and 35 age-, sex-, and education-matched controls. The cortical thickness and subcortical volume were calculated using FreeSurfer software. Patients were divided into two subgroups based on the previous number of episodes.

Results: Regional abnormalities in patients with MDD were primarily observed in the frontal-limbic circuits. The negative structural association between the left DLPFC and left amygdala and the positive structural association between the bilateral DLPFC observed in controls were absent in patients with MDD. The medial orbitofrontal cortex and posterior cingulate cortex were thicker in patients with multiple-episode MDD than in patients with first-episode MDD and were positively correlated with disorder duration. No structural alterations were correlated with symptom severity.

Conclusions: These findings may provide structural evidence for deficits in functional networks in MDD and supports an underlying structural mechanism of dysfunction involving top-down or bottom-up processes. Morphological abnormalities in the medial orbitofrontal cortex and posterior cingulate cortex may be critical for the pathophysiological progression of multiple-episode MDD.

Keywords: major depressive disorder, structural covariance, cortical thickness, subcortical volume, dorsolateral prefrontal cortex, amygdala

INTRODUCTION

Many previous anatomical studies have focused on decreases in gray matter volume in patients with major depressive disorder (MDD). The abnormal regions reported in these studies, which are collectively known as cortical-limbic areas include the dorsolateral prefrontal cortex (DLPFC), orbitofrontal cortex (OFC), anterior cingulate cortex (ACC), posterior cingulate cortex (PCC), and amygdala (1, 2). However, these previous findings remain inconclusive (2, 3). Voxel-based morphometry, one of the most common methods used to measure volumetric changes, may actually impair the identification of subtle cortical differences because of heavy smoothing of the images and substantial cortical folding (4). Furthermore, volumetric changes are largely driven by gyrification and cortical surface area rather than cortical thickness (5), and alterations in cortical thickness are more sensitive to disease states than alterations in volume or surface area (6). In contrast to volumetric research, which consistently shows a decreasing trend in gray matter volume in patients with first-episode (FE) MDD (7), other studies have shown an increase in the thickness of several cerebral regions in untreated patients with FE MDD compared to that of controls (8–10). Based on these findings, whether a compensatory mechanism, chronic trajectory or potential age-of-onset effects participate in the pathological processes occurring during the early stage of MDD warrants further examination.

Although MDD has attracted increasing attention from the scientific community and the Chinese government, it is not recognized by most of the public. Even in a general hospital, only approximately 4% of depressed patients are identified by internists (11). Meanwhile, many depressed patients endure the disease for many years and experience multiple episodes (MEs) before seeking treatment because of the stigma and shame associated with depression in traditional Chinese culture. Without treatment, the episodes may continue and be characterized by increasingly serious symptoms. Therefore, the choice of an appropriate therapeutic schedule is more difficult for MEs compared to FEs. However, according to the result of a longitudinal observational study (12), none of the traditional demographic factors (e.g., sex, age, and socioeconomic status), clinical variables (e.g., prior episodes, age-of-onset, and episode severity) or treatment exposure (e.g., the presence or absence of treatment and treatment adequacy) are reliable predictors of recovery or recurrence in patients with MDD. Researchers have focused on examining dynamic neurobiological alterations, such as anatomical and functional deficits, some of which may be more sensitive to recurrence (13, 14). Possible structural differences between patients with FE and ME MDD, which are not clearly explored, may offer new targets for therapeutic intervention.

In the current study, we sought to use whole-brain analysis method and simultaneously attempted to make priori assumptions regarding the locations of structural deficits to systematically evaluate anatomical abnormalities. The treatment-naïve group in our study consisted of currently depressed patients with MDD to exclude the neuroprotective effects of continuous therapy and enable a direct assessment of underlying state-related changes in patients with MDD. Based on the existing literature, we hypothesized that patients with MDD would exhibit both decreased and increased cortical thickness and subcortical volumes in regions such as the DLPFC, OFC, and amygdala, and these regions may not be associated with the severity of current depressive symptoms. We also postulated that patients with ME MDD would exhibit reductions in structural measures compared with patients with FE MDD.

Abbreviations: MDD, major depressive disorder; DLPFC, dorsolateral prefrontal cortex; OFC, orbitofrontal cortex; ACC, anterior cingulate cortex; PCC, posterior cingulate cortex; CA, cornu ammonis; DG, dentate gyrus; FDR, false discovery rate.

MATERIALS AND METHODS

Subjects

Forty-one medication-naïve, middle aged patients with MDD were recruited as potential participants from the outpatient clinic at the Department of Psychology of Southwest Hospital, Chongqing, China. All participants participated in interviews and received independent evaluations by 2 psychologists, including the 24-item Hamilton Rating Depression Scale (HAM-D_{24}) (15), the Self-rating Depression Scale (SDS) (16), and the Self-rating Anxiety Scale (SAS) (17). Depression duration was assessed in an interview using the life-chart methodology. The inclusion criteria for patients were: (1) aged 18–48 years; (2) met the Diagnostic and Statistical Manual of Mental Disorders IV (DSM-IV) diagnostic criteria for MDD; (3) patients were not receiving treatment (not taking antidepressant drugs or engaged in formal psychotherapy) and currently depressed; (4) a total HAM-D_{24} score > 20 (moderate severity); (5) no history of bipolar disorder, schizophrenia, schizoaffective disorder, psychosis, bulimia, seizures, obsessive-compulsive disorder, primary post-traumatic disorder, or a current primary diagnosis of anorexia; (6) no history of alcohol abuse, substance dependence, suicidal behavior, brain injury or any contraindications for MRI; and (7) right-handedness. Thirty-five patients (22 female) met these criteria and were included in the study. Twenty of patients were currently experiencing their first depressive episode. The remaining patients had recovered from their first episode and were in the acute stage of at least their second depressive episode.

We also recruited 35 age-, sex-, and education-matched normal controls (NC) who had no history of drug dependence, psychiatric disease, traumatic brain injury, epilepsy, or chronic medical disease, such as heart failure, and no evidence to suggest an intracranial space-occupying lesion, hemorrhage, infarction, or other major neurological disease. In addition, these controls were right-handed.

All patients included in the study provided written informed consent. The study was approved by the Ethics Committee of the Southwest Hospital.

MRI Acquisition

A Siemens 3.0-Tesla Trio Tim MRI scanner (Siemens AG, Erlangen, Germany) was used to acquire structural images with a standard head coil. The subject was placed in a supine position during image acquisition. The head was fixed with sponge pads to reduce movement, and the subject was asked to keep the head as still as possible during the scan. The following magnetization-prepared rapid gradient echo acquisition parameters were used: repetition time (TR) = 1900 ms; echo time (TE) = 2.52 ms; inversion time (TI) = 1100 ms; flip angle = 9°; field of view (FOV) = 256 × 256 mm; slice thickness = 1 mm; number of slices = 176; and voxel size = 1 × 1 × 1 mm.

MRI Analysis

Structural images were subjected to volume segmentation and cortical surface reconstruction using FreeSurfer software (Massachusetts General Hospital, Boston, MA, U.S., http://surfer.nmr.mgh.harvard.edu). The post-processing procedures have been described in detail in previous studies (18, 19) and primarily consisted of the following steps: Talairach coordinate system conversion, bias-field correction, signal strength standardization, removal of the skull and soft tissues, automated volume partitioning and white matter segmentation, topology correction, and determination of the gray-white matter and leptomeningeal tissue boundaries. Inflated brain surfaces and cortical thicknesses were obtained. These post-processing procedures were performed separately on each cerebral hemisphere. Cortical thickness was defined as the shortest straight-line distance between the pial surface and the gray-white matter boundary. The volumes of subcortical regions, including the thalamus, caudate, putamen, pallidum, and amygdala, were extracted. As researchers are still debating whether hippocampal volumes are reduced in patients with MDD (20–22), we further segmented the hippocampus to determine whether structural variations in hippocampal subfields play a role in patients with MDD. The segmentations of the hippocampus include the fimbria, presubiculum, subiculum, cornu ammonis (CA) 1, CA2/3, CA4/dentate gyrus (DG) fields and the hippocampal fissure (23).

Statistical Analyses

First, we compared the demographic and clinical features and hemispheric cortex measurements between patients with MDD and NCs. The Mann-Whitney U-test or independent sample t-test were used for parameters that were not normally distributed (i.e., age, education level) and parameters with a normal distribution, (e.g., HAM-D_{24} score, SDS score, and SAS score), respectively. The chi-square test was used to assess differences in sex distribution. Differences in cortical thickness between the patients with MDD and NCs were then evaluated using the vertex-wise general linear model and a whole-brain statistical threshold correction was performed using the Monte Carlo simulation method. Statistical significance was set at a cluster-wise corrected P-value < 0.05. The average cortical thickness of the significant clusters was calculated for every subject to obtain a regionally specific comparator. Specifically, eight regions of interest (ROIs), including the bilateral DLPFC, OFC, ACC, and PCC, were created based on the Desikan template (24) and previous research (25) to extract the average cortical thickness. Between-group differences in average cortical thickness of the ROIs were assessed using an independent samples t-test, and differences in subcortical volumes were assessed using the Mann-Whitney U-test. Next, the MDD group was divided into two subgroups according to the number of episodes, i.e., the FE group and the ME group. The differences in average cortical thickness and subcortical volume in all regions observed between the MDD and NC groups in the previous statistical comparison were examined in the FE and ME groups using the independent sample t-test. Finally, correlation analyses were performed to explore the relationships among brain structures and clinical features. Structural covariance was examined with Pearson correlation analysis to determine the structural relationships between the left DLPFC and left amygdala, right DLPFC and right amygdala, left DLPFC and right DLPFC, and left amygdala and right amygdala. Then, Snedecor's method (26) was used to transform r-values to z-values to evaluate the significant differences in correlation coefficients between patients with MDD and NCs. False discovery rate (FDR) correction was applied to between-group analyses and correlation analyses that involved multiple comparisons.

RESULTS

Participants' Characteristics and Hemispheric Measures

Table 1 shows the demographic information, clinical data and hemispheric measurements for the MDD and NC groups. The two groups were matched in terms of age, sex, and education (P > 0.05). As expected, the patients with MDD had higher HAM-D_{24} scores, SDS scores, and SAS scores than the NCs. The patients with MDD showed a nearly significant trend for the increase in the average cortical thickness of the left hemisphere ($t = 1.987$, $P = 0.052$). No significant differences in the average cortical thickness of the right hemisphere and total subcortical volume were observed between the MDD and NC groups.

Surface-Based Cortical Thickness Analysis

A comparison of the cortical thickness between the MDD and NC groups showed relatively symmetrical changes in 16 clusters (**Figure 1** and **Table 2**), with both significant increases and decreases in cortical thickness observed. The largest and most significant increases in thickness were observed in the bilateral insula, superior frontal cortex, middle temporal gyrus, left PCC, caudal middle frontal cortex, precuneus, precentral gyrus, and right entorhinal cortex. The regions with significantly decreased thickness were the bilateral rostral middle frontal cortex, left lingual gyrus, medial orbitofrontal cortex (MOFC), and right pericalcarine cortex (**Figure 1** and **Table 2**).

ROI-Based Cortical Thickness Analysis

Abnormal structural changes in the DLPFC, OFC, ACC, and PCC in patients with MDD have been reported in many structural studies (1, 2). Therefore, we further calculated the average cortical thickness of these cortical areas using the ROI method. The bilateral DLPFC, left ACC, and bilateral PCC were thicker in patients with MDD than in NCs (FDR-corrected $P < 0.05$), and the right OFC was thinner in patients with MDD than in NCs (FDR-corrected $P < 0.05$) (**Figure 2A**).

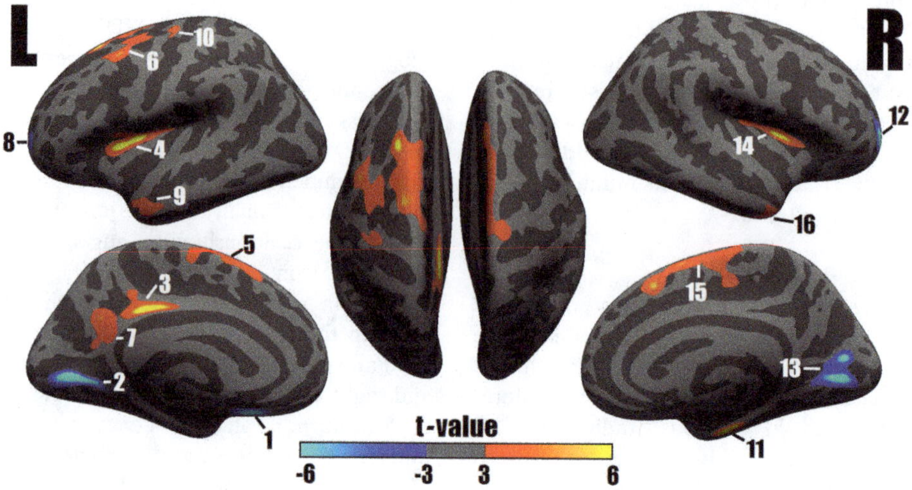

FIGURE 1 | Surface maps of significant differences in cortical thickness between patients with MDD and NCs. As determined by the GLM analysis, differences are presented on an inflated cortical surface (corrected *P*-value < 0.05). Dark gray indicates a gyrus; light gray indicates a sulcus. "L" indicates the lateral, medial and dorsal surfaces of the left hemisphere. "R" indicates the lateral, medial and dorsal surfaces of the right hemisphere. The color bar represents the *t* values from −6 to −3 and 3 to 6. Blue indicates cortical thinning in the MDD group compared with the NC group; a closer proximity to sky blue indicates a greater difference. Red to yellow indicates cortical thickening in the MDD group compared with the NC group; a closer proximity to yellow indicates a greater difference. The numerals refer to the cluster numbers listed in **Table 2**.

TABLE 1 | Demographic features and hemispheric cortex measures.

Characteristic	MDD (n = 35)	NC (n = 35)	Diagnosis effect	*P* value	FE (n = 20)	ME (n = 15)	Diagnosis effect	*P*
DEMOGRAPHIC/CLINICAL CHARACTERISTICS								
Age, years	28.91 ± 1.57	28.11 ± 1.15	$u = -0.218$	0.827	27.40 ± 1.90	30.93 ± 2.64	$t = -1.115$	0.273
Age-of-onset, years	27.00 ± 1.53	–	–	–	26.45 ± 1.92	27.73 ± 2.56	$t = -0.410$	0.684
Sex, female: male	22:13	20:15	$\chi^2 = 0.238$	0.626	13:7	9:6	$\chi^2 = 0.092$	0.762
Education, years	13.71 ± 0.51	13.91 ± 0.61	$u = -0.336$	0.737	13.80 ± 0.66	13.60 ± 0.83	$t = 0.191$	0.850
Duration of disorder, years	1.65 ± 0.26	–	–	–	0.57 ± 0.07	3.10 ± 0.32	$t = -7.737$	<0.0001
HAM-D_{24} score	30.45 ± 0.68	2.54 ± 0.26	$t = 38.142$	<0.0001	28.80 ± 0.97	30.93 ± 1.40	$t = -1.295$	0.204
SAS score	56.49 ± 1.94	27.46 ± 0.27	$t = 14.846$	<0.0001	58.15 ± 2.46	54.20 ± 3.08	$t = 1.014$	0.318
SDS score	61.77 ± 1.57	27.51 ± 0.26	$t = 21.465$	<0.0001	63.30 ± 1.87	60.80 ± 2.42	$t = 0.833$	0.411
HEMISPHERIC CORTEX MEASURES								
Mean cortical thickness of LH, mm	2.56 ± 0.01	2.51 ± 0.02	$t = 1.987$	0.052	2.54 ± 0.02	2.58 ± 0.02	$t = -1.671$	0.104
Mean cortical thickness of RH, mm	2.54 ± 0.01	2.50 ± 0.02	$t = 1.380$	0.174	2.53 ± 0.02	2.56 ± 0.02	$t = -1.107$	0.276
Total subcortical volume of LH, mm^3	25789 ± 368	26330 ± 426	$t = -0.964$	0.339	25628 ± 347	26003 ± 737	$t = -0.460$	0.650
Total subcortical volume of RH, mm^3	24883 ± 387	25244 ± 482	$t = -0.584$	0.561	24719 ± 373	25103 ± 768	$t = -0.451$	0.657

MDD, major depressive disorder; NC, normal control; FE, first episode; ME, multiple episode; HAM-D_{24}, 24-item Hamilton Depression Scale; SAS, Self-rating Anxiety Scale; SDS, Self-rating Depression Scale; LH, left hemisphere; RH, right hemisphere.

Continuous variables are expressed as mean ± SEM.

Significance P-value < 0.05.

To test differences in age, and education between MDD patients and NCs, Mann-Whitney U-test was applied.

To test differences in HAM-D_{24} score, SAS score, SDS score, mean cortical thickness, and total subcortical volume between MDD patients and NCs, independent sample t-test was applied.

To test differences in age, age of onset, education, duration of disorder, HAM-D24 score, SAS score, SDS score, mean cortical thickness, and total subcortical volume between FE and ME groups, independent sample t-test was applied.

To test the distribution of female/male chi-square test was computed.

Subcortical Volume Analysis

Compared to the NC group, the MDD group showed lower volumes in the left pallidum (FDR-corrected $P < 0.05$). Greater subcortical volumes were detected in the bilateral amygdala (FDR-corrected $P < 0.05$) (**Figure 2B**).

In the hippocampal subfields analysis, no significant differences in the volumes of any of the seven hippocampal

TABLE 2 | Surface-based cluster summary of significant cortical changes in patients with MDD.

Cluster Number	*t*-value Max	Size (mm^2)	MNI coordinates of peak vertex			CWP	CWPLow	CWPHi	Anatomical location
			X	*Y*	*Z*				
LH									
1	−7.834	222.51	−5.9	21.3	−20.8	0.0193	0.0169	0.0219	Medial orbitofrontal cortex
2	−7.395	711.89	−6.5	−74.1	4.3	0.0002	<0.0001	0.0004	Lingual gyrus
3	7.150	369.94	−5.0	−32.6	33.2	0.0004	<0.0001	0.0008	Posterior cingulate cortex
4	7.001	553.11	−30.7	9.5	9.4	0.0002	<0.0001	0.0004	Insula
5	6.577	1409.82	−23.0	23.3	54.5	0.0002	<0.0001	0.0004	Superior frontal cortex
6	5.481	652.21	−39.2	7.7	52.9	0.0002	<0.0001	0.0004	Caudal middle frontal cortex
7	5.283	435.36	−8.7	−58.6	26.8	0.0002	<0.0001	0.0004	Precuneus
8	−5.114	304.83	−22.1	52.0	−3.8	0.0030	0.0020	0.0040	Rostral middle frontal cortex
9	4.600	400.80	−55.0	−0.0	−29.4	0.0002	<0.0001	0.0004	Middle temporal cortex
10	3.930	211.57	−34.8	−20.0	64.9	0.0232	0.0205	0.0260	Precentral gyrus
RH									
11	8.020	233.78	22.5	−12.4	−30.5	0.0140	0.0118	0.0161	Entorhinal cortex
12	−7.518	680.38	23.2	51.3	−0.6	0.0002	<0.0001	0.0004	Rostral middle frontal cortex
13	−7.217	1061.45	8.1	−74.3	5.0	0.0002	<0.0001	0.0004	Pericalcarine cortex
14	6.449	312.31	33.2	2.8	11.6	0.0018	0.0010	0.0026	Insula
15	5.843	1098.42	8.2	17.9	49.1	0.0002	<0.0001	0.0004	Superior frontal cortex
16	5.058	334.41	44.7	−0.5	−33.0	0.0016	0.0010	0.0024	Middle temporal cortex

CWP, cluster wise P-value; MNI, Montreal Neurological Institute; LH, left hemisphere; RH, right hemisphere.
CWPLow and CWPHi: 90% confidence interval for CWP.

subfields were found between the MDD and NC groups (FDR-corrected $P > 0.05$) (**Figure 2C**).

Subgroup Analysis

As shown in **Table 1**, no differences in sex, age, age-of-onset, education, HAM-D_{24} score, SAS score, SDS score, hemispheric cortical thickness or subcortical volume were observed between the subgroups (FE vs. ME). No significant differences in subcortical volumes were observed in the subgroup comparison of FE and ME MDD patients. Surprisingly, cluster 1 and cluster 3 were thicker in the ME group than in the FE group (FDR-corrected $P < 0.05$). The peak vertexes of clusters 1 and 3 are located in the MOFC and PCC, respectively.

Correlation Analysis

Among the clinical characteristics, only a significant positive correlation between the SAS score and SDS score ($r = 0.589$, $P << 0.0001$) was detected.

In patients with MDD, no changes in cortical thickness, or subcortical volume in clusters or areas were significantly correlated with symptom severity (using the HAM-D_{24}, SDS, and SAS scores). However, the average cortical thickness of clusters 1 and 3 showed positive correlations with disease duration in the MDD group (FDR-corrected $P < 0.05$).

Structural covariance analyses were specifically performed among the DLPFC and amygdala in the MDD and NC groups. In NCs, the left DLPFC—left amygdala and the right DLPFC—right amygdala showed significantly negative correlations; the left DLPFC—right DLPFC and the left amygdala—right amygdala showed significantly positive correlations. In the patients with MDD, only the left amygdala—right amygdala showed a significantly positive association (**Table 3**). Using Snedecor's method (26), we further found differences in the correlation coefficients (*r*-values) of the left DLPFC—left amygdala and the left DLPFC—right DLPFC between the MDD and NC groups (**Table 3**).

DISCUSSION

Consistent with our hypotheses, prominent thickening and thinning was observed in specific cortical regions in patients with MDD. Although significant differences in cortical thickness at the hemispheric level were not observed, patients with MDD had a nearly significant trend toward an increase in the average cortical thickness of the left hemisphere. Thus, cortical thickening and not thinning might distinguish the groups. Subcortical regions also showed volumetric abnormalities in both directions in the MDD group; however, the total subcortical volume did not display any significantly changes. Therefore, the volumetric changes in subcortical regions at the hemispheric level were relatively balanced.

Based on the results of our study, altered cortical thickness and subcortical volumes of brain regions, such as the precentral gyrus, rostral middle frontal cortex, superior frontal cortex, MOFC, insula, amygdala, ACC, entorhinal cortex, and pallidum, are involved the five frontal-basal ganglia circuits (27, 28) (the motor circuit, oculomotor circuit, dorsolateral prefrontal circuit, orbitofrontal circuit and anterior cingulate circuit). These frontal-basal ganglia circuits play important roles in

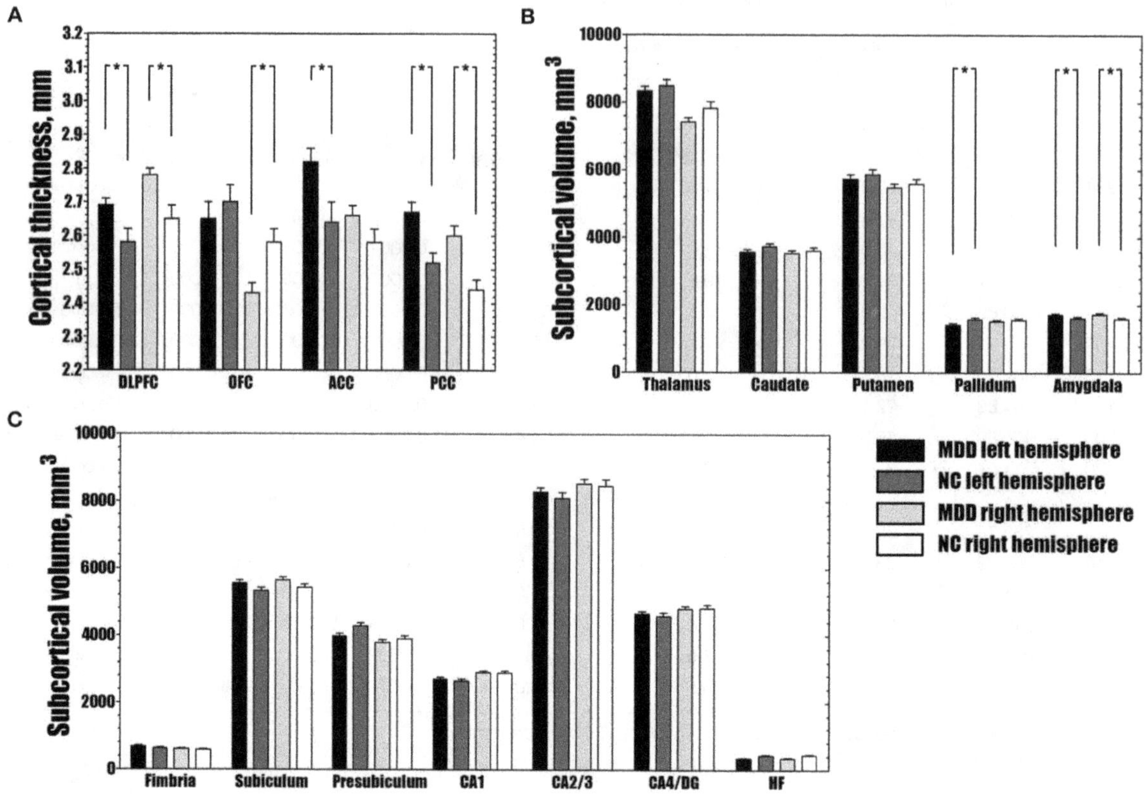

FIGURE 2 | Differences in average cortical thickness **(A)**, subcortical volume **(B)** and volume of hippocampal subfields **(C)** between the MDD and NC groups. **(A)** The MDD group shows greater average cortical thickness in the bilateral DLPFC, left ACC and bilateral PCC, and smaller average cortical thickness in the right OFC than the NC group (FDR-corrected $P < 0.05$). **(B)** The MDD group has a larger bilateral amygdala and smaller left pallidum than the NC group (FDR-corrected $P < 0.05$). **(C)** No significant differences were observed in the volumes of hippocampal subfields between the MDD and NC groups (FDR-corrected $P > 0.05$). The error bars indicate standard errors. *FDR-corrected $P < 0.05$. MDD, major depressive disorder; NC, normal controls; DLPFC, dorsolateral prefrontal cortex; OFC, orbitofrontal cortex; ACC, anterior cingulate cortex; PCC, posterior cingulate cortex; CA, cornu ammonis; DG, dentate gyrus; HF, hippocampal fissure; FDR, false discovery rate.

motor activity and human behavior. The dorsolateral prefrontal circuit mainly mediates executive function, and dysfunction of this circuit may produce impairments in retrieving remote memories, managing actions according to an external stimulus, altering behaviors appropriately, and mental flexibility. Subjects with dysfunction of the orbitofrontal circuit and anterior cingulate circuit exhibit personality changes including behavioral disinhibition, emotional lability, and reduced motivation (28). These regionally specific characteristics of structural changes in our study convincingly supported that MDD could involve deficits in neural networks across the whole brain. Grieve et al. (2) also found widespread gray matter volume reductions in a large sample of MDD patients. However, some participants in their study may have had a history of antidepressants uses, which could have an important impact on brain structures. It should be noted that cortical volume is composed of cortical surface area and cortical thickness, and decreased cortical volume could be coupled with increased cortical thickness.

Unlike the distributed cluster results, even when no statistical differences in regional areas were present between the two groups, the average cortical thickness could be significantly changed due to the accumulation of minor alterations. Therefore, comparison of the average cortical thickness of a brain subarea can reflect integral alterations in this area. Thus, we measured the average cortical thickness of the DLPFC, OFC, ACC, and PCC, which play key roles in the frontal-basal ganglia circuits. Our results demonstrated that the right OFC thickness and the left pallidum volume were decreased, while the thickness of the bilateral DLPFC, left ACC and bilateral PCC and the volume of bilateral amygdala were increased in patients with MDD. The OFC connects the frontal monitoring systems (e.g., the DLPFC) to the limbic system (e.g., cingulate, amygdala) (29), and the pallidum is involved in the five parallel frontal-basal ganglia circuits (28). Therefore, one possible explanation for these alterations could be dysfunction of the OFC and pallidum, which might lead to abnormalities in connectivity among cortical-limbic areas. Without sufficient inhibitory control, the amygdala activity in depressed patients is usually increased in response to emotional stimuli (30). To compensate for this less efficient self-regulation, the DLPFC and cingulate are recruited to a greater degree. Such a compensatory mechanism was found in remitted MDD patients who had a thicker PCC than non-remitting patients (4).

TABLE 3 | Comparison results of correlation coefficients of the DLPFC-amygdala between MDD and NC groups.

	Correlation analysis				*Z*	FDR-corrected *P*
	MDD		NC			
	r	FDR-corrected *P*	*r*	FDR-corrected *P*		
L DLPFC - L amygdala	0.084	0.632	−0.466	0.007	2.357	0.037
R DLPFC - R amygdala	−0.326	0.112	−0.346	0.042	0.09	0.928
L DLPFC - R DLPFC	0.281	0.136	0.884	<0.0001	−4.42	<0.0001
L amygdala - R amygdala	0.760	<0.0001	0.808	<0.0001	−0.5	0.823

MDD, major depressive disorder; NC, normal control; FDR, false discovery rate; L, left; R, right; DLPFC, dorsolateral prefrontal cortex.

The altered relationship among the DLPFC and amygdala was an another critical factor underlying the impairment in functional connectivity in patients with MDD. Although the thickness of the bilateral DLPFC and the volume of the left amygdala were greater, the negative relationship between the left DLPFC and left amygdala and the positive relationship between the left DLPFC and right DLPFC were absent, suggesting that the inverse reciprocity between the ipsilateral DLPFC and amygdala and the synergistic pattern between the bilateral DLPFC in patients with MDD were impaired. Cognitive-control and emotional-processing circuitry usually work in opposition to each other, and disharmony between the two areas may also be present in normal individuals, such as adolescents. Because different cerebral regions follow unique maturational trajectories during brain growth and development, with cortical maturity lagging behind that of subcortical region (31), healthy adolescents often exhibit impetuous but deficient top-down (cortical-to-limbic) cognitive control or intensive bottom-up (limbic-to-cortical) emotional processing (32). However, resting-state fMRI studies have found that adolescents with MDD may show decreased bottom-up connectivity or an increased imbalance in resting-state functional activity in frontal-subcortical circuits (32, 33). In a study on adult subjects (34), patients with depression showed enhanced amygdala responses and failure to recruit the DLPFC when exposed to affective distracters during cognitive tasks. As shown in another study (35), depressed individuals showed a positive association between the prefrontal cortex and amygdala during an affective task, and an opposite association was observed in controls. However, antidepressant treatment can reverse the functional patterns and connectivity impairments of depression by decreasing limbic activity in response to a negative stimulus and increasing cortical-limbic connectivity (36, 37). Similarly, chronic therapies with different antidepressants can block or reverse neuronal atrophy and cell loss in several cerebral regions such as prefrontal cortex and amygdala through increasing expression of neurotrophic factors (38). In a longitudinal study (39), remitted patients who received intensive antidepressant therapy showed a pattern of increasing cortical thickness in the OFC, DLPFC and inferior temporal gyrus over follow-up. These findings indicated that dysregulation of bottom-up emotional processing and top-down cognitive control are crucial features underlying the pathophysiology of MDD and that these features can explain why depressed individuals tend toward the processing of negative emotion such as fear, sadness or anxiety (40). Therefore, our work provides further evidence for a potential morphological basis of disorganized regional interactions in cortical-limbic circuits in patients with MDD.

Few structural MRI studies have analyzed hippocampal subregions in untreated patients with MDD. A meta-analysis (41) confirmed that only patients with MDD who with a disease duration longer than 2 years or more than 1 disease episode displayed smaller hippocampal volume than controls. The mean duration of MDD in patients in our study was approximately 1.65 years, which could explain why we could not find significant differences in hippocampal subfield volumes. Travis et al. (42) and Na et al. (43) also did not find differences in hippocampal subfield volumes between MDD patients and controls. However, they found correlations between volumes of specific hippocampal subregions and glucocorticoid receptor methylation and cortisol levels were altered in patients with MDD. Therefore, the structural pathophysiological process of hippocampal subregions in MDD patients whose disorder duration is less than 2 years or that in FE patients need to be further explored.

Another important goal of this study was to assess morphometric changes in patients with MDD who experienced multiple depressive episodes but were never treated. Although the main cortical change in patients with MDD has been consistently shown to be a reduction in the thickness (8, 21, 44) or volume (2, 3, 7, 22, 45), an increasing number of studies have recently reported increases in cortical thickness in untreated patients with FE MDD (9, 10, 46). Our results further verify that cortical thickness is also increased in untreated patients with ME MDD. The increased cortical thickness may reflect the early course of a chronic pathological trajectory that will eventually result in reduction of cortical volume (8). However, it may be a result of the compensatory response of plastic neurons, glia or neuropils. Considering that no difference in age was found between the FE and ME groups in our study, theoretically, the FE patients would have a later age-of-onset than ME patients, which might impact cortical thickness. However, the two groups did not show a significant difference in age-of-onset, possibly due to the relatively small sample size. Regardless of the mechanism, these changes may be related to inflammation, the hypothalamic-pituitary (HPA)-axis, or neurogenesis (9, 47, 48). Additionally, the severity of depression was not greater in the participants with

ME MDD than in patients with FE MDD, and MEs may lead to thickening of the MOFC and PCC. Moreover, cortical thickness and subcortical volume did not exhibit significant changes as depressive symptoms increased in the patients with MDD, which is consistent with previous studies (2, 46, 49). Nevertheless, the left MOFC and PCC displayed positive relationships with the disease duration. Therefore, dynamic cerebral morphometry may be a more reliable and continuous measure of disease progression in patients with MDD than traditional demographic and clinical variables.

Increases in the thickness of the MOFC and PCC in patients with ME MDD may reveal pivotal pathophysiological mechanisms of the ME process. Patients with MDD often show an increase in self-focused behaviors. The self-reflective function of the MOFC and PCC was proven to have two dissociated components using functional techniques. Specifically, the MOFC is related to a more inward-directed focus (e.g., hope and aspirations), whereas the PCC is related to a more outward-directed, social focus (e.g., duties and obligations) (50). In task-negative networks, Zhou et al. (51) observed increased functional connectivity of the MOFC and PCC in patients with MDD, which may reflect a potential basis for the negative bias in emotional processing. According to the results of a resting-state fMRI study, functional dysconnectivity is linked to local cortical thinning in patients with MDD (44). Therefore, we speculate that reinforced connectivity may be associated with increased thickness of the MOFC and PCC, but this hypothesis requires further verification.

Several limitations of this study should be noted. First, our sample size was relatively small, so any morphometric abnormalities that we identified must be interpreted with caution. A larger number of patients might be useful in obtaining more robust results. Second, this study was a cross-sectional investigation, and potential variations in the duration of illness should be studied longitudinally in future studies. Third, the actual number of depressive episodes was not recorded in the present study; thus, we were unable to assess any relationships between structural changes and the number of depressive episodes. Furthermore, although none of the depressed participants had received treatment, some results may be exaggerated or hidden because patients with FE and ME MDD were combined for certain analyses. Further studies that combine other neuroimaging methods, such as resting-state fMRI and DTI, are needed to explore the associations between the functional and structural changes that underlie impairments in top-down and bottom-up regulation in patients with MDD.

In conclusion, the present study complements and extends previous anatomical studies of patients with MDD through a surface-based approach and shows that structural alterations in untreated patients with MDD are primarily located in the frontal-basal ganglia circuits, which may provide a structural evidence for deficits in functional networks involved in MDD. The finding of a lack of correlation within DLPFC and amygdala in patients with MDD supports an underlying structural mechanism for dysregulation of top-down or bottom-up processes. Moreover, dynamic changes in morphology were observed during the progression of MDD, which may be a more reliable measure than traditional clinical variables, and alterations in the MOFC and PCC may represent a critical pathophysiological mechanism in the progression of ME MDD. These findings contribute to improving our understanding of the neurobiology and pathophysiology of MDD and offer potential targets for the development of more effective treatments for this condition.

AUTHOR CONTRIBUTIONS

HL and WQ designed experiments. SR, QT, and ZZ carried out experiments. ZZ, SR, YW, CL, and QH analyzed imaging results. ZZ and HL wrote the manuscript. All authors contributed to manuscript revision, read and approved the submitted version.

FUNDING

This study was funded by the National Nature Science Foundation of China (grant No. 81171283) and the Innovative Talents Project of Southwest Hospital (grant No. SWH2015QN12).

ACKNOWLEDGMENTS

We thank all the individuals who participated in this study.

REFERENCES

1. Bora E, Fornito A, Pantelis C, Yucel M. Gray matter abnormalities in Major Depressive Disorder: a meta-analysis of voxel based morphometry studies. *J Affect Disord* (2012) 138:9–18. doi: 10.1016/j.jad.2011.03.049
2. Grieve SM, Korgaonkar MS, Koslow SH, Gordon E, Williams LM. Widespread reductions in gray matter volume in depression. *Neuroimage Clin.* (2013) 3:332–9. doi: 10.1016/j.nicl.2013.08.016
3. Vasic N, Wolf ND, Grön G, Sosic-Vasic Z, Connemann BJ, Sambataro F, et al. Baseline brain perfusion and brain structure in patients with major depression: a multimodal magnetic resonance imaging study. *J Psychiatry Neurosci Jpn* (2015) 40:412. doi: 10.1503/jpn.140246
4. Jarnum H, Eskildsen SF, Steffensen EG, Lundbye-Christensen S, Simonsen CW, Thomsen IS, et al. Longitudinal MRI study of cortical thickness, perfusion, metabolite levels in major depressive disorder. *Acta Psychiatr Scand.* (2011) 124:435–46. doi: 10.1111/j.1600-0447.2011.01766.x
5. Hogstrom LJ, Westlye LT, Walhovd KB, Fjell AM. The structure of the cerebral cortex across adult life: age-related patterns of surface area, thickness, gyrification. *Cereb Cortex* (2013) 23:2521–2530. doi: 10.1093/cercor/bhs231
6. Meyer M, Liem F, Hirsiger S, Jancke L, Hanggi J. Cortical surface area and cortical thickness demonstrate differential structural asymmetry in auditory-related areas of the human cortex. *Cereb Cortex* (2014) 24:2541–52. doi: 10.1093/cercor/bht094
7. Zhang H, Li L, Wu M, Chen Z, Hu X, Chen Y, et al. Brain gray matter alterations in first episodes of depression: A meta-analysis of whole-brain studies. *Neurosci Biobehav Rev.* (2016) 60:43–50. doi: 10.1016/j.neubiorev.2015.10.011

8. Van EP, Van WG, Katzenbauer M, Groen W, Tepest R, Fernández G, et al. Paralimbic cortical thickness in first-episode depression: evidence for trait-related differences in mood regulation. *Am J Psychiatry* (2013) 170:1477–86. doi: 10.1176/appi.ajp.2013.121 21504
9. Qiu L, Lui S, Kuang W, Huang X, Li J, Li J, et al. Regional increases of cortical thickness in untreated, first-episode major depressive disorder. *Transl Psychiatry* (2014) 4:e378. doi: 10.1038/tp.2014.18
10. Yang XH, Wang Y, Huang J, Zhu CY, Liu XQ, Cheung EF, et al. Increased prefrontal and parietal cortical thickness does not correlate with anhedonia in patients with untreated first-episode major depressive disorders. *Psychiatry Res Neuroimaging* (2015) 234:144–51. doi: 10.1016/j.pscychresns.2015.09.014
11. Qin X, Wang W, Jin Q, Ai L, Li Y, Dong G, et al. Prevalence and rates of recognition of depressive disorders in internal medicine outpatient departments of 23 general hospitals in Shenyang, China. *J Affect Disord* (2008) 110:46–54. doi: 10.1016/j.jad.2007.12.237
12. Kovacs M, Obrosky S, George C. The course of major depressive disorder from childhood to young adulthood: Recovery and recurrence in a longitudinal observational study. *J Affect Disord.* (2016) 203:374. doi: 10.1016/j.jad.2016.05.042
13. Post RM, Fleming J, Kapczinski F. Neurobiological correlates of illness progression in the recurrent affective disorders. *J Psychiatr Res.* (2012) 46:561–73. doi: 10.1016/j.jpsychires.2012.02.004
14. Farb N.a.S., Irving JA, erson AK, Segal ZV. A Two-Factor Model of Relapse/Recurrence Vulnerability in Unipolar Depression. *J Abnorm Psychol.* (2015) 124:38–53. doi: 10.1037/abn0000031
15. Hamilton M. A rating scale for depression. *J Neurol Neurosurg Psychiatry* (1960) 23:56–62. doi: 10.1136/jnnp.23.1.56
16. Zung WW. A Self-Rating Depression Scale. *Arch Gen Psychiatry* (1965) 12:63–70. doi: 10.1001/archpsyc.1965.01720310065008
17. Zung WW. A rating instrument for anxiety disorders. *Psychosomatics* (1971) 12:371–379 doi: 10.1016/S0033-3182(71)71479-0
18. Dale AM, Fischl B, Sereno MI. Cortical surface-based analysis. I. Segmentation and surface reconstruction. *Neuroimage* (1999) 9:179. doi: 10.1006/nimg.1998.0395
19. Fischl B, Dale AM. Measuring the thickness of the human cerebral cortex from magnetic resonance images. *Proc Natl Acad Sci USA.* (2000) 97:11050–5. doi: 10.1073/pnas.200033797
20. Cole J, Costafreda SG, Mcguffin P, Fu CH. Hippocampal atrophy in first episode depression: a meta-analysis of magnetic resonance imaging studies. *J Affect Disord* (2011) 134:483–7. doi: 10.1016/j.jad.2011.05.057
21. Lim HK, Jung WS, Ahn KJ, Won WY, Hahn C, Lee SY, et al. Regional cortical thickness and subcortical volume changes are associated with cognitive impairments in the drug-naive patients with late-onset depression. *Neuropsychopharmacol Offic Public Am Coll Neuropsychopharmacol.* (2012) 37:838–49. doi: 10.1038/npp.2011.264
22. Han KM, Choi S, Jung J, Na KS, Yoon HK, Lee MS, et al. Cortical thickness, cortical and subcortical volume, white matter integrity in patients with their first episode of major depression. *J Affect Disord.* (2014) 155:42. doi: 10.1016/j.jad.2013.10.021
23. Van Leemput K, Bakkour A, Benner T, Wiggins G, Wald LL, Augustinack J, et al. Automated segmentation of hippocampal subfields from ultra-high resolution *in vivo* MRI. *Hippocampus* (2009) 19:549–57. doi: 10.1002/hipo.20615
24. Desikan RS, Ségonne F, Fischl B, Quinn BT, Dickerson BC, Blacker D, et al. An automated labeling system for subdividing the human cerebral cortex on MRI scans into gyral based regions of interest. *Neuroimage* (2006) 31:968. doi: 10.1016/j.neuroimage.2006.01.021
25. Shirer WR, Ryali S, Rykhlevskaia E, Menon V, Greicius MD. Decoding subject-driven cognitive states with whole-brain connectivity patterns. *Cereb Cortex* (2012) 22:158–65. doi: 10.1093/cercor/bhr099
26. Snedecor GG, Cochran W. *Statistical Methods, 8th Edn.* Ames: Iowa State University Press (1989).
27. Alexander GE, Delong MR, Strick PL. Parallel organization of functionally segregated circuits linking basal ganglia and cortex. *Annu Rev Neurosci.* (1986) 9:357. doi: 10.1146/annurev.ne.09.030186.002041
28. Tekin S, Cummings JL. Frontal–subcortical neuronal circuits and clinical neuropsychiatry : An update. *J Psychosomatic Res.* (2002) 53:647–54. doi: 10.1016/S0022-3999(02)00428-2
29. Elliott R, Dolan RJ, Frith CD. Dissociable functions in the medial and lateral orbitofrontal cortex: evidence from human neuroimaging studies. *Cereb Cortex* (2000) 10:308–17. doi: 10.1093/cercor/10.3.308
30. Pulcu E, Lythe K, Elliott R, Green S, Moll J, Deakin JF, et al. Increased amygdala response to shame in remitted major depressive disorder. *PLoS ONE* (2013) 9:e86900. doi: 10.1371/journal.pone.0086900
31. Gogtay N, Giedd JN, Lusk L, Hayashi KM, Greenstein D, Vaituzis AC, et al. Dynamic mapping of human cortical development during childhood through early adulthood. *Proc Natl. Acad Sci USA.* (2004) 101:8174. doi: 10.1073/pnas.0402680101
32. Jiao Q, Ding J, Lu G, Su L, Zhang Z, Wang Z, et al. Increased Activity Imbalance in Fronto-Subcortical Circuits in Adolescents with Major Depression. *PLoS ONE* (2011) 6:e25159. doi: 10.1371/journal.pone.00 25159
33. Musgrove DR, Eberly LE, Klimes-Dougan B, Basgoze Z, Thomas KM, Mueller BA, et al. Impaired bottom-up effective connectivity between amygdala and subgenual anterior cingulate cortex in unmedicated adolescents with major depression: results from a dynamic causal modeling analysis. *Brain Connect* (2015) 5:608–19. doi: 10.1089/brain.2014.0312
34. Fales CL, Barch DM, Rundle MM, Mintun MA, Snyder AZ, Cohen JD, et al. Altered emotional interference processing in affective and cognitive-control brain circuitry in major depression. *Biol Psychiatry* (2008) 63:377–84. doi: 10.1016/j.biopsych.2007.06.012
35. Johnstone T, Van Reekum CM, Urry HL, Kalin NH, Davidson RJ. Neurobiology of disease failure to regulate: counterproductive recruitment of top- down prefrontal-subcortical circuitry in major depression. *J Neurosci Offic J Soc Neurosci.* (2007) 27:8877–84. doi: 10.1523/JNEUROSCI.2063-07.2007
36. Mayberg HS, Liotti M, Brannan SK, Mcginnis S, Mahurin RK, Jerabek PA, et al. Reciprocal limbic-cortical function and negative mood: converging PET findings in depression and normal sadness. *Am J Psychiatry* (1999) 156:675–82.
37. Rigucci S, Serafini G, Pompili M, Kotzalidis GD, Tatarelli R. Anatomical and functional correlates in major depressive disorder: the contribution of neuroimaging studies. *World J Biol Psychiatry* (2010) 11:165–80. doi: 10.3109/15622970903131571
38. Duman RS, Monteggia LM. A neurotrophic model for stress-related mood disorders. *Biol Psychiatry* (2006) 59:1116–27. doi: 10.1016/j.biopsych.2006.02.013
39. Phillips JL, Batten LA, Tremblay P, Aldosary F, Blier P. A prospective, longitudinal study of the effect of remission on cortical thickness and hippocampal volume in patients with treatment-resistant depression. *Int J Neuropsychopharmacol.* (2015) 18:pyv037. doi: 10.1093/ijnp/pyv037
40. Drevets WC. Neuroimaging and neuropathological studies of depression: implications for the cognitive-emotional features of mood disorders. *Curr Opin Neurobiol.* (2001) 11:240–9. doi: 10.1016/S0959-4388(00) 00203-8
41. Mckinnon MC, Yucel K, Nazarov A, Macqueen GM. A meta-analysis examining clinical predictors of hippocampal volume in patients with major depressive disorder. *J Psychiatry Neurosci.* (2009) 34:41–54.
42. Travis SG, Coupland NJ, Hegadoren K, Silverstone PH, Huang Y, Carter R, et al. Effects of cortisol on hippocampal subfields volumes and memory performance in healthy control subjects and patients with major depressive disorder. *J Affect Disord* (2016) 201:34–41. doi: 10.1016/j.jad.2016.04.049
43. Na KS, Chang HS, Won E, Han KM, Choi S, Tae WS, et al. Association between glucocorticoid receptor methylation and hippocampal subfields in major depressive disorder. *PLoS ONE* (2014) 9:e85425. doi: 10.1371/journal.pone.0085425
44. Van Tol MJ, Li M, Metzger CD, Hailla N, Horn DI, Li W, et al. Local cortical thinning links to resting-state disconnectivity in major depressive disorder. *Psychol Med.* (2014) 44:2053–65. doi: 10.1017/S0033291713002742
45. Andreescu C, Butters MA, Begley A, Rajji T, Wu M, Meltzer CC, et al. Gray matter changes in late life depression–a structural MRI analysis. *Neuropsychopharmacology* (2008) 33:2566–72. doi: 10.1038/sj.npp.1301655

46. Reynolds S, Carrey N, Jaworska N, Langevin LM, Yang XR, Macmaster FP. Cortical thickness in youth with major depressive disorder. *BMC Psychiatry* (2014) 14:83. doi: 10.1186/1471-244X-14-83
47. Liberto CM, Albrecht PJ, Herx LM, Yong VW, Levison SW. Pro-regenerative properties of cytokine-activated astrocytes. *J Neurochem.* (2004) 89:1092–1100. doi: 10.1111/j.1471-4159.2004.02420.x
48. Ohira K, Takeuchi R, Shoji H, Miyakawa T. Fluoxetine-Induced Cortical Adult Neurogenesis. *Neuropsychopharmacol Offic Public Am Coll Neuropsychopharmacol.* (2013) 38:909–20. doi: 10.1038/npp.2013.2
49. Tu PC, Chen LF, Hsieh JC, Bai YM, Li CT, Su TP. Regional cortical thinning in patients with major depressive disorder: a surface-based morphometry study. *Psychiatry Res.* (2012) 202:206. doi: 10.1016/j.pscychresns.2011.07.011
50. Johnson MK, Raye CL, Mitchell KJ, Touryan SR, Greene EJ, Nolen-Hoeksema S. Dissociating medial frontal and posterior cingulate activity during self-reflection. *Soc Cogn Affect Neurosci.* (2006) 1:56. doi: 10.1093/scan/nsl004
51. Zhou Y, Yu C, Zheng H, Liu Y, Song M, Qin W, et al. Increased neural resources recruitment in the intrinsic organization in major depression. *J Affect Disord* (2010) 121:220–30. doi: 10.1016/j.jad.2009.05.029

7

Stress Induced Hormone and Neuromodulator Changes in Menopausal Depressive Rats

Simeng Gu[1,2†], Liyuan Jing[2†], Yang Li[2], Jason H. Huang[3,4] and Fushun Wang[2,3*]*

[1] School of Psychology, Jiangsu University Medical Center, Zhenjiang, China, [2] School of Psychology, Institute of Emotional Studies, Nanjing University of Chinese Medicine, Nanjing, China, [3] Department of Neurosurgery, Baylor Scott & White Health, Temple, TX, United States, [4] Department of Surgery, Texas A&M University, Temple, TX, United States

***Correspondence:**
Jason H. Huang
Jason.huang@bswhealth.org
Fushun Wang
13814541138@163.com

†These authors have contributed equally to this work.

Objective: Previously, we showed that neuromodulators are important factors involved in depression, here we aim to further investigate the interactions between neuromodulators and sex hormone involved in menopause related depression in rats.

Methods: Menopausal depression was made with bilateral ovariectomies in female SD rats followed by chronic mild unpredictable stress treatment for 21 days. Thirty six rats were randomly divided into four groups: sham surgery group, sham/stress group, surgery group, surgery/stress group. Then open-field locomotor scores and sucrose intake were employed to observe behavior changes. The levels of norepinephrine (NE), dopamine (DA), serotonin (5-HT) in the cerebral spinal fluid and serum adrenocorticotropic hormone (ACTH), cortisone were determined with High-performance liquid chromatography (HPLC). Serum estradiol (E2), follicle-stimulating hormone (FSH), and luteinizing hormone (LH) were measured with radioimmunoassay.

Results: The open-field locomotor scores and sucrose intake were significantly decreased after the surgery and stress treatment ($p < 0.01$). The Serum E_2 level decreased significantly after the surgery ($p < 0.01$), but serum LH, FSH levels increased significantly in the surgery group than the sham surgery group ($p < 0.01$). The cortisone levels increased significantly in sham/stress group than that in the sham surgery group during the first 2 weeks at stressful treatment, but decrease afterwards. The monoamine levels in the surgery/stress group were much lower than those in the sham surgery group ($p < 0.01$). The correlation analysis found that LH and FSH are related more to the neurotransmitter release than E_2.

Conclusion: Ovary removal rats showed depression-like behaviors, with LH and FSH increase and monoamine decrease, and the levels of these monoamines in the stress treated groups changed only after the stressful treatment. The LH, FSH hormone increasing might be the reason for the lower monoamine release, which in turn might be the reason for depressed syndromes in the menopause. The cortisone and ACTH in the serum in the surgery/stress group were much higher than that in the sham surgery group.

Keywords: ACTH, cortisone, menopausal, LH, FSH, monoamine, depression

INTRODUCTION

Major depressive disorder is a leading cause of disability worldwide, and affects more than 17% of the populations, making it one of the most prevalent health-related causes of human suffering (1, 2). However, the mechanisms of depression are far from clear (3), the most widely accepted theory about the mechanism of depression points to the monoamine neurotransmitters, including norepinephrine (NE), serotonin (5-HT), and dopamine (DA) (4–6). The 5-HT and NE reuptake inhibitors and selective 5-HT reuptake inhibitors are considered to be the first choice of treatment for depression (2, 7–9). Even though compelling evidence from genetic studies and pharmacological studies points to dysfunction of the central monoamine network in depression (10), many other hormones or neuromodulators might be involved too, such as hypothalamus-pituitary-axis (HPA) hormones (1) and sex hormones (11).

Depression occurrence in female patients are twice as many as male patients (12), which suggested that depression is related to sex hormone (13, 14). In addition, menopause depression is a well-known symptom for menopausal period (15, 16), which is due to the ovarian dysfunction 1 year after menopause (17). The major symptom of menopause depression is similar to that of major depression (18, 19). However, after decades of accumulated research, the existence of a menopause-associated depression is still controversial. The confusion is attributed to insufficient knowledge on the women's "vulnerability" to depression in the midlife years (19). Here we screened the chronic changes of hormones and neurotransmitters after artificial removal ovaries in adult rats, trying to see how the hormone changes and their interaction with monoamine neurotransmitters. This study would help us clarify the relationship between sex hormones and neurotransmitters.

MATERIALS AND METHODS

Animals

Thirty six female Sprague-Dawley (SD) rats with body weight averaged (470 ± 20) g, at the age about 1 years old, were purchased from Academy of Military Medical Sciences (Beijing, China). They were randomly divided into 4 groups: sham surgery group (faked surgery with no stress), sham/stress group (faked surgery with stress), surgery group (surgery with no stress treatment), surgery/stress group (surgery with stress treatment), with 9 rats in each group. The animals were treated as shown before: 9 rats in the sham surgery group were treated with sham surgery (only open the abdomen), 9 rats in the sham/stress group were treated with sham surgery and stress, 9 rats in the surgery group were only treated with surgery to remove the ovaries but no stress, 9 rats in the surgery/stress group were treated with surgery and stress. After 1 week's recovery from the surgery, the animals were treated with chronic unpredictable mild stress for 3 weeks. All the procedures were approved by the Institution of Animal Care and Use Committee of Nanjing University of Chinese Medicine.

Instrument

US thermo microplate reader, which was used to read the radioimmunoassay; KH30R desktop high-speed refrigerated centrifuge, low temperature ultracentrifuge, which are used for taking up serum, are provided by the central laboratory. 3200 ATRAP high-performance ligquid chromatography (HPLC) tandem mass spectrometer (ABI, USA), equipped with atomospheric pressure chemical ionization sources (LC-APCI-MS/MS).

Animal Surgery/Control

Ovary Removal

Rat in the two surgery groups were given "ovariectomy," and the rats in the sham surgery groups were just given surgery to open the belly. Surgical procedure: the surgery was performed in a super-clean bench, and the rats were given 100 $mg.kg^{-1}$ ketamine to induce anesthesia and fixed on a hard plate with supine position. Seventy-five percentage alcohol was used to clean the skin of surgery place. A marker was made in the rat 1 cm below the ribs, and 2 cm outside the spine and the soft tissue was sectioned separately. The peripheral blood vessels were ligated, and both sides of ovaries were removed, and finally the uterus was removed, and the skin was sutured, and the rats were put in one cage to be fed separately. It usually took 15 min for the surgery, and all the rats survived after the surgery. The method of determining successful ovariectomy is the vaginal epithelium keratosis test: 5 days continuous monitoring the rat vagina did not find the estrous cycle.

Chronic Unpredictable Mild Stress

All rats were housed in a single cage after the surgery, and after 7 days' recovery from surgery, they were treated with random chronic unavoidable stresses for 21 days. Stress treatment lasted for the 2 h, which includes 36 V AC electric shock foot (every 1 min stimulated 1 times; each time lasted 10 s, a total of 30 times), 4°C cold water swimming 5 min, 45°C heat stress 5 min, 15 min shaking (1 times/s), rat cage tilted 45° for 12 h, clip tail (1 min), wet bedding 10 h, empty bottle for 1 h, each stimulus applied for 2 times. Rats in stress group were treated with stress continuously for 21 days after the surgery.

Behavioral Observation Indicators

Open-Field Test

Every 7th day after the surgery, the animals were tested with "open-field test," which was done in an open box as reported before (20), with the height to be 40 cm, and both the length and width to be 80 cm. The bottom surface was marked with white lines which divided into 25 large areas. The horizontal activity of rats was measured by the number of bottom blocks, 1 grid is 1 point, and the vertical activity points were measured as the number of upright, from the rat's front feet left the bottom to lay down their feet. Testing was performed for 5 min in a well-illuminated transparent acrylic cage, and the rats were gently placed in the center and left to explore the area for 5 min. The digitized image of the path taken by each animal was tracked by a camera, and the total locomotor activity was analyzed using

ANY-maze software. The testing apparatus was cleaned with 70% ethanol and then dried between each test.

Sucrose Intake Test

Sucrose intake test was carried out on the 7th day after surgery. Each rat was given 133 mL of 1% sucrose solution after 24 h fasting and the amount of sucrose solution consumed by rats was calculated.

Hormones and Neurotransmitters Measurement

Estradiol (E2), luteinizing hormone (LH) and follicle-stimulating hormone (FSH) were measured every 7th day from the blood serum from the caudal vein. At about 10 O'clock every morning on the 7th day, 500 μl blood was driven from the caudal vein from each animal with a 1 ml syringe, which was washed with 100 μl 0.9% NaCl and 12500 U heparin inside. The supernatant was ready to be used for the radioimmunoassay after the blood was centrifuged. The content of E2 (estradiol), LH (luteinizing hormone) and FSH (follicle-stimulating hormone) were determined by radioimmunoassay. RIA kit used was bought from the United States Depp Company. Specific operation was carried out according to the instructions. The ACTH and cortisone in the serum were measured with a 3200 ATRAP high-performance liquid chromatography (HPLC) tandem mass spectrometer (ABI, USA), equipped with atmospheric pressure chemical ionization sources (LC-APCI-MS/MS). The neurotransmitter measurement in the cerebral spinal fluid was also done with HPLC. The cerebral spinal fluid (CSF) was dilated with a pump to inject artificial CSF to the brain and the CSF pumped out was used in a HPLC to measure NE, DA and serotonin (21). The monoamine levels were assessed by comparing the reference standard with respective peak area and elution time of the samples using a calibration curve for each monoamine neurotransmitter. After the chronic stress and the behavior test, the animals were decapitated under anesthesia with isoflurane (2%).

Statistical Processing Method

SPSS20.0 software was used for statistical analysis, and the data were used in the form of $\bar{x} \pm s$. Analysis of variance (ANOVA) and repeated measured ANVOA were used to compare the difference between groups.

RESULTS

Body Weight

The body weight was measured before the surgery and also on the 7th day after surgery. **Table 1** shows that the body weights of the animals in each group decreased than those in the sham surgery group, and the body weights of the rats in the sham/stress and surgery/stress groups were significantly lower than those in the sham surgery group ($p < 0.01$, One-Way ANOVA, **Table 1**), but there was no significant difference between the sham surgery group and surgery group ($p > 0.05$, One-Way ANOVA,).

TABLE 1 | Stress on body weight of rats with menopausal depression ($x \pm s$, g).

Group	Sham surgery	Sham/stress	Surgery	Surgery/stress
Before castration	474.53 ± 11.49	475.29 ± 8.15	479.15 ± 9.94	473.49 ± 8.75
After castration	471.32 ± 9.34	456.31 ± 9.43*	462.69 ± 8.28	447.73 ± 7.15*

*$p < 0.01$, One-way ANOVA.

Behavioral Assessment

The results showed that there was no significant difference before the surgery or stressful treatment in the behavior tests among the surgery groups (One-way ANOVA, $p > 0.05$, **Figure 1**). But the scores of vertical movement and horizontal movement in the surgery groups decreased gradually than those in the sham surgery group (repeated measures one-way ANOVA, Normality test passed $p = 0.031$; and the differences among the four different treated groups were significantly higher, and they were dependent on the time). We next compared the four different treated groups, and found that the movements in surgery and stress treated groups were different from that of the sham group, (*$p < 0.01$, **$p < 0.001$, One-way ANOVA comparisons between the four groups on the same 7th days), but there was no significant difference between the sham + stress group and surgery only group.

Sucrose Intake

The rats in the castration group consumed less sucrose than those in the sham surgery only group ($p < 0.001$, One-way ANOVA comparisons between the four groups on the 7th days; **Figure 2**). The sucrose consumption in the stress + surgery group was even lower than that in the stress and sham surgery group ($p < 0.001$, One-way ANOVA). Repeated measure one-way ANOVA was done to find that Normality test passed $p = 0.086$; and there is significant difference among the four different treated groups, especially the surgery + stress group compared with the sham surgery with no stress treatment group.

Monoamine Neurotransmitters and Hormones

The levels of neurotransmitters norepinephrine (NE), dopamine (DA) and serotonin (5-HT) in the CSF and cortisone in the serum were tested with high performance liquid chromatography (HPLC). Repeated measure one-way ANOVA was done in NE, DA, 5-HT and cortisone group respectively; and there were significant differences among the four different treated groups, especially the surgery + stress group compared with the sham surgery with no stress treatment group). We next compared the four different treated groups, and found that the concentrations of NE, DA, 5-HT and cortisone in surgery and stress treated groups were different from the sham group, starting from the first week stress treatment (*$p < 0.01$, **$p < 0.001$, One-way ANOVA comparisons between the four groups on the same 7th days). The levels of NE and cortisone in the CSF increased significantly lower in the surgery groups compared with the sham surgery group, and the concentration of DA and 5-HT

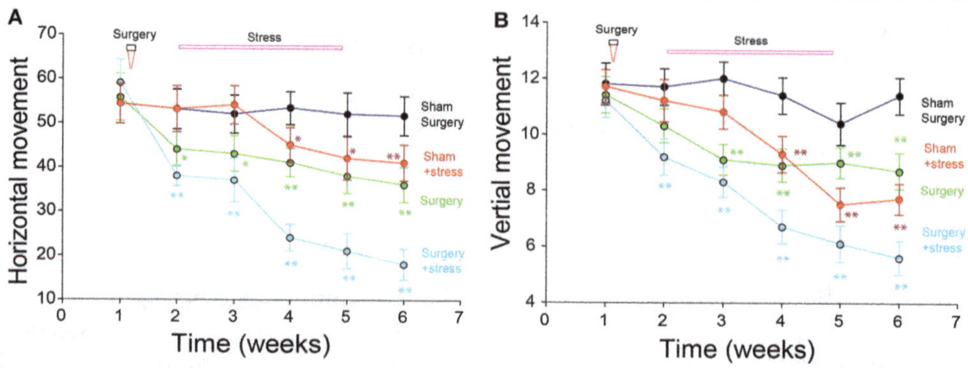

FIGURE 1 | Open box movement changes after surgery and stress treatment. **(A)** Both the stress and surgery decreased the horizontal movement. **(B)** Both the stress and surgery decreased the vertical movement (*$p < 0.01$, **$p < 0.001$, repeat measure one-way ANOVA comparisons between the four groups on the 7th days).

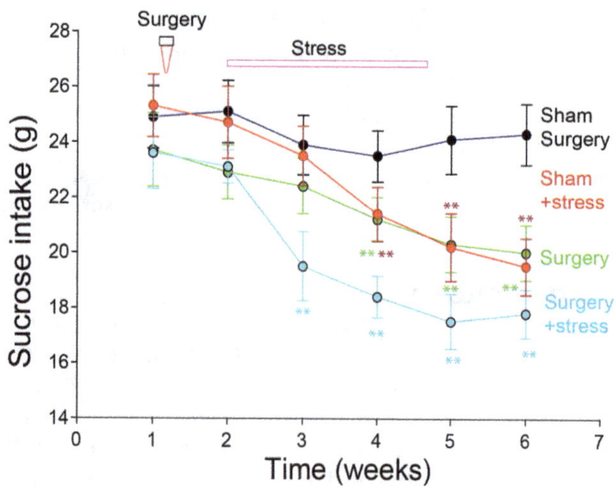

FIGURE 2 | Sucrose intake in rats with menopausal depression (*$p < 0.01$, **$p < 0.001$, repeated measure one-way ANOVA comparisons between the four groups on the 7th days).

increased significantly in the surgery groups starting from the first week stress treatment. The cortisone levels in the serum in the sham/stress group were much higher than that in the sham surgery group. And the levels of these monoamines in the stress treated groups changed only after the stressful treatment (*$p < 0.01$, **$p < 0.001$, repeated measure one-way ANOVA comparisons between the four groups; **Figure 3**).

Sex Hormones

The levels of estradiol in the serum of the surgery group were significantly lower than those in the sham surgery group (repeated measure one-way ANOVA, $p < 0.01$; **Figure 4**), but they were not different between the sham surgery and sham surgery/stress group or surgery group with surgery/stress group. The levels of serum luteinizing hormone and follicle-stimulating hormone in the two stressful groups were significantly higher than those in the sham surgery group (repeated measure one-way ANOVA, $p < 0.01$). The level of serum ACTH was significantly higher in the stressful treatment group than that in sham surgery group (repeated measure one-way ANOVA, $p < 0.01$).

Correlation Between Sex Hormones and Neurotransmitters

The correlation between the levels of sex hormones and neurotransmitters was analyzed, and we found that there was little correlation between estradiol in the serum with the neurotransmitter, but the correlations were significantly high in the two stress treated groups (**Table 2**).

DISCUSSION

The pathological mechanism of depression is far from clear (3, 22), and is a hot topic for neuroscience research (23, 24). We have reported before that patients with depression in the brain showed monoamine neurotransmitter changes and neurological dysfunction in the cortex and the hippocampus (1, 2). However, there are many other hormones that also involved (22), such as hormones released from hypothalamus-pituitary-axis (HPA) (25, 26). In this study, we probed into the role of sex hormones in the depression, because clinical data showed that the occurrence of depression in female patients are twice as many as male patients (25), which suggested that estradiol might induce depression (27). However, it seems contradictory that depression is a well-known symptom for perimenopausal period, which suggested that lack of estradiol will induce depression (28). Here, we used ovariectomized female SD rats to stop the estradiol release, and found that these rats were much easier to get depressed at chronic mild stress. On the contrary to decreases in estradiol release, LH and FSH levels are greatly increased, possibly due the removal of feedback inhibition of estradiol (29). In addition, the correlation analysis found that LH and FSH are positively correlated with the changes of stress hormones such as cortisone and ACTH. Therefore the LH and FSH increase might be the reason for depression. As far as we know, this study might be the first to directly measure the chronic changes of the sex hormones

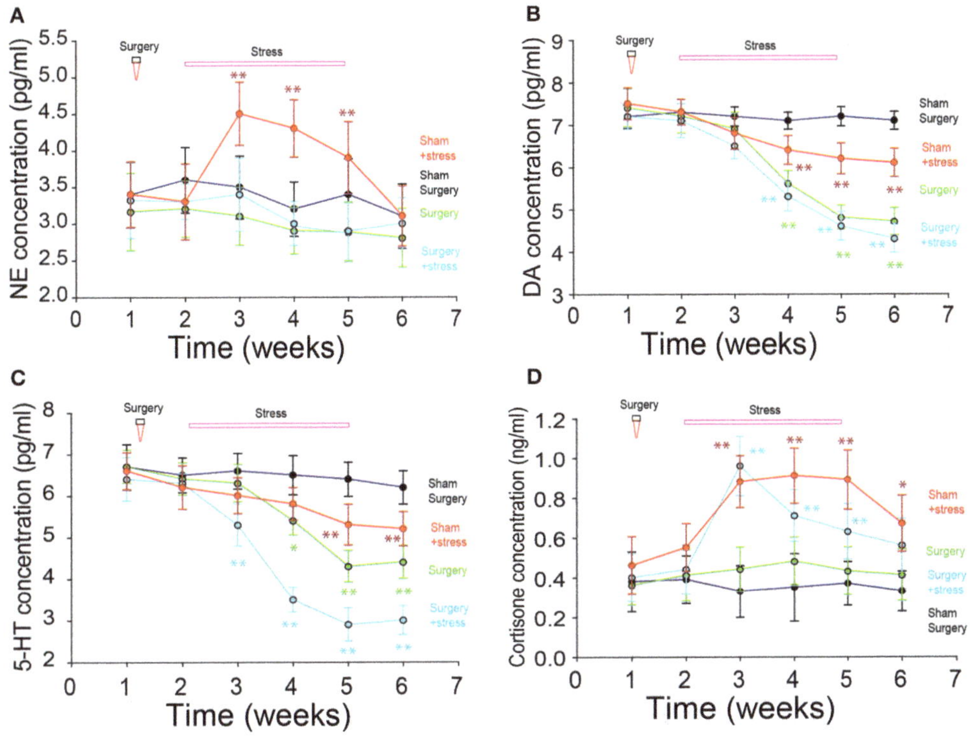

FIGURE 3 | Neuromodulator changes in rats with menopausal depression. **(A)** Norepinephrine (NE) changes did not change much among the groups ($P > 0.05$, One-way ANOVA). **(B)** Dopamine (DA) decreased significantly after the stress and surgery treatment. **(C)** 5-HT decreased significantly after the stress and surgery treatment. **(D)** Cortisone increased significantly in the stress treatment groups ($^*p < 0.01$, $^{**}p < 0.001$, repeat measure one-way ANOVA comparisons between the four groups on the 7th days).

and also neurotransmitters after ovary removal and also chronic stress.

The Stress Related Hormones Increased Together With LH and FSH

In addition to LH and FSH, the cortisone level also increased after the ovary removal, especially in the face of stressful situations. Consistent with our reports, abnormal cortisone release following stress has been reported (30). ACTH and cortisone, which are part of HPA axis (Hypothalamus-pituitary-adrenal axis) are stressful hormones (30). The positive correlation between LH and FSH together with cortisone and ACTH suggests that LH and FSH are related to stress. LH, FSH and ACTH are all released from anterior pituitary gland, which are regulated by neurons in the hypothalamus, which in turn are negatively controlled by estradiol. There is also the possibility for LH and ACTH to coordinate with each other to enhance the stressful reactions, which might be reason for the menopause depression. If so, it is easy to understand women's prone to depression. Consistent with the increase of LH and FSH after ovariectomization, who are also increased in the menopause patients (31, 32). LH release surges up during ovulation in the menstrual cycle, and LH detection is used to detect ovulation, which occurs about 24–48 h after the LH surge. LH surge up during ovulation in the menstrual cycle and also after menopause might be the reason for depression.

The Stress Related Norepinephrine Also Increased Together With LH and FSH

In addition to ACTH and cortisone, NE also increased after stressful treatment and ovariectomization. It is easy to understand the increase of cortisone, which is the downward pathway for ACTH. But how does NE release was affected is not clear. There is also the possibility that HPA axis affects NE release. Maybe, LH can also directly affect the brain functions (32), many papers have focused on the effects of estradiol on the monoamine release or up-take (33). Estradiol has profound effects on brain chemistry, structure, and function and is trophic for regions such as the pre-frontal cortex and hippocampus that are critical to affect emotional regulation (34). LH was recently reported as a candidate for its role in the mental disorders (12, 35).

The Reward Related DA and 5-HT Neurotransmitter Release Are Negatively Correlated With LH and FSH

Contrary to increases of NE and ACTH release, DA and 5-HT releases decreased significantly. DA and 5-HT are important neurotransmitters in the brain, and low level of either DA or 5-HT has proved to be related to depression (7, 36–38). DA is the

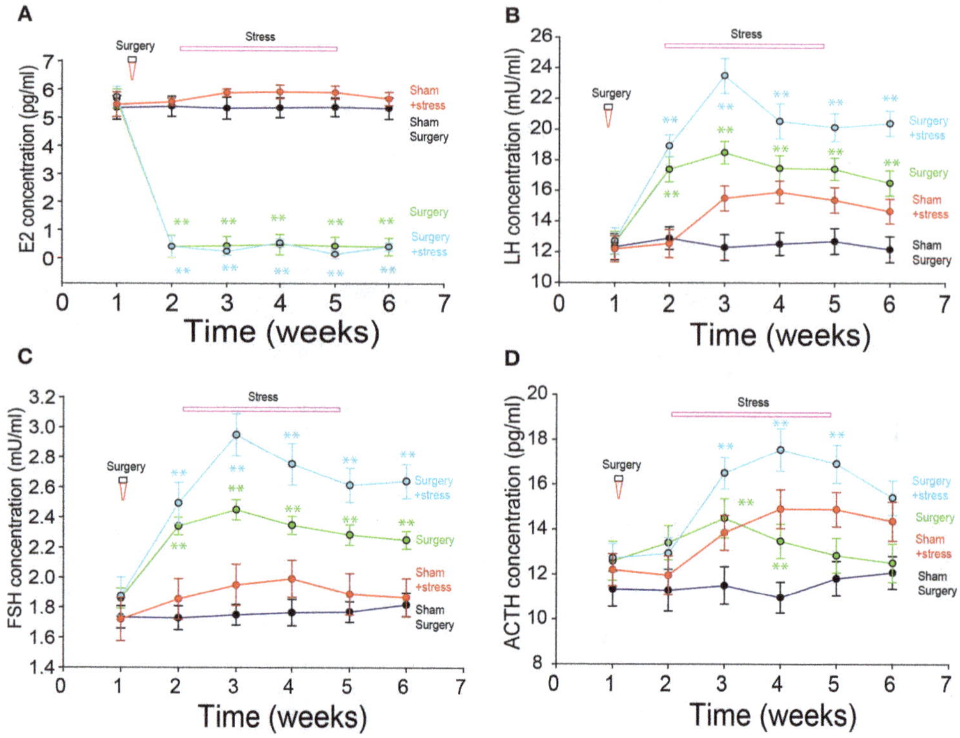

FIGURE 4 | The sex hormone changes after bilateral ovariectomies. **(A)** Estradiol changes among the groups. **(B)** Luteinizing hormone (LH) changes among the groups. **(C)** Follicle-stimulating hormone (FSH) changes among the groups. **(D)** ACTH changes among the groups. (*$p < 0.01$, **$p < 0.001$, repeated measure one-way ANOVA comparisons between the four groups on the 7th days).

TABLE 2 | Correlations between sex hormones with neuromodulators.

Group	Estradiol	LH	FSH
NE	0.12	0.54	0.50
DA	0.07	−0.34	−0.36
5-HT	0.14	−0.28	−0.27
Cortisone	0.16	0.65	0.68
ACTH	0.04	0.72	0.76

neurotransmitter for reward (39), and low level of DA function can lead to depression (40, 41). The serotonin transporter ensures the recapture of serotonin and is the pharmacological target of selective serotonin reuptake inhibitor (SSRI) antidepressants (42). Our data found that both DA and 5-HT releases are negatively correlated with LH release after ovariectomization, which further support the role of LH in depression. The reason might be that the projections from neurons in hypothalamus inhibits the DA release (43–45), or 5-HT release. Another possible way is that estradiol and LH might directly affect the DA neurons (38). Sure there might be interactions between monoamine neurons and hypothalamus (46). However, our data showed that the LH increase seems to start at the first 7th days, while the DA and 5-HT release decrease tops at the 3rd 7th days, which suggested that LH increase might be the cause for the DA and 5-HT decrease.

In all, perimenopause and postmenopause provide a natural laboratory for the study of sex hormone on depression (16). With the aging of our society, women living at least a third of their lives in the postmenopausal state, determining the long-term health effects of hormonal fluctuations has become a major women's health concern.

AUTHOR CONTRIBUTIONS

FW and JH designed the experiments. SG, LJ, and YL performed the experiments. SG and LJ did the data analysis. FW and JH wrote the paper.

ACKNOWLEDGMENTS

This work was supported, in part, by NIH R01 NS067433, Scott & White Plummer Foundation Grant, National Science Foundation in China 816280007, Jiangsu Specially Appointed Professorship Foundation, Jiangsu Nature Foundation BK20151565, Jiangsu Traditional Chinese Medicine Foundation ZD201501, Jiangsu Six Talent Peak project 2015YY006 and University Science Research Project of Jiangsu Province (17KJD310001).

REFERENCES

1. Wang F, Pan F, Lee L. A. Huang, J. H. Stress induced neuroplasticity and mental disorders. *Neural Plast.* (2017) 2017:9634501. doi: 10.1155/2017/9634501
2. Gu S, Wang W, Wang F. Huang, J. H. Neuromodulator and Emotion Biomarker for Stress Induced Mental Disorders. *Neural Plast.* (2016) 2016:2609128. doi: 10.1155/2016/2609128
3. Malinow, R. Depression: Ketamine steps out of the darkness. *Nature* (2016) 533:477–8. doi: 10.1038/nature17897
4. Moeller SJ, Parvaz MA, Shumay E, Wu S, Beebe-Wang N, Konova AB, et al. Monoamine polygenic liability in health and cocaine dependence: imaging genetics study of aversive processing and associations with depression symptomatology. *Drug Alcohol Depend* (2014) 140:17–24. doi: 10.1016/j.drugalcdep.2014.04.019
5. Hamon M, Blier, P. Monoamine neurocircuitry in depression and strategies for new treatments. *Prog Neuro-Psychopharmacol Biol Psychiatry* (2013) 45:54–63. doi: 10.1016/j.pnpbp.2013.04.009.
6. Marshe VS,. Maciukiewicz M, Rej S, Tiwari AK, Sibille E, Blumberger DM et al. Norepinephrine transporter gene variants and remission from depression with venlafaxine treatment in older adults. *Am J Psychiatry* (2017) 174:468–75. doi: 10.1176/appi.ajp.2016.16050617.
7. Muhammed K, Manohar S, Ben Yehuda M, Chong TT-J, Tofaris G, Lennox G, et al. Reward sensitivity deficits modulated by dopamine are associated with apathy in Parkinson's disease. *Brain* (2016) 139:2706–21. doi: 10.1093/brain/aww188
8. Zheng Z, Gu S, Lei Y, Lu S, Wang W, Li Y, et al. Safety needs mediate stressful events induced mental disorders. *Neural Plast.* (2016) 2016:8058093. doi: 10.1155/2016/8058093
9. Zahavi AY, Sabbagh MA, Washburn D, Mazurka R, Bagby RM, Strauss J, et al. Serotonin and dopamine gene variation and theory of mind decoding accuracy in major depression: a preliminary investigation. *PLoS ONE* (2016) 11:e0150872. doi: 10.1371/journal.pone.0150872
10. Wright B, Alexander D, Aghahoseini A, York Surgical Outcomes Research Team. Does preoperative depression and/or serotonin transporter gene polymorphism predict outcome after laparoscopic cholecystectomy? *BMJ Open* (2016) 6:e007969. doi: 10.1136/bmjopen-2015-007969
11. Freeman EW. Associations of depression with the transition to menopause. *Menopause* (2010) 17, 823–7. doi: 10.1097/gme.0b013e3181db9f8b
12. Blair J. A. Palm R, Chang J, McGee H, Zhu X, Wang X, et al. Luteinizing hormone downregulation but not estrogen replacement improves ovariectomy-associated cognition and spine density loss independently of treatment onset timing. *Horm Behav.* (2016) 78:60–66. doi: 10.1016/j.yhbeh.2015.10.013
13. Reding KM, Schmidt PJ, Rubinow DR. Perimenopausal depression and early menopause: cause or consequence? *Menopause* (2017) 24:1333–5. doi: 10.1097/GME.0000000000001016
14. Schmidt P. J. Ben Dor R, Martinez PE, Guerrieri GM, Harsh VL, Thompson K, et al. Effects of Estradiol Withdrawal on Mood in Women With Past Perimenopausal Depression: A Randomized Clinical Trial. *JAMA Psychiatry* (2015) 72:714–26. doi: 10.1001/jamapsychiatry.2015.0111
15. Perich T, Ussher J. Meade T. Menopause and illness course in bipolar disorder: A systematic review. *Bipolar Disord.* (2017) 19:434–43. doi: 10.1111/bdi.12530
16. Gordon JL, Rubinow DR, Eisenlohr-Moul TA, Xia K, Schmidt PJ, Girdler SS. Efficacy of transdermal estradiol and micronized progesterone in the prevention of depressive symptoms in the menopause transition: a randomized clinical trial. *JAMA Psychiatry* (2018) 5:149–57. doi: 10.1001/jamapsychiatry.2017.3998
17. Zahn R, Lythe KE, Gethin JA,Green S, Deakin JF, Workman C, et al. Negative emotions towards others are diminished in remitted major depression. *Eur Psychiatry* (2015) 30:448–53. doi: 10.1016/j.eurpsy.2015.02.005
18. Stone EA, Quartermain D, Lin Y, Lehmann ML. Central alpha1-adrenergic system in behavioral activity and depression. *Biochem Pharmacol.* (2007) 73:1063–75. doi: 10.1016/j.bcp.2006.10.001
19. Soares CN. Menopause and depression: keep your eye on the long run. *Menopause* (2016) 23:1272–4. doi: 10.1097/GME.0000000000000791
20. Xue W, Wang W, Gong T, Zhang H, Tao W, Xue L, et al. PKA-CREB-BDNF signaling regulated long lasting antidepressant activities of Yueju but not ketamine. *Sci Rep.* (2016) 6:26331. doi: 10.1038/srep26331
21. Simeng G, Wendong D, Fushun, W. Effects of maternal deprivation at different lactation period on depression behavior and brain catecholamine of rats offsprings. *Chin J Behav Med Brain Sci.* (2014) 23:394–7.
22. Wang, P. Li H, Barde S, Zhang MD, Sun J, Wang T et al. Depression-like behavior in rat: Involvement of galanin receptor subtype 1 in the ventral periaqueductal gray. *Proc Natl Acad Sci U S A.* (2016) 113:E4726–35. doi: 10.1073/pnas.1609198113
23. Yang Y, Cui Y, Sang K, Dong Y, Ni Z, Ma S, et al. Ketamine blocks bursting in the lateral habenula to rapidly relieve depression. *Nature* (2018) 554:317–22. doi: 10.1038/nature25509
24. Cui Y, Yang Y, Ni Z, Dong Y, Cai G, Foncell A, et al. Astroglial Kir4.1 in the lateral habenula drives neuronal bursts in depression. *Nature* (2018) 554:323–7. doi: 10.1038/nature25752
25. Goel N, Innala L, Viau V. Sex differences in serotonin (5-HT) 1A receptor regulation of HPA axis and dorsal raphe responses to acute restraint. *Psychoneuroendocrinology* (2014) 40:232–41. doi: 10.1016/j.psyneuen.2013.11.020
26. Fox, ME, Studebaker RI, Swofford NJ, Wightman RM. Stress and drug dependence differentially modulate norepinephrine signaling in animals with varied HPA axis function. *Neuropsychopharmacology* (2015) 40:1752–61. doi: 10.1038/npp.2015.23
27. Chhibber A, Woody SK, Karim Rumi MA, Soares MJ, Zhao L. Estrogen receptor beta deficiency impairs BDNF-5-HT2A signaling in the hippocampus of female brain: a possible mechanism for menopausal depression. *Psychoneuroendocrinology* (2017) 82:107–16. doi: 10.1016/j.psyneuen.2017.05.016
28. Whedon JM, KizhakkeVeettil A, Rugo NA, Kieffer KA. Bioidentical estrogen for menopausal depressive symptoms: a systematic review and meta-analysis. *J Womens Health* (2017) 26:18–28. doi: 10.1089/jwh.2015.5628
29. Kornstein SG, Young EA, Harvey AT, Wisniewski SR, Barkin JL, Thase ME, et al. The influence of menopause status and postmenopausal use of hormone therapy on presentation of major depression in women. *Menopause* (2010) 17:828–39. doi: 10.1097/gme.0b013e3181d770a8
30. Walter EE, Fernandez F, Snelling M, Barkus E. Stress induced cortisol release and schizotypy. *Psychoneuroendocrinology* (2018) 89:209–15. doi: 10.1016/j.psyneuen.2018.01.012
31. Roelfsema F, Pijl H, Keenan DM, Veldhuis JD. Diminished adrenal sensitivity and ACTH efficacy in obese premenopausal women. *Eur J Endocrinol.* (2012) 167:633–42. doi: 10.1530/EJE-12-0592
32. Kok P, Kok SW, Buijs MM, Westenberg JJ, Roelfsema F, Frölich M, et al. Enhanced circadian ACTH release in obese premenopausal women: reversal by short-term acipimox treatment. *Am J Physiol Endocrinol Metab.* (2004) 287:E848–56. doi: 10.1152/ajpendo.00254.2004
33. Epperson CN, Kim DR, Bale TL. Estradiol modulation of monoamine metabolism: one possible mechanism underlying sex differences in risk for depression and dementia. *JAMA Psychiatry* (2014) 71:869–70. doi: 10.1001/jamapsychiatry.2014.729
34. Shanmugan S, Epperson CN. Estrogen and the prefrontal cortex: towards a new understanding of estrogen's effects on executive functions in the menopause transition. *Hum Brain Mapp.* (2014) 35:847–65. doi: 10.1002/hbm.22218
35. Blair JA, Bhatta S, McGee H, Casadesus G. Luteinizing hormone: Evidence for direct action in the CNS. *Horm Behav.* (2015) 76:57–62. doi: 10.1016/j.yhbeh.2015.06.020
36. Wang L, Zhou C, Zhu D, Wang X, Fang L, Zhong J, et al. Serotonin-1A receptor alterations in depression: a meta-analysis of molecular imaging studies. *BMC Psychiatry* (2016) 16:319. doi: 10.1186/s12888-016-1025-0
37. Taylor AE, Munafo MR. Triangulating meta-analyses: the example of the serotonin transporter gene, stressful life events and major depression. *BMC Psychol.* (2016) 4:23. doi: 10.1186/s40359-016-0129-0
38. Pascucci T, Ventura R, Latagliata EC, Cabib S, Puglisi-Allegra S. The medial prefrontal cortex determines the accumbens dopamine response to stress through the opposing influences of norepinephrine and dopamine. *Cereb Cortex* (2007) 17:2796–804. doi: 10.1093/cercor/bhm008

39. Howe MW, Tierney PL, Sandberg SG, Phillips PE, Graybiel AM. Prolonged dopamine signalling in striatum signals proximity and value of distant rewards. *Nature* (2013) 500:575–9. doi: 10.1038/nature12475
40. Tye SJ, Miller AD, Blaha CD. Ventral tegmental ionotropic glutamate receptor stimulation of nucleus accumbens tonic dopamine efflux blunts hindbrain-evoked phasic neurotransmission: implications for dopamine dysregulation disorders. *Neuroscience* (2013) 252:337–45. doi: 10.1016/j.neuroscience.2013.08.010
41. Tye KM, Mirzabekov JJ, Warden MR, Ferenczi EA, Tsai H-C, Finkelstein J, et al. Dopamine neurons modulate neural encoding and expression of depression-related behaviour. *Nature* (2013) 493:537–41. doi: 10.1038/nature11740
42. Baudry A, Mouillet-Richard S, Schneider B, Launay JM, Kellermann O. miR-16 targets the serotonin transporter: a new facet for adaptive responses to antidepressants. *Science* (2010) 329:1537–41. doi: 10.1126/science.1193692
43. Nieh EH, Vander Weele CM, Matthews GA, Presbrey KN, Wichmann R, Leppla CA, et al. Inhibitory input from the lateral hypothalamus to the ventral tegmental area disinhibits dopamine neurons and promotes behavioral activation. *Neuron* (2016) 90:1286–98. doi: 10.1016/j.neuron.2016.04.035
44. Sharpe MJ, Marchant NJ, Whitaker LR, Richie CT, Zhang YJ, Campbell EJ, et al. Lateral hypothalamic GABAergic neurons encode reward predictions that are relayed to the ventral tegmental area to regulate learning. *Curr Biol.* (2017) 27:2089–100 e2085. doi: 10.1016/j.cub.2017.06.024
45. Morales M, Margolis EB. Ventral tegmental area: cellular heterogeneity, connectivity and behaviour. *Nat Rev Neurosci.* (2017) 18:73–85. doi: 10.1038/nrn.2016.165
46. Chauhan NR, Kapoor M, Prabha Singh L, Gupta RK, Chand Meena R, Tulsawani R, et al. Heat stress-induced neuroinflammation and aberration in monoamine levels in hypothalamus are associated with temperature dysregulation. *Neuroscience* (2017) 358:79–92. doi: 10.1016/j.neuroscience.2017.06.023

8

A Conscious Resting State fMRI Study in SLE Patients without Major Neuropsychiatric Manifestations

Shuang Liu[1,2†], *Yuqi Cheng*[2,3†], *Zhongqi Xie*[1], *Aiyun Lai*[1], *Zhaoping Lv*[1], *Yueyin Zhao*[1], *Xiufeng Xu*[3], *Chunrong Luo*[4], *Hongjun Yu*[4], *Baoci Shan*[5], *Lin Xu*[6] *and Jian Xu*[1,2*]

[1] *Department of Rheumatology and Immunology, First Affiliated Hospital of Kunming Medical University, Kunming, China,* [2] *Yunnan Key Laboratory of Laboratory Medicine, Kunming, China,* [3] *Department of Psychiatry, First Affiliated Hospital of Kunming Medical University, Kunming, China,* [4] *Magnetic Resonance Imaging Center, The First Hospital of Kunming, Kunming, China,* [5] *Key Laboratory of Nuclear Analysis, Institute of High Energy Physics, Chinese Academy of Sciences, Beijing, China,* [6] *Key Laboratory of Animal Models and Human Disease Mechanisms, Kunming Institute of Zoology, Chinese Academy of Sciences, Kunming, China*

***Correspondence:**
Jian Xu
casxujian@163.com

† These authors have contributed equally to this work

Neuropsychiatric systemic lupus erythematosus (NPSLE) is one of the main causes of death in patients with systemic lupus erythematosus (SLE). Signs and symptoms of NPSLE are heterogeneous, and it is hard to diagnose, and treat NPSLE patients in the early stage. We conducted this study to explore the possible brain activity changes using resting state functional magnetic resonance imaging (rs-fMRI) in SLE patients without major neuropsychiatric manifestations (non-NPSLE patients). We also tried to investigate the possible associations among brain activity, disease activity, depression, and anxiety. In our study, 118 non-NPSLE patients and 81 healthy controls (HC) were recruited. Rs-fMRI data were used to calculate the regional homogeneity (ReHo) in all participants. We found decreased ReHo values in the fusiform gyrus and thalamus and increased ReHo values in the parahippocampal gyrus and uncus. The disease activity was positively correlated with ReHo values of the cerebellum and negatively correlated with values in the frontal gyrus. Several brain areas showed correlations with depressive and anxiety statuses. These results suggested that abnormal brain activities might occur before NPSLE and might be the foundation of anxiety and depression symptoms. Early detection and proper treatment of brain dysfunction might prevent the progression to NPSLE. More studies are needed to understand the complicated underlying mechanisms.

Keywords: systemic lupus erythematosus patients without major neuropsychiatric manifestations (non-NPSLE patients), resting-state functional magnetic resonance imaging (rs-fMRI), regional homogeneity (ReHo), disease activity, anxiety, depression

INTRODUCTION

Systemic lupus erythematosus (SLE) is an autoimmune disease with multiorgan involvement and several typical autoantibodies. Central nervous system (CNS) involvement is common. Patients with neuropsychiatric signs and symptoms are classified as neuropsychiatric SLE (NPSLE) patients. NPSLE patients show poor prognosis, low quality of life and high mortality. In 1999, the American College of Rheumatology (ACR) defined 19 typical neuropsychiatric symptoms such as cerebrovascular disease (CVD), seizures, anxiety, and cognitive dysfunction (1). While obvious NPSLE symptoms such as CVD and seizures are well-recognized by doctors, subtle ones such as anxiety and mild cognitive dysfunction are underestimated. Early detection and interventions are very important for those patients. Clinical psychiatric evaluations, such as the Hamilton Anxiety Scale (HAMA) and the Hamilton Depression Scale (HAMD), are widely used in patients with anxiety and depressive disorders. Conventional magnetic resonance imaging (MRI) is used to evaluate structural abnormalities, and functional MRI (fMRI) is used to evaluate brain activity. Task-related fMRI and conscious resting state fMRI (rs-fMRI) are used to reveal different aspects of brain function.

In this study, we examined SLE patients without major neuropsychiatric manifestations or abnormal conventional MRI as non-NPSLE patients. We used conscious rs-fMRI to explore the possible changes of brain activity and tried to find the associations among brain activity, disease activity, and depression, and anxiety statuses.

MATERIALS AND METHODS

Subjects

SLE patients in the inpatient and outpatient divisions of the Rheumatology and Immunology Department of First Affiliated Hospital of Kunming Medical University, a member unit of the Chinese SLE Treatment and Research Group (CSTAR), were recruited in this study from August of 2003 to August of 2015. All participants went through a standardized protocol and were evaluated by the same investigators throughout the course of the study. Before enrollment in the study, each participant provided written informed consent after receiving a complete description of the study. This research protocol was approved by the Institutional Review Board of Kunming Medical University, Yunnan Province, PR China (ClinicalTrials.gov: NCT00703742).

The inclusion criteria were as follows: (1) patients diagnosed as SLE according to the 1997 revised American College of Rheumatology (ACR) criteria for the classification of SLE (2) (2) patients between the ages of 15 and 60; and (3) patients or statutory guardians willing to attend this study and give written informed consent.

The exclusion criteria were as follows: (1) patients fitting the ACR diagnostic criteria for rheumatoid arthritis, systemic sclerosis, Sjögren's syndrome (primary or secondary) or other connective tissue diseases and drug-induced SLE; (2) patients with organic brain or neurological disorders that would disturb the structure or diffusion imaging of the brain (i.e., history of head trauma, Parkinson's disease or seizures); (3) patients with major active psychiatric manifestations, such as obvious disorganized behaviors and conscious disturbances; (4) patients with a history of substance abuse; (5) patients who were pregnant or suspected to be pregnant; (6) patients with contraindication to MRI, such as claustrophobia or cardiac pacemakers; (7) patients with serious clinical conditions that could cause cerebral atrophy, such as a history of arterial hypertension, diabetes mellitus, stroke or renal insufficiency; and (8) patients with structural abnormities of the brain identified by conventional T1- and T2-weighted MRI.

All of the recruited 118 SLE patients received the full sets of laboratory tests, disease activity evaluations, psychiatric evaluations, general questionnaires, and MRI scans. In addition, 81 healthy controls (HC) with age and gender matched were recruited. A rheumatologist and a neurologist performed the complete general physical examinations, including neurological examinations to all subjects to exclude major disorders. Psychiatric symptoms were screened by a psychiatrist using the Structured Clinical Interview for the Diagnostic and Statistical Manual of Mental Disorders (DSM)-IV Non-Patient Version (SCID-NP). All participants were right-handed Chinese Han people.

Clinical Features of SLE Patients

Gender and age were recorded for all participants. All of the clinical manifestations and laboratory test findings were recorded for each of the SLE patients. The disease activity was measured by the SLE disease activity index (SLEDAI) on the same day as the MRI scan. Active disease status was defined as a SLEDAI score of higher than nine (3, 4). The depression status was evaluated by HAMD, and the anxiety status was evaluated by HAMA. Patients were diagnosed with depression when the HAMD scores were $\geq$ 17 and were diagnosed with anxiety when the HAMA scores $\geq$ 14. All participants were right-handed as assessed by the Edinburgh Handedness Inventory (5). All clinical data were collected on the MRI examination day.

MRI Images Acquisition

The MRI images acquisition was performed by an experienced neuroradiologist. The MRI sequences were performed on all participants by using a 1.5T clinical MRI scanner manufactured by General Electric (GE) Company (Twin speed, Milwaukee, WI, USA), which was equipped with a birdcage head coil. Supportive foam pads were used to minimize the head movement. A rapid sagittal localizer scan was acquired to confirm the alignment. Normal T1 and T2 MRI scans were taken to exclude obvious structural abnormalities.

A set of conscious rs-fMRI scans was taken on each participant according to the standard protocols. Each participant was required to keep quiet and sober without active and intentional thinking. We used a gradient echo type echo planar imaging (GRE-EPI) technique with the following parameters: repetition time (TR) = 2,000 ms, echo time (TE) = 40 ms, matrix size = 64 × 64, thickness = 5 mm with an interslice gap of 1 mm, field of view = 240 mm, flip angle = 90°, number of excitation (NEX) 2.00, time point = 160. The whole-brain images were acquired in axial planes parallel to the anterior commissure-posterior commissure line. For each participant, 24 continuous slices were acquired and the total fMRI scan time was 320 s. All of the images were re-evaluated for imaging quality by the neuroradiologist.

Data Processing

The Digital Imaging and Communications in Medicine (DICOM) image data were processed via the MRIcro software (version 1.40, Chris Rorden's Neuropsychology Laboratory, University of South Carolina, Columbia, SC, USA; http://www.mricro.com). All data were analyzed via statistical parametric mapping (SPM) 8 (Wellcome Department of Cognitive Neurology, Institute of Neurology, London, UK; http://www.fil.

ion.ucl.ac.uk/) based on MATLAB 7.1 (The MathWorks, Inc. Natick, MA, USA). The images of the first 10 time points were discarded to allow the subjects to adapt to the MRI scanner and to minimize the effects of magnetic inhomogeneity. The remaining images were corrected for slice-time and head movement. Each individual image was normalized and transformed into the standardized Montreal Neurological Institute (MNI) template. Then, the images were resampled at the 3 × 3 × 3 mm scale. A filter with a full-width at half maximum (FWHM) of 10 mm was used to remove the noise for each normalized image. A bandpass filter with a range of 0.01–0.08 Hz was applied to reduce the effects of low-frequency drift and high-frequency respiratory or cardiac noises.

Analysis of Regional Homogeneity (ReHo)

We used the Resting-State fMRI Data Analysis Toolkit (REST) (http://www.restfmri.net) to calculate the Kendall's coefficient concordance (KCC) value for each voxel. Then, we obtained the ReHo values to provide a voxel-based measurement of the brain activity. We used two-sample *t*-tests to analyze the differences in ReHo values between the SLE and HC groups with a false discovery rate (FDR) correction ($p < 0.05$, cluster > 34 voxels). We also analyzed the correlations between ReHo values and SLEDAI, HAMA and HAMD scores with a false discovery rate (FDR) correction ($p < 0.05$, cluster > 34 voxels). The differences between the demographic characteristics of the SLE and HC groups were analyzed by SPSS 20.0 (IBM Inc. Armonk, NY, USA). The results were statistically significant when $p < 0.05$. All of the statistical tests were two-sided.

RESULTS

Demographic and Clinical Information

The mean age of the 118 SLE patients was 28.6 years old (standard deviation (*SD*) = 7.7). The mean disease duration of SLE patients was 19.2 months (*SD* = 20.8). The age and gender were comparable between the SLE and HC group. Detailed results are shown in **Table 1**.

TABLE 1 | Demographic and clinical characteristics of SLE and HC groups.

	SLE ($n = 118$)	HC ($n = 81$)	t	p
Age (year, Mean ± SD)	28.6 ± 7.7	29.0 ± 7.9	−0.375	0.708
Female /Male	98/20	67/14	0.004	0.951
Disease duration (m, Mean ± SD)	19.2 ± 20.8	NA		
SLEDAI (Mean ± SD)	10.3 ± 6.8	NA		
HAMA (Mean ± SD)	7.1 ± 5.3	NA		
HAMD (Mean ± SD)	8.9 ± 5.8	NA		

SLE, systemic lupus erythematosus; HC, healthy control; SD, standard deviation; NA, not applicable; SLEDAI, SLE disease activity index; HAMA, Hamilton Anxiety Scale; HAMD, Hamilton Depression Scale.

The ReHo Value Differences Between the SLE and HC Groups

In the study, four SLE patients and six HC subjects were excluded due to brain movement if the translation exceeded 2 mm or if the rotation exceeded 2. Data from the remaining 114 SLE patients and 75 HC subjects were analyzed. The average head motion assessed by the mean framewise displacement (FD)_Jenkinson index between the two groups were comparable (0.0475 ± 0.0235 vs. 0.0547 ± 0.0273, $p = 0.066$) (6).

In the conscious resting state, the ReHo values increased in areas including the left parahippocampal gyrus and right uncus. Brain areas with decreased ReHo values included the right fusiform gyrus and left thalamus. Detailed results are shown in **Table 2** and **Figure 1**.

Correlations Between the ReHo Values and Disease Activity and Depressive and Anxiety Statuses

Brain areas that showed positive correlations with SLEDAI included: the right cerebellum anterior lobe, left cerebellum posterior lobe, and right superior temporal gyrus. Brain areas that showed negative correlations with SLEDAI were the right medial and inferior frontal gyrus. Detailed results are shown in **Table 3** and **Figure 2**.

Brain areas which showed negative correlations with HAMA included: the left paracentral lobule, left postcentral gyrus, right precuneus, and left superior temporal gyrus. Detailed results are shown in **Table 4** and **Figure 3**.

Brain areas that showed negative correlations with HAMD included: the right cuneus, left postcentral gyrus, right superior temporal gyrus, and right fusiform gyrus. Detailed results are shown in **Table 5** and **Figure 4**.

DISCUSSION

Conventional MRI and fMRI are widely used in evaluations of the brain structure and activity, respectively. Functional MRI has been used to reveal brain activities, such as working memory, depression and anxiety status, both in the normal population and in patients with several types of diseases (7, 8). As a non-invasive imaging technique, fMRI is widely used in the early diagnosis, differential diagnosis, and monitoring of neuropsychiatric diseases. Since the Ogawa team reported the blood oxygenation level dependent (BOLD) method, it has been used for the detection of regional neural activity, in task-related situations and in the conscious resting state (9). The regional homogeneity (ReHo) method is used to evaluate the regional brain synchronization by measuring the time series of a given voxel and its nearby voxels in the conscious resting state. ReHo values reflect regional brain synchronization, and increased or decreased values may represent abnormal regional brain activity (10).

TABLE 2 | ReHo values in non-NPSLE patients.

Versus HC	Brain area	Cluster size (voxel)	MNI coordinate (peak value)			*T*-value (peak value)	Effect size
			X	Y	Z		
Increased	Left parahippocampal gyrus	135	−24	−6	−18	5.97	0.41
	Right uncus	232	27	3	−21	5.44	0.48
Decreased	Right fusiform gyrus	143	21	−60	−12	−4.54	−0.34
	Left thalamus	208	−3	−27	9	−5.57	−0.43

HC, healthy control; MNI, Montreal Neurological Institute.

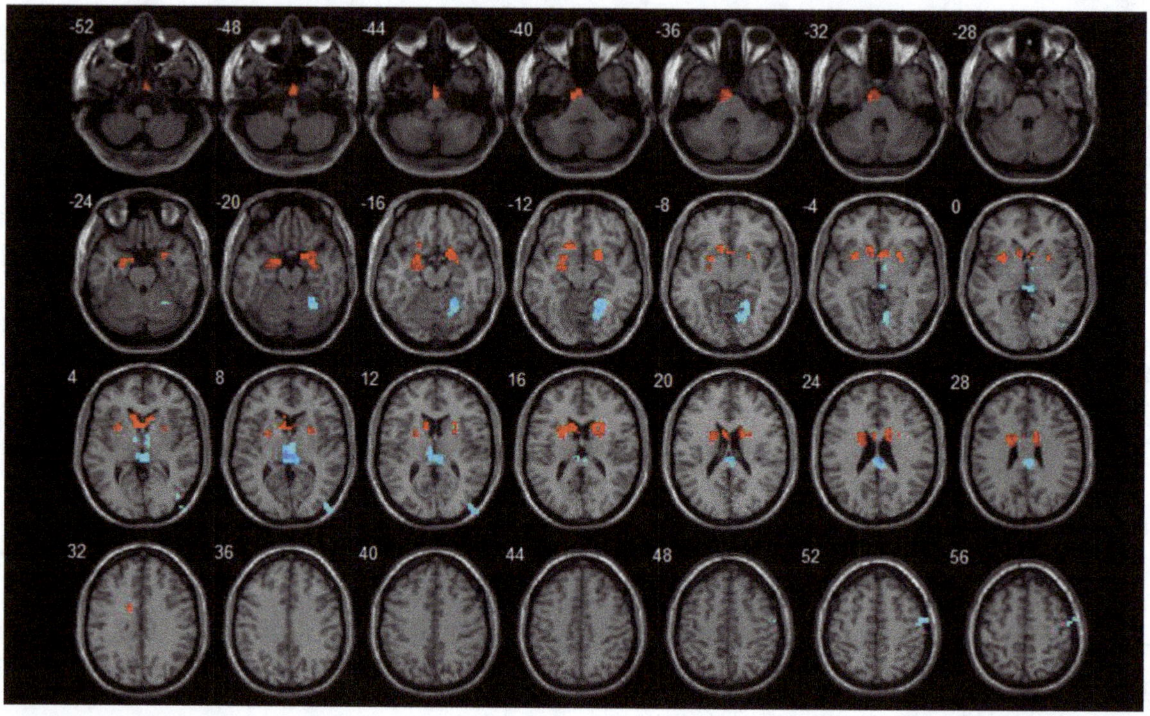

FIGURE 1 | ReHo value differences between SLE and HC groups ($p < 0.05$). Red spots show areas with increased ReHo values in SLE patients, while blue ones show those with decreased ReHo values.

In task-related fMRI studies, the participants showed high activation of target brain regions with relatively less disturbance. Task-related fMRI has been used in SLE patients to evaluate their brain activations, including motor function, working memory, and emotional activities. Rocca et al. found that NPSLE patients had more movement-associated brain activations than did the HC group in the motor function test. There were also strong correlations between the activations and the extent and severity of brain damages (11). Fitzgibbon et al. (12) found greater activations in the frontoparietal lobe of NPSLE patients than that of the HC group in working memory tasks, which might suggest brain dysfunction and the recruitment of extra brain areas, such as for compensation. Mackay et al. found that SLE patients with short disease durations showed more cortical activations in working memory tasks and fearful paradigms than did patients with long disease durations. This finding suggests that compensation could occur in a relatively short time, and long-term disease might result in severe neural damage and low activations (13). Conscious rs-fMRI could reveal the resting state brain function or brain networks. The default mode network (DMN) is a network of brain areas including the posterior cingulate cortex (PCC), the ventral anterior cingulate cortex (ACC), and other brain areas. It is the network for self-related cognitive activity and monitoring of the internal mental landscape. It is activated during the conscious resting state and is deactivated during complicated tasks (14–20). Lin et al. (21) found that non-NPSLE patients showed higher brain activations in the DMN and in the cerebellum and that the activations of the cerebellum were positively correlated with disease activities. Recently, Nystedt et al. (22) found that SLE patients with or without neuropsychiatric manifestations had brain connectivity changes in the DMN and other related brain

TABLE 3 | Correlations of ReHo values between brain areas and SLEDAI.

Correlations	Brain area	Cluster size (voxel)	MNI coordinate (peak value)			T value (peak value)
			X	Y	Z	
Positive	Right cerebellum anterior lobe	57	9	−51	−12	4.08
	Left cerebellum posterior lobe	44	−24	−63	−54	3.32
	Right superior temporal gyrus	34	54	−21	0	3.92
Negative	Right medial frontal gyrus	73	6	57	0	−3.87
	Right inferior frontal gyrus	47	30	18	−21	−3.69
		34	48	45	6	−4.34

MNI, Montreal Neurological Institute.

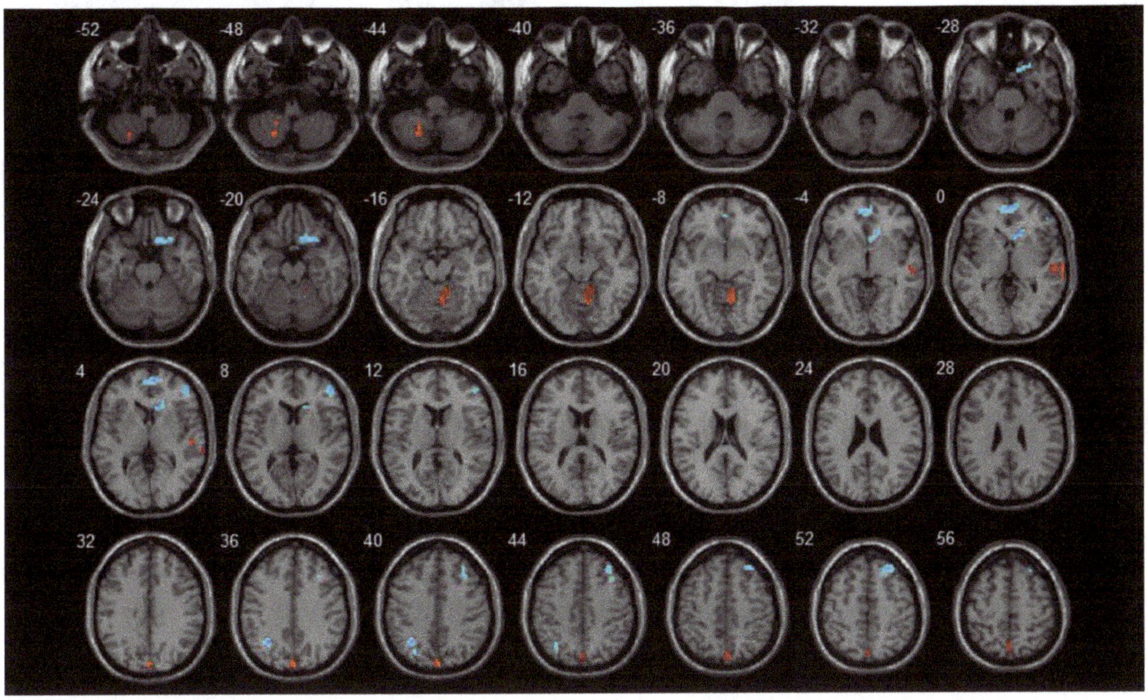

FIGURE 2 | Correlations between ReHo values and disease activity ($p < 0.05$). Red spots show areas with positive correlations with SLEDAI, while blue ones show areas with negative correlations.

areas, and these changes might reveal both brain damage and compensations.

Several studies have proven that in SLE patients, brain dysfunction could occur before structural changes, and the kinds of brain damage detected by different imaging methods were quite different in patients with or without neuropsychiatric symptoms (23–27). Therefore, we conducted this study to find possible brain dysfunction by conscious rs-fMRI and explored their associations with disease activity, depression and anxiety status in a relatively large sample of non-NPSLE patients.

We found that the ReHo values of non-NPSLE patients were decreased in brain areas including the fusiform gyrus and thalamus, and there was a negative correlation between the fusiform gyrus and the HAMD score. The fusiform gyrus is mainly involved in the visual recognition network. It is associated with emotional face and character processing, visual attention and learning process (28, 29). Mak et al. found that the fusiform gyrus showed decreased activities in non-NPSLE patients during the executive function test (30). A recent study showed cortical thickness reductions in the fusiform gyrus and in the lingual gyrus and abnormal resting-state functional connectivity (RSFC) in non-NPSLE patients. It suggested that cortical abnormalities might affect brain functional connectivity in non-NPSLE patients (31). These findings are consistent with our finding. The thalamus is crucial as a relay station in the brain. It can relay information between the subcortex and the cortex for most sensory systems. The increased activities of the thalamus in the resting state were reported in major depressive patients

TABLE 4 | Correlations of ReHo values between brain areas and HAMA.

Correlations	Brain area	Cluster size (voxel)	MNI coordinate (peak value)			*T*-value (peak value)
			X	Y	Z	
Negative	Left paracentral lobule	36	−6	−39	60	−3.49
	Left postcentral gyrus	98	−36	−36	69	−4.07
	Right precuneus	59	6	−84	45	−3.53
	Left superior temporal gyrus	106	−51	−45	18	−4.10

MNI, Montreal Neurological Institute.

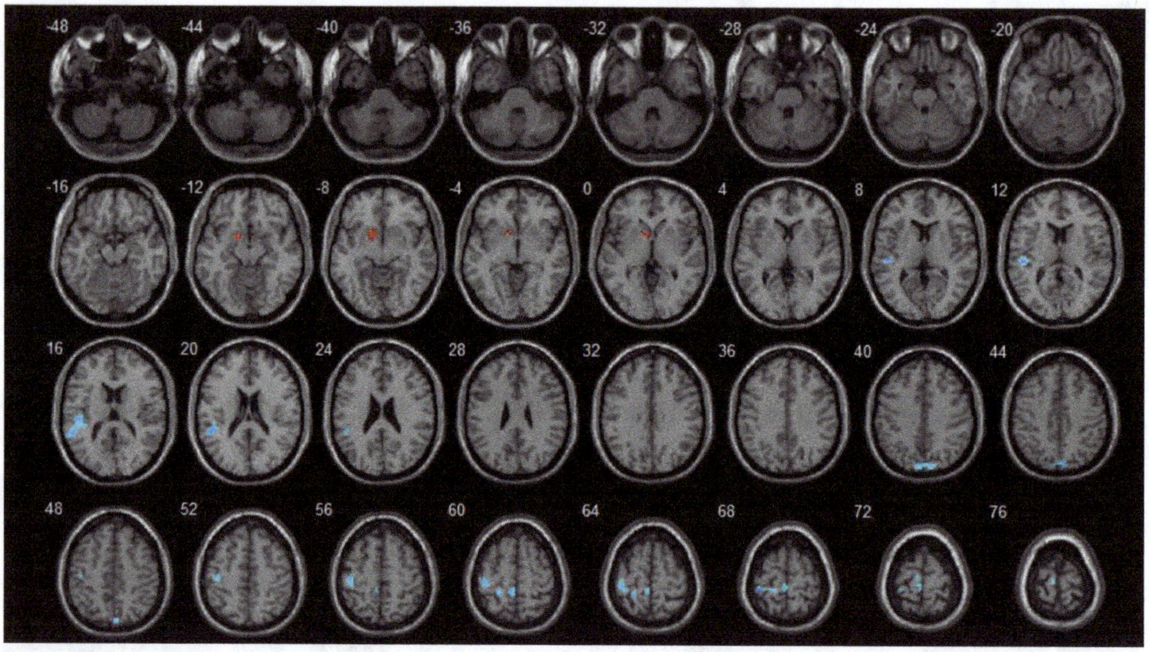

FIGURE 3 | Correlations between ReHo values and HAMA scores ($p < 0.05$). Blue spots show areas with negative correlations with HAMA.

(29, 32). Nystedt et al. found hyperconnectivity of the thalamus in non-NPSLE patients, which might suggest a compensatory mechanism (22).

Increased ReHo values in the left parahippocampal gyrus and in the right uncus were found. They are both part of the limbic lobe, which also consists of the hippocampus, the cingulate gyrus, and so on. In another study, we found decreased bilateral hippocampal volume and density in non-NPSLE patients (unpublished results). In a comprehensive perspective, these results might suggest structural damage and functional compensatory mechanisms in the limbic lobe. The limbic lobe is involved in several brain activities, including motivation, emotion, learning, and the memory process. NPSLE patients with greater hippocampus activity and hippocampal functional connectivity were found to have better learning efficiency (33). It was reported that SLE patients without cognitive impairments had increased activity in the hippocampus, and the compensation of the brain function was decreased as the disease eventually progressed (34). As we mentioned earlier, Rocca et al. found that there were positive correlations between the activations and brain damage in NPSLE patients (11). This finding might suggest that there was a compensatory mechanism during the early stage of SLE, and the brain function was eventually damaged during the advanced stage (22).

Our study showed a positive correlation between disease activity and the cerebellum, which might suggest a compensatory mechanism. Ren et al. found that the activity of the cortico-basal ganglia-thalamic-cortical circuit and amygdala-hippocampus coupling was decreased, while an increased cerebellar-frontal activity could compensate for the brain function in cognitive tasks in non-NPSLE patients (35). Lin et al. also found a positive correlation between the cerebellar activity and the SLEDAI score during the resting stage in non-NPSLE patients. They considered that the cerebellum could be part of the executive control network and related to the pathogenesis of NPSLE (21).

We found that the right medial and inferior frontal gyrus were both negatively correlated with the SLEDAI score. The frontal gyrus is the center of emotional regulation and voluntary

TABLE 5 | Correlations of ReHo values between brain areas and HAMD.

Correlations	Brain area	Cluster size (voxel)	MNI coordinate (peak value)			*T*-value (peak value)
			X	Y	Z	
Negative	Right cuneus	46	24	−87	33	−3.36
	Left postcentral gyrus	35	−42	−27	63	−3.40
	Right superior temporal gyrus	39	54	−36	12	−3.81
	Right fusiform gyrus	36	48	−66	−18	−3.72

MNI, Montreal Neurological Institute.

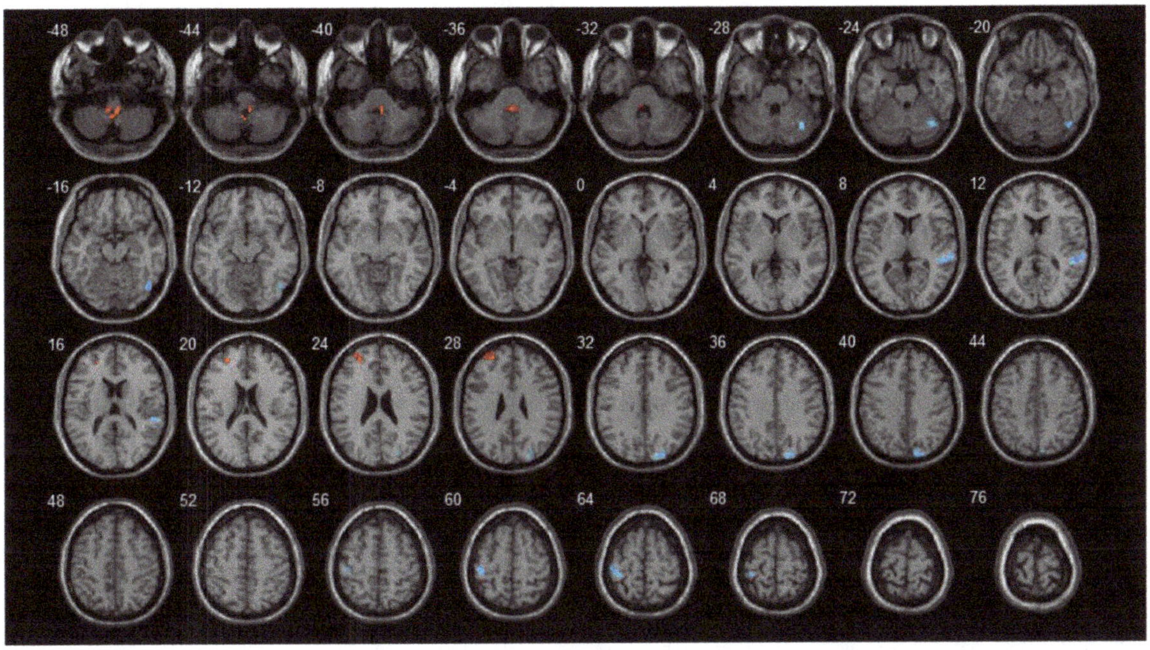

FIGURE 4 | Correlations between ReHo values and HAMD scores ($p < 0.05$). Blue spots showed areas with negative correlation with HAMD.

movement. Fitzgibbon et al. found fronto-parietal cortex hyperactivation and positive correlations with disease activities in NPSLE patients in working memory tasks (12), whereas Hou et al. found similar results in non-NPSLE patients during the resting state (36). Rocca et al. found activations in the frontal and parietal lobes in NPSLE patients during motor tasks. There were positive correlations between the activation of sensorimotor areas and the extent and severity of brain damage (11). We failed to find this compensation effect and found quite opposite results. One possible explanation is that our participants had a relatively short disease duration and we had a larger sample. The frontal gyrus may play a complicated role in SLE patients, and more studies are needed to elucidate the exact role.

The HAMA and HAMD scores were negatively correlated with similar brain areas, including the left paracentral lobule and postcentral gyrus, the right precuneus and cuneus, and the bilateral superior temporal gyrus. The postcentral gyrus is the primary somatosensory cortex, and the paracentral lobule controls motor and sensory innervations. The precuneus is involved in the episodic memory, visuospatial processing, and self-consciousness. The cuneus is involved in basic visual processing. The superior temporal gyrus contains the primary auditory cortex and Wernicke's area, which is involved in the comprehension of language. The abnormal brain activities in the precuneus, cuneus and superior temporal gyrus of SLE patients were reported in previous studies (11, 21, 30, 37). However, the correlations between depression and the anxiety status within these areas in SLE patients were not reported previously. More studies are needed to confirm our finding and to explore the underlying mechanism.

There are still some flaws in our study. One is that we only used ReHo values to reflect the brain activity, because there were other available methods, such as the amplitude of low frequency fluctuations (ALFF). Zou et al. found that the reliability of ReHo values was good with standard protocols including nuisance correction, enough scan durations, and fast sampling rates (38). In our study, we considered the ReHo value to be feasible for reflecting the brain activity.

We found that the brain areas with decreased ReHo values were in the fusiform gyrus and thalamus, while the areas with increased ReHo values were in the limbic lobe. We found that SLEDAI showed a positive correlation with brain areas in the cerebellum and a negative correlation with brain areas in the frontal gyrus. Several brain areas showed negative correlations with depression and anxiety statuses. These results gave us some clues on how the brain synchronization changes in non-NPSLE patients. Early detection and proper treatment of brain dysfunction might prevent progression to NPSLE. More studies are needed to reveal the underlying mechanisms.

AUTHOR CONTRIBUTIONS

SL and YC were responsible for the management of the research and writing the article. ZX, AL, ZL, and YZ were responsible for recruiting and following up the patients. CL and HY were responsible for doing MRI. XX, BS, and LX were responsible for the consultation of the research. JX was responsible for the whole research and article.

ACKNOWLEDGMENTS

We thank all of the volunteers who participated in this study. We thank Doctor Daying Feng of the Department of Rheumatology and Immunology of First Affiliated Hospital of Kunming Medical University, for recruiting the volunteers.

This work is supported by grants from National Natural Science Foundation of China (81160379, 81460256, 81560233, 81501406, and 81760296), the Funding of Yunnan Provincial Health Science and Technology Plan (2014NS171, 2016NS026, 2017NS051, 2018NS0133 and 2018NS0134), Yunnan Provincial Fund for High Level Reserve Talents in Health Science (H-2017068), The Hundred-Talent Program of Kunming Medical University (60117190457), Innovative Research Team of Kunming Medical University (CXTD201613), Yunnan Provincial Fund for Preparatory Young Leaders in Academia and Technology (2015HB071), the Funding of Ministry of Science and Technology of Yunnan Province (2014HC018), the Funding of Yunnan Provincial Department of Education, and Yunnan Applied Basic Research Projects-Union Foundation [2017FE467, 2017FE467 (−138)].

REFERENCES

1. The American College of Rheumatology nomenclature and case definitions for neuropsychiatric lupus syndromes. *Arthritis Rheum.* (1999) 42:599–608. doi: 10.1002/1529-0131(199904)42:4<599::AID-ANR2>3.0.CO;2-F
2. Hochberg MC. Updating the American College of Rheumatology revised criteria for the classification of systemic lupus erythematosus. *Arthritis Rheum.* (1997) 40:1725. doi: 10.1002/1529-0131(199709)40:9<1725::AID-ART29>3.0.CO;2-Y
3. Bombardier C, Gladman DD, Urowitz MB, Caron D, Chang CH. Derivation of the SLEDAI. A disease activity index for lupus patients. The committee on prognosis studies in SLE. *Arthritis Rheum.* (1992) 35:630–40.
4. Gladman DD, Ibañez D, Urowitz MB. Systemic lupus erythematosus disease activity index 2000. *J Rheumatol.* (2002) 29:288–91.
5. Oldfield RC. The assessment and analysis of handedness: the Edinburgh inventory. *Neuropsychologia* (1971) 9:97–113. doi: 10.1016/0028-3932(71)90067-4
6. Jenkinson M, Bannister P, Brady M, Smith S. Improved optimization for the robust and accurate linear registration and motion correction of brain images. *Neuroimage* (2002) 17:825–41. doi: 10.1006/nimg.2002.1132
7. Lueken U, Straube B, Yang Y, Hahn T, Beesdo-Baum K, Wittchen HU, et al. Separating depressive comorbidity from panic disorder: a combined functional magnetic resonance imaging and machine learning approach. *J Affect Disord.* (2015) 184:182–92. doi: 10.1016/j.jad.2015.05.052
8. Ragland JD, Ranganath C, Phillips J, Boudewyn MA, Kring AM, Lesh TA, et al. Cognitive control of episodic memory in schizophrenia: differential role of dorsolateral and ventrolateral prefrontal cortex. *Front Hum Neurosci.* (2015) 9:604. doi: 10.3389/fnhum.2015.00604
9. Ogawa S, Lee TM, Kay AR, Tank DW. Brain magnetic resonance imaging with contrast dependent on blood oxygenation. *Proc Natl Acad Sci USA.* (1990) 87:9868–72.
10. Zang Y, Jiang T, Lu Y, He Y, Tian L. Regional homogeneity approach to fMRI data analysis. *Neuroimage* (2004) 22:394–400. doi: 10.1016/j.neuroimage.2003.12.030
11. Rocca MA, Agosta F, Mezzapesa DM, Ciboddo G, Falini A, Comi G, et al. An fMRI study of the motor system in patients with neuropsychiatric systemic lupus erythematosus. *Neuroimage* (2006) 30:478–84. doi: 10.1016/j.neuroimage.2005.09.047
12. Fitzgibbon BM, Fairhall SL, Kirk IJ, Kalev-Zylinska M, Pui K, Dalbeth N, et al. Functional MRI in NPSLE patients reveals increased parietal and frontal brain activation during a working memory task compared with controls. *Rheumatology* (2008) 47:50–3. doi: 10.1093/rheumatology/kem287
13. Mackay M, Bussa MP, Aranow C, Ulug AM, Volpe BT, Huerta PT, et al. Differences in regional brain activation patterns assessed by functional magnetic resonance imaging in patients with systemic lupus erythematosus stratified by disease duration. *Mol Med.* (2011) 17:1349–56. doi: 10.2119/molmed.2011.00185
14. Mazoyer B, Zago L, Mellet E, Bricogne S, Etard O, Houdé O, et al. Cortical networks for working memory and executive functions sustain the conscious resting state in man. *Brain Res Bull.* (2001) 54:287–98. doi: 10.1016/S0361-9230(00)00437-8
15. Binder JR, Frost JA, Hammeke TA, Bellgowan PS, Rao SM, Cox RW. Conceptual processing during the conscious resting state. A functional MRI study. *J Cogn Neurosci.* (1999) 11:80–95.
16. Gusnard DA, Raichle ME, Raichle ME. Searching for a baseline: functional imaging and the resting human brain. *Nat Rev Neurosci.* (2001) 2:685–94. doi: 10.1038/35094500
17. Laureys S, Goldman S, Phillips C, Van Bogaert P, Aerts J, Luxen A, et al. Impaired effective cortical connectivity in vegetative state: preliminary investigation using PET. *Neuroimage* (1999) 9:377–82. doi: 10.1006/nimg.1998.0414
18. Menon V. Large-scale brain networks and psychopathology: a unifying triple network model. *Trends Cogn Sci.* (2011) 15:483–506. doi: 10.1016/j.tics.2011.08.003
19. Bressler SL, Menon V. Large-scale brain networks in cognition: emerging methods and principles. *Trends Cogn Sci.* (2010) 14:277–90. doi: 10.1016/j.tics.2010.04.004
20. Greicius MD, Krasnow B, Reiss AL, Menon V. Functional connectivity in the resting brain: a network analysis of the default mode hypothesis. *Proc Natl Acad Sci USA.* (2003) 100:253–8. doi: 10.1073/pnas.0135058100
21. Lin Y, Zou QH, Wang J, Wang Y, Zhou DQ, Zhang RH, et al. Localization of cerebral functional deficits in patients with non-neuropsychiatric systemic lupus erythematosus. *Hum Brain Mapp.* (2011) 32:1847–55. doi: 10.1002/hbm.21158
22. Nystedt J, Mannfolk P, Jönsen A, Bengtsson A, Nilsson P, Sundgren PC, et al. Functional connectivity changes in systemic lupus erythematosus: a resting-state study. *Brain Connect.* (2018) 8:220–34. doi: 10.1089/brain.2017.0557

23. Kozora E, Arciniegas DB, Filley CM, Ellison MC, West SG, Brown MS, et al. Cognition, MRS neurometabolites, and MRI volumetrics in non-neuropsychiatric systemic lupus erythematosus: preliminary data. *Cogn Behav Neurol.* (2005) 18:159–62. doi: 10.1097/01.wnn.0000181543.05064.4b
24. Appenzeller S, Carnevalle AD, Li LM, Costallat LT, Cendes F. Hippocampal atrophy in systemic lupus erythematosus. *Ann Rheum Dis.* (2006) 65:1585–9. doi: 10.1136/ard.2005.049486
25. Appenzeller S, Bonilha L, Rio PA, Min LL, Costallat LT, Cendes F. Longitudinal analysis of gray and white matter loss in patients with systemic lupus erythematosus. *Neuroimage* (2007) 34:694–701. doi: 10.1016/j.neuroimage.2006.09.029
26. Castellino G, Govoni M, Padovan M, Colamussi P, Borrelli M, Trotta F. Proton magnetic resonance spectroscopy may predict future brain lesions in SLE patients: a functional multi-imaging approach and follow up. *Ann Rheum Dis.* (2005) 64:1022–7. doi: 10.1136/ard.2004.026773
27. Zhang L, Harrison M, Heier LA, Zimmerman RD, Ravdin L, Lockshin M, et al. Diffusion changes in patients with systemic lupus erythematosus. *Magn Reson Imaging* (2007) 25:399–405. doi: 10.1016/j.mri.2006.09.037
28. Caspers J, Zilles K, Amunts K, Laird AR, Fox PT, Eickhoff SB. Functional characterization and differential coactivation patterns of two cytoarchitectonic visual areas on the human posterior fusiform gyrus. *Hum Brain Mapp.* (2014) 35:2754–67. doi: 10.1002/hbm.22364
29. Fusar-Poli P, Placentino A, Carletti F, Landi P, Allen P, Surguladze S, et al. Functional atlas of emotional faces processing: a voxel-based meta-analysis of 105 functional magnetic resonance imaging studies. *J Psychiatry Neurosci.* (2009) 34:418–32.
30. Mak A, Ren T, Fu EH, Cheak AA, Ho RC. A prospective functional MRI study for executive function in patients with systemic lupus erythematosus without neuropsychiatric symptoms. *Semin Arthritis Rheum.* (2012) 41:849–58. doi: 10.1016/j.semarthrit.2011.11.010
31. Niu C, Tan X, Liu X, Han K, Niu M, Xu J, et al. Cortical thickness reductions associate with abnormal resting-state functional connectivity in non-neuropsychiatric systemic lupus erythematosus. *Brain Imaging Behav.* (2018) 12:674–84. doi: 10.1007/s11682-017-9729-4
32. Greicius MD, Flores BH, Menon V, Glover GH, Solvason HB, Kenna H, et al. Resting-state functional connectivity in major depression: abnormally increased contributions from subgenual cingulate cortex and thalamus. *Biol Psychiatry* (2007) 62:429–37. doi: 10.1016/j.biopsych.2006.09.020
33. Shapira-Lichter I, Vakil E, Litinsky I, Oren N, Glikmann-Johnston Y, Caspi D, et al. Learning and memory-related brain activity dynamics are altered in systemic lupus erythematosus: a functional magnetic resonance imaging study. *Lupus* (2013) 22:562–73. doi: 10.1177/0961203313480399
34. Buckner RL, Andrews-Hanna JR, Schacter DL. The brain's default network: anatomy, function, and relevance to disease. *Ann NY Acad Sci.* (2008) 1124:1–38. doi: 10.1196/annals.1440.011
35. Ren T, Ho RC, Mak A. Dysfunctional cortico-basal ganglia-thalamic circuit and altered hippocampal-amygdala activity on cognitive set-shifting in non-neuropsychiatric systemic lupus erythematosus. *Arthritis Rheum.* (2012) 64:4048–59. doi: 10.1002/art.34660
36. Hou J, Lin Y, Zhang W, Song L, Wu W, Wang J, et al. Abnormalities of frontal-parietal resting-state functional connectivity are related to disease activity in patients with systemic lupus erythematosus. *PLoS ONE* (2013) 8:e74530. doi: 10.1371/journal.pone.0074530
37. DiFrancesco MW, Holland SK, Ris MD, Adler CM, Nelson S, DelBello MP, et al. Functional magnetic resonance imaging assessment of cognitive function in childhood-onset systemic lupus erythematosus: a pilot study. *Arthritis Rheum.* (2007) 56:4151–63. doi: 10.1002/art.23132
38. Zuo XN, Xu T, Jiang L, Yang Z, Cao XY, He Y, et al. Toward reliable characterization of functional homogeneity in the human brain: preprocessing, scan duration, imaging resolution and computational space. *Neuroimage* (2013) 65:374–86. doi: 10.1016/j.neuroimage.2012.10.017

9

EEG Microstates Indicate Heightened Somatic Awareness in Insomnia: Toward Objective Assessment of Subjective Mental Content

Yishul Wei[1], Jennifer R. Ramautar[1], Michele A. Colombo[1,2,3], Bart H. W. te Lindert[1] and Eus J. W. Van Someren[1,4,5]*

[1] Department of Sleep and Cognition, Netherlands Institute for Neuroscience (NIN), An Institute of the Royal Netherlands Academy of Arts and Sciences, Amsterdam, Netherlands, [2] Bernstein Center Freiburg and Faculty of Biology, University of Freiburg, Freiburg, Germany, [3] Centre for Chronobiology, Psychiatric Hospital of the University of Basel (UPK), Basel, Switzerland, [4] Department of Psychiatry, Amsterdam UMC, Vrije Universiteit Amsterdam, Amsterdam, Netherlands, [5] Department of Integrative Neurophysiology, Center for Neurogenomics and Cognitive Research (CNCR), Amsterdam Neuroscience, Vrije Universiteit Amsterdam, Amsterdam, Netherlands

***Correspondence:**
Eus J. W. Van Someren
e.j.w.someren@vu.nl

People with Insomnia Disorder (ID) not only experience abundant nocturnal mentation, but also report altered spontaneous mental content during daytime wakefulness, such as an increase in bodily experiences (heightened somatic awareness). Previous studies have shown that resting-state EEG can be temporally partitioned into quasi-stable microstates, and that these microstates form a small number of canonical classes that are consistent across people. Furthermore, the microstate classes have been associated with individual differences in resting mental content including somatic awareness. To address the hypothesis that altered resting mental content in ID would be reflected in an altered representation of the corresponding EEG microstates, we analyzed resting-state high-density EEG of 32 people with ID and 32 age- and sex-matched controls assessed during 5-min eyes-closed wakefulness. Using data-driven topographical k-means clustering, we found that 5 microstate classes optimally explained the EEG scalp voltage map sequences across participants. For each microstate class, 3 dynamic features were obtained: mean duration, frequency of occurrence, and proportional coverage time. People with ID had a shorter mean duration of class C microstates, and more frequent occurrence of class D microstates. The finding is consistent with previously established associations of these microstate properties with somatic awareness, and increased somatic awareness in ID. EEG microstate assessment could provide objective markers of subjective experience dimensions in studies on consciousness during the transition between wake and sleep, when self-report is not possible because it would interfere with the very process under study. Addressing somatic awareness may benefit psychotherapeutic treatment of insomnia.

Keywords: high-density EEG, resting state, microstate, insomnia disorder, wakefulness, mental content, somatic awareness, electrical neuroimaging

INTRODUCTION

Insomnia Disorder (ID) is a chronic disorder characterized by both nighttime and daytime symptoms. Nighttime symptoms include difficulty falling asleep, frequent or prolonged awakenings during the night, and early morning awakening. Daytime symptoms refer to fatigue, impaired concentration, mood disturbances, or other subjective complaints on daytime functioning (1). The maintenance of insomnia symptoms is likely to involve a host of cognitive factors including various forms of spontaneous mental activity as well as dysfunctional beliefs and attentional biases (2–4). A recent study found that people suffering from ID markedly differ from those without sleep complaints in several dimensions of spontaneous awareness, thoughts, and feelings (5) quantified using the Amsterdam Resting State Questionnaire (ARSQ) (6). The neural bases of the altered cognitive processes in ID are currently not well understood. As subjective mental states are increasingly viewed as arising from the interactions between distributed brain networks (7–9), studying the collective dynamic organization of brain network activity might reveal key mechanisms underlying the altered awareness, thoughts, feelings, and other mental states in ID.

Electroencephalography (EEG) is a relatively cost-efficient and non-disruptive means to measure brain activity and has been widely utilized in research on mental processes. EEG microstate analysis is a particularly valuable methodology for quantifying the rapid dynamics of large-scale brain networks not captured by the limited temporal resolution of functional magnetic resonance imaging (fMRI) (10, 11). EEG microstates are defined as quasi-stable scalp voltage configurations which on average last for tens of milliseconds. Transitions between microstates are assumed to reflect dynamic activation of distributed brain networks at sub-second timescales (12, 13). Resting-state EEG microstates during eyes-closed wakefulness are most commonly grouped into 4 classes (conventionally labeled as microstate classes A, B, C, and D) through topographical clustering techniques (10), although in a recent study up to 7 distinct microstate classes were identified (14). Combined EEG-fMRI has been utilized to confirm that the blood-oxygen-level dependent (BOLD) correlates of the 4 canonical microstate classes exhibit spatial patterns of well-known resting-state networks (15). Specifically, intra-individual fluctuations of class A, B, C, and D microstates were linked to activation of the "auditory," "visual," "salience," and "attention" networks, respectively. In addition, studies using electric source imaging have provided complementary information about the neural substrates of EEG microstates, such as sources common to all microstates which cannot be detected with BOLD fMRI (14, 16).

Although EEG microstates have been hypothesized to represent the building blocks of mentation, or "atoms of thoughts and emotions" (17), efforts to directly test the relationship between microstate properties and subjective mental content have only recently emerged. An experimental study adopting a within-subjects task manipulation reported increased presence of class A and B microstates while participants were engaged in visual and verbal thinking tasks, respectively (18). A second study correlated microstate properties during the eyes-closed resting state with each dimension of the ARSQ across participants (19). The most robust finding of this study was a negative association between the proportional coverage time of class C microstates and the "somatic awareness" dimension of the ARSQ. The mean duration of class C microstates also showed a negative association with somatic awareness. In addition, the proportional coverage time and mean duration of class B microstates were positively associated with the "comfort" dimension of the ARSQ. Properties of class D microstates showed rather nonspecific associations with multiple ARSQ dimensions, while those of class A microstates were not systematically associated with any specific ARSQ dimension.

Given these observed associations between subjective mental content and microstate properties during the eyes-closed wake resting state, we hypothesized that people with ID would exhibit altered microstate dynamics in line with their altered resting mental content (5). The present study utilized 256-channel high-density EEG (HD-EEG) in a sample of 32 patients and 32 matched controls to verify the hypothesis. To our knowledge, this is the first study on EEG microstate dynamics in ID.

MATERIALS AND METHODS

Participants and EEG Recordings

We analyzed resting-state HD-EEG recordings of 32 people meeting the DSM-5 (20) criteria for ID (25 female, age range 21–67 y) and 32 age- and sex-matched controls (CTRL) without sleep complaints (26 female, age range 22–70 y) from a previously reported study (21). Participants were recruited through advertisement and the Netherlands Sleep Registry and were screened by telephone followed by a face-to-face structured interview. Exclusion criteria for all participants were: (1) diagnosed sleep apnea, restless legs syndrome, narcolepsy, or other somatic, neurological, or psychiatric disorders; (2) use of sleep medications within the prior 2 months; (3) overt shifted or irregular sleep–wake rhythms, assessed using 1 week of actigraphy (Actiwatch AW4, Cambridge Neurotechnology Ltd., Cambridge, United Kingdom or GENEActiv Sleep, Activinsights Ltd., Kimbolton, United Kingdom) supplemented by sleep diaries; (4) scores above the minimal to mild range of anxiety or depression symptom severity, as evaluated by either the Hospital Anxiety and Depression Scale (HADS) (22), or the Beck Anxiety Inventory (BAI) (23) and Beck Depression Inventory (BDI-IA) (24). Furthermore, all patients had Insomnia Severity Index (ISI) (25) scores above 10, and all controls had ISI scores less than 8. The study was approved by the ethics committee of the VU University Medical Center, Amsterdam, The Netherlands. All participants provided written informed consent.

HD-EEG was acquired in a laboratory setting using a 256-channel HydroCel Geodesic Sensor Net (Electrical Geodesic Inc., Eugene, OR) connected to a Net Amps 300 amplifier (input impedance: 200 MΩ, A/D converter: 24 bits), with the ground electrode placed at the centro-parietal midline and reference at the vertex. Electrode impedances were kept below 100 kΩ. Signals were online band-pass filtered between 0.1–100 Hz and digitized at 1000 Hz.

Protocol

On the recording days, participants were asked to refrain from alcohol and drugs, as well as to limit consumption of caffeinated beverages to a maximum of 2 cups, which were allowed only before noon. Wake resting-state HD-EEG was recorded during the evening (between 19:00 and habitual bedtime) while the participant was seated upright. The original protocol consisted of eyes-open (EO) followed by eyes-closed (EC) conditions of 5-min duration each (21). Vigilance level was monitored in real-time during recording by laboratory staff. In the occasional cases where signs of falling asleep were observed (e.g., slow eye movements, attenuation of alpha waves), the participant was alerted and recording of the 5-min assessment was restarted. Since so far validation of the reliability of microstate properties has been carried out only in EC (11), and only the links between mental content and microstate properties during EC have been demonstrated (18, 19), we here restricted analyses to the EC data.

EEG Preprocessing

Preprocessing and signal analyses were performed in MATLAB 8.3 (The Mathworks Inc., Natick, MA). EEG data were preprocessed using the MEEGPIPE toolbox (https://github.com/meegpipe/meegpipe). The preprocessing procedure involved several automatic and manual steps as detailed previously (21). Briefly, voltage drifts within channels were estimated by local polynomial approximation (26) and subtracted. The signals were downsampled to 250 Hz and band-pass filtered at 0.5–62.5 Hz. Modified z-score (27) criteria applied to the standard deviation, range, and gradient of the voltage signals were used to marked noisy EEG channels and sporadic noisy segments. Noisy channels were linearly interpolated from neighboring channels. Sporadic noisy segments were excluded from analyses. The remaining segments were submitted to independent component decomposition (28). Components of power-line noise, eye movement, pulse wave, and cardiac field artifacts were identified through visual inspection of their time courses and topographical distribution and projected out of the data. The total duration of artifact-free data did not differ between groups (mean $\pm$ standard deviation: ID $= 289.4 \pm 50.2$ s, CTRL $= 289.2 \pm 21.4$ s, $p = 0.98$).

Microstate Analysis

The method for identifying the microstate classes closely followed previous studies that used the same 256-channel HydroCel Geodesic Sensor Net (29, 30). The preprocessed EEG signals from 204 electrodes overlying the scalp area (excluding electrodes at the cheeks and the nape) were further band-pass filtered at 1–40 Hz and re-referenced to the common average. Momentary topographies at the local maxima of the global field power (GFP) were submitted to k-means clustering based on their absolute spatial correlations (ignoring polarity differences). The k-means clustering routine was run multiple times for each participant with the pre-defined number of clusters varying from 3 to 11. The optimal number of clusters for each individual, k_i^*, was then determined by the Krzanowski–Lai criterion which identifies the point of maximal normalized curvature on the dispersion curve (31). The normalized cluster-mean topographies from all participants were then submitted to group-level k-means clustering, which was also run multiple times with the pre-defined number of clusters varying from 3 to 11. A constraint was imposed such that the k_i^* clusters from an individual had to be assigned to $\min\left(k_i^*, k\right)$ distinct group-level classes, where k is the pre-defined number of group-level clusters (viz. classes) in a particular run. Finally, the Krzanowski–Lai criterion was applied again to determine the optimal number of group-level clusters, k^*.

The average topographies of the group-level microstate classes were fitted back to individual EEG recordings competitively. Each momentary topography at the GFP local maxima was assigned to the microstate class with which the highest absolute spatial correlation was attained. Consecutive GFP local maxima assigned to the same microstate class were merged into one microstate, with start and end times of each microstate defined as midpoints to the neighboring GFP local maxima (11, 18). Microstates whose start or end times could not be estimated (i.e., those at the very beginning and very end of the recording and those bordering noisy segments) were omitted from analyses. From the resulting sequences of alternating microstates, we calculated the following standard dynamic features for each microstate class for each participant (11, 12, 19): (1) Mean Duration—the mean duration in milliseconds of the microstates of a particular class. (2) Frequency of Occurrence—the number of microstates of a particular class per second. (3) Proportional Coverage Time—the percentage of time spent in a particular microstate class.

It has been suggested that fitting microstate classes only at the GFP local maxima, thus ignoring the fine-grained dynamics between GFP local maxima, might be suboptimal (13). However, we found that almost perfectly correlated feature values were produced by fitting microstate classes either only at the GFP local maxima or at every timeframe (**Supplementary Table 1**). In other words, fitting microstate classes at either timescale provides essentially equivalent information, at least as far as the dynamic features we studied here are concerned.

Statistical Analyses

Randomized permutation tests for topographical differences (conventionally referred to as TANOVA) (11, 31) were used to compare microstate topographies between ID and CTRL. Group differences in microstate dynamic features (mean duration, frequency of occurrence, and proportional coverage time for each class) were expressed in Cohen's d and their significance was further assessed by means of linear regression modeling with two-tailed Wald z-tests, performed using R (32). Linear mixed-effects regression models with Gaussian random effects (33) were set up for mean duration and frequency of occurrence and Dirichlet regression (34, 35) for proportional coverage time, as the latter better models compositional data which sum up to 100% within each participant.[1] All regression models included age and sex as covariates in addition to group contrasts and the within-subjects factor (microstate class). In total, $3k^*$ group effects were tested (3 dynamic features for each of the

[1] In particular, the proportional coverage time correlates mostly negatively between microstate classes, while the mean duration, as well as frequency of occurrence, correlates positively between microstate classes.

TABLE 1 | Characteristics of participants (mean ± standard deviation).

	Control (n = 32)	Insomnia disorder (n = 32)	p
Age, y	46.8 ± 15.0	48.5 ± 14.1	0.64
Sex, female/male	26/6	25/7	1
ISI	2.00 ± 1.97	17.19 ± 3.75	< 0.0001
BAI	2.00 ± 2.33	6.42 ± 4.93	0.06
BDI-IA	2.00 ± 1.85	4.75 ± 3.84	0.11
HADS—Anxiety	4.33 ± 2.10	5.75 ± 2.38	0.06
HADS—Depression	1.88 ± 1.65	3.60 ± 3.30	0.09

ISI, Insomnia Severity Index; BAI, Beck Anxiety Inventory; BDI-IA, Beck Depression Inventory IA; HADS, Hospital Anxiety and Depression Scale.
p-values are determined by Fisher exact test for sex and by Wilcoxon rank-sum tests for the other variables.

k^* identified microstate classes). Following Rieger et al. (36), the group contrasts for proportional coverage time were not considered independent tests because the values of proportional coverage time could be deduced from mean duration and frequency of occurrence. Therefore, the p-value threshold $\frac{0.05}{(2k^*)}$ for controlling the family-wise error rate (FWER) was employed.

RESULTS

Demographic and Clinical Characteristics

Demographic and clinical characteristics of patients and controls are summarized in **Table 1**. As expected, patients had significantly higher ISI scores and tended to report higher BAI, BDI-IA, and HADS scores than controls.

Microstate Topographies

At the individual level, the Krzanowski–Lai criterion suggested 4–6 as the optimal number of clusters for all participants (mean ± standard deviation: ID = 4.38 ± 0.55, CTRL = 4.31 ± 0.47, p = 0.63). At the group level, the Krzanowski–Lai criterion suggested a 5-class model as optimal either for ID, for CTRL, or for all participants combined. **Figure 1** shows the overall dispersion (i.e., within-cluster global dissimilarity) for different numbers of group-level clusters, as well as the corresponding mean percentages of global variance explained when the cluster topographies were fitted back to the GFP local maxima in individual EEG recordings. The global explained variance derived from the optimal 5-class model did not differ significantly between the two groups (mean ± standard deviation: ID = 65.68 ± 8.57 %, CTRL = 66.16 ± 6.77 %, p = 0.80).[2]

Figure 2 shows the average topographies for the 5 identified microstate classes in both groups. The average topographies for 4 of the identified classes resemble the 4 canonical microstate topographies reported in previous studies and are labeled hereafter as microstate classes A, B, C, and D accordingly. The 5th microstate class resembles microstate class E identified by Custo et al. (14) in a large sample and therefore we also label it as microstate class E. Permutation TANOVA performed separately for each microstate class revealed that the microstate topographies significantly differed between the two groups for microstate class A (p = 0.04) but not for the other classes (all p > 0.15).

Microstate Dynamics

The mean and standard deviation of mean duration, frequency of occurrence, and proportional coverage time for each microstate class for each group are presented in **Table 2**. Linear mixed-effects regression indicated group differences in the mean duration of class C microstates (group effect ± standard error = −7.61 ± 2.68 ms, z = −2.84, p = 0.0045) and the frequency of occurrence of class D microstates (group effect ± standard error = 0.62 ± 0.26 s^{-1}, z = 2.38, p = 0.018) were significant at the p < 0.05 level, albeit only the former had a p-value below the FWER-controlling threshold (0.05/10 = 0.005). Both differences had medium unadjusted effect sizes (Cohen's d = −0.57 and 0.47, respectively). Other group effects on mean duration or frequency of occurrence did not reach significance (all p > 0.18). Dirichlet regression revealed no significant group effect on proportional coverage time for any of the microstate classes (all p > 0.10), although the differences for microstate classes C and D were of medium unadjusted effect sizes (Cohen's d = −0.42 and 0.51, respectively).

DISCUSSION

The current study systematically examined the dynamics of brain electric microstates characterizing the resting-state high-density electroencephalograms of people suffering from Insomnia Disorder and matched healthy controls. Using a data-driven approach, we identified 5 representative microstate classes, similar to those found in previous studies. Between-group comparison showed specifically that the mean duration of class C microstates in ID is shortened, and moreover indicated that class D microstates occur more frequently in ID.

Previous investigations on resting-state EEG microstates predominantly fixed the number of microstate classes at 4 without verifying it with objective model selection criteria [reviewed in (10, 13)]. We applied the Krzanowski–Lai criterion to a hierarchical clustering procedure to determine the optimal number of microstate classes, an approach taken by some HD-EEG microstate studies (30, 37). A recent study with a large sample size used a much more complicated criterion to determine the number of clusters and found a total number of 7 microstate classes at the group level (14), among which the 5 classes with the greatest amounts of global explained variance resemble the 5 microstate classes we identified. This would suggest that the 5 topographies (labeled as microstate classes A, B, C, D, and E) indeed occurred in a sufficient proportion of the participants, whereas additional microstate

[2]We here report global explained variance calculated according to the formula given in Murray et al. (31). Studies that explicitly mentioned to have used the same formula reported a similar amount of global variance explained by the microstates (11, 30). However, when we examined the source code of a few open source software packages for microstate analysis, we found that the implementation therein deviates from this definition. The difference in definition may be one of the reasons accounting for the discrepancy between studies regarding the global variance explained by 4 microstate classes which has been recently noted (13).

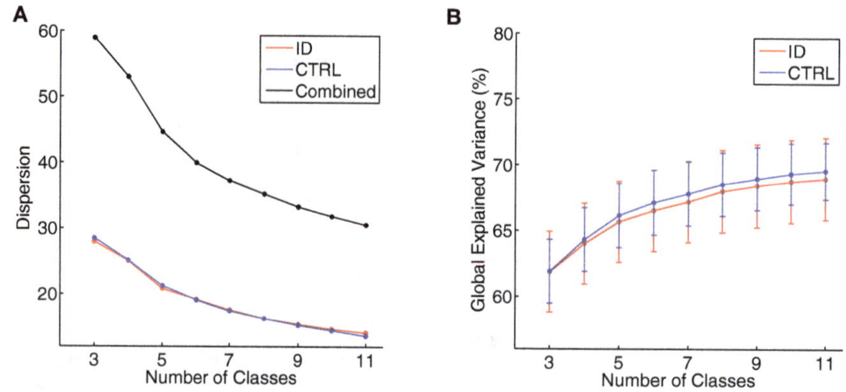

FIGURE 1 | (A) Group-level dispersion (i.e., within-cluster global dissimilarity) for 3- to 11-class models, displayed separately for people with Insomnia Disorder (ID, red line), healthy controls (CTRL, blue line), and all participants combined (black line). **(B)** Mean percentages of global variance explained by all microstate classes when microstate topographies resulting from 3- to 11-class models were fitted back to individual EEG data, displayed separately for people with Insomnia Disorder (ID, red line) and healthy controls (CTRL, blue line). Error bars indicate 95% confidence intervals.

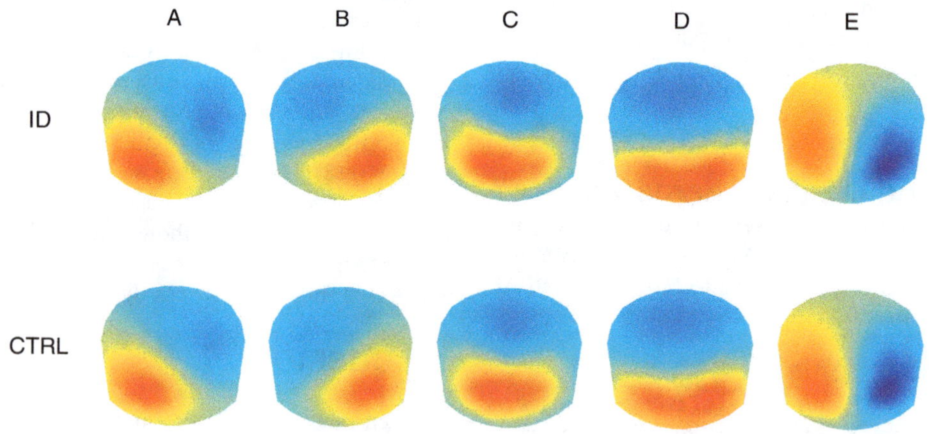

FIGURE 2 | Average topographic maps for the 5 optimal microstate classes **(A–E)** in people with Insomnia Disorder (ID) and healthy controls (CTRL). Note that by convention microstate labeling only depends on the spatial configuration while the absolute voltage and polarity are ignored.

clusters might be too idiosyncratic to be reliably detected with our smaller sample size. Due to the competitive fitting procedure in microstate analysis, adding or removing a microstate class may substantially affect the resulting dynamic features. Comparing results between studies that use different model orders might thus not be tenable. To address this concern, we performed additional sensitivity analysis adopting the conventional 4-class model (**Supplementary Figure 1**). It could be shown that different methodologies did not substantially affect the observed group differences of medium effect sizes (**Supplementary Table 2**). This allows us to interpret the functional significance of the current findings within the context of previous studies.

EEG microstates have been widely regarded as the "atoms" of conscious mentation (10, 13, 17). Since we did not collect data on subjective mental content, we could only speculate the functional relevance of our results by comparing with previous studies on subjective mental content in ID assessed with the ARSQ (5) and on the associations between microstate properties and ARSQ scores (19). The study by Pipinis et al. found a robust negative correlation across people between the proportional coverage time of class C microstates and somatic awareness, whereas a similar but slightly weaker negative correlation with somatic awareness was also reported for the mean duration of class C microstates (19). Further stepwise regression showed that a combination of the proportional coverage time of class C microstates and the frequency of occurrence of class D microstates optimally explained inter-individual variation in somatic awareness (19). Thus, among the dimensions of spontaneous mental content differing between people suffering from ID and people without sleep complaints (5), the current findings regarding class C and D microstates may be particularly relevant to elevated somatic awareness in ID.

Moreover, the salience network, commonly associated with microstate class C, has been implicated in a wide range of interoceptive and emotional experiences as well as in salience filtering, autonomic processing, and executive control

TABLE 2 | Microstate dynamic features (mean ± standard deviation).

	Microstate class	Control (n = 32)	Insomnia disorder (n = 32)	Cohen's d	p
Mean Duration (ms)	A	53.88 ± 7.84	51.45 ± 8.62	−0.30	0.45
	B	57.55 ± 11.02	53.54 ± 7.89	−0.42	0.18
	C	60.71 ± 16.74	52.69 ± 11.09	−0.57	0.0045
	D	60.40 ± 10.60	62.67 ± 15.43	0.17	0.31
	E	50.47 ± 7.58	47.30 ± 6.69	−0.44	0.30
Frequency of Occurrence (1/s)	A	3.42 ± 0.87	3.64 ± 0.80	0.26	0.47
	B	3.71 ± 0.45	3.89 ± 0.86	0.26	0.56
	C	3.67 ± 1.18	3.51 ± 1.41	−0.12	0.47
	D	3.80 ± 1.61	4.45 ± 1.09	0.47	0.018
	E	3.07 ± 0.77	3.02 ± 0.89	−0.05	0.78
Proportional Coverage Time (%)	A	18.04 ± 3.47	18.63 ± 4.65	0.14	0.66
	B	21.11 ± 3.92	20.50 ± 4.08	−0.15	0.50
	C	22.70 ± 10.47	18.74 ± 8.51	−0.42	0.10
	D	22.93 ± 9.92	28.02 ± 9.88	0.51	0.44
	E	15.23 ± 3.42	14.11 ± 4.14	−0.29	0.34

p-values are determined by linear mixed-effects (for mean duration and frequency of occurrence) and Dirichlet (for proportional coverage time) regression models with Wald z-tests.

(38–40). The fronto-parietal network, commonly associated with microstate class D, comprises systems typically involved in orienting and/or stimulus-driven shifts of attention (41, 42). It is therefore reasonable that the coordination between these networks implements key mechanisms whereby sensory stimuli arising from the body are gated into awareness. In sum, these converging lines of evidence suggest that the abnormal microstate dynamic patterns we find in people with ID could possibly underpin the heightened level of somatic awareness, which may in turn underlie their heightened somatization complaints (43–45).

Our findings appear consistent with a growing number of resting-state fMRI studies showing aberrations involving the salience and attention networks in ID (46–50). We note that resting-state fMRI and EEG microstates provide complementary insights into brain network functioning: Resting-state fMRI usually studies the correlation strength within or between networks, while EEG microstates give information about their temporal activity patterns. Caveats in light of recent research, however, need to be mentioned in regard to interpreting the neural substrates of the current results. First, there is still an ongoing debate on whether EEG microstates represent time periods during which the associated networks are activated or inhibited (13, 14, 16). Second, the above discussion has followed the majority of previous works on EEG microstates by interpreting the functional roles of the microstate classes with reference to their intra-individual BOLD correlates in distinct brain networks reported in a simultaneous EEG-fMRI study (15). On the other hand, because intra-individual and inter-individual variations in microstate properties can be driven by different mental processes (18), other neural sources might be responsible for the observed differences (14, 16).

Although TANOVA suggested significant between-group topographical differences for microstate class A, the spatial correlations between the average topographies of the two groups were high for all microstate classes (Pearson r = 0.996, 0.998, 0.997, 0.998, and 0.997 for microstate classes A, B, C, D, and E, respectively). To further explore the topographical differences for microstate class A, electrode-wise t-tests were carried out. Results indicated that group differences were mainly circumscribed to the left lateral parietal region, where the normalized absolute voltage was lower in ID. This finding might reflect subtly but systematically different network activity between the groups contributed by regional sources within a largely intact distributed network.

The stringent selection criteria the current study employed ensured that anxiety and depression symptom severity for all participants was below clinical thresholds, although it could still be observed that people with ID tended to report higher levels of anxiety and depression than CTRL. Of note, among the instruments we used to assess anxiety and depression, the BDI-IA includes items on sleep and fatigue which overlap with ID symptomology. The group differences are in line with previous studies showing that people with ID and no depression or anxiety disorders are likely to report mild levels of depression and anxiety (51, 52), and in line with recently found strong genetic correlations of insomnia with both anxiety and depression (53, 54). Curiously few studies have investigated EEG microstate alterations in depression and anxiety disorders. One study found an increased mean duration and more proportional coverage time of class A microstates as well as reduced frequency of occurrence of class C microstates in patients with panic disorder (55). These effects differ from the ones we here report for ID. An early study focused on EEG microstates in depression (56). The methodology of this study deviates substantially from contemporary microstate analysis, making the results difficult to be compared with. More research is needed in order to better disentangle how microstate properties are related to depression, anxiety, and insomnia.

EEG microstate analysis may serve as a valuable paradigm for future investigations on nocturnal mentation in ID. Previous studies have shown that insomnia severity is associated with the frequency of thought-like nocturnal mentation (57) which might be experienced as wakefulness (58). It is still unclear, however, whether (and how) distinct nocturnal thought content contributes differentially to the experience of insomnia (59, 60). While self-report provides a more direct assessment of mental content, it bears challenging methodological limitations for nocturnal mentation. Real-time reporting would interfere with the very process of sleep initiation or maintenance under study, while responses collected after a night of sleep are prone to forgetting or recall bias. In comparison, using EEG to assess the neural correlates of mentation is less disruptive and not hampered by these limitations. It awaits future investigations to validate the value of EEG microstate features and other possible neural correlates of momentary mental content in evaluating the content of nocturnal mentation, and in bridging the gaps in current understanding of ID.

CONCLUSIONS

The current study assessed, for the first time, resting-state EEG microstate dynamics in people with Insomnia Disorder as compared to matched healthy controls. It is found that ID is especially associated with a shorter mean duration of class C microstates and more frequent occurrence of class D microstates. These microstate alterations may underlie heightened somatic awareness in ID. Properties of EEG microstates are promising objective markers of mental content and could facilitate future investigations on nocturnal mentation or the subjective experience during the transition between wake and sleep or other conditions where self-report of mental content is not possible or desirable. Addressing somatic awareness could benefit psychotherapeutic treatment of insomnia, and the development of effective strategies to do so could profit from assessment of EEG microstate properties as possible biomarkers of somatic awareness.

AUTHOR CONTRIBUTIONS

JR, MC, and BtL collected the data. YW, MC, and BtL prepared and organized data in digital formats. YW and MC performed the analysis. EV supervised the project. YW wrote the manuscript. All authors participated in the revision of the manuscript.

FUNDING

Research leading to these results has received funding from the Bial Foundation grants 252/12 and 190/16, the Netherlands Organization of Scientific Research (NWO) grant VICI-453.07.001, and the European Research Council Advanced Grant 671084 INSOMNIA.

REFERENCES

1. Morin CM, Drake CL, Harvey AG, Krystal AD, Manber R, Riemann D, et al. Insomnia disorder. *Nat Rev Dis Prim.* (2015) 1:15026. doi: 10.1038/nrdp.2015.26
2. Harvey AG. A cognitive model of insomnia. *Behav Res Ther.* (2002) 40:869–93. doi: 10.1016/S0005-7967(01)00061-4
3. Espie CA, Broomfield NM, MacMahon KMA, Macphee LM, Taylor LM. The attention-intention-effort pathway in the development of psychophysiologic insomnia: a theoretical review. *Sleep Med Rev.* (2006) 10:215–45. doi: 10.1016/j.smrv.2006.03.002
4. Hiller RM, Johnston A, Dohnt H, Lovato N, Gradisar M. Assessing cognitive processes related to insomnia: a review and measurement guide for Harvey's cognitive model for the maintenance of insomnia. *Sleep Med Rev.* (2015) 23:46–53. doi: 10.1016/j.smrv.2014.11.006
5. Palagini L, Cellini N, Mauri M, Mazzei I, Simpraga S, Dell'Osso L, et al. Multiple phenotypes of resting-state cognition are altered in insomnia disorder. *Sleep Health* (2016) 2:239–45. doi: 10.1016/j.sleh.2016.05.003
6. Diaz BA, Van Der Sluis S, Benjamins JS, Stoffers D, Hardstone R, Mansvelder HD, et al. The ARSQ 2.0 reveals age and personality effects on mind-wandering experiences. *Front Psychol.* (2014) 5:271. doi: 10.3389/fpsyg.2014.00271
7. Barrett LF. The future of psychology: connecting mind to brain. *Perspect Psychol Sci.* (2009) 4:326–39. doi: 10.1111/j.1745-6924.2009.01134.x
8. Christoff K, Irving ZC, Fox KCR, Spreng RN, Andrews-Hanna JR. Mind-wandering as spontaneous thought: a dynamic framework. *Nat Rev Neurosci.* (2016) 17:718–31. doi: 10.1038/nrn.2016.113
9. Kucyi A. Just a thought: how mind-wandering is represented in dynamic brain connectivity. *Neuroimage* (2018) doi: 10.1016/j.neuroimage.2017.07.001. [Epub ahead of print].
10. Khanna A, Pascual-Leone A, Michel CM, Farzan F. Microstates in resting-state EEG: current status and future directions. *Neurosci Biobehav Rev.* (2015) 49:105–13. doi: 10.1016/j.neubiorev.2014.12.010
11. Khanna A, Pascual-Leone A, Farzan F. Reliability of resting-state microstate features in electroencephalography. *PLoS ONE* (2014) 9:e114163. doi: 10.1371/journal.pone.0114163
12. Koenig T, Prichep L, Lehmann D, Sosa PV, Braeker E, Kleinlogel H, et al. Millisecond by millisecond, year by year: normative EEG microstates and developmental stages. *Neuroimage* (2002) 16:41–8. doi: 10.1006/nimg.2002.1070
13. Michel CM, Koenig T. EEG microstates as a tool for studying the temporal dynamics of whole-brain neuronal networks: a review. *Neuroimage* (2018) doi: 10.1016/j.neuroimage.2017.11.062. [Epub ahead of print].
14. Custo A, Van Der Ville D, Wells WM, Tomescu MI, Brunet D, Michel CM. Electroencephalographic resting-state networks: source localization of microstates. *Brain Connect.* (2017) 7:671–82. doi: 10.1089/brain.2016.0476
15. Britz J, Van De Ville D, Michel CM. BOLD correlates of EEG topography reveal rapid resting-state network dynamics. *Neuroimage* (2010) 52:1162–70. doi: 10.1016/j.neuroimage.2010.02.052
16. Milz P, Pascual-Marqui RD, Achermann P, Kochi K, Faber PL. The EEG microstate topography is predominantly determined by intracortical sources in the alpha band. *Neuroimage* (2017) 162:353–61. doi: 10.1016/j.neuroimage.2017.08.058

17. Lehmann D. Consciousness: microstates of the brain's electric field as atoms of thought and emotion. In: Pereira A Jr, Lehmann D, editors. *The Unity of Mind, Brain and World: Current Perspectives on a Science of Consciousness.* Cambridge: Cambridge University Press (2013). p. 191–218.
18. Milz P, Faber PL, Lehmann D, Koenig T, Kochi K, Pascual-Marqui RD. The functional significance of EEG microstates—associations with modalities of thinking. *Neuroimage* (2016) 125:643–56. doi: 10.1016/j.neuroimage.2015.08.023
19. Pipinis E, Melynyte S, Koenig T, Jarutyte L, Linkenkaer-Hansen K, Ruksenas O, et al. Association between resting-state microstates and ratings on the Amsterdam Resting-State Questionnaire. *Brain Topogr.* (2017) 30:245–8. doi: 10.1007/s10548-016-0522-2
20. American Psychiatric Association. *Diagnostic and Statistical Manual of Mental Disorder* 5th ed. Washington, DC: American Psychiatric Publishing (2013).
21. Wei Y, Ramautar JR, Colombo MA, Stoffers D, Gómez-Herrero G, van der Meijden WP, et al. I keep a close watch on this heart of mine: increased interoception in insomnia. *Sleep* (2016) 39:2113–24. doi: 10.5665/sleep.6308
22. Zigmond AS, Snaith RP. The hospital anxiety and depression scale. *Acta Psychiatr Scand.* (1983) 67:361–70. doi: 10.1111/j.1600-0447.1983.tb09716.x
23. Beck AT, Epstein N, Brown G, Steer RA. An inventory for measuring clinical anxiety: psychometric properties. *J Consult Clin Psychol.* (1988) 56:893–7. doi: 10.1037/0022-006X.56.6.893
24. Beck AT, Steer RA. *Manual for the Beck Depression Inventory.* San Antonio, TX: Psychological Corporation (1993).
25. Bastien CH, Vallières A, Morin CM. Validation of the Insomnia Severity Index as an outcome measure for insomnia research. *Sleep Med.* (2001) 2:297–307. doi: 10.1016/S1389-9457(00)00065-4
26. Katkovnik V, Egiazarian K, Astola J. *Local Approximation Techniques in Signal and Image Processing.* Bellingham, WA: SPIE Press (2006). p. 553.
27. Iglewicz B, Hoaglin DC. *How to Detect and Handle Outliers.* Milwaukee, WI: ASQC Quality Press (1993). (The ASQC Basic References in Quality Control: Statistical Techniques Vol. 16).
28. Jung T-P, Makeig S, Humphries C, Lee T-W, McKeown MJ, Iragui V, et al. Removing electroencephalographic artifacts by blind source separation. *Psychophysiology* (2000) 37:163–78. doi: 10.1111/1469-8986.3720163
29. Tomescu MI, Rihs TA, Becker R, Britz J, Custo A, Grouiller F, et al. Deviant dynamics of EEG resting state pattern in 22q11.2 deletion syndrome adolescents: a vulnerability marker of schizophrenia? *Schizophr Res.* (2014) 157:175–81. doi: 10.1016/j.schres.2014.05.036
30. Gschwind M, Hardmeier M, Van De Ville D, Tomescu MI, Penner I-K, Naegelin Y, et al. Fluctuations of spontaneous EEG topographies predict disease state in relapsing-remitting multiple sclerosis. *NeuroImage Clin.* (2016) 12:466–77. doi: 10.1016/j.nicl.2016.08.008
31. Murray MM, Brunet D, Michel CM. Topographic ERP analyses: a step-by-step tutorial review. *Brain Topogr.* (2008) 20:249–64. doi: 10.1007/s10548-008-0054-5
32. R Core Team. *R: A Language and Environment for Statistical Computing.* Vienna: R Foundation for Statistical Computing (2015).
33. Bates D, Mächler M, Bolker B, Walker S. Fitting linear mixed-effects models using lme4. *J Stat Softw.* (2015) 67:1. doi: 10.18637/jss.v067.i01
34. Gueorguieva R, Rosenheck R, Zelterman D. Dirichlet component regression and its applications to psychiatric data. *Comput Stat Data Anal.* (2008) 52:5344–55. doi: 10.1016/j.csda.2008.05.030
35. Maier MJ. *DirichletReg: Dirichlet Regression for Compositional Data in R.* Vol. 125, Research Report Series/Department of Statistics and Mathematics. WU Vienna University of Economics and Business (2014).
36. Rieger K, Diaz Hernandez L, Baenninger A, Koenig T. 15 years of microstate research in schizophrenia—where are we? A meta-analysis. *Front Psychiatry* (2016) 7:22. doi: 10.3389/fpsyt.2016.00022
37. Hatz F, Hardmeier M, Bousleiman H, Rüegg S, Schindler C, Fuhr P. Reliability of functional connectivity of electroencephalography applying microstate-segmented versus classical calculation of phase lag index. *Brain Connect.* (2016) 6:461–9. doi: 10.1089/brain.2015.0368
38. Medford N, Critchley HD. Conjoint activity of anterior insular and anterior cingulate cortex: awareness and response. *Brain Struct Funct.* (2010) 214:535–49. doi: 10.1007/s00429-010-0265-x
39. Menon V. Large-scale brain networks and psychopathology: a unifying triple network model. *Trends Cogn Sci.* (2011) 15:483–506. doi: 10.1016/j.tics.2011.08.003
40. Uddin LQ. Salience processing and insular cortical function and dysfunction. *Nat Rev Neurosci.* (2015) 16:55–61. doi: 10.1038/nrn3857
41. Vossel S, Geng JJ, Fink GR. Dorsal and ventral attention systems: distinct neural circuits but collaborative roles. *Neuroscience* (2014) 20:150–9. doi: 10.1177/1073858413494269
42. Petersen SE, Posner MI. The attention system of the human brain: 20 years after. *Annu Rev Neurosci.* (2012) 35:73–89. doi: 10.1146/annurev-neuro-062111-150525
43. Hammad MA, Barsky AJ, Regestein QR. Correlation between somatic sensation inventory scores and hyperarousal scale scores. *Psychosomatics* (2001) 42:29–34. doi: 10.1176/appi.psy.42.1.29
44. Zhang J, Lam S-P, Li SX, Tang NL, Yu MWM, Li AM, et al. Insomnia, sleep quality, pain, and somatic symptoms: sex differences and shared genetic components. *Pain* (2012) 153:666–73. doi: 10.1016/j.pain.2011.12.003
45. Wei Y, Blanken TF, Van Someren EJW. Insomnia really hurts: effect of a bad night's sleep on pain increases with insomnia severity. *Front Psychiatry* (2018) 9:377. doi: 10.3389/fpsyt.2018.00377
46. Tagliazucchi E, Van Someren EJW. The large-scale functional connectivity correlates of consciousness and arousal during the healthy and pathological human sleep cycle. *Neuroimage* (2017) 160:55–72. doi: 10.1016/j.neuroimage.2017.06.026
47. Li S, Tian J, Li M, Wang T, Lin C, Yin Y, et al. Altered resting state connectivity in right side frontoparietal network in primary insomnia patients. *Eur Radiol.* (2018) 28:664–72. doi: 10.1007/s00330-017-5012-8
48. Dong X, Qin H, Wu T, Hu H, Liao K, Cheng F, et al. Rest but busy: aberrant resting-state functional connectivity of triple network model in insomnia. *Brain Behav.* (2018) 8:e00876. doi: 10.1002/brb3.876
49. Li Z, Chen R, Guan M, Wang E, Qian T, Zhao C, et al. Disrupted brain network topology in chronic insomnia disorder: a resting-state fMRI study. *NeuroImage Clin.* (2018) 18:178–85. doi: 10.1016/j.nicl.2018.01.012
50. Liu X, Zheng J, Liu B-X, Dai X-J. Altered connection properties of important network hubs may be neural risk factors for individuals with primary insomnia. *Sci Rep.* (2018) 8:5891. doi: 10.1038/s41598-018-23699-3
51. Carney CE, Ulmer C, Edinger JD, Krystal AD, Knauss F. Assessing depression symptoms in those with insomnia: an examination of the Beck Depression Inventory second edition (BDI-II). *J Psychiatr Res.* (2009) 43:576–82. doi: 10.1016/j.jpsychires.2008.09.002
52. Carney CE, Moss TG, Harris AL, Edinger JD, Krystal AD. Should we be anxious when assessing anxiety using the Beck Anxiety Inventory in clinical insomnia patients? *J Psychiatr Res.* (2011) 45:1243–9. doi: 10.1016/j.jpsychires.2011.03.011
53. Hammerschlag AR, Stringer S, de Leeuw CA, Sniekers S, Taskesen E, Watanabe K, et al. Genome-wide association analysis of insomnia complaints identifies risk genes and genetic overlap with psychiatric and metabolic traits. *Nat Genet.* (2017) 49:1584–92. doi: 10.1038/ng.3888
54. Jansen PR, Watanabe K, Stringer S, Skene N, Bryois J, Hammerschlag AR, et al. Genome-wide analysis of insomnia (N=1,331,010) identifies novel loci and functional pathways. *bioRxiv 214973* (2018). doi: 10.1101/214973
55. Kikuchi M, Koenig T, Munesue T, Hanaoka A, Strik W, Dierks T, et al. EEG microstate analysis in drug-naive patients with panic disorder. *PLoS ONE* (2011) 6:e22912. doi: 10.1371/journal.pone.0022912
56. Strik WK, Dierks T, Becker T, Lehmann D. Larger topographical variance and decreased duration of brain electric microstates in depression. *J Neural Transm.* (1995) 99:213–22. doi: 10.1007/BF01271480
57. Wassing R, Benjamins JS, Dekker K, Moens S, Spiegelhalder K, Feige B, et al. Slow dissolving of emotional distress contributes to hyperarousal. *Proc Natl Acad Sci USA.* (2016) 113:2538–43. doi: 10.1073/pnas.1522520113

58. Feige B, Nanovska S, Baglioni C, Bier B, Cabrera L, Diemers S, et al. Insomnia—perchance a dream? Results from a NREM/REM sleep awakening study in good sleepers and patients with insomnia. *Sleep* (2018) 41:zsy032. doi: 10.1093/sleep/zsy032
59. Fichten CS, Libman E, Creti L, Amsel R, Sabourin S, Brender W, et al. Role of thoughts during nocturnal awake times in the insomnia experience of older adults. *Cognit Ther Res.* (2001) 25:665–92. doi: 10.1023/A:1012963121729
60. Alapin I, Libman E, Bailes S, Fichten CS. Role of nocturnal cognitive arousal in the complaint of insomnia among older adults. *Behav Sleep Med.* (2003) 1:155–70. doi: 10.1207/S15402010BSM0103_3

10

Enhanced Network Efficiency of Functional Brain Networks in Primary Insomnia Patients

Xiaofen Ma[1], Guihua Jiang[1], Shishun Fu[1], Jin Fang[1], Yunfan Wu[1], Mengchen Liu[1], Guang Xu[2] and Tianyue Wang[1]*

[1] Department of Medical Imaging, Guangdong Second Provincial General Hospital, Guangzhou, China, [2] Department of Neurology, Guangdong Second Provincial General Hospital, Guangzhou, China

***Correspondence:**
Guihua Jiang
mayuqin2004@163.com

Accumulating evidence from neuroimaging studies suggests that primary insomnia (PI) affects interregional neural coordination of multiple interacting functional brain networks. However, a complete understanding of the whole-brain network organization from a system-level perspective in PI is still lacking. To this end, we investigated in topological organization changes in brain functional networks in PI. 36 PI patients and 38 age-, sex-, and education-matched healthy controls were recruited. All participants underwent a series of neuropsychological assessments and resting-state functional magnetic resonance imaging scans. Individual whole-brain functional network were constructed and analyzed using graph theory-based network approaches. There were no significant differences with respect to age, sex, or education between groups ($P > 0.05$). Graph-based analyses revealed that participants with PI had a significantly higher total number of edges ($P = 0.022$), global efficiency ($P = 0.014$), and normalized global efficiency ($P = 0.002$), and a significantly lower normalized local efficiency ($P = 0.042$) compared with controls. Locally, several prefrontal and parietal regions, the superior temporal gyrus, and the thalamus exhibited higher nodal efficiency in participants with PI ($P < 0.05$, false discovery rate corrected). In addition, most of these regions showed increased functional connectivity in PI patients ($P < 0.05$, corrected). Finally, altered network efficiency was correlated with neuropsychological variables of the Epworth Sleepiness Scale and Insomnia Severity Index in patients with PI. PI is associated with abnormal organization of large-scale functional brain networks, which may account for memory and emotional dysfunction in people with PI. These findings provide novel implications for neural substrates associated with PI.

Keywords: primary insomnia, brain network, default mode network, small-world efficiency, resting-state magnetic resonance imaging

INTRODUCTION

Primary insomnia (PI) is one of the most prevalent chronic sleep disorders. PI refers to difficulty falling asleep or maintaining sleep for at least 1 month. It is associated with sequelae of daytime impairment or clinically significant distress, and it is not attributable to a medical, psychiatric, or environmental cause (1, 2). According to epidemiological reports, 10% of the adult population experiences chronic insomnia, and PI is estimated to occur in 25% of all people with chronic insomnia worldwide (3). Moreover, the rate of PI continues to grow globally with increasing industrialization, urbanization, and work pressures (3). PI results in daytime fatigue, mood disruption, and cognitive impairments, which can lead to various psychiatric and cognitive disorders (e.g., depressive and anxiety disorders) (4, 5). In addition, PI can negatively affect social productivity and life quality, as well as increase accident risk and health-care utilization (6, 7). However, despite the adverse socioeconomic impact of PI, the neurobiological causes and consequences of the disorder are not fully understood.

Recent advances of neuroimaging techniques have provided powerful tools with which to investigate the neurobiological mechanisms of insomnia. To date, many studies have used different neuroimaging modalities to examine insomnia-related alterations in brain structure, function, and metabolism. For example, using structural magnetic resonance imaging (MRI), brain atrophy is consistently observed with PI in a specific set of regions such as the hippocampus (8, 9) and frontoparietal cortex (10, 11). However, functional studies based on functional MRI (fMRI) and positron emission tomography frequently report insomnia-related increases in multiple regions of spontaneous brain activity and metabolism, which may be due to compensatory adaption (12–15). In addition to local alterations, given the interconnected nature of the human brain, an increasing number of studies have begun to examine abnormal interregional functional integration in insomnia. Killgore and colleagues tested the sensory–motor network in patients with sleep dysfunction and found that difficulty in falling asleep was associated with increased functional connectivity between the primary visual cortex and other sensory regions such as the primary auditory cortex, olfactory cortex, and supplementary motor area (16). Chen et al. studied the inner relationship between the salience network and emotional regions in patients with insomnia and found that these patients have increased functional connectivity between the insula and salience network (17). Furthermore, elevated functional connectivity between the insula and emotional circuit (cingulate cortex, thalamus, and precuneus) has been observed in PI (18). Taken together, these studies suggest that PI can be viewed as a global rather than focal disorder that affects interregional neural coordination of multiple rather than single functional systems.

Human whole-brain networks can be mapped from different modalities of non-invasive neuroimaging techniques such as resting-state fMRI (R-fMRI). R-fMRI is a promising tool for mapping intrinsic brain connectivity networks and has been widely applied to various brain disorders (19). These networks can be further characterized by graph-based approaches by mathematically modeling them as graphs composed of nodes interconnected by edges. With the graph-based approaches, several features are consistently found in healthy brain networks, such as small-worldness (20), modularity (21), and hubs (22). Moreover, accumulating evidence suggests that abnormalities in these configurations are largely responsible for cognitive and behavioral dysfunctions in various brain disorders (23, 24), However, to date, few studies have examined whether and how PI alters whole-brain network organization from a system-level perspective of network segregation and integrity.

In this study, we used graph-based approaches to investigate topological abnormalities of functional brain networks in individuals with PI and to examine clinical correlates of the alterations. Among numerous graph theory-based measures, we exclusively focused on small-world organization because it is one of the most widely used models for human brain network studies (20). The small-world model, which was originally proposed in terms of parameters of clustering coefficient and characteristic path length (25), is an attractive model to characterize brain networks because the combination of high local clustering and short path length supports the two fundamental organizational principles in the brain: functional segregation and functional integration. Subsequently, the small-world theory is expanded based on two biologically more sensible measures: efficiency and cost (26). Compared with conventional clustering coefficient and characteristic path length measures, the combination of efficiency and cost has a number of technical and conceptual advantages since it can (i) represent how efficiently a network exchanges information at local and global levels with a single measure, (ii) examine the economical small-world properties of a network in the sense of providing high global and local efficiency of parallel information processing at low wiring costs, and (iii) deal with disconnected and/or non-sparse graphs (26, 27). To this end, we collected R-fMRI data from 36 patients with PI and 38 age-, sex-, and education-matched healthy controls (HCs). We then constructed individual functional brain networks by calculating interregional functional connectivity of spontaneous blood oxygen level dependent (BOLD) time series signals among 246 regions of interest (ROIs). Next, graph theory-based approaches were used to topologically characterize the resultant networks at global and nodal levels. Finally, PI-related network alterations were statistically inferred using a nonparametric permutation test and correlated with the results of patient neuropsychological assessment.

MATERIALS AND METHODS

Subjects

Patients with PI were recruited from the Department of Neurology at Guangdong No. 2 Provincial People's Hospital in Guangzhou, China from April 2014 to April 2016. The diagnosis of PI was made according to the Diagnostic and Statistical Manual of Mental Disorders, version 5. The exclusion criteria included (i) insomnia secondary to severe mental diseases (e.g., depression, anxiety, or epilepsy), (ii) other sleep disorders, (iii) history of serious organic disease including significant head trauma or loss of consciousness >30 min, (iv) history of medication treatment for insomnia, (v) history of alcohol, drug, or tobacco abuse, (vi) intense signal on conventional T1- and T2-FLAIR MRI, and (vii) female patients who were pregnant, nursing, or menstruating. We enrolled patients with PI who had all of the following symptoms according to the Pittsburgh Sleep Quality Index (PSQI) (28) and the Insomnia Severity Index (ISI) (29): early awakening, difficulty falling asleep, and difficulty maintaining sleep. In total, 36 patients with PI (12 men; mean age = 38.67 ± 9.53 years) were included in this study. By means of advertisements, we also recruited 38 age-, sex-, and education-matched HCs from the local community (12 men; mean age = 37.79 ± 9.92 years). HCs were included in the study according to the following criteria: (i) good sleep quality and an ISI score <7, (ii) no brain lesions or prior substantial head trauma as verified by conventional T1- or T2-FLAIR MRI, and (iii) no history of psychiatric or neurological diseases. All participants were right handed as assessed using the Edinburgh Handedness Inventory (30). This study was approved by the Ethics Committee of Guangdong No. 2 Provincial People's Hospital, and all participants provided informed written consent before MR scanning.

Neuropsychological Assessment

Each participant underwent a series of neuropsychological assessments to evaluate their sleep situation and mental status, including the PSQI, the Epworth Sleepiness Scale (ESS) (31), the ISI, the Self-rating Anxiety Scale (SAS) (32), and the Self-rating Depression Scale (SDS) (32).

Data Acquisition

All participants were scanned using a 3.0-T Ingenia MRI scanner (Philips Healthcare, The Netherlands) at the Department of Medical Imaging of Guangdong No. 2 Provincial People's Hospital. During R-fMRI data acquisition, participants were asked to lie quietly with their eyes closed and not think of anything specific or fall asleep while inside the scanner. The detailed acquisition parameters were as follows: repetition time (TR) = 2,000 ms, echo time (TE) = 35 ms, flip angle (FA) = 90°, slice thickness = 3.6 mm with a 0.7-mm gap, matrix = 64 × 64, field of view (FOV) = 230 mm × 230 mm, and 35 transverse planes parallel to the AC–PC line. The R-fMRI scan lasted for 8 min, and a total of 240 volumes were obtained for each participant. In addition, individual high-resolution anatomical images were acquired using a T1-weighted three-dimensional volumetric magnetization-prepared rapid acquisition gradient-echo sequence: 185 axial slices, TR = 8.4 ms, TE = 3.9 ms, FA = 8°, slice thickness = 1.0 mm, no gap, matrix = 256 × 256, and FOV = 256 mm × 256 mm.

Data Preprocessing

Data preprocessing was performed using the GRETNA toolbox based on the SPM12 package (http://www.fil.ion.ucl.ac.uk/spm/software/spm12/) and included (i) removal of the first 10 volumes to allow for T1 equilibration effects, (ii) realignment to correct for spatial displacements due to head motion, (iii) spatial normalization into the Montreal Neurological Institute space *via* segmentation of structural images, (iv) removal of linear trend, (v) temporal band-pass filtering (0.01–0.08 Hz), and (vi) nuisance regression of white matter signals, cerebrospinal fluid signals, and 24-parameter head-motion profiles (33). Participants with head motion >2 mm or >2° in any direction were excluded. There were no significant differences in the maximum, root mean square, and mean framewise displacement of head motion profiles between groups (all $P > 0.05$). The white matter and cerebrospinal fluid signals were derived by averaging signals within white matter and cerebrospinal fluid masks, respectively, in terms of prior probability maps in SPM12 (threshold = 0.8). We did not regress out global signals because this is a controversial preprocessing step for R-fMRI studies (34).

Network Construction

We constructed individual functional brain networks in a manner similar to previous studies (35–38). Briefly, we first parceled the cerebrum into 246 ROIs based on a prior brain atlas (39). We then calculated the mean BOLD signal time series for each ROI by averaging the signals across all voxels in that region. Next, the resultant mean time series were correlated with each other to generate a 246 × 246 correlation matrix for each participant. To denoise spurious interregional correlations in the results correlation matrices, we retained only those correlations whose corresponding P-values passed through a statistical threshold ($P < 0.05$, Bonferroni-corrected over connections). Such a significance level-based thresholding procedure effectively avoids erroneous evaluations of network topology (40). Finally, negative correlations were excluded due to their ambiguous interpretation (41–43) and detrimental effects on test–retest reliability (44).

Network Analysis

For the brain networks constructed above, we calculated several graph-based metrics to characterize their topological organization at different levels, including global small-world network efficiency (global efficiency, local efficiency, normalized global efficiency, and normalized local efficiency) and local nodal centrality (nodal efficiency). We briefly explain these metrics below in the context of a weighted network G with N nodes and K edges.

Small-World Efficiency

Efficiency is a biologically relevant metric to describe brain networks from the perspective of parallel information propagation and exchange (26, 27) and can be calculated at both global and local levels. Mathematically, global efficiency is defined as:

$$E_{\text{glob}}(G) = \frac{1}{N(N-1)} \sum_{i \neq j \in G} \frac{1}{d_{ij}} \tag{1}$$

where d_{ij} is the shortest path length between node i and node j in G and is calculated as the smallest sum of edge lengths throughout all possible paths from node i and node j. The length of an edge was designated as the reciprocal of the edge weight (i.e., correlation coefficient), which can be interpreted as a functional distance that a high correlation coefficient corresponds to a short functional distance. Global efficiency measures the ability of parallel information transmission over the network. The local efficiency of G is measured as:

$$E_{\text{loc}}(G) = \frac{1}{N} \sum_{i \in G} E_{\text{glob}}(G_i) \tag{2}$$

where $E_{\text{glob}}(G_i)$ is the global efficiency of G_i, the subgraph composed of the neighbors of node i (i.e., nodes linked directly to node i). Local efficiency measures the fault tolerance of the network, indicating the capability of information exchange for each subgraph when the index node is eliminated.

To determine whether brain networks had a small-world organization, local efficiency and global efficiency were normalized *via* dividing them by the corresponding mean derived from 100 random networks that preserved the same number of nodes, edges, and degree distributions as the real brain networks (45–47). Typically, a network with approximately equal global efficiency and larger local efficiency than matched random networks (i.e., normalized global efficiency ~1 and normalized local efficiency >1) is said to be a small-world network (25).

Nodal Centrality

We calculated nodal efficiency to capture the centrality of individual nodes in a network. The nodal efficiency of a given node i is calculated as (27):

$$e_i = \frac{1}{N-1} \sum_{j \neq i \in G} \frac{1}{d_{ij}}. \quad (3)$$

Nodal efficiency measures the ability of information propagation between a node and the remaining nodes in the network. A node with high nodal efficiency indicates high capability of information transmission with other nodes and can therefore be categorized as a hub.

Statistical Analysis

Between-Group Differences in Demographic and Neuropsychological Data

For demographic and clinical variables, between-group differences were examined using two-sample, two-tailed t-tests. These variables included age, education, and neuropsychological measurement scores (PSQI, ESS, ISI, SAS, and SDS). In addition, we used a two-tailed chi-square test to determine between-group differences in sex data.

Between-Group Differences in Network Organization

Between-group differences in network properties (global efficiency, local efficiency, normalized global efficiency, normalized local efficiency, and nodal efficiency) were determined by nonparametric permutation tests. Briefly, for each network metric, we first calculated the between-group difference in the mean values. An empirical distribution of the difference was then obtained by randomly reallocating all values into two groups and recalculating the mean differences between the two randomized groups (10,000 permutations). The 95th percentile points of the empirical distribution were used as critical values in a one-tailed test of whether the observed group differences could occur by chance. For comparisons of nodal efficiency, the false discovery rate (FDR) procedure was used to correct for multiple comparisons. Given the marginally significant between-group difference in education, we reanalyzed the above comparisons and obtained largely comparable results (data not shown).

Between-Group Differences in Functional Connectivity

To examine between-group differences in interregional functional connectivity, a network-based statistic (NBS) method (48) was followed. Briefly, a primary threshold ($P < 0.05$) was applied to the t-values (246 × 246 matrix) derived from an edge-by-edge between-group comparison of interregional functional connectivity (two-sample t-test). Among the resultant suprathreshold connections, we identified all connected components and recorded their size (i.e., number of links). To estimate the significance of each identified component, a null distribution of the connected component size was empirically derived using a permutation approach (10,000 permutations). For each permutation, all participants were randomly divided into two groups, and the same primary threshold (i.e., $P < 0.05$) was used to filter suprathreshold links in the comparison between the two randomized groups. The size of the maximal connected component among these links was recorded to form the null distribution. Finally, for any connected component of size M that was observed in the comparison of the right grouping, the corrected P value was determined by calculating the proportion of the 10,000 permutations for which the maximal connected component was larger than M. Notably, only connections that were positive in >85% of all participants were included in NBS analysis.

Brain–Behavior Relationships

For network metrics that showed significant PI-related alterations, partial correlation analyses were used to assess their relationships with neuropsychological measurements (PSQI, ESS, ISI, SAS, and SDS) and disease duration in the PI group. Effects of age, sex, and education were controlled during the correlation analysis. For the correlation analyses, we did not perform multiple correlation correction given the exploratory nature of this pilot study.

RESULTS

Demographic and Clinical Characteristics

Demographic, neuropsychological, and clinical characteristics of participants are shown in **Table 1**. The HC and PI groups showed no significant between-group differences in age (P = 0.699), sex (P = 0.872), or education (P = 0.054). The average disease duration for participants in the PI group was 28.61 months. As expected, patients with PI had higher PSQI, ISI, SAS, and SDS scores than the controls ($P < 0.001$) (**Table 1**).

TABLE 1 | Demographic, neuropsychological, and clinical characteristics of the participants.

	PI (n = 36)	HCs (n = 38)	P value
Age (years)	38.67 ± 9.53	37.79 ± 9.92	0.699
Gender (M/F)	12/24	12/26	0.872
Education (years)	10.06 ± 3.81	11.66 ± 3.20	0.054
PSQI	11.75 ± 3.78	1.68 ± 1.90	<0.001
ISI	17.28 ± 6.70	1.39 ± 2.40	<0.001
SAS	53.97 ± 10.12	42.45 ± 6.39	<0.001
SDS	52.92 ± 9.25	39.55 ± 10.58	<0.001
ESS	11.00 ± 4.63	–	–
Duration (months)	28.61 ± 43.58	–	–

PI, primary insomnia; HCs, healthy controls; M, male; F, female; PSQI, Pittsburgh Sleep Quality Index; ISI, Insomnia Severity Index; SAS, Self-rating Anxiety Scale; SDS, Self-rating Depression Scale; ESS, Epworth Sleepiness Scale.

Altered Small-World Efficiency in PI

The mean correlation matrices of the PI and HC groups are shown in **Figure 1**. We first examined the largest component size of each individual network. We found that networks of 30 HCs and 29 PI patients had no isolated nodes, and networks of all the other participants had one isolated node. Patients with PI had significantly more connections in their whole-brain networks compared with HCs (network density = 0.192 ± 0.056 and 0.222 ± 0.071 for the HC and PI groups, respectively; $P = 0.022$). Network efficiency analysis indicated that the functional brain networks of both groups exhibited small-world organization, as characterized by normalized local efficiency >1 (HC group: 1.270 ± 0.125; PI group: 1.221 ± 0.117) and normalized global efficiency approximately equal to 1 (HC group: 0.940 ± 0.019; PI group: 0.954 ± 0.022). Nevertheless, further statistical comparisons revealed that patients with PI had significantly higher global efficiency ($P = 0.014$) and normalized global efficiency ($P = 0.002$) as well as lower normalized local efficiency ($P = 0.042$) in comparison with HCs (**Figure 1**).

Altered Nodal Centrality in PI

The PI group had significantly increased nodal efficiency for 21 regions ($P < 0.05$, FDR corrected) compared with the HC group (**Figure 2**). These regions predominately encompassed the superior frontal gyrus, middle frontal gyrus, superior temporal gyrus, cingulate gyrus/precuneus, thalamus, superior parietal lobule, and supramarginal gyrus.

Altered Functional Connectivity in PI

We identified one connected component that exhibited increased functional connectivity among participants with PI as compared with HCs ($P = 0.044$, corrected) (**Table 2**; **Figure 3**). The component included 22 nodes and 27 edges and mainly involved the parietal and prefrontal regions and the insula. It is worth mentioning that most of the regions showing increased nodal efficiency, as described earlier, were included in this component. No components showed significantly decreased functional connectivity in a comparison between PI patients and HCs.

Brain–Behavior Relationship

Among patients with PI, ESS scores exhibited significant negative correlations with the total number of edges ($r = -0.358$; $P = 0.041$) and global efficiency ($r = -0.375$; $P = 0.031$) and a significant positive correlation with normalized local efficiency ($r = 0.430$; $P = 0.013$) (**Figure 4**). In addition, a significant negative correlation was found between ISI scores and normalized local efficiency ($r = -0.354$; $P = 0.044$) (**Figure 4**). No significant correlations were found between other network measures and neuropsychological variables (all $P > 0.05$).

DISCUSSION

In this study, we examined the topology of functional brain networks in patients with PI by graph theory-based analysis of R-fMRI. Our results suggest that patients with PI had overly connected functional brain networks as characterized by increased global network efficiency and increased nodal centrality as well as elevated interregional functional connectivity of regions, mainly in the default mode network (DMN) and emotional circuit. Moreover, altered network architecture was related to patient neuropsychological performance. These findings may contribute to a better understanding of the neurobiological mechanisms underlying PI.

The human brain is a complex, interconnected network that continuously integrates information across multiple sensory systems. Numerous studies suggest that its powerful performance originates mainly from a nontrivial topological wiring diagram such as efficient small-world architecture (19, 49, 50). In this study, we found that patients with PI exhibited the increased overall connectivity in their functional brain networks is consistent with previous studies reporting increased functional connectivity and structural connectivity in PI (18, 51, 52). Increased overall connectivity could also explain why increased

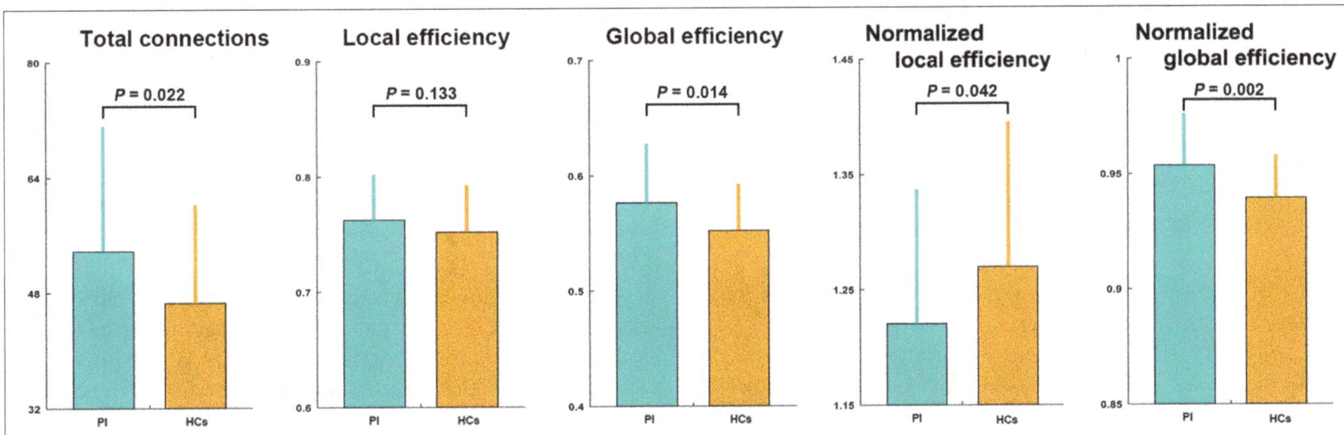

FIGURE 1 | Between-group differences in total number of connections and network efficiency of functional brain networks. Patients with PI had significantly higher total connections ($P = 0.022$), global efficiency ($P = 0.014$), and normalized global efficiency ($P = 0.002$), and lower normalized local efficiency ($P = 0.042$) compared with controls. Error bars denote mean and SD. PI, primary insomnia; HCs, healthy controls.

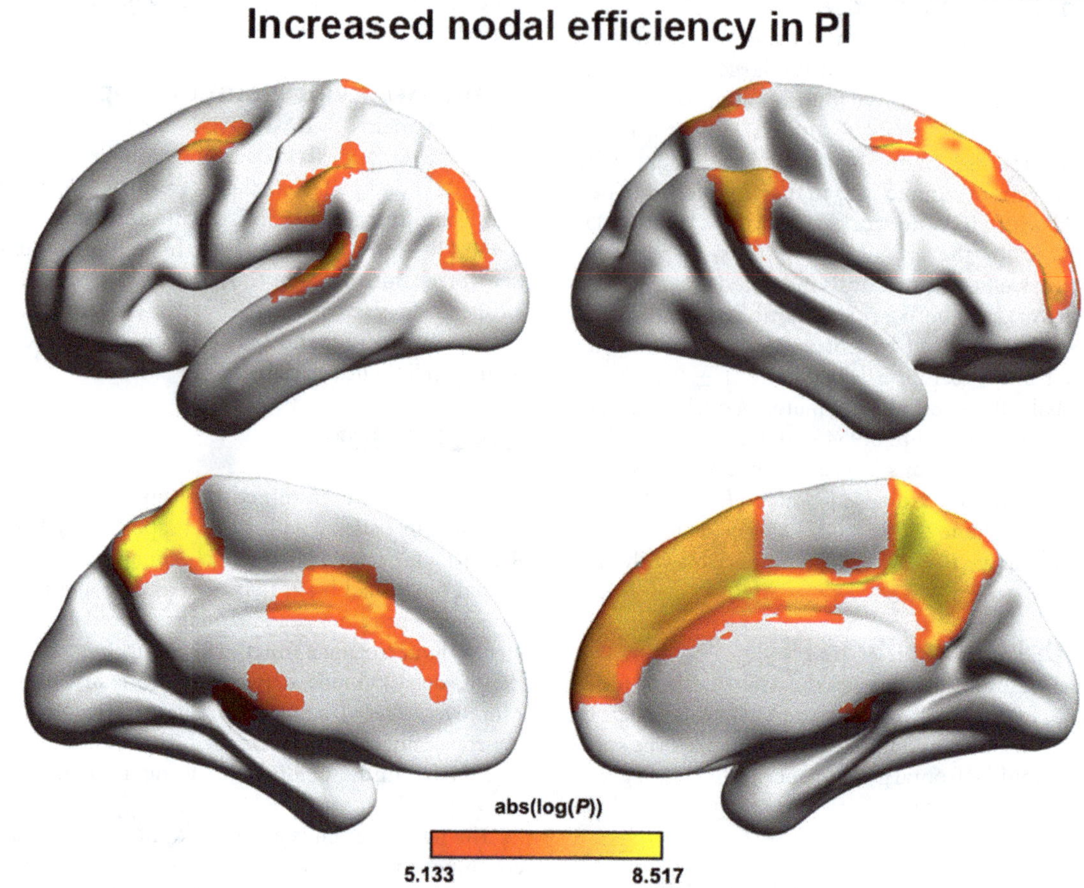

FIGURE 2 | Between-group differences in regional nodal efficiency. Warm color regions show significantly increased nodal efficiency of several prefrontal and parietal regions, the superior temporal gyrus, and the thalamus in patients with PI ($P < 0.05$, corrected). PI, primary insomnia.

global efficiency was observed in patients with PI because more connections (i.e., larger network density) might result in more routing paths and therefore more efficient information propagation and exchanges. However, after normalization by matched random networks, global efficiency was still larger in patients with PI than in the controls. This suggests that increased global efficiency of functional brain networks in patients with PI is not entirely due to more connections but instead may reflect an intrinsic alteration in brain wiring patterns. Global efficiency is mainly reflects integrative information processing across brain remote regions that constitutes the basis of cognitive processing (53). Thus, the observed increase of global efficiency implies a hyperactive functional integration of patient brains. This is supported by our findings of increased nodal efficiency and functional connectivity for numerous regions in patients with PI. We discuss the PI-related increases in detail below.

In addition to increased global efficiency, participants with PI had decreased normalized local efficiency which may be explained by impaired functional segregation of patient brains (26). As normal brain function requires an optimal balance between local specialization and global integration, the combination of increased global efficiency and decreased normalized local efficiency indicates a disruption in the normal balance and suggests a tendency toward random network configuration of functional brain networks in patients with PI.

Interestingly, we found that increased overall connectivity and altered network efficiency were related to behavioral disturbances, as indicated by the ESS and ISI scores of patients with PI. ESS is a validated questionnaire that is widely used to assess subjective sleepiness and sleep propensity. Existing evidence suggests that different levels of complaints of daytime sleepiness are broadly experienced by people with insomnia (54). The ISI is a brief instrument that was designed to assess severity of both nighttime and daytime components of insomnia (31). Thus, our results suggest that topological alterations of functional brain networks may account for excessive daytime sleepiness and sleep dysfunction among people with PI.

After examining PI-related network alterations globally, we also investigated PI-related alterations in regional nodal centrality and interregional functional connectivity. At the nodal level, multiple regions that showed increased nodal efficiency were mainly in the DMN (e.g., precuneus, prefrontal cortex, and superior parietal lobule) and emotional circuit (e.g., cingulate cortex, thalamus, and frontal gyrus) in participants with PI. Nodal efficiency measures the extent of information exchange between a given node and all other nodes in a network and therefore

TABLE 2 | Connections showing increased functional connectivity in the PI patients.

Region A			Region B			
Abbr	**Name**	**MNI**	**Abbr**	**Name**	**MNI**	***P* value**
SFG_R_7_5	Superior frontal gyrus	[7, −4, 60]	STG_L_6_3	Superior temporal gyrus	[−50, −11, 1]	0.0445
SPL_L_5_1	Superior parietal lobule	[−16, −60, 63]	SPL_R_5_1	Superior parietal lobule	[19, −57, 65]	0.0408
SPL_L_5_1	Superior parietal lobule	[−16, −60, 63]	SPL_L_5_2	Superior parietal lobule	[−15, −71, 52]	0.0087
SPL_L_5_2	Superior parietal lobule	[−15, −71, 52]	SPL_R_5_2	Superior parietal lobule	[19, −69, 54]	0.0059
PrG_L_6_5	Precentral gyrus	[−52, 0, 8]	IPL_L_6_6	Supramarginal gyrus	[−53, −31, 23]	0.0438
IPL_L_6_3	Supramarginal gyrus	[−51, −33, 42]	IPL_L_6_6	Supramarginal gyrus	[−53, −31, 23]	0.0060
SPL_L_5_2	Superior parietal lobule	[−15, −71, 52]	Pcun_L_4_1	Precuneus	[−5, −63, 51]	0.0023
SPL_R_5_2	Superior parietal lobule	[19, −69, 54]	Pcun_R_4_1	Precuneus	[6, −65, 51]	0.0207
PCL_R_2_1	Paracentral lobule	[10, −34, 54]	Pcun_L_4_2	Precuneus	[−8, −47, 57]	0.0151
PCL_R_2_1	Paracentral lobule	[10, −34, 54]	Pcun_R_4_2	Precuneus	[7, −47, 58]	0.0417
SPL_R_5_2	Superior parietal lobule	[19, −69, 54]	Pcun_R_4_2	Precuneus	[7, −47, 58]	0.0282
Pcun_L_4_2	Precuneus	[−8, −47, 57]	Pcun_R_4_2	Precuneus	[7, −47, 58]	0.0442
PrG_L_6_5	Precentral gyrus	[−52, 0, 8]	INS_L_6_5	Rostrodorsal posterior insula	[−38, −8, 8]	0.0242
PoG_L_4_2	Postcentral gyrus	[−56, −14, 16]	INS_L_6_6	Caudoventral anterior insula	[−38, 5, 5]	0.0334
INS_L_6_1	Caudodorsal posterior insula	[−36, −20, 10]	INS_L_6_6	Caudoventral anterior insula	[−38, 5, 5]	0.0021
INS_L_6_5	Rostrodorsal posterior insula	[−38, −8, 8]	INS_L_6_6	Caudoventral anterior insula	[−38, 5, 5]	0.0002
STG_L_6_3	Superior temporal gyrus	[−50, −11, 1]	CG_L_7_5	Cingulate gyrus	[−5, 7, 37]	0.0252
IPL_L_6_6	Supramarginal gyrus	[−53, −31, 23]	CG_L_7_5	Cingulate gyrus	[−5, 7, 37]	0.0154
PCL_R_2_1	Paracentral lobule	[10, −34, 54]	CG_L_7_6	Cingulate gyrus	[−7, −23, 41]	0.0049
Pcun_L_4_2	Precuneus	[−8, −47, 57]	CG_L_7_6	Cingulate gyrus	[−7, −23, 41]	0.0014
Pcun_R_4_2	Precuneus	[7, −47, 58]	CG_L_7_6	Cingulate gyrus	[−7, −23, 41]	0.0046
CG_L_7_5	Cingulate gyrus	[−5, 7, 37]	CG_L_7_6	Cingulate gyrus	[−7, −23, 41]	0.0420
CG_R_7_5	Cingulate gyrus	[4, 6, 38]	CG_L_7_6	Cingulate gyrus	[−7, −23, 41]	0.0170
PCL_R_2_1	Paracentral lobule	[10, −34, 54]	CG_R_7_6	Cingulate gyrus	[6, −20, 40]	0.0062
Pcun_L_4_2	Precuneus	[−8, −47, 57]	CG_R_7_6	Cingulate gyrus	[6, −20, 40]	0.0089
Pcun_R_4_2	Precuneus	[7, −47, 58]	CG_R_7_6	Cingulate gyrus	[6, −20, 40]	0.0048
CG_L_7_6	Cingulate gyrus	[−7, −23, 41]	CG_R_7_6	Cingulate gyrus	[6, −20, 40]	0.0197

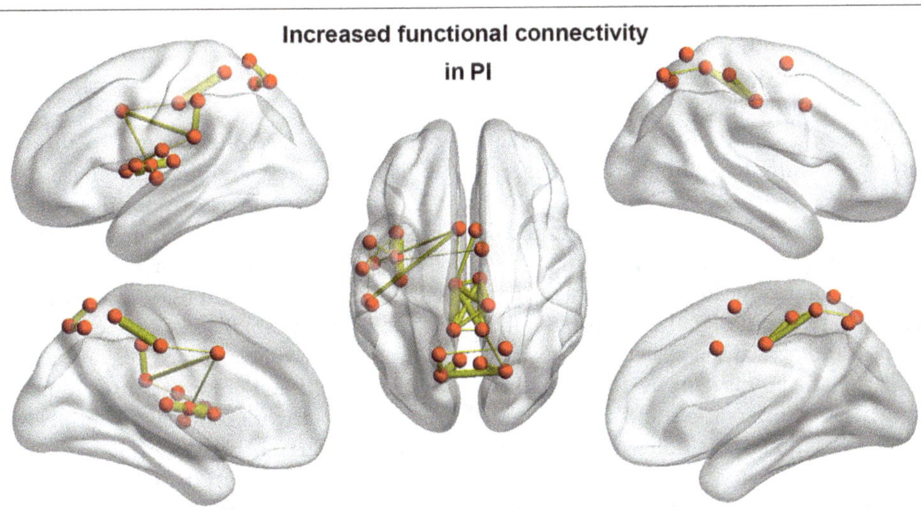

FIGURE 3 | Between-group differences in functional connectivity. Patients with PI showed significantly increased functional connectivity that mainly involved the parietal and prefrontal regions and the insula. Line width is proportional to the significance level of the between-group difference. PI, primary insomnia.

reflects the importance or information load of the node (27). Thus, increased nodal efficiency indicates higher information flow of these regions in patient brains. This is consistent with our findings that most of these regions exhibited increased functional connectivity in patients with PI. Interestingly, these regions are largely comparable to those reported to show hypermetabolism in patients with insomnia (12), which is also in agreement with recent findings that functional connectivity is closely coupled with metabolism (55, 56). Future studies are warranted to examine to what extent increased functional connectivity reflects hypermetabolism in PI.

The DMN includes a set of anatomically and functionally interconnected regions that are involved in a wide spectrum of cognitive processing. It is active when individuals are engaged

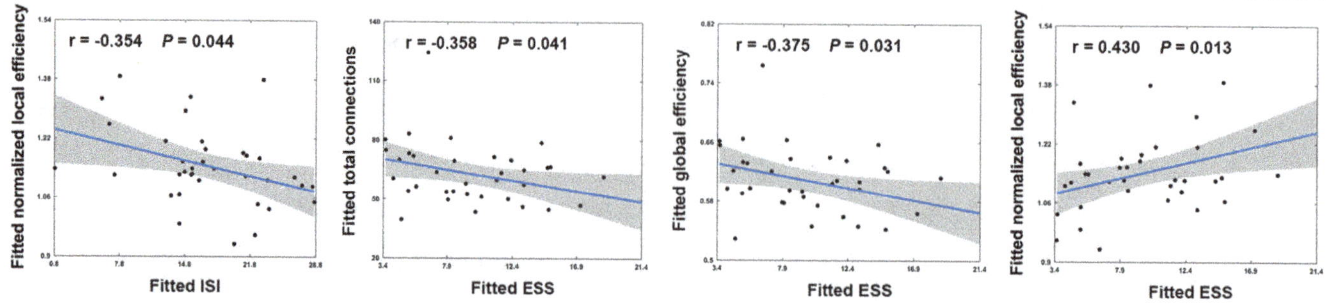

FIGURE 4 | Scatter plots showing significant correlations between network measures and neuropsychological variables in patients with PI. Effects of age, sex, and education were controlled during the correlation analyses. Thus, the fitted values (i.e., the observed network measures and neuropsychological variables minus the estimated effects of age, sex, and education) that are plotted reflect the "true" relationships. ISI, Insomnia Severity Index; ESS, Epworth Sleepiness Scale.

in internally focused tasks such as memory or self-relevant mental processing (57, 58). Using independent component analysis, a previous study found that people with insomnia had increased connectivity of the DMN (59), which is consistent with our findings. Intriguingly, we found that the DMN components affected by PI largely overlapped with the core regions of the mentalizing network (e.g., the medial prefrontal cortex and posterior cingulate cortex/precuneus), which is a subnetwork of the DMN that is typically activated when individuals are engaged in a working memory task (60–62). Clinically, working memory deterioration is the most common symptom of daytime dysfunction in PI (63, 64) and is one of the most apparent and arguably easiest to detect neural markers of PI (65, 66). Based on these findings, we hypothesize that increased nodal efficiency and functional connectivity of DMN regions in PI, particularly the mentalizing network, may reflect a compensatory mechanism of the brain to maintain normal working memory-related processing by adding or establishing new connections.

In addition to the DMN, increases in PI-related nodal efficiency occur in the emotional circuit. The emotional circuit mainly includes the amygdala, prefrontal lobe, thalamus, insular lobe, and cingulate cortex (67). Specifically, the prefrontal lobe and thalamus are central to the perception system and form a channel of prefrontal cortex–thalamus–corpus striatum that cumulatively allows for effective integration and handling of emotional regulation (68). Psychometric studies have demonstrated that emotional hyperarousal may be a primary neural mechanism underlying emotional regulation dysfunction (e.g., anxiety or depression) in patients with PI (69, 70). Similarly, numerous neuroimaging studies have reported overactivity of emotional processing-related brain regions (e.g., prefrontal lobe, thalamus, and insula) in PI (13, 15, 18). Furthermore, electrophysiological studies have found decreased levels of γ-aminobutyric acid in emotion-related regions of PI patients (71). The present findings are consistent with those of previous studies and provide further evidence for the emotional hyperarousal hypothesis from the perspective of functional integration. We hypothesize that increased efficiency in emotional regions may underlie emotional dysfunction frequently observed in PI.

Currently, the relationship between insomnia and emotional dysfunction is not fully understood. Previous studies indicate that sleep disturbances have detrimental effects on physical health and are thought to be a risk factor for development and maintenance of mood and anxiety disorders (72–75). Thus, high levels of anxiety and depression are frequently evident in patients with insomnia (76), and high rates of sleep disturbances are observed in patients with anxiety or depressive disorders (77). There are several possible explanations for the interrelationship between anxiety/depression and insomnia. One possibility is that they are simply comorbid, which may be explained by common maintenance mechanisms. Indeed, when we examined relationships between PSQI and ISI scores and scores from SAS and SDS, high positive correlations were found (all $r > 0.5$, $P < 0.001$). A second possibility is that insomnia is epiphenomenal to anxiety and depression or that anxiety and depression are epiphenomenal to insomnia. A third possibility is that anxiety and depression are risk factors for insomnia (78–81). In summary, insomnia and emotional dysfunction are tightly coupled and require further study. Notably, we did not observe significant correlations between increased nodal efficiency and SAS and SDS scores of PI patients, possibly due to the relatively small sample size.

Together, we determined that PI is associated with a hyperactive functional brain connectome as characterized by increased network efficiency and elevated functional connectivity. Currently, the biological mechanism underlying this hyperconnectivity is not fully understood, although it is a common phenomenon in brain disorders (82). Given the high plasticity and compensatory mechanisms of the human brain, one possible interpretation is that the brains of people with PI require ongoing recruitment of available detour paths to maintain normal function by adaptively adjusting regional connectivity profiles in response to pathological attacks and damage caused by the disease (83). More recently, a review indicated that this hyperconnectivity may be optimally expressed by increasing connections through the most central and metabolically efficient regions (84). This is consistent with our findings that increased PI-related efficiency and connectivity were mainly located in the DMN and emotional circuit, which are frequently reported to serve as highly connected hubs in the brain (22). Future studies may provide deeper insights into such hyperconnectivity by combining fMRI with other imaging techniques (e.g., structural and metabolic imaging) and biochemical techniques.

There are several further considerations that merit mention for this pilot study. First, the sample size was relatively small. Therefore, reproducibility of the current findings should be examined in a large cohort of patients. Second, the SDS and SAS scores of patients with PI were still higher than those of participants in the control group. In addition, we found increased functional connectivity of the emotional circle in the PI group. Thus, altered connectivity patterns among participants with PI may not be due to insomnia alone but may also result from secondary mood changes. Further studies are needed to clarify this point. Third, because of the cross-sectional design of this study, we cannot address the temporal relationship between functional brain networks reorganization and progression of PI. Longitudinal studies are needed to illuminate this important issue. Finally, functional brain networks arise from underlying structural pathways (85, 86). Although a recent diffusion tensor imaging study demonstrated abnormalities in several specific neural tracts in PI (87), whole-brain structural networks in PI remain largely unknown.

In summary, from the viewpoint of system-level network separation and integration, this study provides the first evidence for an aberrant functional connectome in PI, which is characterized by increased nodal centrality and interregional functional connectivity in the DMN and emotional circuit. These findings provide novel implications for neural substrates associated with PI.

AUTHOR CONTRIBUTIONS

GJ and XM designed experiments. XM, SF, and JF carried out experiments and analyzed experimental results. XM wrote the manuscript. JF assisted with statistical analysis. YW, ML, and TW assisted with carrying out experiments.

ACKNOWLEDGMENTS

The authors would like to express their appreciation to Dr. Xiaopeng Zong of the Department of Radiology and BRIC, University of North Carolina at Chapel Hill, Chapel Hill, NC, for technical support and constructive advices. We also thank all patients and volunteers for participating in this study. This work was funded by the National Natural Science Foundation of China (grant numbers: 81471639, 81771807), the Science and Technology Planning Project of Guangdong Province (grant number: 2017A020215077), and the science foundation of Guangdong Second Provincial General hospital (grant number: YQ2015-001).

REFERENCES

1. Edinger JD, Bonnet MH, Bootzin RR, Doghramji K, Dorsey CM, Espie CA, et al. Derivation of research diagnostic criteria for insomnia: report of an American academy of sleep medicine work group. *Sleep* (2004) 27:1567–96. doi:10.1093/sleep/27.8.1567
2. Roth T. Comorbid insomnia: current directions and future challenges. *Am J Manag Care* (2009) 15(Suppl):S6–13.
3. Roth T, Roehrs T. Insomnia: epidemiology, characteristics, and consequences. *Clin Cornerstone* (2003) 5:5–15. doi:10.1016/S1098-3597(03)90031-7
4. Taylor DJ, Lichstein KL, Durrence HH, Reidel BW, Bush AJ. Epidemiology of insomnia, depression, and anxiety. *Sleep* (2005) 28:1457–64. doi:10.1093/sleep/28.11.1457
5. Baglioni C, Battagliese G, Feige B, Spiegelhalder K, Nissen C, Voderholzer U, et al. Insomnia as a predictor of depression: a meta-analytic evaluation of longitudinal epidemiological studies. *J Affect Disord* (2011) 135:10–9. doi:10.1016/j.jad.2011.01.011
6. Roth T. Insomnia: definition, prevalence, etiology, and consequences. *J Clin Sleep Med* (2007) 3:S7–10.
7. Leger D, Bayon V. Societal costs of insomnia. *Sleep Med Rev* (2010) 14:379–89. doi:10.1016/j.smrv.2010.01.003
8. Riemann D, Voderholzer U, Spiegelhalder K, Hornyak M, Buysse DJ, Nissen C, et al. Chronic insomnia and MRI-measured hippocampal volumes: a pilot study. *Sleep* (2007) 30:955–8. doi:10.1093/sleep/30.8.955
9. Winkelman JW, Benson KL, Buxton OM, Lyoo IK, Yoon S, O'Connor S, et al. Lack of hippocampal volume differences in primary insomnia and good sleeper controls: an MRI volumetric study at 3 Tesla. *Sleep Med* (2010) 11:576–82. doi:10.1016/j.sleep.2010.03.009
10. Altena E, Vrenken H, Van Der Werf YD, van den Heuvel OA, Van Someren EJ. Reduced orbitofrontal and parietal gray matter in chronic insomnia: a voxel-based morphometric study. *Biol Psychiatry* (2010) 67:182–5. doi:10.1016/j.biopsych.2009.08.003
11. Joo EY, Noh HJ, Kim JS, Koo DL, Kim D, Hwang KJ, et al. Brain gray matter deficits in patients with chronic primary insomnia. *Sleep* (2013) 36:999–1007. doi:10.5665/sleep.2796
12. Nofzinger EA, Buysse DJ, Germain A, Price JC, Miewald JM, Kupfer DJ. Functional neuroimaging evidence for hyperarousal in insomnia. *Am J Psychiatry* (2004) 161:2126–8. doi:10.1176/appi.ajp.161.11.2126
13. Dai XJ, Peng DC, Gong HH, Wan AL, Nie X, Li HJ, et al. Altered intrinsic regional brain spontaneous activity and subjective sleep quality in patients with chronic primary insomnia: a resting-state fMRI study. *Neuropsychiatr Dis Treat* (2014) 10:2163–75. doi:10.2147/NDT.S69681
14. Li C, Ma X, Dong M, Yin Y, Hua K, Li M, et al. Abnormal spontaneous regional brain activity in primary insomnia: a resting-state functional magnetic resonance imaging study. *Neuropsychiatr Dis Treat* (2016) 12:1371–8. doi:10.2147/NDT.S109633
15. Wang T, Li S, Jiang G, Lin C, Li M, Ma X, et al. Regional homogeneity changes in patients with primary insomnia. *Eur Radiol* (2016) 26:1292–300. doi:10.1007/s00330-015-3960-4
16. Killgore WD, Schwab ZJ, Kipman M, Deldonno SR, Weber M. Insomnia-related complaints correlate with functional connectivity between sensory-motor regions. *Neuroreport* (2013) 24:233–40. doi:10.1097/WNR.0b013e32835edbdd
17. Chen MC, Chang C, Glover GH, Gotlib IH. Increased insula coactivation with salience networks in insomnia. *Biol Psychol* (2014) 97:1–8. doi:10.1016/j.biopsycho.2013.12.016
18. Wang T, Yan J, Li S, Zhan W, Ma X, Xia L, et al. Increased insular connectivity with emotional regions in primary insomnia patients: a resting-state fMRI study. *Eur Radiol* (2017) 27:3703–9. doi:10.1007/s00330-016-4680-0
19. Wang J, Zuo X, He Y. Graph-based network analysis of resting-state functional MRI. *Front Syst Neurosci* (2010) 4:16. doi:10.3389/fnsys.2010.00016
20. Liao X, Vasilakos AV, He Y. Small-world human brain networks: perspectives and challenges. *Neurosci Biobehav Rev* (2017) 77:286–300. doi:10.1016/j.neubiorev.2017.03.018

21. Sporns O, Betzel RF. Modular brain networks. *Annu Rev Psychol* (2016) 67:613–40. doi:10.1146/annurev-psych-122414-033634
22. Van den Heuvel MP, Sporns O. Network hubs in the human brain. *Trends Cogn Sci* (2013) 17:683–96. doi:10.1016/j.tics.2013.09.012
23. Bassett DS, Bullmore ET. Human brain networks in health and disease. *Curr Opin Neurol* (2009) 22:340–7. doi:10.1097/WCO.0b013e32832d93dd
24. Xia M, He Y. Magnetic resonance imaging and graph theoretical analysis of complex brain networks in neuropsychiatric disorders. *Brain Connect* (2011) 1:349–65. doi:10.1089/brain.2011.0062
25. Watts DJ, Strogatz SH. Collective dynamics of 'small-world' networks. *Nature* (1998) 393:440–2. doi:10.1103/PhysRevE.91.052815
26. Latora V, Marchiori M. Efficient behavior of small-world networks. *Phys Rev Lett* (2001) 87:198701. doi:10.1103/PhysRevLett.87.198701
27. Achard S, Bullmore E. Efficiency and cost of economical brain functional networks. *PLoS Comput Biol* (2007) 3:e17. doi:10.1371/journal.pcbi.0030017
28. Buysse DJ, Reynolds CF III, Monk TH, Berman SR, Kupfer DJ. The Pittsburgh sleep quality index: a new instrument for psychiatric practice and research. *Psychiatry Res* (1989) 28:193–213. doi:10.1016/0165-1781(89)90047-4
29. Bastien CH, Vallieres A, Morin CM. Validation of the Insomnia Severity Index as an outcome measure for insomnia research. *Sleep Med* (2001) 2:297–307. doi:10.1016/S1389-9457(00)00065-4
30. Oldfield RC. The assessment and analysis of handedness: the Edinburgh inventory. *Neuropsychologia* (1971) 9:97–113. doi:10.1016/0028-3932(71)90067-4
31. Doneh B. Epworth Sleepiness Scale. *Occup Med (Lond)* (2015) 65:508. doi:10.1093/occmed/kqv042
32. Gainotti G, Cianchetti C, Taramelli M, Tiacci C. The guided self-rating anxiety-depression scale for use in clinical psychopharmacology. *Act Nerv Super (Praha)* (1972) 14:49–51.
33. Friston KJ, Williams S, Howard R, Frackowiak RS, Turner R. Movement-related effects in fMRI time-series. *Magn Reson Med* (1996) 35:346–55. doi:10.1002/mrm.1910350312
34. Murphy K, Fox MD. Towards a consensus regarding global signal regression for resting state functional connectivity MRI. *Neuroimage* (2017) 154:169–73. doi:10.1016/j.neuroimage.2016.11.052
35. Wang J, Zuo X, Dai Z, Xia M, Zhao Z, Zhao X, et al. Disrupted functional brain connectome in individuals at risk for Alzheimer's disease. *Biol Psychiatry* (2013) 73:472–81. doi:10.1016/j.biopsych.2012.03.026
36. Liu F, Guo W, Fouche JP, Wang Y, Wang W, Ding J, et al. Multivariate classification of social anxiety disorder using whole brain functional connectivity. *Brain Struct Funct* (2015) 220:101–15. doi:10.1007/s00429-013-0641-4
37. Ma X, Jiang G, Li S, Wang J, Zhan W, Zeng S, et al. Aberrant functional connectome in neurologically asymptomatic patients with end-stage renal disease. *PLoS One* (2015) 10:e0121085. doi:10.1371/journal.pone.0121085
38. Wang J, Wang X, He Y, Yu X, Wang H, He Y. Apolipoprotein E epsilon4 modulates functional brain connectome in Alzheimer's disease. *Hum Brain Mapp* (2015) 36:1828–46. doi:10.1002/hbm.22740
39. Fan L, Li H, Zhuo J, Zhang Y, Wang J, Chen L, et al. The Human Brainnetome Atlas: a new brain atlas based on connectional architecture. *Cereb Cortex* (2016) 26:3508–26. doi:10.1093/cercor/bhw157
40. Toppi J, De Vico Fallani F, Vecchiato G, Maglione AG, Cincotti F, Mattia D, et al. How the statistical validation of functional connectivity patterns can prevent erroneous definition of small-world properties of a brain connectivity network. *Comput Math Methods Med* (2012) 2012:130985. doi:10.1155/2012/130985
41. Fox MD, Zhang D, Snyder AZ, Raichle ME. The global signal and observed anticorrelated resting state brain networks. *J Neurophysiol* (2009) 101:3270–83. doi:10.1152/jn.90777.2008
42. Murphy K, Birn RM, Handwerker DA, Jones TB, Bandettini PA. The impact of global signal regression on resting state correlations: are anti-correlated networks introduced? *Neuroimage* (2009) 44:893–905. doi:10.1016/j.neuroimage.2008.09.036
43. Weissenbacher A, Kasess C, Gerstl F, Lanzenberger R, Moser E, Windischberger C. Correlations and anticorrelations in resting-state functional connectivity MRI: a quantitative comparison of preprocessing strategies. *Neuroimage* (2009) 47:1408–16. doi:10.1016/j.neuroimage.2009.05.005
44. Wang JH, Zuo XN, Gohel S, Milham MP, Biswal BB, He Y. Graph theoretical analysis of functional brain networks: test-retest evaluation on short- and long-term resting-state functional MRI data. *PLoS One* (2011) 6:e21976. doi:10.1371/journal.pone.0021976
45. Maslov S, Sneppen K. Specificity and stability in topology of protein networks. *Science* (2002) 296:910–3. doi:10.1126/science.1065103
46. Milo R, Shen-Orr S, Itzkovitz S, Kashtan N, Chklovskii D, Alon U. Network motifs: simple building blocks of complex networks. *Science* (2002) 298:824–7. doi:10.1126/science.298.5594.824
47. Liu F, Zhuo C, Yu C. Altered cerebral blood flow covariance network in schizophrenia. *Front Neurosci* (2016) 10:308. doi:10.3389/fnins.2016.00308
48. Zalesky A, Fornito A, Harding IH, Cocchi L, Yucel M, Pantelis C, et al. Whole-brain anatomical networks: does the choice of nodes matter? *Neuroimage* (2010) 50:970–83. doi:10.1016/j.neuroimage.2009.12.027
49. Bullmore E, Sporns O. Complex brain networks: graph theoretical analysis of structural and functional systems. *Nat Rev Neurosci* (2009) 10:186–98. doi:10.1038/nrn2575
50. He Y, Evans A. Graph theoretical modeling of brain connectivity. *Curr Opin Neurol* (2010) 23:341–50. doi:10.1097/WCO.0b013e32833aa567
51. Li Y, Wang E, Zhang H, Dou S, Liu L, Tong L, et al. Functional connectivity changes between parietal and prefrontal cortices in primary insomnia patients: evidence from resting-state fMRI. *Eur J Med Res* (2014) 19:32. doi:10.1186/2047-783X-19-32
52. Zhao L, Wang E, Zhang X, Karama S, Khundrakpam B, Zhang H, et al. Cortical structural connectivity alterations in primary insomnia: insights from MRI-based morphometric correlation analysis. *Biomed Res Int* (2015) 2015:817595. doi:10.1155/2015/817595
53. Sporns O, Zwi JD. The small world of the cerebral cortex. *Neuroinformatics* (2004) 2:145–62. doi:10.1385/NI
54. Gumenyuk V, Belcher R, Drake CL, Roth T. Differential sleep, sleepiness, and neurophysiology in the insomnia phenotypes of shift work disorder. *Sleep* (2015) 38:119–26. doi:10.5665/sleep.4336
55. Liang X, Zou Q, He Y, Yang Y. Coupling of functional connectivity and regional cerebral blood flow reveals a physiological basis for network hubs of the human brain. *Proc Natl Acad Sci U S A* (2013) 110:1929–34. doi:10.1073/pnas.1214900110
56. Tomasi D, Wang GJ, Volkow ND. Energetic cost of brain functional connectivity. *Proc Natl Acad Sci U S A* (2013) 110:13642–7. doi:10.1073/pnas.1303346110
57. Buckner RL, Andrews-Hanna JR, Schacter DL. The brain's default network: anatomy, function, and relevance to disease. *Ann N Y Acad Sci* (2008) 1124:1–38. doi:10.1196/annals.1440.011
58. Zuo N, Song M, Fan L, Eickhoff SB, Jiang T. Different interaction modes for the default mode network revealed by resting state functional magnetic resonance imaging. *Eur J Neurosci* (2016) 43:78–88. doi:10.1111/ejn.13112
59. Kaufmann T, Elvsashagen T, Alnaes D, Zak N, Pedersen PO, Norbom LB, et al. The brain functional connectome is robustly altered by lack of sleep. *Neuroimage* (2016) 127:324–32. doi:10.1016/j.neuroimage.2015.12.028
60. Atique B, Erb M, Gharabaghi A, Grodd W, Anders S. Task-specific activity and connectivity within the mentalizing network during emotion and intention mentalizing. *Neuroimage* (2011) 55:1899–911. doi:10.1016/j.neuroimage.2010.12.036
61. Meyer ML, Lieberman MD. Social working memory: neurocognitive networks and directions for future research. *Front Psychol* (2012) 3:571. doi:10.3389/fpsyg.2012.00571
62. Muscatell KA, Morelli SA, Falk EB, Way BM, Pfeifer JH, Galinsky AD, et al. Social status modulates neural activity in the mentalizing network. *Neuroimage* (2012) 60:1771–7. doi:10.1016/j.neuroimage.2012.01.080
63. McCall WV. A psychiatric perspective on insomnia. *J Clin Psychiatry* (2001) 62(Suppl 10):27–32.
64. Buysse DJ, Thompson W, Scott J, Franzen PL, Germain A, Hall M, et al. Daytime symptoms in primary insomnia: a prospective analysis using ecological momentary assessment. *Sleep Med* (2007) 8:198–208. doi:10.1016/j.sleep.2006.10.006
65. Costa A, Peppe A, Dell'Agnello G, Carlesimo GA, Murri L, Bonuccelli U, et al. Dopaminergic modulation of visual-spatial working memory in Parkinson's disease. *Dement Geriatr Cogn Disord* (2003) 15:55–66. doi:10.1159/000067968
66. Espie CA, Kyle SD, Hames P, Cyhlarova E, Benzeval M. The daytime impact of DSM-5 insomnia disorder: comparative analysis of insomnia subtypes from the Great British sleep survey. *J Clin Psychiatry* (2012) 73:e1478–84. doi:10.4088/JCP.12m07954
67. Phillips ML, Drevets WC, Rauch SL, Lane R. Neurobiology of emotion perception I: the neural basis of normal emotion perception. *Biol Psychiatry* (2003) 54:504–14. doi:10.1016/S0006-3223(03)00168-9

68. Frith CD, Frith U. Interacting minds – a biological basis. *Science* (1999) 286:1692–5. doi:10.1126/science.286.5445.1692
69. Baglioni C, Spiegelhalder K, Lombardo C, Riemann D. Sleep and emotions: a focus on insomnia. *Sleep Med Rev* (2010) 14:227–38. doi:10.1016/j.smrv.2009.10.007
70. Riemann D, Spiegelhalder K, Feige B, Voderholzer U, Berger M, Perlis M, et al. The hyperarousal model of insomnia: a review of the concept and its evidence. *Sleep Med Rev* (2010) 14:19–31. doi:10.1016/j.smrv.2009.04.002
71. Plante DT, Jensen JE, Schoerning L, Winkelman JW. Reduced gamma-aminobutyric acid in occipital and anterior cingulate cortices in primary insomnia: a link to major depressive disorder? *Neuropsychopharmacology* (2012) 37:1548–57. doi:10.1038/npp.2012.4
72. Leger D, Guilleminault C, Bader G, Levy E, Paillard M. Medical and socio-professional impact of insomnia. *Sleep* (2002) 25:625–9. doi:10.1093/sleep/25.6.621
73. Gregory AM, Caspi A, Eley TC, Moffitt TE, Oconnor TG, Poulton R. Prospective longitudinal associations between persistent sleep problems in childhood and anxiety and depression disorders in adulthood. *J Abnorm Child Psychol* (2005) 33:157–63. doi:10.1007/s10802-005-1824-0
74. Mellman TA. Sleep and anxiety disorders. *Psychiatr Clin North Am* (2006) 29:1047–1058; abstract x. doi:10.1016/j.psc.2006.08.005
75. LeBlanc M, Beaulieu-Bonneau S, Merette C, Savard J, Ivers H, Morin CM. Psychological and health-related quality of life factors associated with insomnia in a population-based sample. *J Psychosom Res* (2007) 63:157–66. doi:10.1016/j.jpsychores.2007.03.004
76. Charon F, Dramaix M, Mendlewicz J. Epidemiological survey of insomniac subjects in a sample of 1,761 outpatients. *Neuropsychobiology* (1989) 21:109–10. doi:10.1159/000118562
77. Weyerer S, Dilling H. Prevalence and treatment of insomnia in the community: results from the upper Bavarian field study. *Sleep* (1991) 14:392–8.
78. Ohayon MM, Roth T. Place of chronic insomnia in the course of depressive and anxiety disorders. *J Psychiatr Res* (2003) 37:9–15. doi:10.1016/S0022-3956(02)00052-3
79. Jansson M, Linton SJ. The role of anxiety and depression in the development of insomnia: cross-sectional and prospective analyses. *Psychol Health* (2006) 21:383–97. doi:10.1080/14768320500129015
80. Johnson EO, Roth T, Breslau N. The association of insomnia with anxiety disorders and depression: exploration of the direction of risk. *J Psychiatr Res* (2006) 40:700–8. doi:10.1016/j.jpsychires.2006.07.008
81. Morphy H, Dunn KM, Lewis M, Boardman HF, Croft PR. Epidemiology of insomnia: a longitudinal study in a UK population. *Sleep* (2007) 30:274–80.
82. Hillary FG, Roman CA, Venkatesan U, Rajtmajer SM, Bajo R, Castellanos ND. Hyperconnectivity is a fundamental response to neurological disruption. *Neuropsychology* (2015) 29:59–75. doi:10.1037/neu0000110
83. Huang Q, Zhang R, Hu X, Ding S, Qian J, Lei T, et al. Disturbed small-world networks and neurocognitive function in frontal lobe low-grade glioma patients. *PLoS One* (2014) 9:e94095. doi:10.1371/journal.pone.0094095
84. Hillary FG, Grafman JH. Injured brains and adaptive networks: the benefits and costs of hyperconnectivity. *Trends Cogn Sci* (2017) 21:385–401. doi:10.1016/j.tics.2017.03.003
85. Honey CJ, Sporns O, Cammoun L, Gigandet X, Thiran JP, Meuli R, et al. Predicting human resting-state functional connectivity from structural connectivity. *Proc Natl Acad Sci U S A* (2009) 106:2035–40. doi:10.1073/pnas.0811168106
86. Hermundstad AM, Bassett DS, Brown KS, Aminoff EM, Clewett D, Freeman S, et al. Structural foundations of resting-state and task-based functional connectivity in the human brain. *Proc Natl Acad Sci U S A* (2013) 110:6169–74. doi:10.1073/pnas.1219562110
87. Li S, Tian J, Bauer A, Huang R, Wen H, Li M, et al. Reduced integrity of right lateralized white matter in patients with primary insomnia: a diffusion-tensor imaging study. *Radiology* (2016) 280:520–8. doi:10.1148/radiol.2016152038

11

Alteration of Brain Structure with Long-Term Abstinence of Methamphetamine by Voxel-Based Morphometry

Zhixue Zhang[1,2†], *Lei He*[1†], *Shucai Huang*[3], *Lidan Fan*[1], *Yining Li*[1], *Ping Li*[2], *Jun Zhang*[4], *Jun Liu*[1*] *and Ru Yang*[1*]

[1] Department of Radiology, The Second Xiangya Hospital, Central South University, Changsha, China, [2] Department of Radiology, The First Hospital of Hunan University of Chinese Medicine, Changsha, China, [3] Department of Psychiatry, The Fourth People's Hospital of Wuhu, Wuhu, China, [4] Hunan Judicial Police Academy, Changsha, China

***Correspondence:**
Jun Liu
junliu123@csu.edu.cn
Ru Yang
yr_smu@126.com

† These authors have contributed equally to this work

Background: A large portion of previous studies that have demonstrated brain gray matter reduction in individuals who use methamphetamine (MA) have focused on short-term abstinence, but few studies have focused on the effects of long-term abstinence of methamphetamine on brain structures.

Materials and Methods: Our study includes 40 healthy controls and 44 abstinent methamphetamine-dependent (AMD) subjects who have abstained for at least 14 months. For every AMD subject, the age when they first used MA, the total time of MA use, the frequency of MA use in the last month before abstinence, the duration of abstinence and the craving score were recorded. Here we used magnetic resonance imaging (MRI) to measure the gray matter volume (GMV) of each subject with voxel-based morphometry method. Two-sample t-test (AlphaSim corrected) was performed to obtain brain regions with different gray matter volume (GMV) between groups. In addition, partial correlation coefficients adjusted for age, years of education, smoking, and drinking were calculated in the AMD group to assess associations between the mean GMV values in significant clusters and variables of MA use and abstinence.

Results: Compared with the healthy control group, AMD group showed increased gray matter volumes in the bilateral cerebellum and decreased volumes in the right calcarine and right cuneus. Moreover, GMV of left cerebellum are positively correlated with the duration of abstinence in the AMD group ($p = 0.040$, $r = 0.626$).

Conclusions: The present study showed that the gray matter volume in some brain regions is abnormal in the AMD subjects with long-term abstinence. Changes in gray matter volume of visual and cognitive function regions suggested that these areas play important roles in the progress of MA addiction and abstinence. In addition, positive correlation between GMV of the left cerebellum crus and duration of abstinence suggested that prolonged abstinence is beneficial to cognitive function recovery.

Keywords: addiction, methamphetamine, long-term abstinence, voxel-based morphometry, gray matter volume

INTRODUCTION

Methamphetamine is a highly addictive psychostimulant drug that principally affects the monoamine neurotransmitter systems of the brain and results in feelings of alertness, increased energy and euphoria (1–3). This drug has become a global public health problem due to its ease of production and has more rapid onset and serious neurotoxic effects compared with other traditional drugs (4, 5). World Drug Report 2018 (6) described that up to 2016, about 31 million drug users have shown to have problematic use of drugs. In China, it is reported that there are 2.5 million people that have problematic use of illicit drugs. Synthetic drugs remain the major source of abuse. Among the various drugs seized, methamphetamine and related products account for 31.6%, which is much higher than 10.6% for heroin and 8.1% for ketamine. As a consequence, methamphetamine abuse and related substances have become a serious health crisis (7). Methamphetamine abuse can cause various physical illnesses and psychotic disorders (8–11). Worse of all, even after undergoing substance abuse treatment, patients often relapse when they encounter stress and other high risk environments that may trigger drug use (12–14).

Researches have shown that methamphetamine abuse causes comprehensive changes to brain structures and functions (15–17). After a period of abstinence, brain structure and metabolism can be restored and improved to a certain extent (18–20). Among various methods to investigate brain changes, voxel-based morphometry (VBM) is an automated and efficient tool for whole-brain analysis to detect structural differences. This method is sensitive to subtle brain alterations in gray matter. VBM was developed to detect group differences in the relative concentration of gray matter tissues across the whole brain in a voxel-wise manner. Comparing with traditional morphometric approaches which rely on measuring brain volumes manually, it provides more rapid results and is used for various brain regions (21). Hence, it has been widely used in studies on psychiatric disorders including chemical substance addiction (22, 23). For example, Hanlon and Canterberry (24) indicated that the duration of abstinence was associated with increased gray matter volume (GMV) in the dorsolateral prefrontal cortex, posterior cingulate cortex, and superior parietal lobe by studying about 40 male cocaine abusers. A study on alcohol abstinent patients has shown that abstinence therapy is beneficial for the recovery of GMV in the frontal lobe (25). However, these studies using the VBM method mainly focused on short-term abstinence and results from various studies are inconsistent (26–28).

To investigate brain structure with long-term abstinence could further illuminate the nature of drug relapse, thus conducive to improve long-term abstinence treatment efficacy and rehabilitation programs. Yang et al. (29) utilized a non-human primate model of addiction and showed that neurochemical changes associated with long-term drug use do not persist after prolonged abstinence, suggesting therapeutic effects of long-term abstinence. Wang et al. (30) found that thalamic metabolism was recovered and was associated with improved performance in motor and verbal memory tasks in five long-term abstinent MA abusers. However, these studies which focused on long-term abstinence are either based on small samples or on non-human primate.

In order to overcome shortcomings of the related studies mentioned above, in this study, relatively larger samples (44 AMD subjects and 40 healthy controls) with a long abstinence duration (14–25 month) were collected to investigate the volume changes on gray matter of AMD patients compared with healthy controls (HC) using the VBM method.

MATERIALS AND METHODS

Subjects

Our study includes 44 AMD subjects and 40 healthy control subjects. All AMD subjects are from Pingtang Mandatory Detoxification in Changsha City, Hunan Province. They all were diagnosed using the Diagnostic and Statistical Manual on Mental Disorders (DSM-V) and after that had received a long-term (14–25 month) compulsory abstinence. During abstinence, the participants were treated with medicine, education, and physical exercise and didn't show any significant abstinence symptoms. Inclusion criteria for all subjects included males, ranging in age from 18 to 45 years old, graduated from at least elementary school, normal visual acuity with or without lens correction, normal hearing, and right handed. Exclusion criteria included diseases that affect cognitive function such as head trauma history, cerebrovascular disease, epilepsy, severe mental illness, severe heart, liver, kidney diseases, drug use in the past 6 months, other substance use or dependence except nicotine in the past 5 years, contraindications to MR examination such as claustrophobia. In addition, for every AMD subject, the age when they first used MA, the total time of MA use, the frequency of MA use in the last month before abstinence, the abstinence duration, and the craving score were recorded.

The research protocol was approved by the Ethics Committee of the Second Xiangya Hospital, Central South University. All subjects volunteered to participate in this study and signed the informed consent form. Confidentiality of personal information and freedom to withdraw from the study were guaranteed.

MR Imaging Acquisition

All MRI data were acquired on a 3T Siemens Skyra MRI scanner (Magnetom Skyra, Siemens, Germany) equipped with a 32-channel head coil. The MRI scanning included T1-weight imaging (T1WI), T2-weight imaging (T2WI), and fluid attenuated inversion recovery (FLAIR) sequences. Each scan included a high-resolution T1-weighted anatomical magnetically prepared rapid acquisition gradient echo (3D MPRAGE) sequence with the following parameters: TR = 2,000 ms, TE = 2.6 ms, TI = 900 ms, flip angle = 8°, 176 slices, slice thickness = 1 mm, slice spacing = 1 mm, FOV = 256 × 256 mm^2, acquisition matrix = 256 × 256, voxel size = 1 × 1 × 1 mm^3. Subjects were placed in a supine position with foam padding between their head and the head coil to minimize head motions.

Voxel-Based Morphometry (VBM)

The quality of the T1-weighted images was visually checked for artifacts, structural abnormalities, and apparent head motion and no subject was excluded. Images were processed with Voxel-based Morphometry 8 (VBM8) toolbox (http://dbm.neuro.uni-jena.de/vbm/). Brain images were bias corrected, segmented and spatially normalized to the standard Montreal Neurological Institute (MNI) space. To preserve the actual gray matter values locally, segmented gray matter images were then modulated by a procedure in which the intensity value of each voxel was multiplied by the local value of the Jacobian determinants. Finally, the modulated gray matter volume were smoothed with an 8 mm full-width at half maximum (FWHM) Gaussian kernel.

Statistical Analysis

Demographics were compared between the groups with SPSS 21.0. Patients with AMD and healthy control groups were compared on age and the years of education using two-sample t-test; smoking and drinking using chi-square test, and the significance level was set to $p < 0.05$.

Voxel-wise GMV differences between two groups were computed using two-sample t-test with individual's total GMV, age, gender, and education as covariates. The group GMV difference was corrected for multiple comparisons to a significant level of $p < 0.05$ by combining the individual voxel $p < 0.01$ and cluster size >603 voxels. This correction was confined within a whole brain mask and was determined by Monte Carlo simulations using the DPABI AlphaSim program. On regions showed significantly different GMV between AMD group and healthy group, partial correlation coefficients adjusted for age, years of education, smoking, and drinking were calculated in AMD group to assess association between the mean GMV difference and their age when they first used MA, the total time of MA use, the frequency of MA use in the last month before abstinence, the abstinence duration and the craving score. Significance level was set to $p < 0.05$.

RESULTS

Demographics and Clinical Characteristics of the Participants

Forty-four AMD subjects and forty healthy subjects are included in this study. There is no significant difference between AMD group and HC group in age (mean ± SD) (33.1 ± 6.8 for AMD group; 34.3 ± 7.5 for HC group; $t = 0.760$, $p = 0.450$), the years of education (8.7 ± 2.2 for AMD group; 9.5 ± 2.3 for HC group; $t = 1.656$, $p = 0.102$), smoking (43 of 44 AMD subjects smoke; 38 of 40 HC subjects smoke; $\chi^2 = 0.007$, $p = 0.933$) and drinking (16 of 44 AMD subjects drink; 8 of 40 HC subjects drink; $\chi^2 = 2.006$, $p = 0.157$) as showed in **Table 1**.

VBM Results

Group differences are shown in **Tables 2, 3** and **Figure 1**. In comparison with HC group, the significant GMV reductions in AMD group were around right calcarine and right cuneus. In contrast, the significant GMV increases in AMD group are around the left cerebellum and right cerebellum.

TABLE 1 | Demographic information and characterization.

Group	*N*	Age/year	Education/year	Smoke		Drink	
				Yes	No	Yes	No
AMD	44	33.1 ± 6.8	8.7 ± 2.2	43	1	6	28
HC	40	34.3 ± 7.5	9.5 ± 2.3	38	2	8	32
		$t = 0.760$	$t = 1.656$	$\chi^2 = 0.007$		$\chi^2 = 2.006$	
p		0.450[a]	0.102[a]	0.933[b]		0.157[b]	

[a] *Two-sample t-test.*
[b] *Chi-square test.*
Significant level was set at $p < 0.05$. There are no statistically significant differences between AMD and HC group based on demographic information and characterization. N, number of participants; AMD, abstinent methamphetamine-dependent; HC, healthy control.

TABLE 2 | Regions with reduced GMV in AMD group compared with HC group.

Brain region (AAL)	Peak *t*-value	Cluster size (voxels)	Peak MNI coordinates		
			X	Y	Z
Calcarine_R	−3.7848	846	27	−70.5	9
Cuneus_R	−3.7277	1,240	7.5	−75	22.5

Statistical threshold was $p < 0.05$ corrected for multiple comparisons by AlphaSim. A combination threshold of voxels' $p < 0.01$ and cluster size >603 voxels was considered significant; Coordinates are located in Montreal Neurological Institute (MNI) space; L, left hemisphere, R, right hemisphere; AAL, Anatomic-Automatic-Labeling template.

TABLE 3 | Regions with increased GMV in AMD group compared with HC group.

Brain region (AAL)	Peak *t*-value	Cluster size (voxels)	Peak MNI coordinates		
			X	Y	Z
Cerebelum_Crus1_L	3.6753	858	−48	−67.5	−22.5
Cerebelum_Crus1_R	3.9336	1,455	58.5	−63	−31.5

Statistical threshold was $p < 0.05$ corrected for multiple comparisons by AlphaSim. A combination threshold of voxels' $p < 0.01$ and cluster size >603 voxels was considered significant; Coordinates are located in Montreal Neurological Institute (MNI) space; L, left hemisphere, R, right hemisphere; AAL, Anatomic-Automatic-Labeling template.

Correlation Analyses

The length of abstinent duration of AMD subjects is positively correlated with GMV in left cerebellum crus as showed in **Figure 2** ($p = 0.040$, $r = 0.626$). However, no other significant correlation was found in the AMD group.

DISCUSSION

In our study, we compared GMV between abstinent methamphetamine-dependent group and healthy control group using VBM. We found that AMD group showed significant increased GMV in the bilateral cerebellum crus, and decreased GMV in the right calcarine and right cuneus. In addition, in the AMD group, duration of abstinence is positively correlated with GMV in the left cerebellum crus.

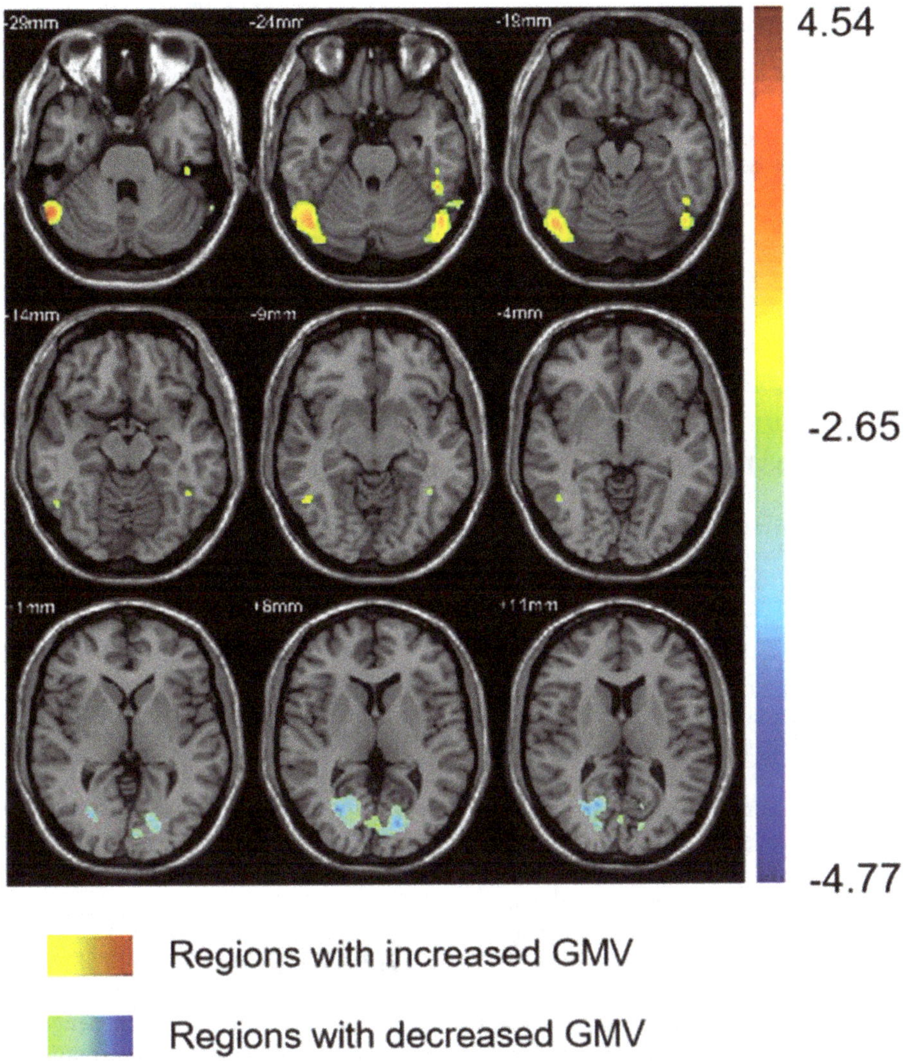

FIGURE 1 | Regions with different GMV in AMD group compared with HC group. GMV, gray matter volume; AMD, abstinent methamphetamine-dependent; HC, healthy control.

Numerous studies have confirmed drug abuse reduces volume of the cerebellum (31–33). Studies showed that the cerebellum is involved in the procedure of addiction, such as memory, predictive power, and executive control ability (34). Researches have shown that cerebellum crus is associated with cognitive and emotional function (35–37). In our study, the volume of bilateral cerebellar crus was increased in AMD group, which is consistent with previous studies. Kühn et al. (38) confirmed that cerebellar gray matter volume is negatively correlated with the degree of nicotine dependence. Schwartz et al. (39) found that patients with heroin dependence had an increased density of gray matter after 2 months of withdrawal, associated with cognitive, memory, and mood improvements, and with decreased levels of craving for drugs. A spectroscopy study on the abstinence of methamphetamine found that abstinence therapy contributes to the normalization of cerebellar neurometabolites (29). Therefore, we speculated that increased GMV of the cerebellum founded in our study may indicate partial recovery of cerebellar function in AMD patients. Importantly, we also found that the duration of abstinence was positively correlated with the left cerebellar volume, which may suggest that the long-term abstinence is beneficial for cerebellum recovery. Moreover, as the left cerebellar volume GMV increases over abstinence time, we inferred that this increase is probably associated with abstinence instead of addiction.

The cortex around the calcarine fissure is the primary visual cortex, which accepts direct projection from the retina to recognize text, identify objects, determine the relationship between objects, distance difference, recent memory, and so on (40, 41). Neuroimaging studies often report that the activity in visual areas is significantly associated with drug cues exposure, treatment effect of drug abuse and prediction

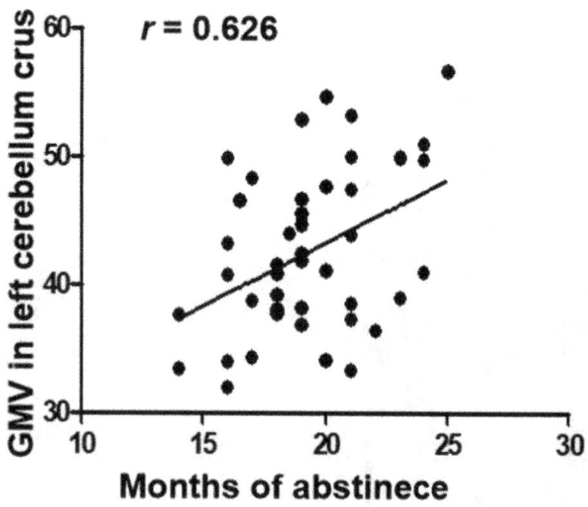

FIGURE 2 | Correlations between duration of abstinence and GMV in the left cerebellum crus in AMD subjects. GMV, gray matter volume; AMD, abstinent methamphetamine-dependent.

of relapse. It has shown that neural circuitry of addiction, consistently discriminates drug cues from neutral cues in substance dependence. A study by Helenna et al. based on VBM, found that visual associated cortices showed decreasing trends of cortical gray matter volumes on methamphetamine abusers, which may contribute to psychiatric symptoms (42). Our result that the volume of the visual cortex of AMD group decreased implies that drug cue-induced craving, which is one of the most robust factors to continued use and relapse across substances (43), is significant among methamphetamine abuser after long-term abstinence.

In our study, the AMD group also showed decreases in right cuneus volumes. The cuneus is involved in visual processing (44) and associated with cessation outcomes (43). A VBM study (45) on smokers showed that compared to relapsers, quitters had significantly smaller GMV in their right cuneus. Therefore, it is possible that the decreased GMV of cuneus has an impact on abstinence and relapse.

STRENGTH AND LIMITATIONS

The current study investigated AMD subjects' brain alterations after long-term abstinence. To the best of our knowledge, this is the first study to reveal brain gray matter alterations after an extended abstinence duration. Changes on visual and cognitive function regions suggest that these areas play important roles in the progress of MA addiction and abstinence.

There are several limitations in this study. (1) This is a cross-sectional study, the image data of AMD subjects before abstinence was not collected. As a result, the causal link of abnormal gray matter volume and the abstinence status was not determined. (2) Most of the subjects and controls have a history of smoking. The effect of smoking on the gray matter volume of the brain has been confirmed in the literature (46). Although smoking status is a covariate in this study, the influence of smoking on brain structure cannot be completely excluded. Further study with non-smoking subgroups would help to address this issue. (3) There are no female subjects in this study. The sex differences in the brain can influence the responses to drugs of abuse, progressive changes in the brain after exposure to drugs of abuse and whether addiction results from drug-taking experiences (47). For example, women exhibit more rapid escalation from casual drug taking to addiction, exhibit a greater withdrawal response with abstinence, and tend to exhibit greater vulnerability than men in terms of treatment outcome (48). Therefore, our results are only applicable in male subjects.

In summary, based on the VBM analysis, this study found gray matter changes in the bilateral cerebellar crus, the right calcarine and right cuneus in methamphetamine-dependent subjects with long-term abstinence. In addition, the volume of left cerebellum was positively correlated with abstinent duration, suggesting that prolonged abstinence may be beneficial to cognitive function recovery. This study provides an imaging basis for revealing the neural mechanism of long-term abstinence of methamphetamine.

AUTHOR CONTRIBUTIONS

JL and JZ conceptualized and designed the research. PL, SH, LF, and YL performed the experiments. RY undertook the statistical analysis. ZZ, LH, and YJ wrote the first draft of the manuscript. ZZ and RY contributed to the final manuscript. All authors critically reviewed content and approved final version for publication.

FUNDING

National Natural Science Foundation of China, Grant Number: 81671671. Natural Science Foundation of Hunan Province, China, Grant Number: 2015JJ4081. The National Key Research and Development Program of China (Grant number: 2016YFC0800908).

REFERENCES

1. Kamei H, Nagai T, Nakano H, Togan Y, Takayanagi M, Takahashi K, et al. Repeated methamphetamine treatment impairs recognition memory through a failure of novelty-induced ERK1/2 activation in the prefrontal cortex of mice. *Biol Psychiatry* (2006) 59:75–84. doi: 10.1016/j.biopsych.2005.06.006
2. Gold MS, Kobeissy FH, Wang KK, Merlo LJ, Bruijnzeel AW, Krasnova IN, et al. Methamphetamine- and trauma-induced brain injuries: comparative cellular and molecular neurobiological substrates. *Biol Psychiatry* (2009) 66:118–27. doi: 10.1016/j.biopsych.2009.02.021
3. Panenka WJ, Procyshyn RM, Lecomte T, MacEwan GW, Flynn SW, Honer WG, et al. Methamphetamine use: a comprehensive review of molecular,

preclinical and clinical findings. *Drug Alcohol Depend.* (2013) 129:167–79. doi: 10.1016/j.drugalcdep.2012.11.016

4. Var SR, Day TR, Vitomirov A, Smith DM, Soontornniyomkij V, Moore DJ, et al. Mitochondrial injury and cognitive function in HIV infection and methamphetamine use. *AIDS* (2016) 30:839–48. doi: 10.1097/QAD.0000000000001027
5. Darke S, Kaye S, Duflou J. Methamphetamine-related death is an under-addressed public health problem. *Addiction* (2017) 112:2204–5. doi: 10.1111/add.14035
6. UNODC. *World Drug Report* (2018).
7. NNCC. *Annual Report on Drug Control in China* (2016).
8. Gonzalez R, Rippeth JD, Carey CL, Heaton RK, Moore DJ, Schweinsburg BC, et al. Neurocognitive performance of methamphetamine users discordant for history of marijuana exposure. *Drug Alcohol Depend.* (2004) 76:181–90. doi: 10.1016/j.drugalcdep.2004.04.014
9. Woods SP, Rippeth JD, Conover E, Gongvatana A, Gonzalez R, Carey CL, et al. Deficient strategic control of verbal encoding and retrieval in individuals with methamphetamine dependence. *Neuropsychology* (2005) 19:35–43. doi: 10.1037/0894-4105.19.1.35
10. Cruickshank CC, Dyer KR. A review of the clinical pharmacology of methamphetamine. *Addiction* (2009) 104:1085–99. doi: 10.1111/j.1360-0443.2009.02564.x
11. London ED, Kohno M, Morales AM, Ballard ME. Chronic methamphetamine abuse and corticostriatal deficits revealed by neuroimaging. *Brain Res.* (2015) 1628(Pt A):174–85. doi: 10.1016/j.brainres.2014.10.044
12. Volkow ND, Wang GJ, Telang F, Fowler JS, Logan J, Childress AR, et al. Cocaine cues and dopamine in dorsal striatum: mechanism of craving in cocaine addiction. *J Neurosci.* (2006) 26:6583–8. doi: 10.1523/JNEUROSCI.1544-06.2006
13. McKetin R, Najman JM, Baker AL, Lubman DI, Dawe S, Ali R, et al. Evaluating the impact of community-based treatment options on methamphetamine use: findings from the Methamphetamine Treatment Evaluation Study (MATES). *Addiction* (2012) 107:1998–2008. doi: 10.1111/j.1360-0443.2012.03933.x
14. Brecht ML, Herbeck D. Time to relapse following treatment for methamphetamine use: a long-term perspective on patterns and predictors. *Drug Alcohol Depend.* (2014) 139:18–25. doi: 10.1016/j.drugalcdep.2014.02.702
15. Chang L, Cloak C, Patterson K, Grob C, Miller EN, Ernst T. Enlarged striatum in abstinent methamphetamine abusers: a possible compensatory response. *Biol Psychiatry* (2005) 57:967–74. doi: 10.1016/j.biopsych.2005.01.039
16. Ernst T, Chang L. Adaptation of brain glutamate plus glutamine during abstinence from chronic methamphetamine use. *J Neuroimmune Pharmacol.* (2008) 3:165–72. doi: 10.1007/s11481-008-9108-4
17. Groman SM, Lee B, Seu E, James AS, Feiler K, Mandelkern MA, et al. Dysregulation of D(2)-mediated dopamine transmission in monkeys after chronic escalating methamphetamine exposure. *J Neurosci.* (2012) 32:5843–52. doi: 10.1523/JNEUROSCI.0029-12.2012
18. Brooks SJ, Burch KH, Maiorana SA, Cocolas E, Schioth HB, Nilsson EK, et al. Psychological intervention with working memory training increases basal ganglia volume: a VBM study of inpatient treatment for methamphetamine use. *Neuroimage Clin.* (2016) 12:478–91. doi: 10.1016/j.nicl.2016.08.019
19. Choi JK, Lim G, Chen YI, Jenkins BG. Abstinence to chronic methamphetamine switches connectivity between striatal, hippocampal and sensorimotor regions and increases cerebral blood volume response. *Neuroimage* (2018) 174:364–79. doi: 10.1016/j.neuroimage.2018.02.059
20. Stock AK, Radle M, Beste C. Methamphetamine-associated difficulties in cognitive control allocation may normalize after prolonged abstinence. *Progr Neuro-Psychopharmacol Biol Psychiatry* (2019) 88:41–52. doi: 10.1016/j.pnpbp.2018.06.015
21. Ashburner J, Friston KJ. Voxel-based morphometry—the methods. *Neuroimage* (2000) 11:805–21. doi: 10.1006/nimg.2000.0582
22. Morales AM, Lee B, Hellemann G, O'Neill J, London ED. Gray-matter volume in methamphetamine dependence: cigarette smoking and changes with abstinence from methamphetamine. *Drug Alcohol Depend.* (2012) 125:230–8. doi: 10.1016/j.drugalcdep.2012.02.017
23. Hartwell EE, Moallem NR, Courtney KE, Glasner-Edwards S, Ray LA. Sex differences in the association between internalizing symptoms and craving in methamphetamine users. *J Addict Med.* (2016) 10:395–401. doi: 10.1097/ADM.0000000000000250
24. Hanlon CA, Canterberry M. The use of brain imaging to elucidate neural circuit changes in cocaine addiction. *Substance Abuse Rehabil.* (2012) 3:115–28. doi: 10.2147/SAR.S35153
25. Durazzo TC, Mon A, Gazdzinski S, Yeh PH, Meyerhoff DJ. Serial longitudinal magnetic resonance imaging data indicate non-linear regional gray matter volume recovery in abstinent alcohol-dependent individuals. *Addict Biol.* (2015) 20:956–67. doi: 10.1111/adb.12180
26. Hser YI, Hoffman V, Grella CE, Anglin MD. A 33-year follow-up of narcotics addicts. *Arch Gen Psychiatry* (2001) 58:503–8. doi: 10.1001/archpsyc.58.5.503
27. Jan RK, Lin JC, Miles SW, Kydd RR, Russell BR. Striatal volume increases in active methamphetamine-dependent individuals and correlation with cognitive performance. *Brain Sci.* (2012) 2:553–72. doi: 10.3390/brainsci2040553
28. Li Q, Li W, Wang H, Wang Y, Zhang Y, Zhu J, et al. Predicting subsequent relapse by drug-related cue-induced brain activation in heroin addiction: an event-related functional magnetic resonance imaging study. *Addict Biol.* (2015) 20:968–78. doi: 10.1111/adb.12182
29. Yang S, Belcher AM, Chefer S, Vaupel DB, Schindler CW, Stein EA, et al. Withdrawal from long-term methamphetamine self-administration 'normalizes' neurometabolites in rhesus monkeys: a (1) H MR spectroscopy study. *Addict Biol.* (2015) 20:69–79. doi: 10.1111/adb.12078
30. Wang GJ, Volkow ND, Chang L, Miller E, Sedler M, Hitzemann R, et al. Partial recovery of brain metabolism in methamphetamine abusers after protracted abstinence. *Am J Psychiatry* (2004) 161:242–8. doi: 10.1176/appi.ajp.161.2.242
31. Nurmedov S, Metin B, Ekmen S, Noyan O, Yilmaz O, Darcin A, et al. Thalamic and cerebellar gray matter volume reduction in synthetic cannabinoids users. *Eur Addict Res.* (2015) 21:315–20. doi: 10.1159/000430437
32. Vnukova M, Ptacek R, Raboch J, Stefano GB. Decreased central nervous system Grey Matter Volume (GMV) in smokers affects cognitive abilities: a systematic review. *Med Sci Monit.* (2017) 23:1907–15. doi: 10.12659/MSM.901870
33. Zhou D, Rasmussen C, Pei J, Andrew G, Reynolds JN, Beaulieu C. Preserved cortical asymmetry despite thinner cortex in children and adolescents with prenatal alcohol exposure and associated conditions. *Hum Brain Mapp.* (2018) 39:72–88. doi: 10.1002/hbm.23818
34. Moulton EA, Elman I, Becerra LR, Goldstein RZ, Borsook D. The cerebellum and addiction: insights gained from neuroimaging research. *Addict Biol.* (2014) 19:317–31. doi: 10.1111/adb.12101
35. Buckner RL, Krienen FM, Castellanos A, Diaz JC, Yeo BT. The organization of the human cerebellum estimated by intrinsic functional connectivity. *J Neurophysiol.* (2011) 106:2322–45. doi: 10.1152/jn.00339.2011
36. Leggio M, Olivito G. Topography of the cerebellum in relation to social brain regions and emotions. *Handb Clin Neurol.* (2018) 154:71–84. doi: 10.1016/B978-0-444-63956-1.00005-9
37. Schmahmann JD. The cerebellum and cognition. *Neurosci Lett.* (2018) 688:62–75. doi: 10.1016/j.neulet.2018.07.005
38. Kühn S, Romanowski A, Schilling C, Mobascher A, Warbrick T, Winterer G, et al. Brain grey matter deficits in smokers: focus on the cerebellum. *Brain Struct Funct* (2012) 217:517–22. doi: 10.1007/s00429-011-0346-5
39. Schwartz DL, Mitchell AD, Lahna DL, Luber HS, Huckans MS, Mitchell SH, et al. Global and local morphometric differences in recently abstinent methamphetamine-dependent individuals. *Neuroimage* (2010) 50:1392–401. doi: 10.1016/j.neuroimage.2010.01.056
40. Nordahl TE, Salo R, Natsuaki Y, Galloway GP, Waters C, Moore CD, et al. Methamphetamine users in sustained abstinence: a proton magnetic resonance spectroscopy study. *Arch Gen Psychiatry* (2005) 62:444–52. doi: 10.1001/archpsyc.62.4.444
41. Shmuel A, Leopold DA. Neuronal correlates of spontaneous fluctuations in fMRI signals in monkey visual cortex: implications for functional connectivity at rest. *Hum Brain Mapp.* (2008) 29:751–61. doi: 10.1002/hbm.20580

42. Nakama H, Chang L, Fein G, Shimotsu R, Jiang CS, Ernst T. Methamphetamine users show greater than normal age-related cortical gray matter loss. *Addiction* (2011) 106:1474–83. doi: 10.1111/j.1360-0443.2011.03433.x
43. Hanlon CA, Dowdle LT, Naselaris T, Canterberry M, Cortese BM. Visual cortex activation to drug cues: a meta-analysis of functional neuroimaging papers in addiction and substance abuse literature. *Drug Alcohol Depend.* (2014) 143:206–12. doi: 10.1016/j.drugalcdep.2014.07.028
44. Fink GR, Halligan PW, Marshall JC, Frith CD, Frackowiak RS, Dolan RJ. Where in the brain does visual attention select the forest and the trees? *Nature* (1996) 382:626–8. doi: 10.1038/382626a0
45. Froeliger B, Kozink RV, Rose JE, Behm FM, Salley AN, McClernon FJ. Hippocampal and striatal gray matter volume are associated with a smoking cessation treatment outcome: results of an exploratory voxel-based morphometric analysis. *Psychopharmacology* (2010) 210:577–83. doi: 10.1007/s00213-010-1862-3
46. Sharma A, Brody AL. *In vivo* brain imaging of human exposure to nicotine and tobacco. *Handb Exp Pharmacol.* (2009) 192:145–71. doi: 10.1007/978-3-540-69248-5_6
47. Becker JB, McClellan ML, Reed BG. Sex differences, gender and addiction. *J Neurosci Res.* (2017) 95:136–47. doi: 10.1002/jnr.23963
48. Becker JB. Sex differences in addiction. *Dialogues Clin Neurosci* (2016) 18:395–402.

12

Craving Responses to Methamphetamine and Sexual Visual Cues in Individuals with Methamphetamine Use Disorder After Long-Term Drug Rehabilitation

Shucai Huang[1], *Zhixue Zhang*[2], *Yuanyuan Dai*[1], *Changcun Zhang*[3], *Cheng Yang*[4,5], *Lidan Fan*[2], *Jun Liu*[2], *Wei Hao*[4,5] *and Hongxian Chen*[4,5*]

[1] *Department of Psychiatry, The Fourth People's Hospital of Wuhu, Wuhu, China,* [2] *Department of Medical Imaging, The Second Xiangya Hospital, Central South University, Changsha, China,* [3] *Pingtang Isolated Compulsory Drug Rehabilitation Center in Hunan Province, Changsha, China,* [4] *Department of Psychiatry, The Second Xiangya Hospital, Central South University, Changsha, China,* [5] *Hunan Key Laboratory of Psychiatry and Mental Health, Chinese National Clinical Research Center on Mental Disorders (Xiangya), Chinese National Technology Institute on Mental Disorders, Mental Health Institute of the Second Xiangya Hospital, Central South University, Changsha, China*

***Correspondence:**
Hongxian Chen
shenhx2018@csu.edu.cn

Studies utilizing functional magnetic resonance imaging (fMRI) cue-reactivity paradigms have demonstrated that short-term abstinent or current methamphetamine (MA) users have increased brain activity in the ventral striatum, caudate nucleus and medial frontal cortex, when exposed to MA-related visual cues. However, patterns of brain activity following cue-reactivity in subjects with long-term MA abstinence, especially long-term compulsory drug rehabilitation, have not been well studied. To enrich knowledge in this field, functional brain imaging was conducted during a cue-reactivity paradigm task in 28 individuals with MA use disorder following long-term compulsory drug rehabilitation, and 27 healthy control subjects. The results showed that, when compared with controls, individuals with MA use disorder displayed elevated activity in the bilateral medial prefrontal cortex (mPFC) and right lateral posterior cingulate cortex in response to MA-related images. Additionally, the anterior cingulate region of mPFC activation during the MA-related cue-reactivity paradigm was positively correlated with craving alterations and previous frequency of drug use. No significant differences in brain activity in response to pornographic images were found between the two groups. Compared to MA cues, individuals with MA use disorder had increased activation in the occipital lobe when exposed to pornographic cues. In conclusion, the present study indicates that, even after long-term drug rehabilitation, individuals with MA use disorder have unique brain activity when exposed to MA-related cues. Additionally, our results illustrate that the libido brain response might be restored, and that sexual demand might be more robust than drug demand, in individuals with MA use disorder following long-term drug rehabilitation.

Keywords: methamphetamine, long-term drug rehabilitation, cue-reactivity, fMRI, medial prefrontal cortex

INTRODUCTION

Methamphetamine (MA) is an amphetamine-type stimulant that is often used as a recreational drug. It enters the central nervous system (CNS) quickly, resulting in the rapid onset of euphoria, which further motivates drug abuse [1]. In 2014, over 35 million individuals abused amphetamine and methamphetamine worldwide. MA abuse has become a serious public health problem for countries around the world, particularly in China [2]. Since 2016, the number of synthetic drug (MA mainly) users has dramatically increased to 1.51 million, accounting for 60.5% of all registered illicit drug users in China. Furthermore, approximately 360,000 first-time synthetic drug users were recorded in 2016, accounting for 81% of all first-time illicit drug users that year [3].

Drug addiction is a chronic disease characterized by a high rate of relapse [4]. In China, for example, the relapse rate for heroin users, within 2 years of abstinence, is over 90% [5, 6]. Limited data from two follow-up studies demonstrated that the relapse rate in individuals abusing MA, within 1 year following drug rehabilitation, was at least 50% [7, 8]. Drug cravings are very important in the etiology of psychostimulant use relapse [9]. It has been reported that MA cravings decrease within 2 months of abstinence [10]; however, detailed characteristics of MA cravings, including the relationship between the duration of rehabilitation and craving levels, in MA use disorder remain understudied [11].

In recent years, the use of functional magnetic resonance imaging (fMRI) cue-reactivity paradigms has greatly expanded our understanding of the neurobiology underlying addiction and relapse, by providing an opportunity to test the mechanisms by which interventions influence behavior [12]. Recent studies utilizing these techniques have shown that patients with MA use disorder have elevated drug cravings and increased brain activation in interconnected limbic regions (i.e., ventral striatum, cingulate cortex, caudate nucleus, orbitofrontal cortex and medial prefrontal cortex (mPFC) when exposed to drug-related visual cues [13, 14]. However, the patterns of brain activation, following the presentation of MA-related cues, are still poorly understood in long-term abstinent MA abusers.

Reward-related behaviors can be divided into two categories: (1) natural rewards caused by eating, sexual opportunity, and other behaviors in favor of survival and reproduction; (2) drug-related rewards caused by the powerful motivational effects of psychoactive substances on natural reward circuits, which are not necessary for survival and reproduction. It is well accepted that pleasure caused by addictive drug use tends to be more rapid, more robust, and longer lasting than natural rewards. It is also known that the euphoric effects of different addictive drugs are diverse, depending on their respective pharmacological mechanisms. Results from an fMRI study suggested that, when compared with healthy controls, both current heroin users and ex-heroin users were less responsive to sexual cues, but had increased activation in the prefrontal and temporal cortex when exposed to drug cues [15]. Unlike opiates, MA use probably does not lead to robust pleasure, as some people use MA to improve their own sexual performance [16, 17]. As a result of different biological mechanisms, the cortical response to drug and sexual cues in individuals with MA use disorder might be different from those of opiate users. However, empirical evidence is still lacking.

In this study, we attempted to explore the patterns of cortical activation in the brains of individuals with long-term MA abstinence when exposed to drug- and sexual-related visual cues using fMRI cue-reactivity paradigms. In light of the high relapse rate in MA use disorder, we hypothesized that (1) cravings in individuals with MA use disorder would still be intense following at least 16 months of drug rehabilitation, and (2) drug-related cues might arouse cravings accompanied by specific brain region activation.

MATERIALS AND METHODS

Subjects

This was a case-control study. Participants included 28 long-term abstinent MA addicts and 27 age-matched healthy volunteers.

Participants with long-term MA abstinence were recruited from the Pingtang Isolated Compulsory Drug Rehabilitation Center in Hunan Province. For the convenience of presenting uniform pornographic images in the fMRI cue-reactivity paradigm, only males were included in the study. Further inclusion criteria were: aged between 18 and 45 years; of Han Chinese ethnicity; right-handedness; meeting Diagnostic and Statistical Manual of Mental Disorders (DSM-IV) criteria for MA dependence, as determined by interviews conducted using the Chinese version of the Structured Clinical Interview for DSM-IV axis I disorders, research version for patients (SCID-I/P) [18]; a history of MA use > twice per week and for >2 years; a duration of drug abstinence >16 months. Exclusion criteria were: illiteracy; a lifetime diagnosis of substance dependence other than MA and nicotine; current or past major medical, neurological or axis I psychiatric disorders; current use of psychotropic medications or intravenous drugs; learning disabilities or CNS disease; a history of head injury with skull fracture or loss of consciousness of 10 min or more; homosexuality; and contraindications for MRI.

Healthy controls were local residents, who were male, 18–45 years old, of Han Chinese ethnicity, and right-handed. Those who were current or past MA users, met DSM-IV criteria for any axis I, major medical, and/or neurological disorders were excluded.

All subjects were required to abstain from alcohol and/or other potential psychoactive substances for at least 48 h prior to scanning. Meanwhile, all healthy volunteers were required to abstain from all sexual behavior for at least 3 days prior to scanning.

All study procedures were conducted in accordance with the ethical standards of the 1975 Helsinki Declaration. The ethical review board of the Second Xiangya Hospital of Central South University approved all study procedures. All participants were fully informed about research procedures and signed informed consent.

Measures

Urine screening was conducted to detect the current use of MA, ketamine, opiates, and cocaine prior to the interview and MRI scan. All clinical interviews were conducted by an experienced psychiatrist. The self-rated questionnaires and SCID-I/P were used to collect demographic and drug use information, and to make diagnoses of psychiatric disorders, respectively. The Edinburgh Handedness Inventory [19] was employed to determine the handedness of all participants. MA craving scores and sexual behavior were assessed on a 0–10 visual analog scale (VAS) [20] (0 for the weakest craving and 10 for the strongest craving) prior to and immediately following each MRI scan.

Procedure

Task Design

The cue-reactivity paradigm was utilized to carry out this study. The cue-reactivity paradigm has been widely used to assess the involvement of neurobiological pathways in the processes underlying cravings for alcohol, nicotine, cocaine, and opioids [12]. The cue-induced MRI scanning procedure was designed based on previous reports by George et al. [21], Myrick et al. [22], and Myrick [23], with minor modifications. Briefly, as illustrated in **Figure 1**, a 450-s sequence for cue-image presentation, consisting of six epochs, was designed. The duration of each epoch was 75 s and contained three 20-s blocks and a 15-s rest. The 20-s blocks presented MA-related, pornographic and neutral images, respectively. The 15-s rest displayed a crosshair. Each 20-s block contained five different images, each displayed for 4 s. A total of 30 MA-related images, 30 sex-related images, and 30 neutral images were presented during the MRI scan, and each image was unique. In order to control for time and order effects across subjects, the order of the images, the blocks within the epoch, and the epochs were all randomly presented [21–23].

All MA-related images, which fall into MA samples, drug paraphernalia and simulation scenarios, were authentic and shot using an SLR camera by researchers. MA samples were provided by the pharmacology laboratory of the Hunan Public Security Bureau. Drug paraphernalia and simulation scenarios of drug use were self-developed and modified after testing by individuals with MA use disorder from the Xinkaipu Isolated Compulsory Drug Rehabilitation Center. Pornographic images were Asian related and high definition (HD). Neutral images were acquired from the internet, including images of artifacts and neutral daily actions. All images were scaled to the same size, resolution and hue through the use of Photoshop (Adobe, San Jose, California) software.

The reliability of all images in the present study were tested preliminarily, and results showed that all images had satisfactory reliability. Each MA-related image was scored (0–10) by 156 individuals with MA use disorder from the Xinkaipu Isolated Compulsory Drug Rehabilitation Center, according to their subjective feelings. We then selected 30 of the 150 images in accordance with the scores. Finally, these 30 images were screened by another 100 individuals with MA use disorder, and the results showed that the recognition rate of these images was 100%. Pornographic and neutral images were checked in the same way as described above. The validity of these images was not tested due to a lack of reference images.

The task paradigm was created and presented in E-prime 2.0 software (http://www.pstnet.com/eprime.cfm) on a computer which was connected to MRI-compatible nonferro-magnetic goggles. Pupil trajectory of all participants was recorded using a mini camera located in the goggles. Participants were required to press a button, which was connected to a computer, when they saw the images clearly. Reaction time (RT), i.e., time taken to press the button, was recorded. A RT longer than 2 s for each image was disqualified and this data was removed from the analysis. The action of planning and pressing is related to executive function, which affects other functional activity in the brain. Therefore, functional image data at the corresponding time points of button pressing were excluded from the analyses.

Functional MRI Data Acquisition

Scanning was conducted in a 3.0 Tesla Siemens scanner (Allegra; Siemens Medical System, Erlangen, Germany) equipped with a standard head volume coil. For fMRI scanning, whole brain echo-planar images were acquired using a T2 weighted gradient echo sequence with blood oxygen level-dependent (BOLD) contrast: repetition time (TR) = 2,000 ms, echo time (TE) = 30 ms, flip = 80°, field of view (FOV) = 220 mm × 220 mm, voxel size = 3.4 mm × 3.4 mm × 4.0 mm, slice thickness = 4 mm, gap = 1 mm, matrix = fMRI scanning 64 × 64, number of slice = 36. The total time of the fMRI scan was 450 s. Earplugs, and cushions placed around the head were used for sound insulation and to control head movement, respectively.

Statistical Analyses

Demographics and Behavioral Data Analysis

Comparisons of demographic and behavioral data between MA users and healthy controls were performed with either independent-sample t-tests (continuous variables) or χ^2 tests (categorical variables). Comparisons of increased craving scores (ICS) before and after scanning were performed using paired-sample t-tests. SPSS 18.0 software (SPSS, Chicago, Illinois) was used for all analyses. The level of statistical significance was set at $P < 0.05$ (two-sided).

fMRI Data Analysis

Functional images were transferred into an appropriate format for analysis with the Statistical Parametric Mapping 8 software package (SPM 8, http://www.fil.ion.ucl.ac.uk/spm/software/spm8/). First, all functional images were realigned to the first volume of each session as a reference. After this realignment, data sets were selected on the basis of their quality (scan stability), as demonstrated by small motion correction. The realigned images were then stereotactically normalized into a standard resolution of 3 × 3 × 3 mm voxels using the Montreal Neurological Institute (MNI) EPI template in SPM 8, and subsequently smoothed with a 6-mm full-width at half-maximum (FWHM) Gaussian kernel. In the first level of statistical analysis, predetermined conditions effecting entire functional brain volume were analyzed using a boxcar function, convolved with the modeled hemodynamic response function, as the general linear model. Contrast maps were obtained which reflected the differences between MA vs. neutral control, sex vs. neutral control, MA vs. rest, sex vs. rest, and MA vs. sex for each individual. The resulting first level contrast images were entered into second level (random effects)

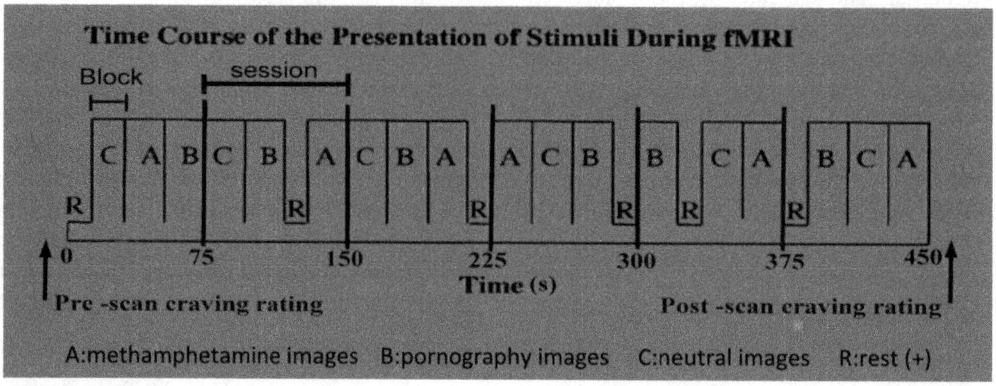

FIGURE 1 | Procedure of fMRI cue-reactivity paradigms in this study.

analyses for between-group comparisons. We included age, education, nicotine and RT as covariates in the second level model. To assess the effects of stress, one-sample t-tests were performed in all subjects and in each group. Imaging results were corrected using a family-wise error rate for comparisons (significance at $p < 0.05$) [24, 25].

As we had no priori hypotheses for the activity of brain regions, one-sample t-test contrasts between MA vs. neutral control (and sex vs. neutral control) were performed for each group, using whole brain analysis with a statistical threshold of $P_{FWEcor} < 0.05$ and $k = 30$ voxels. Two-sample t-tests were adopted to detect the main differences between the MA group and the control group.

The voxel locations of significant MA or pornographic cues activated in two groups ($P_{FWEcor} < 0.05$ and $k = 30$ voxels) were used to create masks for time course extraction, and 6-mm radius spherical regions of interest (ROI) were used to create masks. Using the masks, averaged time courses of multi voxels were calculated from each individual data with MarsBar 0.44 (http://marsbar.sourceforge.net/) and log-roi-batch v2.0 (http://www.aimfeld.ch/) [24].

Correlation Analysis Between MA-Related Variables and Activation Level of ROIs

Correlations between activation level of ROI and clinical features of MA abuse, including years of age and education, age of starting MA use, duration (months) of MA use, dosage (g) of MA per time, frequency of MA use, craving score when using MA, smoking status, craving score before/after scanning and ICS, were calculated by Pearson correlation. Two-tailed levels of significance ($P < 0.05$) were used.

RESULTS

Demographic and Behavioral Data

There were no significant differences in age and education status between the two groups. Detailed information on demographics and past drug use characteristics of individuals with MA use disorder and healthy controls are displayed in **Table 1**.

TABLE 1 | Demographics and drug use characteristics of subjects with MA use disorder and control subjects.

	Subjects with MA use disorder	Healthy control subjects
Cases	**28**	**27**
DEMOGRAPHICS		
Age (years)	31.68 ± 7.06	33.93 ± 7.21
Education (years)	8.96 ± 2.03	10.04 ± 3.03
Male (%)	28 (100%)	27 (100%)
Right-handed (%)	28 (100%)	27 (100%)
MA USE VARIABLES		
Age of first use	25.18 ± 7.14	–
Range (years)	15–40	–
Duration of drug use (months)	59.96 ± 32.98	–
Range (months)	24–190	–
Previous frequency of drug use (days per year)	222.71 ± 114.41	–
Range (days per year)	72–365	–
Duration of abstinence (months)	18.50 ± 2.64	–
Range (months)	16–24	–
OTHER DRUGS EVER USED		
Alcohol (%)	13 (46.42%)	12 (44.44%)
Cigarette[a]	28 (100%)	17 (62.96%)
Ketamine[b]	14 (50%)	–
Ecstasy[b]	3 (10.71%)	–
Marijuana[b]	1 (3.57%)	–

The results were presented as mean ± SD.
[a] Significantly different from control group, $P \leq 0.01$.
[b] Recreational use, the frequency of drug use was <25 times during the participants' lifetime.

Subjective drug craving scores in the MA group were significantly higher after, than prior to, scanning [1.16 ($SD = 1.27$) vs. 0.39 ($SD = 0.62$), $t = 5.03$, df $= 27$, $P < 0.01$]. In contrast, drug craving scores in the control group were 0 at all times of the study.

Subjective sex craving scores in the MA group were significantly higher after, than prior to, scanning [5.43 (*SD* = 1.94) vs. 2.51 (*SD* = 1.43), $t = 11.40$, df = 27, $P < 0.01$]. Additionally, sex craving scores in the control group were significantly higher after, than prior to, scanning [4.67 (*SD* = 1.71) vs. 2.25 (*SD* = 1.22), $t = 9.43$, df = 26, $P < 0.01$]. Nevertheless, no significant differences were found between the two groups in subjective sex craving scores (before: $t = 0.72$, df = 53, $P = 0.47$, after: $t = 1.54$, df = 53, $P = 0.13$, ICS: $t = 1.37$, df = 53, $P = 0.18$).

After scanning, subjective craving scores for sex were significantly higher than craving scores for drugs in the MA group ($t = 9.77$, df = 54, $P < 0.01$).

fMRI Data

Compared with the control group, there was a significantly elevated response to MA-related cues in the mPFC and right lateral posterior cingulate cortex, relative to the baseline control condition in the MA group (**Figure 2**, **Table 2**).

Bilateral mPFC, and the occipital and temporal gyrus were activated significantly in both the MA and control groups, when exposed to pornographic images (**Figure 3**). However, no significant differences in brain activity, in response to sex-related cues, were detected between the two groups.

When compared to MA-related image cues, individuals with MA use disorder had elevated left lateral occipital and bilateral temporal gyrus responses, but no reduction in brain activity, when exposed to pornographic image cues (**Figure 4**, **Table 3**).

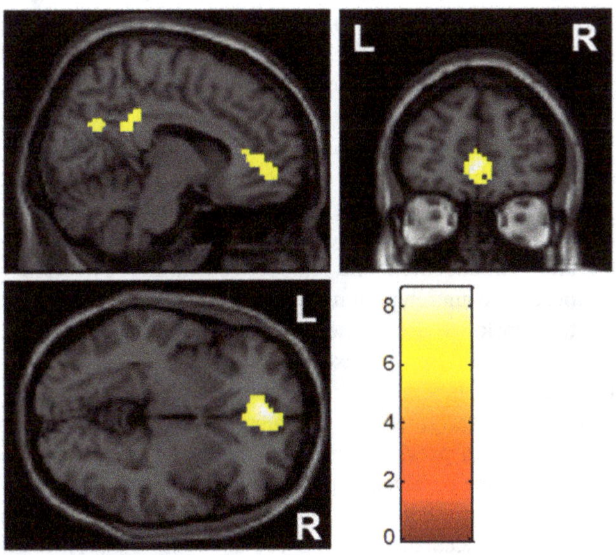

FIGURE 2 | Group comparisons of brain activation when exposed to MA-related images ($p < 0.05$, family-wise error rate corrected).

Correlation Between Demographic or Behavioral Variables and the Activation Level of ROIs

Brain regions displaying significant activation to MA-related image cues in MA groups (including bilateral mPFC, occipital and temporal gyrus) were selected as the functional ROIs. Correlations between the activation level of these selected ROIs and years of age, years of education, age of starting MA use, duration (months) of MA use, dosage (g) of MA use per time, previous frequency of drug use, craving score when MA using, craving score for MA before/after scanning, and ICS in patients with MA use disorder were examined. The activation level of the left lateral anterior cingulate region of the mPFC was positively correlated with previous frequency of MA use ($r = 0.419$, $P = 0.027$) and ICS for MA ($r = 0.463$, $P = 0.013$) (**Figure 5**). We did not find any other significant correlations between variables of MA use and activation levels of ROIs.

Meanwhile, brain regions which were significantly activated in response to sex-related images in both groups (including bilateral mPFC, occipital and temporal gyrus) were selected as functional ROIs. The correlations between the activation level of these ROIs and craving scores sex before/after scanning and ICS in all participants were examined. The activation level in a part of the mPFC was positively correlated with ICS for sex ($r = 0.385$, $P < 0.01$) (**Figure 3**). We did not find any other significant correlations between variables of subjective craving for sex and activation levels of selected ROIs.

DISCUSSION

Studies of fMRI cue-reactivity paradigms in nicotine [26], alcohol [22], cocaine [27], and MA [14] dependence have identified two interacting circuits that are involved in the process of cue-induced craving: (1) a reward circuit including the nucleus accumbens, ventral tegmental area, amygdala, thalamus, hippocampus and mPFC cortex; (2) a visual attention and planning circuit including the occipital cortex, parietal cortex, and the frontal cortex [28]. Consistent with previous studies, we also found that participants with long-term MA abstinence had

TABLE 2 | Brain regions significantly activated by MA-related images in individuals with MA use disorder when compared with healthy controls.

Region	Hemisphere	Montreal neurological institute coordinate			Voxels	*t*	P(FWE correction)
		X	*Y*	*Z*			
Medial prefrontal cortex	Inter	0	48	−3	267	8.60	<0.001
Posterior cingulate cortex	Right	9	−45	27	36	5.95	0.006

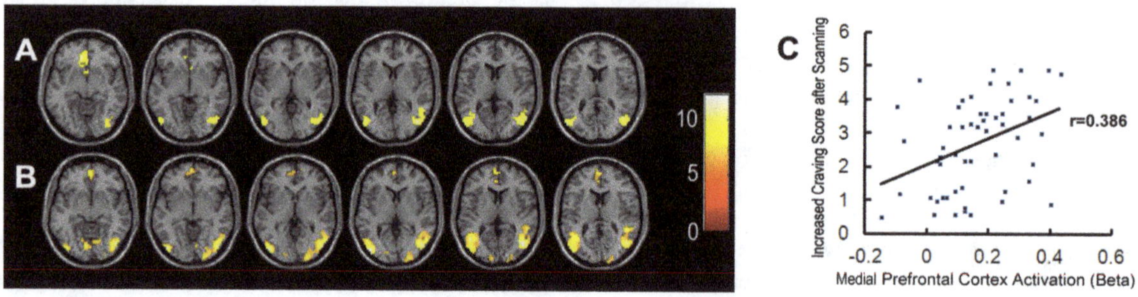

FIGURE 3 | Brain activation when exposed to pornographic images. **(A)** Shows significant activation in brain regions in the healthy control group ($n = 27$). **(B)** Shows significant activation in brain regions in the MA group ($n = 28$). **(C)** Shows the correlation between activation in the medial prefrontal cortex and craving scores for sex in all participants.

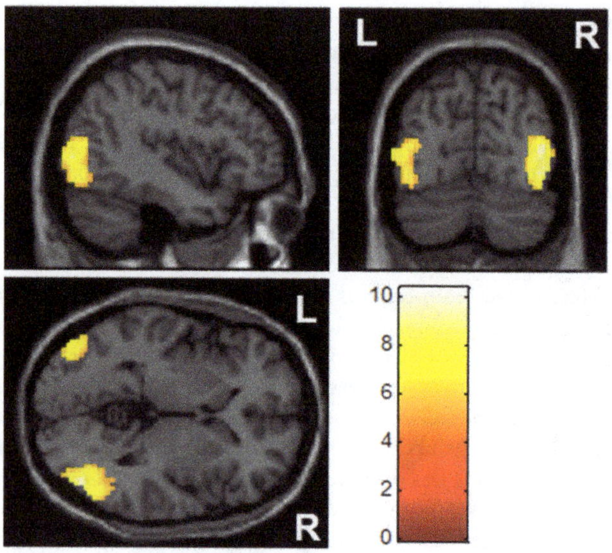

FIGURE 4 | Comparison of brain activation between pornographic images and MA-related images. The bilateral occipital cortex was significantly activated by pornographic images when compared with MA-related images in the MA group ($p < 0.05$, family-wise error rate corrected).

significantly increased brain activation in the mPFC (including ACC) and posterior cingulate gyrus when exposed to MA cues, compared to healthy controls. This indicates that MA-related cues may trigger cravings through the reward circuit, and get more attention via the planning circuit in individuals with MA use disorder after long-term drug abstinence. These findings support the theory that ordinary long-term abstinence may not completely improve the extraordinary brain response to MA-related cues, in individuals with MA use disorder.

Previous studies have shown that the mPFC is involved in drug cravings, compulsive seeking behavior and relapse, and that individuals with dysfunction in the ACC of the mPFC display reduced impulse control and enhanced drug-seeking behaviors [29–31]. In our present study, we further found that the activation in the ACC region of the mPFC, when exposed to drug-related cues, was positively correlated with the previous frequency of MA use and ICS in individuals with MA use disorder. This suggests that the responsivity in the ACC region of the mPFC to drug cues could partly reflect a previous history of MA abuse and a current degree of cravings for individuals with MA use disorder. Accordingly, we speculate that the drug-cue-induced activation in the ACC region of the mPFC is a potential predictor of previous MA abuse and current craving level. Additionally, we found that few patients with MA use disorder had aspiration to get rid of drug abuse (7/28). This might be one of the important reasons explaining how the significant increase in the ACC region of the mPFC activity remained in these individuals after long-term abstinence. This is consistent with the results of a previous investigation [27] which demonstrated that drug-cue-induced activation in the middle frontal gyrus was negatively correlated with the level of willingness and motivation to abstain from drug. Therefore, we propose that the lack of motivation to quit for these individuals might be an important risk factor in relapse, and that intensive psychotherapies focusing on drug rehabilitation motivation enhancement and relapse prevention are necessary in the process of drug rehabilitation.

In this work, we also found that pornographic cues produced no significant differences, except for a notable increase in the activity in some areas of occipital lobe, when compared with the activation following MA-related cues in the MA group. It has been reported in previous studies that similar cortical areas in the occipital lobe involved in the processes of visual information, and sensory representation of visual stimulation is processed in these lobes according to the previous experiences, leading to instinctive attention biases to specific visual representation [32, 33]. Therefore, our results might suggest that the brains of individuals with MA use disorder are more interested in sexual visual stimulation, rather than drug-related visual cues, with long-term drug abstinence, which are supported faintly by significantly higher subjective craving scores for sex than drugs in the MA group. This speculation needs to be verified by more rigorous studies.

It has been reported that MA use can improve sexual performance as a result of increased pleasure and extended sexual intercourse, resulting from a transient increase in the release of monoamine neurotransmitters and androgens [16, 17].

TABLE 3 | Brain regions significantly activated by pornographic images when compared with MA-related images in the MA group.

Region	Hemisphere	Montreal neurological institute coordinate			Voxels	*t*	P(FWE correction)
		X	*Y*	*Z*			
Inferior occipital gyrus	Right	45	−78	−6	479	7.65	<0.001
Middle occipital gyrus	Left	−42	−81	3	243	6.77	<0.001

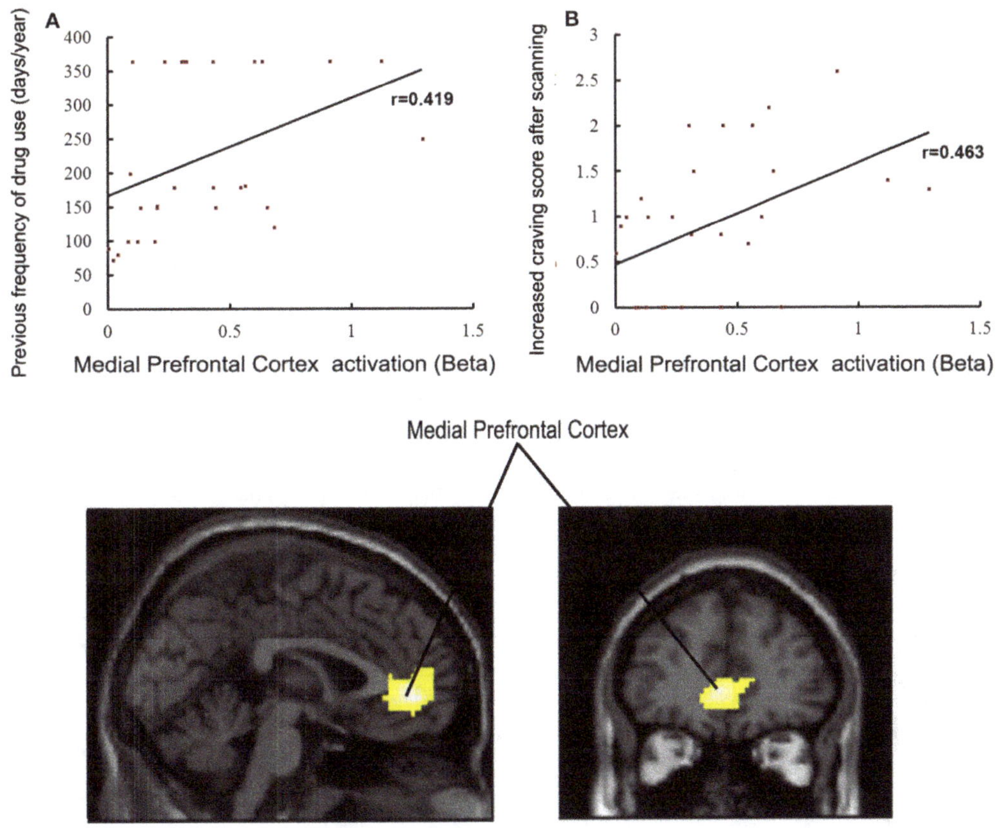

FIGURE 5 | (A) Correlations between activation in the medial prefrontal cortex and previous frequency of drug use in MA group ($p < 0.05$). **(B)** Correlations between activation in the medial prefrontal cortex and craving scores for drugs in the MA group ($p < 0.05$).

However, there is evidence that chronic MA exposure reduces sexual motivation in a dose-dependent manner in humans and experimental animals due to chronic neurotoxicity, monoamine neurotransmitter attenuation, and regulation disorder of androgens, and that these effects of MA probably do not last following drug abstinence due to the recovery of androgens and monoamine neurotransmitters to some extent [34–36]. Consistent with these studies, the final finding of our study is that no significant differences existed in individuals with MA use disorder after long-term drug abstinence in both subjective craving scores and brain responses to pornographic cues, when compared with healthy controls. This demonstrates that the libido of the participants may have been restored. Conversely, a significant reduction in activation of the prefrontal cortex of individuals with heroin use disorder, when exposed to pornographic cues, has been reported in one previous study [15]. These differences of brain activation in response to sexual cues in individuals with different drug use disorders are very interesting.

Several limitations need to be noted when interpreting the results of this study. First, our work is a cross-sectional comparison only, and we could not collect MRI data from these individuals prior to abstinence. Therefore, we could not compare the brain response to related cues before and after abstinence. In addition, due to cultural traditions and stigma of drug abuse, it was difficult to recruit individuals with MA use disorder after long-term voluntary drug abstinence. Therefore, it is not possible for us to compare the differences in cue-induced brain activity between compulsory and voluntary abstinence. Third, the individuals with MA use disorder that we recruited were all from compulsory drug rehabilitation centers. These participants might report a lower level of drug cravings for some reasons; this might introduce bias to the results of the correlation analyses.

In summary, our study reveals patterns of brain activity following exposure to different image cues (neutral, drug, and sex) in healthy controls and individuals with MA use disorder after long-term drug rehabilitation. Extremely enhanced activation remained in the mPFC and posterior cingulate cortex following drug-related cues in individuals who underwent long-term drug rehabilitation. Meanwhile, our results also suggest that the drug-cue-induced activation in the ACC region of the mPFC is positively correlated with a previous history of MA use and the current degree of cravings in individuals with long-term drug abstinence. Additionally, the present study found no significant difference in both subjective craving scores and brain responses to pornographic cues in patients with long-term MA abstinence, when compared with healthy controls. However, a remarkable increase in the activation of some areas involved in the processing of visual information in the occipital lobe, induced by pornographic cues, was found when comparing the brain activation following MA-related cues. This indicates that the brain response to libido might be restored, and the sexual demand might be more robust than drug demand, in individuals with MA use disorder after long-term drug abstinence.

AUTHOR CONTRIBUTIONS

SH, HC, and WH conceptualized and designed the research; ZZ, JL, and CY performed the experiments; SH and LF undertook the statistical analysis; SH and WH wrote the first draft of the manuscript; HC and WH contributed to the final manuscript. All authors critically reviewed content and approved final version for publication.

FUNDING

This work was supported by National Basic Research Program of China (2015CB553504) to WH and National Research Program of China (2016YFC0800908-Z02) to HC.

REFERENCES

1. Vearrier D, Greenberg MI, Miller SN, Okaneku JT, Haggerty DA. Methamphetamine: history, pathophysiology, adverse health effects, current trends, and hazards associated with the clandestine manufacture of methamphetamine. *Dis Mon.* (2012) **58**:38–89. doi: 10.1016/j.disamonth.2011.09.004
2. United Nations Office on Drugs and Crime (UNODC). *World Drug Report 2016*. Vienna (2016).
3. China National Narcotics Control Commission (NNCC). *Annual Report on Drug Control in China*. Beijing (2016).
4. Weiss F. Neurobiology of craving, conditioned reward and relapse. *Curr. Opin Pharmacol.* (2005) **5**:9–19. doi: 10.1016/j.coph.2004.11.001
5. Sullivan SG, Wu Z. Rapid scale up of harm reduction in China. *Int J Drug Policy* (2007) **18**:118–28. doi: 10.1016/j.drugpo.2006.11.014
6. Wang H. An analysis of relapse factors of opioid addicts. *Chin J Drug Abuse Prev Treat.* (2004) **10**:85–7. doi: 10.3390/ijerph13020177
7. Brecht ML, Herbeck D. Time to relapse following treatment for methamphetamine use: a long-term perspective on patterns and predictors. *Drug Alcohol Depend.* (2014) **139**:18–25. doi: 10.1016/j.drugalcdep.2014.02.702
8. Zang CY. Special follow-up study of relapse factors in addicts after being released from compulsory detoxification centers. *Justice China* (2015) **1**:81–6.
9. Galloway GP, Singleton EG. How long does craving predict use of methamphetamine? Assessment of use one to seven weeks after the assessment of craving: craving and ongoing methamphetamine use. *Subst Abuse* (2009) **1**:63–79.
10. Urschel HR, Hanselka LL, Gromov I, White L, Baron M. Open-label study of a proprietary treatment program targeting type A gamma-aminobutyric acid receptor dysregulation in methamphetamine dependence. *Mayo Clin Proc.* (2007) **82**:1170–8. doi: 10.4065/82.10.1170
11. Shen W, Liu Y, Li L, Zhang Y, Zhou W. Negative moods correlate with craving in female methamphetamine users enrolled in compulsory detoxification. *Subst Abuse Treat Prev Policy* (2012) **7**:44. doi: 10.1186/1747-597X-7-44
12. Courtney KE, Schacht JP, Hutchison K, Roche DJ, Ray LA. Neural substrates of cue reactivity: association with treatment outcomes and relapse. *Addict Biol.* (2016) **21**:3–22. doi: 10.1111/adb.12314
13. Yin JJ, Ma SH, Xu K, Wang ZX, Le HB, Huang JZ, et al. Functional magnetic resonance imaging of methamphetamine craving. *Clin Imaging* (2012) **36**:695–701. doi: 10.1016/j.clinimag.2012.02.006
14. Malcolm R, Myrick H, Li X, Henderson S, Brady KT, George MS. Regional Brain activity in abstinent methamphetamine dependent males following cue exposure. *J Drug Abuse* (2016) **2**:16. doi: 10.21767/2471-853X.100016
15. Jiang YL, Tian W, Lu G, Rudd JA, Lai KF, Yeung LY, et al. Patterns of cortical activation following motor tasks and psychological-inducing movie cues in heroin users: an fMRI study. *Int J Psychiatry Med.* (2014) **247**:5–40. doi: 10.2190/PM.47.1.c
16. Shoptaw S. Methamphetamine use in urban gay and bisexual populations. *Top HIV Med.* (2006) **14**:84–7.
17. Hosseinifard SM, Ahmadian A, Smaeelifar N. The Synergistic (MARATHON) Effect of combined methamphetamine with sexual stimulant drugs on increasing the likelihood of high-risk sexual behaviors. *Addict Health* (2014) **6**:112–8.
18. First MB. *Structured Clinical Interview for DSM-IV-TR Axis I Disorders, Patient Edition*. New York, NY: Biometrics Research, New York State Institute (2002).
19. Oldfield RC. The assessment and analysis of handedness: the Edinburgh inventory. *Neuropsychologia* (1971) **9**:97–113. doi: 10.1016/0028-3932(71)90067-4
20. Mottola CA. Measurement strategies: the visual analogue scale. *Decubitus* (1993) **6**:56–8.
21. George MS, Anton RF, Bloomer C, Teneback C, Drobes DJ, Lorberbaum JP, et al. Activation of prefrontal cortex and anterior thalamus in alcoholic subjects on exposure to alcohol-specific cues. *Arch Gen Psychiatry* (2001) **58**:345–52. doi: 10.1001/archpsyc.58.4.345
22. Myrick H, Anton RF, Li X, Henderson S, Drobes D, Voronin K, et al. Differential brain activity in alcoholics and social drinkers to alcohol cues: relationship to craving. *Neuropsychopharmacol.* (2004) **29**:393–402. doi: 10.1038/sj.npp.1300295
23. Myrick H, Anton RF, Li X, Henderson S, Randall PK, Voronin K. Effect of naltrexone and ondansetron on alcohol cue-induced activation of the ventral striatum in alcohol-dependent people. *Arch Gen Psychiatry* (2008) **65**:466–75. doi: 10.1001/archpsyc.65.4.466
24. Ming Q, Zhong X, Zhang X, Pu W, Dong D, Jiang Y, et al. State-independent and dependent neural responses to psychosocial stress in current and remitted depression. *Am J Psychiatry* (2017) **174**:971–9. doi: 10.1176/appi.ajp.2017.16080974
25. Nichols TE, Das S, Eickhoff SB, Evans AC, Glatard T, Hanke M, et al. *Best Practices in Data Analysis and Sharing in Neuroimaging Using MRI.* OHBM COBIDAS Report v1.0 (2016).
26. Brody AL, Mandelkern MA, London ED, Childress AR, Lee GS, Bota RG, et al. Brain metabolic changes during cigarette craving. *Arch Gen Psychiatry* (2002) **59**:1162–72. doi: 10.1001/archpsyc.59.12.1162
27. Prisciandaro JJ, McRae-Clark AL, Myrick H, Henderson S, Brady KT. Brain activation to cocaine cues and motivation/treatment status. *Addict Biol.* (2014) **19**:240–9. doi: 10.1111/j.1369-1600.2012.00446.x

28. Due DL, Huettel SA, Hall WG, Rubin DC. Activation in mesolimbic and visuospatial neural circuits elicited by smoking cues: evidence from functional magnetic resonance imaging. *Am J Psychiatry* (2002) **159**:954–60. doi: 10.1176/appi.ajp.159.6.954
29. Fineberg NA, Potenza MN, Chamberlain SR, Berlin HA, Menzies L, Bechara A, et al. Probing compulsive and impulsive behaviors, from animal models to endophenotypes: a narrative review. *Neuropsychopharmacology* (2010) **35**:591–604. doi: 10.1038/npp.2009.185
30. Kalivas PW, Volkow ND. The neural basis of addiction: a pathology of motivation and choice. *Am J Psychiatry* (2005) **162**:1403–13. doi: 10.1176/appi.ajp.162.8.1403
31. Brewer JA, Potenza MN. The neurobiology and genetics of impulse control disorders: relationships to drug addictions. *Biochem Pharmacol.* (2008) **75**:63–75. doi: 10.1016/j.bcp.2007.06.043
32. Serences JT. Value-based modulations in human visual cortex. *Neuron* (2008) **60**:1169–81. doi: 10.1016/j.neuron.2008.10.051
33. Luijten M, Veltman DJ, van den Brink W, Hester R, Field M, Smits M, et al. Neurobiological substrate of smoking-related attentional bias. *Neuroimage* (2011) **54**:2374–81. doi: 10.1016/j.neuroimage.2010.09.064
34. Frohmader KS, Bateman KL, Lehman MN, Coolen LM. Effects of methamphetamine on sexual performance and compulsive sex behavior in male rats. *Psychopharmacology* (2010) **212**:93–104. doi: 10.1007/s00213-010-1930-8
35. Bolin BL, Akins CK. Methamphetamine impairs sexual motivation but not sexual performance in male Japanese quail. *Exp Clin Psychopharmacol.* (2009) **17**:10–20. doi: 10.1037/a0014505
36. Frohmader KS. *Effects of Methamphetamine on Sexual Behavior*. The University of Western Ontario (2011).

Metabolites Alterations in the Medial Prefrontal Cortex of Methamphetamine Users in Abstinence: A ^{1}H MRS Study

Qiuxia Wu[1,2,3,4,5,6,7], *Chang Qi*[1,2,3,4,5,6], *Jiang Long*[1,2,3,4,5,6], *Yanhui Liao*[1,2,3,4,5,6], *Xuyi Wang*[1,2,3,4,5,6], *An Xie*[8], *Jianbin Liu*[8], *Wei Hao*[1,2,3,4,5,6], *Yiyuan Tang*[7], *Baozhu Yang*[9], *Tieqiao Liu*[1,2,3,4,5,6*] and *Jinsong Tang*[1,2,3,4,5,6]

[1] *Department of Psychiatry, The Second Xiangya Hospital, Central South University, Changsha, China,* [2] *Mental Health Institute, The Second Xiangya Hospital, Central South University, Changsha, China,* [3] *Chinese National Clinical Research Center on Mental Disorders, Second Xiangya Hospital, Central South University, Changsha, China,* [4] *National Clinical Research Center on Mental Disorders, Changsha, China,* [5] *National Technology Institute on Mental Disorders, Changsha, China,* [6] *Hunan Key Laboratory of Psychiatry and Mental Health, Changsha, China,* [7] *Department of Psychological Sciences, Texas Tech University, Lubbock, TX, United States,* [8] *Department of Radiology, Hunan Provincial People's Hospital, Changsha, China,* [9] *Department of Psychiatry, Yale University School of Medicine, New Haven, CT, United States*

***Correspondence:**
Tieqiao Liu
liutieqiao123@csu.edu.cn

Background: The medial prefrontal cortex (mPFC) contains various neurotransmitter systems and plays an important role in drug use. Broad body of literature on how methamphetamine (MA) affects the structure and metabolism in the animal's mPFC is emerging, while the effects on metabolites of mPFC among human is still unclear. In this study, proton magnetic resonance spectroscopy (^{1}H MRS) was used to measure metabolites of mPFC in methamphetamine dependent subjects.

Methods: Sixty-one subjects with a history of MA dependence (fulfiled the Diagnostic and Statistical Manual of Mental Disorders, fourth edition criteria) and 65 drug-naïve control subjects (age19–45) completed ^{1}H MRS scans using 3.0T Siemens MRI scanner. Single voxel spectra were acquired from the mPFC bilaterally using a point resolved spectroscopy sequence (PRESS). The ^{1}H MRS data were automatically fit with linear combination model for quantification of metabolite levels of n-acetyl-aspartate (NAA), myo-inositol (ml), glycerophosphocholine plus phosphocholine(GPC+PC), phosphocreatine plus creatine (PCr+Cr), and glutamate (Glu). Metabolite levels were reported as ratios to PCr+Cr.

Results: The MA group showed a significant reduction in NAA/PCr+Cr ratio and elevation in Glu/PCr+Cr ratio and ml/PCr+Cr ratio, compared with healthy control. No significant correlation was found between metabolite ratios and MA use variables.

Conclusions: MA use is associated with a significant increased Glu/PCr+Cr ratio, ml/PCr+Cr ratio and reduced NAA/PCr+Cr ratio in the mPFC of MA dependence subjects. These findings suggest that Glu may play a key role in MA induced neurotoxicity.

Keywords: methamphetamine, mPF, NAA/PCr+Cr, Glu/PCr+Cr, ml/PCr+Cr, ^{1}H MRS

INTRODUCTION

Methamphetamine is one of the most consumed amphetamine-type stimulants (ATS) worldwide. According to the World Drug Report 2017 (1), global methamphetamine seizures reached a new peak of 132 tons, increased 21% than previous year, accounting for 60–80% of ATS seizures annually. As MA use is spreading and the treatment demand is growing, evidence on effective treatment is scarce while MA represents the greatest global health burden among ATS (1). There is abundant evidence that MA cause long-lasting impairment to the brain both in preclinical and clinical research. In preclinical studies, chronic MA exposure activated microglials (2) and astrocytes, and increased inflammatory mediators and other oxidative stress related factors (3). While in human neuroimaging studies demonstrated that chronic MA use leads to serious brain changes, including dopaminergic (4, 5), monoaminergic (6), and serotoninergic (7, 8) neurotransmitter system, cerebral glucose metabolism (9, 10), structure and integrity (9–11).

^{1}H magnetic resonance spectroscopy (^{1}H MRS) provides an invasive method to explore the metabolites in the brain. Previous ^{1}H MRS research on MA dependent (MAD) subjects shows alterations in n-acetyl-aspartate (NAA) (12–18), choline (Cho) (12, 13, 16, 17, 19), myo-inositol (mI) (13, 14), and glutamate (Glu) or Glx (meaning glutamate+glutamine) (15, 20) concentrations or the ratios of these metabolites to creatine (Cr). Most of these studies focused on anterior cingulate (12, 16–18), basal ganglia (13, 19), frontal gray (13) and white matter (13–15) , with less evidence in the medial prefrontal cortex (mPFC).

The mPFC is a terminal region of the mesocorticolimbic dopamine system which has been reported to modulate reward seeking behavior (21, 22) and is associated with drug addiction (23). The functional connectivity of the mPFC is decreased in various mental disorders (24–26), including addiction (27, 28). Previous studies suggested ATS dependent subjects have smaller volume (29–31) and decreased gray matter density (32) in the mPFC. To date, there is no report on measuring metabolite levels in the mPFC in MA users relative to healthy subjects. The mPFC contains pyramidal glutamatergic neurons that project to numerous regions (33) and repeated amphetamine administration alters a-amino-3-hydroxy-5-methylisoxazole-4-propionic acid (AMPA) receptor subunits mRNA levels in rat mPFC (34). Thus, metabolite levels in the mPFC may be different between methamphetamine dependent (MAD) subjects and healthy chontrols, especially Glu. In this present study, we performed a semi-quantitative analysis to quantify the levels of NAA, mI, GPC+PC, and Glu of the mPFC in MAD subjects. In this study, we aimed to investigate whether MA use significantly altered metabolite ratios to PCr+Cr in the mPFC. It was hypothesized that first, MA use would be associated with altered metabolite levels in the mPFC, and second, the altered metabolite levels would be significantly correlated with MA use variables, including age of first MA use (years old), duration of MA use (months), and duration of abstinence from MA use (days). In addition, we explored possible relationship between cigarettes smoked per day (CPD), Beck Depression Inventory (BDI) score, State-Trait Anxiety Inventory (STAI) scores and the metabolite levels in MA users.

METHOD

Subjects

The data were collected as a part of the brain imaging study on methamphetamine-induced psychotic symptoms, a study hosted at the Second Xiangya Hospital of Central South University. One hundred and twenty-six subjects (61 MAD subjects and 65 drug-free healthy subjects, age 19–45) were enrolled in this study. Subjects between 18 and 45 years were entitled to participate in the study. MAD volunteers were recruited from The Kangda Voluntary Drug Rehabilitation Centers in Hunan Province. All MA users fulfiled the Diagnostic and Statistical Manual of Mental Disorders, fourth edition (DSM-IV) criteria (35) for lifetime MA dependence assessed by the Structured Clinical Interview (SCID) (36). MAD subjects were excluded if they met criteria for other substance dependence (excluding nicotine dependence) at any time. Subjects were required to abstain from MA for at least 48 h before scanning. Drug free healthy control subjects were recruited from community through advertising. Participants were excluded if they (i) had any general medical condition or neurological disorder, including infectious, hepatic or endocrine disease; (ii) had a history of severe head injury with skull fracture or loss of consciousness of more than 10 min; (iii) had any current or previous psychiatric disorder; (iv) had a family history of psychiatric disorder; (v) women during pregnant or breast-feed stage; (vi) had contraindications for MRI. Two licensed psychiatrist, at MD level, conducted all clinical interviews. Subjects were fully informed about the measurement and MRI scanning in the study. Written informed consent was given by all subjects. This study was approved by the Ethics Committee of the Second Xiangya Hospital, Central South University (No. S095, 2013) and was carried out in accordance with the Declaration of Helsinki. We used the BDI-II to measure the depression symptoms in the last week before undergoing MRI scans. STAI was used to measure anxiety level before MRI scanning (STAI-Y1), and anxiety level as a personal characteristic (STAI-Y2). The demographic characteristic were shown in **Table 1**.

Magnetic Resonance Data Acquisition

Structural MRI and MRS data were acquired with a Siemens Magnetom Trio 3.0 T MR scanner (Siemens, Erlangen, Germany) using an eight-channel standard quadrature headcoil at the Magnetic Resonance Center of Hunan provincial People's Hospital, China. Three-dimensional T1-weighted images were collected using a gradient echo sequence (repetition time = 2,000 ms, echo time = 2.26 ms, field of view= 256 × 256 mm, flip angle = 8°, matrix size =256 × 256, number of slices = 176, slice thickness = 1 mm). Using these images, a single ^{1}H MRS voxel was placed on the corpus callosumand centered on the intrahemispheric fissure, including medial superior frontal gyrus and anterior cingulate cortices, not containing the orbitofrontal cortex (see **Figure 1**). ^{1}H MRS was performed using a short-echo point resolved spectroscopy sequence (PRESS; repetition time = 1,500 ms; echo time = 30 ms;

voxel size 30 × 25 × 30 mm; number of scans = 256, spectral bandwidth = 1,200 Hz, the number of data points = 1,024 points). Water suppression was achieved using a chemical shift selective (CHESS) sequence.

^{1}H MRS spectra were automatically fit with linear combination model (LCModel version 6.3-1B [LCMODEL Inc. CA (37)] at the Second Affiliated Hospital, Shantou University Medical College located in Shantou, Guangdong, China. Metabolite concentration for NAA, PCr+Cr, GPC+PC, mI and Glu were acquired using LCModel software (**Figure 2**). The signal-to-noise ratio (S/N) and full width at half maximum (FWHM) of each spectrum were checked for quality to ensure they were adequate for reliable peak fitting for the metabolites of interest. Only those spectra with FWHM ≤ 0.1 ppm and S/N ≥ 20 were retained. Furthermore, only those metabolite speaks satisfying the LCModel criterion less than 20% of Cramer-Rao lower bound (CRLB) value were reported here. PCr+Cr severs as a reference for other metabolite peaks on the assumption that its concentration is relatively constant. We first observed that there was no absolute PCr+Cr difference prior to forming ratios with respect to PCr+Cr. The common practice of normalization by PCr+Cr removd the across-subject variability, which arises from technical factors, such as coil loading. From these data, the metabolite ratios of NAA/PCr+Cr, mI/PCr+Cr, Glu/PCr+Cr, and GPC+PC/PCr+Cr were reported here.

Segmentation was performed on T1-weighted images using New Segment+DARTEL in Data Processing & Analysis of Brain Imaging (38). Estimation of tissue volume was collected from the normalized gray matter, white matter, and cerebrospinal fluid (CSF) images using custom Matlab (The Mathworks, Inc.) code (http://www.cs.ucl.ac.uk/staff/G.Ridgway/vbm/get_totals.m). GM fractions, WM fractions and CSF fractions in the MAD subjects and controls were shown in **Table 2.** No statistical significance was found between the two groups.

TABLE 1 | Demographics of participants and MA use variables in MRS study.

	Abstinent MAD subjects (N = 61)	Controls (N = 65)	P
Age (range)	29.0 ± 5.8 (19–40)	30.0 ± 6.1 (21–45)	0.38
Gender(female/male)	54/7	53/12	0.33
Education(years)	11.5 ± 2.9	12.4 ± 2.6	0.07
BMI	24.0 ± 3.2	22.8 ± 3.2	0.08
CPD	20 (10, 20)	16 (5, 20)	<0.01
BDI Score	11.0 ± 7.8	4 (0, 8)	<0.01
Total AI Score	75.6 ± 16.0	71.5 ± 16.7	0.17
STAI-Y1	35.0 ± 8.0	33.5 ± 9.9	0.37
STAI-Y2	40.6 ± 9.9	38.0 ± 8.8	0.12
Age started using MA (years old)	23.9 ± 5.7		
Duration of MA use (months)	51.2 ± 26.8		
Abstinence from using MA(days)	42.7 ± 20.9		

Statistical Analysis

Statistical analysis was performed with SPSS 20 (IBM Inc. New York, USA). Assumption of normality of each variable was tested with the Shapiro–Wilk test. Because of non-normality of the data, CPD and BDI scores were compared using a Mann-Whitney U test, and gender with Chi-square test for independence. Metabolite concentrations were reported as mean ± standard deviation. General Linear Model multivariate analysis was used to evaluate group differences in metabolite ratios controlling for CPD and gray matter tissue fraction in the voxle. Correlation analyses between metabolite ratios and each of clinical parameters, including age, months of MA use, days of abstinence, age of onset of MA use, CPD, BDI, total STAI scores, STAI-Y1 score, and STAI-Y2 score were performed using Pearson's or Spearman's correlation analysis, followed by Bonferroni test. Statistical significance was defined at $p < 0.05$, two-tailed.

RESULTS

Demographic Characteristic

The groups did not differ in gender, mean age, BMI, or years of education (**Table 1**). The CPD ($p < 0.01$) in MAD subjects was higher than those in healthy controls. The BDI score ($p < 0.01$) was higher in MAD subjects. There were no

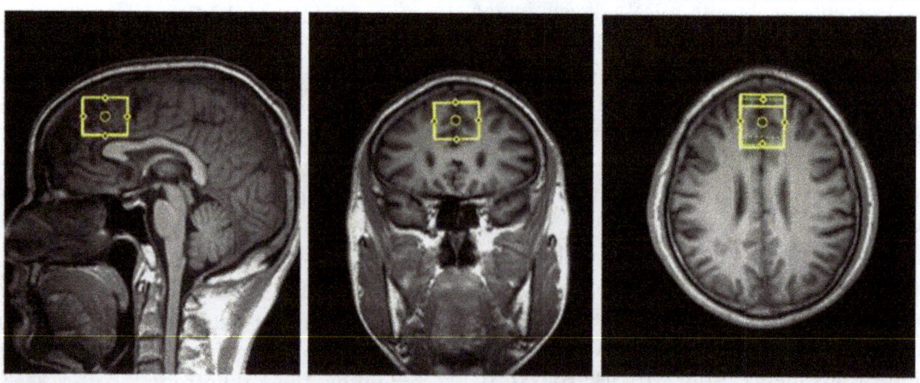

FIGURE 1 | Region of interest in medial prefrontal cortex in coronal, sagittal and transverse views.

significant differences in the total STAI scores ($p = 0.17$), STAI-Y1 ($p = 0.37$), or STAI-Y2 ($p = 0.12$) between the two groups.

Tissue Composition Within Voxels of Interest

Segmentation indicates the fractional contribution of gray matter, white matter and CSF in the MAD group = 44% gray, 30% white and 23% CSF and in healthy control group = 46% gray, 32% white and 23% CSF. No differences in the fractions of gray ($p = 0.06$), white ($p = 0.10$), and CSF ($p = 0.85$) were detected between MAD subjects and controls.

FWHM, S/N, and CRLB Values of MRS Data

There was no difference between the MAD group and control group in FWHM ($p = 0.23$). There was significant difference in S/N between MAD group and healthy control group ($p < 0.01$). There were significant differences between the two groups in CRLB values for NAA ($p < 0.01$), mI ($p < 0.01$), GPC+PC ($p = 0.01$) and Glu ($p < 0.01$) (see **Table 3**).

^{1}H MRS Metabolite Ratios

The MAD group and control group did not differ significantly in absolute PCr+Cr values (mean = 6.47 vs. 6.58, $p = 0.44$), which served as the denominator for the ratios tested. Compared with healthy controls, MAD subjects had significant decreased NAA/PCr+Cr ratios (mean = 1.12 vs. 1.17, $p = 0.02$), increased

TABLE 2 | Tissue fraction of the region of interest in the mPFC.

	Abstinent MAD subjects (*N* = 61)	Controls (*N* = 65)	*P*
Gray matter fraction	0.44 ± 0.08	0.46 ± 0.01	0.06
White matter fraction	0.30 ± 0.06	0.32 ± 0.02	0.10
CSF fraction	0.23 ± 0.05	0.23 ± 0.01	0.85

TABLE 3 | FWHM, S/N, and CRLB values between MAD subjects (n=61) and healthy controls (*n* = 65).

	Abstinent MAD subjects (*N* = 61)	Controls (*N* = 65)	*P*
FWHM(ppm)	0.05 (0.05, 0.06)	0.06 (0.048, 0.067)	0.23
S/N	28.85 ± 5.01	37.91 ± 7.96	<0.01
CRLB values for NAA	0.03 (0.03, 0.04)	0.02 (0.02, 0.03)	<0.01
CRLB values for ml	0.04 (0.03, 0.04)	0.03 (0.03, 0.04)	<0.01
CRLB values for GPC+PC	0.02 (0.02, 0.03)	0.02 (0.02, 0.02)	0.12
CRLB values for Glu	0.06 (0.05, 0.06)	0.05 (0.05, 0.06)	<0.01

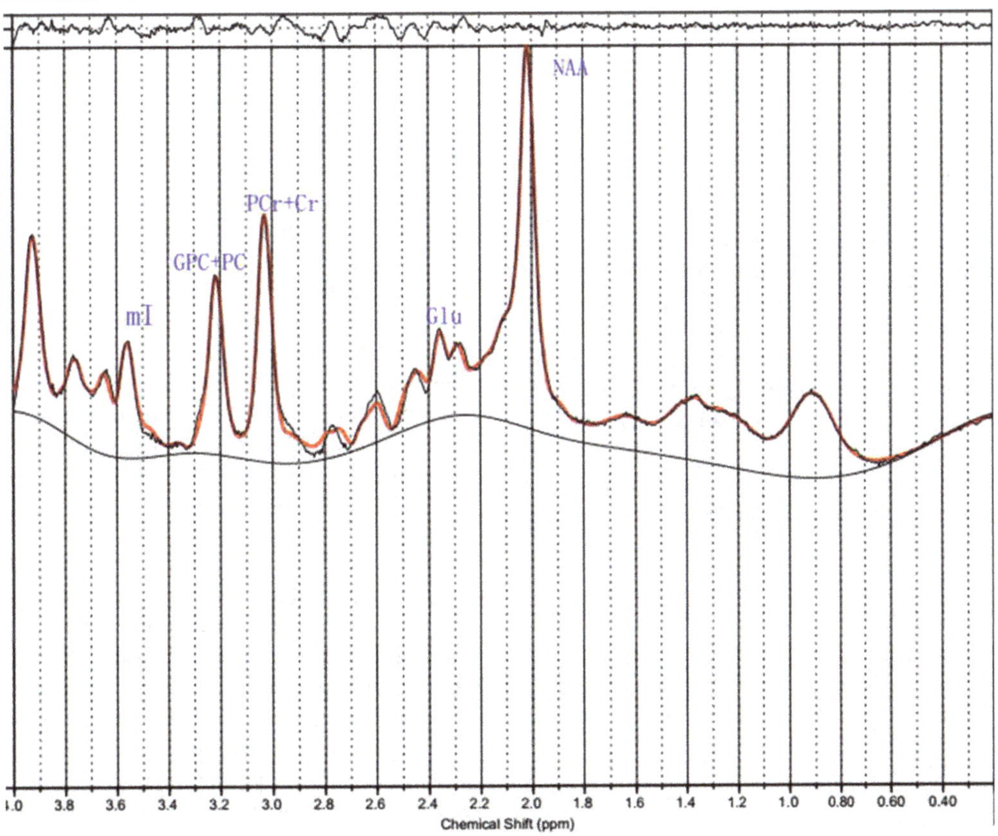

FIGURE 2 | ^{1}H MRS data.Spectra of the unfiltered data superimposed with the LCModel fit.

mI/PCr+Cr ratios (mean = 0.85 vs. 0.80, $p < 0.01$) and Glu/PCr+Cr ratios (mean = 1.03 vs. 0.95, $p < 0.01$) in the mPFC. There was not significant difference in GPC+PC/PCr+Cr between the two groups (mean = 0.27 vs. 0.27, $p = 0.73$) (see **Table 4**).

^{1}H-MRS Metabolite Levels With MA Use, Age, CPD, and Anxiety

For the MA users, there were no significant correlation between ratios of metabolites and MA use variables. There were no significant correlation between age, CPD and metabolite ratios.

DISCUSSION

There was no significant difference in PCr+Cr levels between MAD group and control group, so the differences in NAA/PCr+Cr, mI/PCr+Cr, and Glu/PCr+Cr between groups are probably due to the differences in NAA, mI and Glu levels between groups. The first finding of the present study is that the NAA/PCr+Cr ratio was increased in the mPFC of MAD subjects. Finding the decreased ratio of NAA/PCr+Cr among MAD subjects is consistent with previous studies (12, 16, 18, 39, 40) and as well as other psychiatric disorders (41). NAA is taken as a neuronal marker, and reflects neuronal integrity, viability and number (42). NAA plays a key role in enhancing mitochondrial energy production from Glu (42) and also reflects functional status of neuronal mitochondria (43). The changes of NAA/PCr+Cr may reflect adverse neuron function disorder. Besides, the pathological deletion of dendrite or degeneration of neuron may be related with decreased NAA. The present finding suggests that there is decreased neuronal integrity, viability, number, or mitochondraial dysfunction in the mPFC in MAD individuals, even though they have been abstinent from MA.

The second finding is that the ratio of mI/PCr+Cr was significantly increased in the mPFC of MAD subjects compared with healthy controls. The increased ratio of mI/PCr+Cr in MAD group is in line with previous studies, which were reported in frontal gray matter and white matter of MA users (13, 14, 44). Mostly mI is considered as a marker of glial (45). Some studies suggested that Ins is an osmoregulator (46) and contributes to glucose storage (47) and is a precursor in the PI-cycle second messenger system (47). Elevation of mI may suggest that proliferation of glial cells or inflammation due to the damage of neurons induced by methamphetamine, which is a marker of MA induced neurons damage after NAA decreased. MA has been reported to induced gliosis *in vitro* and in animal experiment. After acute administration of MA to rats (48) and vervet monkeys (49) induced glial activation, and gliosis remains after stopped exposure one and half a year (49).

The final finding is a significant increase in ratios of Glu/PCr+Cr in the mPFC of MAD subjects. The most consistent alteration across MA abuse was reduction in NAA, while change in Glu was inconsistent. Glx and Glu were reported to be lower in the mPFC (39), precuneus, posterior cingulate, and right inferior frontal cortex (20), while Glu was repored to be higher in frontal white matter of abstinent MAD subjects (15). But the Glu levels in the posterior gray matter did not differ with HC (15). In one study, in the frontal gray matter of the MA users, the Glx concentration reduced during early abstinence, reached relatively normal after 1–2 months, and exceeded normal levels in longer-term abstinence (50). In the Crocker's study, the concentration levels of Glu in the MA group was reduced relative to HC and schizophrenia patients (39). In another study, however, Glu levels in the ACC and DLPFC did not differ between MAD subjects and controls (12). Several variables may contribute to these inconsistencies. These studies evaluated different brain regions and used different field strength. Other variables include the length of time using MA, dose, frequency of use, duration of abstinence and the sample size.

This is a relatively large sample study to report of increased ratio of Glu/PCr+Cr in the mPFC among MAD subjects, although preclinical studies have found such findings (51–53). Glu is the major excitatory neurotransmitter, and most of Glu is present intracellularly. Extracellular Glu released from nerve terminals is taken up by Glu receptors and Glu transporters present presynaptically, postsynaptically and extrasynaptically in glial cells, preventing Glu excitotoxicity (54). Glu in the glial cells is converted to glutamine (Gln) through an ATP-dependent process in mitochondria. Gln is subsequently released from the glial cells and taken up by Gln transporters in neurons. Gln in neurons is converted back to Glu. This is the "glutamate–glutamine cycle," which represents 40–50% of the total flux from the TCA cycle (54). Therefore, dysfunction of Glu receptors or Glu transporters may be a possible explanation for elevated Glu concentration in the mPFC. The elevated Glu concentration suggests that the Gln converted from Glu is decreased and decreased activities of glutamateric neurons. Meanwhile the increased extracellular Glu concentration is neurotoxic.

In the research conducted by Sailasuta et al., around 36% of normal glial tricarboxylic acid (TCA) cycle rate was significant reduced in frontal brain of abstinent MA abusers, which may impact the glutamate-glutamine cyle and thus result in accumulation of Glu (55). Therefore, the other possible explanation of the increased Glu concentration in our study is the consequence of dysfunction of glial cells.

Furthermore, the increased extracellular Glu concentration is considered as an important factor of relapse. Glutamateric signal system plays an important role in drug-seeking behavior. It has been reported that the activation of Glu

TABLE 4 | Metabolite concentrations in the mPFC of MAD subjects ($n = 61$) and healthy controls($n = 65$).

	Abstinent MAD subjects ($N = 61$)	Controls ($N = 65$)	P
PCr+Cr	6.47 ± 0.83	6.58 ± 0.70	0.44
NAA/PCr+Cr	1.12 ± 0.08	1.17 ± 0.07	0.01
ml//PCr+Cr	0.85 ± 0.09	0.80 ± 0.09	<0.01
GPC+PC/PCr+Cr	0.27 ± 0.03	0.27 ± 0.03	0.78
Glu/PCr+Cr	1.03 ± 0.15	0.95 ± 0.14	<0.01

transporter (56), or gene expression of the transporter in the nucleus accumbens (57) plays an inhibitory role in MA conditioned place preference (CPP), while mPFC is acritical region for reactivation of the MA-CPP memory (58). Glu released from the mPFC stimulates dopamine release in the ventral tegmental area and the nucleus accumbens (59), while dopaminergic system is considered as primary mechanism initiating drug reinstatement (60). In a preclinical study, the increased expression of the Glu transporter attenuated the MA-CPP, which reduced drug-seeking behavior (61).

Limitations

This study has several limitations. First, most of subjects in this study were men, making it impossible to explore the influence of gender confidently. Second, the characteristics of MAD subjects in this study, including the range of duration of MA use and abstinence, and the drug used in the abstinence would be possible confounding factors. Third, the study is cross-sectional, it is unclear whether alterations in these metabolites would reverse completely during continued abstinence or would persist. Furthermore, MAD subjects had a higher CPD than the controls, and this difference was significant. We noted this difference, controlled this covariate in statistical analysis process and discussed their possible impacts on our MRS results. We concluded that this difference in CPD between the MAD subjects and healthy controls is unlikely to be the reason for the statistically significant alterations of metabolites of the mPFC. Our study is a relatively large sample and we controlled the cigarette smoking when comparing the metabolites. Finally, there were significant differences between MAD subjects and controls in the S/N ratios and CRLB values. But the S/N ratios and CRLB values in both groups characterize relatively good quality of our data. Future studies should include more women MAD subjects, measure alterations longitudinally when MAD subjects using MA (if possible), at the beginning of abstinence, and after longer duration (6–24 months) of abstinence, and match subjects' cigarette smoking.

CONCLUSION

Our findings suggest that the alterations in ratios of Glu/PCr+Cr of the mPFC may underlie the pathophysiology of neurological injury in MA abuse. MA cause the Glu concentration elevation, which has neurotoxicity and may lead to NAA concentration decreased and mI increased. This study implicates that Glu plays an important role in MA dependent disorder, reducing Glu concentration or increasing the activity of Glu receptors in the mPFC may be of great clinical significance in the treatment.

AUTHOR CONTRIBUTIONS

YL, JT, JLi, and TL contributed conception and design of the study. QW, CQ, and AX organized the database. QW performed the statistical analysis and wrote the first draft of the manuscript. JLo, YL, XW, YT, and JT revised the manuscript. TL, BY and WH advised on the statistical analysis, interpretation of findings, and reviewed drafts of the manuscript.

FUNDING

This study was supported by the National Natural Science Foundation of China (Grant No. 81371465 and 81671324 to TL, and 81671325 to YL), Natural Science Foundation of Hunan Province (Grant No. 14JJ4075 to JLo) and Hunan Provincial Innovation Foundation for Postgraduate (Grant No. CX2017B071 to QW).

ACKNOWLEDGMENTS

We acknowledge all the professionals in Kangda Voluntary Drug Rehabilitation Centers who helped a lot in data collection. The authors thank all the subjects who participated in this study.

REFERENCES

1. United Nations Office on Drugs and Crime. *World Drug Report*. United Nations publication, Sales No. 2 E.17.XI.6. (2017).
2. Thomas DM, Walker PD, Benjamins JA, Geddes TJ, Kuhn DM. Methamphetamine neurotoxicity in dopamine nerve endings of the striatum is associated with microglial activation. *J Pharmacol Exp Ther.* (2004) 311:1–7. doi: 10.1124/jpet.104.070961
3. Yamamoto BK, Bankson MG. Amphetamine neurotoxicity: cause and consequence of oxidative stress. *Crit Rev Neurobiol.* (2005) 17:87–117. doi: 10.1615/CritRevNeurobiol.v17.i2.30
4. Sekine Y, Minabe Y, Ouchi Y, Takei N, Iyo M, Nakamura K, et al. Association of dopamine transporter loss in the orbitofrontal and dorsolateral prefrontal cortices with methamphetamine-related psychiatric symptoms. *Am J Psychiatry.* (2003) 160:1699–1701. doi: 10.1176/appi.ajp.160.9.1699
5. Volkow ND, Chang L, Wang GJ, Fowler JS, Leonido-Yee M, Franceschi D, et al. Association of dopamine transporter reduction with psychomotor impairment in methamphetamine abusers. *Am J Psychiatry.* (2001) 158:377–82. doi: 10.1176/appi.ajp.158.3.377
6. McFadden LM, Stout KA, Vieira-Brock PL, Allen SC, Nielsen SM, Wilkins DG, et al. Methamphetamine self-administration acutely decreases monoaminergic transporter function. *Synapse.* (2012) 66:240–5. doi: 10.1002/syn.21506
7. Sekine Y, Ouchi Y, Takei N, Yoshikawa E, Nakamura K, Futatsubashi M, et al. Brain serotonin transporter density and aggression in abstinent methamphetamine abusers. *Arch Gen Sychiatry.* (2006) 63:90–100. doi: 10.1001/archpsyc.63.1.90
8. Kish SJ, Fitzmaurice PS, Boileau I, Schmunk GA, Ang LC, Furukawa Y, et al. Brain serotonin transporter in human methamphetamine users. *Psychopharmacology (Berl).* (2009) 202:649–61. doi: 10.1007/s00213-008-1346-x
9. Volkow ND, Chang L, Wang GJ, Fowler JS, Franceschi D, Sedler MJ, et al. Higher cortical and lower subcortical metabolism in detoxified methamphetamine abusers. *Am J Psychiatry* (2001) 158:383–389. doi: 10.1176/appi.ajp.158.3.383
10. Berman SM, Voytek B, Mandelkern MA, Hassid BD, Isaacson A, MonterossoJ, et al. Changes in cerebral glucose metabolism during early abstinence from chronic methamphetamine abuse. *Mol Psychiatry* (2008) 13:897–908. doi: 10.1038/sj.mp.4002107

11. Chung A, Lyoo IK, Kim SJ, Hwang J, Bae SC, Sung YH, et al. Decreased frontal white-matter integrity in abstinent methamphetamine abusers. *Int J Neuropsychopharmacol.* (2007) 10:765–75. doi: 10.1017/S1461145706007395
12. Howells FM, Uhlmann A, Temmingh H, Sinclair H, Meintjes E, Wilson D, et al. (1)H-magnetic resonance spectroscopy ((1H)-MRS) in methamphetamine dependence and methamphetamine induced psychosis. *Schizophr Res.* (2014) 153:122–8.doi: 10.1016/j.schres.2014.01.029
13. Ernst T, Chang L, Leonido-Yee M, Speck O. Evidence for long-term neurotoxicity associated with methamphetamine abuse: a 1H MRS study. *Neurology* (2000) 54:1344–9. doi: 10.1212/WNL.54.6.1344
14. Sung YH, Cho SC, Hwang J, Kim SJ, Kim H, Bae S, et al. Relationship between N-acetyl-aspartate in gray and white matter of abstinent methamphetamine abusers and their history of drug abuse: a proton magnetic resonance spectroscopy study. *Drug Alcohol Depend.* (2007) 88:28–35. doi: 10.1016/j.drugalcdep.2006.09.011
15. Sailasuta N, Abulseoud O, Hernandez M, Haghani P, Ross BD. Metabolic abnormalities in abstinent methamphetamine dependent subjects. *Subst Abuse.* (2010) 2014:9–20. doi: 10.4137/SART.S4625
16. Nordahl TE, Salo R, Natsuaki Y, Galloway GP, Waters C, Moore CD, et al. Methamphetamine users in sustained abstinence: a proton magnetic resonance spectroscopy study. *Arch Gen Psychiatry.* (2005) 62:444–52. doi: 10.1001/archpsyc.62.4.444
17. Salo R, Nordahl TE, Natsuaki Y, Leamon MH, Galloway GP, Waters C, et al. Attentional control and brain metabolite levels in methamphetamine abusers. *Biol Psychiatry* (2007) 61:1272–80. doi: 10.1016/j.biopsych.2006.07.031
18. Nordahl TE, Salo R, Possin K, Gibson DR, Flynn N, Leamon M, et al. Low N-acetyl-aspartate and high choline in the anterior cingulum of recently abstinent methamphetamine-dependent subjects: a preliminary proton MRS study. *Psychiatry Res.* (2002) 116:43–52. doi: 10.1016/S0925-4927(02)00088-4
19. Sekine Y, Minabe Y, Kawai M, Suzuki K, Iyo M, Isoda H, et al. Metabolite alterations in basal ganglia associated with methamphetamine-related psychiatric symptoms. A proton MRS study. *Neuropsychopharmacology* (2002) 27:453–61. doi: 10.1016/S0893-133X(02)00321-4
20. O'Neill J, Tobias MC, Hudkins M, London ED. Glutamatergic neurometabolites during early abstinence from chronic methamphetamine abuse. *Int J Neuropsychopharmacol.* (2014) 18:pyu059. doi: 10.1093/ijnp/pyu059
21. Kim CK, Ye L, Jennings JH, Pichamoorthy N, Tang DD, Yoo AW, et al. Molecular and circuit-dynamical identification of top-down neural mechanisms for restraint of reward seeking. *Cell* (2017) 170:1013–27.e14. doi: 10.1016/j.cell.2017.07.020
22. Ferenczi EA, Zalocusky KA, Liston C, Grosenick L, Warden MR, Amatya D, et al. Prefrontal cortical regulation of brain wide circuit dynamics and reward-related behavior. *Science* (2016) 351:aac9698. doi: 10.1126/science.aac9698
23. Steketee JD. Neurotransmitter systems of the medial prefrontal cortex: potential role in sensitization to psychostimulants. *Brain Res Rev.* (2003) 41:203–228. doi: 10.1016/S0165-0173(02)00233-3
24. Wang S, Zhang Y, Lv L, Wu R, Fan X, Zhao J, et al. Abnormal regional homogeneity as a potential imaging biomarke for adolescent-onset schizophrenia:a resting-state fMRI study and support vector machine analysis. *Schizophr Res.* (2018) 192:179–84. doi: 10.1016/j.schres.2017.05.038
25. Guo W, Cui X, Liu F, Chen J, Xie G, Wu R, et al. Increased anterior default-mode network homogeneity in first-episode, drug-naive major depressive disorder: a replication study. *J Affect Disord.* (2018) 225:767–72. doi: 10.1016/j.jad.2017.08.089
26. Wu G, Wang Y, Mwansisya TE, Pu W, Zhang H, Liu C, et al. Effective connectivity of the posterior cingulate and medial prefrontal cortices relates to working memory impairment in schizophrenic and bipolar patients. *Schizophr Res.* (2014) 158:85–90. doi: 10.1016/j.schres.2014.06.033
27. Gu H, Salmeron BJ, Ross TJ, Geng X, Zhan W, Stein EA, et al. Mesocorticolimbic circuits are impaired in chronic cocaine users as demonstrated by resting-state functional connectivity. *Neuroimage* (2010) 53:593–601. doi: 10.1016/j.neuroimage.2010.06.066
28. LiaoY, Tang J, Fornito A, Liu T, Chen X, Chen H, et al. Alterations in regional homogeneity of resting-state brain activity in ketamine addicts. *Neurosci Lett.* (2012) 522:36–40. doi: 10.1016/j.neulet.2012.06.009
29. Daumann J, Koester P, Becker B, Wagner D, Imperati D, Gouzoulis-Mayfrank E, et al. Medial prefrontal gray matter volume reductions in users of amphetamine-type stimulants revealed by combined tract-based spatial statistics and voxel-based morphometry. *Neuroimage* (2011) 54:794–801. doi: 10.1016/j.neuroimage.2010.08.065
30. Becker B, Wagner D, Koester P, Tittgemeyer M, Mercer-Chalmers-Bender K, Hurlemann R, et al. Smaller amygdala and medial prefrontal cortex predict escalating stimulant use. *Brain* (2015) 138(Pt 7):2074–86. doi: 10.1093/brain/awv113
31. Aoki Y, Orikabe L, Takayanagi Y, Yahata N, Mozue Y, Sudo Y, et al. Volume reductions in frontopolar and left perisylvian cortices in methamphetamine induced psychosis. *Schizophr Res.* (2013) 147:355–61. doi: 10.1016/j.schres.2013.04.029
32. Kim SJ, Lyoo IK, Hwang J, Chung A, Hoon Sung Y, Kim J, et al. Prefrontal grey-matter changes in short-term and long-term abstinent methamphetamine abusers. *Int J Neuropsychopharmacol.* (2006) 9:221–8. doi: 10.1017/S1461145705005699
33. Sesack SR, Deutch AY, Roth RH, Bunney BS. Topographical organization of the efferent projections of the medial prefrontal cortex in the rat: an anterograde tract-tracing study with Phaseolus vulgaris leucoagglutinin. *J Comp Neurol.* (1989) 290:213–42.
34. Lu W, Chen H, Xue CJ, Wolf ME. Repeated amphetamine administration alters AMPA receptor subunits expression in rat nucleus accumbens and medial prefrontal cortex. *Synapse* (1997) 26:269–80.
35. Spitzer RL, Williams JB, Gibbon M, First MB. The structured clinical interview for DSM-III-R (SCID). I: History, rationale, and description. *Arch Gen Psychiatry.* (1992) 49:624–9.
36. American Psychiatric Association. *Diagnostic and Statistical Manual for Mental Disorders, 4th Edn. (DSM-IV).* Washington, DC: American Psychiatric Association (2000). doi: 10.1176/appi.books.9780890423349
37. Provencher SW. Estimation of metabolite concentrations from localized *in vivo* proton NMR spectra. *Magn Reson Med.* (1993) 30:672–9.
38. Yan CG, Wang XD, Zuo XN, Zang YF. DPABI: Data Processing & Analysis for (Resting-State) Brain Imaging. *Neuroinformatics* (2016) 14:339–51. doi: 10.1007/s12021-016-9299-4
39. Crocker CE, Bernier DC, Hanstock CC, Lakusta B, Purdon SE, Seres P, et al. Prefrontal glutamate levels differentiate early phase schizophrenia and methamphetamine addiction: a (1)H MRS study at 3 Tesla. *Schizophr Res.* (2014) 157:231–7. doi: 10.1016/j.schres.2014.05.004
40. Burger A, Brooks SJ, Stein DJ, Howells FM. The impact of acute and short-term methamphetamine abstinence on brain metabolites: a proton magnetic resonance spectroscopy chemical shift imaging study. *Drug Alcohol Depend.* (2018) 185:226–37. doi: 10.1016/j.drugalcdep.2017.11.029
41. Zong X, Hu M, Li Z, Cao H, He Y, Liao Y, et al. N-acetylaspartate reduction in the medial prefrontal cortex following 8 weeks of risperidone treatment in first-episode drug-naïve schizophrenia patients. *Sci Rep.* (2015) 5:9109. doi: 10.1038/srep09109
42. Moffett JR, Ross B, Arun P, Madhavarao CN, Namboodiri AM. N-Acetylaspartate in the CNS: from neurodiagnostics to neurobiology. *Prog Neurobiol.* (2007) 81:89–131. doi: 10.1016/j.pneurobio.2006.12.003
43. Paslakis G, Träber F, Roberz J, Block W, Jessen F. N-acetyl-aspartate (NAA) as a correlate of pharmacological treatment in psychiatric disorders: a systematic review. *Eur Neuropsychopharmacol.* (2014) 24:1659–75. doi: 10.1016/j.euroneuro.2014.06.004
44. Chang L, Ernst T, Speck O, Grob CS. Additive effects of HIV and chronic methamphetamine use on brain metabolite abnormalities. *Am J Psychiatry* (2005) 162:361–9. doi: 10.1176/appi.ajp.162.2.361
45. Brand A, Richter-Landsberg C, Leibfritz D. Multinuclear NMR studies on the energy metabolism of glial and neuronal cells. *Dev Neurosci.* (1993) 15:289. doi: 10.1159/000111347
46. Nakanishi T, Turner RJ, Burg MB. Osmoregulatory changes in myo-inositol transport by renal cells. *Proc Natl Acad Sci USA.* (1989) 86:6002–6.
47. Ross BD. Biochemical considerations in 1H spectroscopy. Glutamate and glutamine; myo-inositol and related metabolites. *NMR Biomed.* (1991) 4:59–63.
48. Hebert MA, O'Callaghan JP. Protein phosphorylation cascades associated with methamphetamine-induced glial activation. *Ann NY Acad Sci.* (2000) 914:238–62. doi: 10.1111/j.1749-6632.2000.tb05200.x
49. Harveya DC, Lacana G, Taniousa SP, Melega WP. Recovery from methamphetamine induced long-term nigrostriatal dopaminergic

deficits without substantia nigra cell loss. *Brain Res.* (2000) 871:259–70. doi: 10.1016/S0006-8993(00)02439-2

50. Ernst T, Chang L. Adaptation of brain glutamate plus glutamine during abstinence from chronic methamphetamine use. *J Neuroimmune Pharmacol.* (2008) 3:165–72. doi: 10.1007/s11481-008-9108-4
51. Abekawa T, Ohmori T, Koyama T. Effects of repeated administration of a high dose of methamphetamine on dopamine and glutamate release in rat striatum and nucleus accumbens. *Brain Res.* (1994) 643:276–81. doi: 10.1016/0006-8993(94)90033-7
52. Stephans SE, Yamamoto BY. Effect of repeated methamphetamine administrations on dopamine and glutamate efflux in rat prefrontal cortex. *Brain Res.* (1995) 700:99–106. doi: 10.1016/0006-8993(95)00938-M
53. Parsegian A, See RE. Dysregulation of dopamine and glutamate release in the prefrontal cortex and nucleus accumbens following methamphetamine self-administration and during reinstatement in rats. *Neuropsychopharmacology* (2014) 39:811–22. doi: 10.1038/npp.2013.231
54. Danbolt NC. Glutamate uptake. *Prog Neurobiol.* (2001) 65:1–105. doi: 10.1016/S0301-0082(00)00067-8
55. Sailasuta N, Abulseoud O, Harris KC, Ross BD. Glial dysfunction inabstinent methamphetamine abusers. *J Cereb Blood Flow Metab.* (2010) 30:950–60. doi: 10.1038/jcbfm.2009.261
56. Nakagawa T, Fujio M, Ozawa T, Minami M, Satoh M. Effect of MS-153, a glutamate transporter activator, on the conditioned rewarding effects of morphine, methamphetamine and cocaine in mice. *Behav Brain Res.* (2005) 156:233–9. doi: 10.1016/j.bbr.2004.05.029
57. Fujio M, Nakagawa T, Sekiya Y, Ozawa T, Suzuki Y, Minami M, et al.Gene transfer of GLT-1, a glutamate transporter, into the nucleus accumbens shell attenuates methamphetamine- and orphine-induced conditioned place preference in rats. *Eur J Neurosci.* (2005) 22:2744–54. doi: 10.1111/j.1460-9568.2005.04467.x
58. Chiang CY, Cherng CG, Lai YT, Fan HY, Chuang JY, Kao GS, et al. Medial prefrontal cortex and nucleus accumbens core are involved in retrieval of the methamphetamine-associated memory. *Behav Brain Res.* (2009) 197:24–30. doi: 10.1016/j.bbr.2008.07.030
59. Krystal JH, D'Souza DC, Mathalon D, Perry E, Belger A, Hoffman R. NMDA receptor antagonist effects, cortical glutamatergic function, and schizophrenia:toward a paradigm shift in medication development. *Psychopharmacology(Berl).* (2003) 169:215–33. doi: 10.1007/s00213-003-1582-z
60. Willuhn I, Wanat MJ, Clark JJ, Phillips PE. Dopamine signaling in the nucleus accumbens of animals self-administering drugs of abuse. *Curr Top Behav Neurosci.* (2010) 3:29–71. doi: 10.1007/7854_2009_27
61. Abulseoud OA, Miller JD, Wu J, Choi DS, Holschneider DP. Ceftriaxone upregulates the glutamate transporter in medial prefrontal cortex and blocks reinstatement of methamphetamine seeking in a condition place preference paradigm. *Brain Res.* (2012) 1456:14–21. doi: 10.1016/j.brainres.2012.03.045

14

Electrophysiological Evidence for Elimination of the Positive Bias in Elderly Adults with Depressive Symptoms

*Huixia Zhou[1,2], Bibing Dai[1,5], Sonja Rossi[6] and Juan Li[1,2,3,4]**

[1] Center on Ageing Psychology, CAS Key Laboratory of Mental Health, Institute of Psychology, Beijing, China, [2] Department of Psychology, University of Chinese Academy of Sciences, Beijing, China, [3] Magnetic Resonance Imaging Research Center, Institute of Psychology, Chinese Academy of Sciences, Beijing, China, [4] State Key Laboratory of Brain and Cognitive Science, Institute of Biophysics, Chinese Academy of Sciences, Beijing, China, [5] Institute of Psychology, Tianjin Medical University, Tianjin, China, [6] Clinic for Hearing-, Speech- and Voice Disorders, Medical University of Innsbruck, Innsbruck, Austria

Correspondence:
Li Juan
lijuan@psych.ac.cn

Background: Depressed populations demonstrate a greater tendency to have negative interpretations on ambiguous situations. Cognitive theories concerning depression proposed that such a negative bias plays an important role in developing and maintaining depression. There is now fairly consistent evidence arising from different stimuli and assessment methods that depression is featured by such a bias. The current study aimed to explore the neural signatures associated with the interpretation bias in the elderly with depressive symptoms confronted with different facial expressions using event-related brain potentials (ERPs).

Methods: Participants were 14 community-dwelling older adults with depressive symptoms assessed by the Center for Epidemiologic Studies Depression scale scores. We collected event-related potentials of their brain compared to that of 14 healthy aged-matched adults. The late positive potential (LPP) was used to examine cognitive-affective processes associated with judgment of emotional facial expressions between the two groups.

Results: Old adults with depressive symptoms have much smaller amplitude than healthy older adults irrespective of the prime types. When processing the targets, the two groups showed different patterns regarding the LPP. The healthy control group revealed no differences between ambiguous and happy primes, irrespective of whether the targets were sad or happy facial expressions. However, significant differences were found between happy and sad and between ambiguous and sad primes. Such a pattern indicates a positive bias in healthy elderly adults. Regarding the elderly with depressive symptoms, there were no significant differences between ambiguous versus happy, ambiguous versus sad primes, and happy versus sad primes. Concerning reaction times, there was no group difference. Thus, the findings provide some support for cognitive theories of depression.

Conclusion: The current study shows that there is an association between interpretative biases and depressive symptoms in the elderly by using the neuroscientific method of ERPs. The results suggest that ERPs are sensitive to explore the interpretation bias in depressed populations.

Keywords: elderly with depressive symptoms, cognitive theories of depression, positive bias, event-related brain potentials, late positive potential

INTRODUCTION

The predominant symptoms of depression include negative beliefs about the world, the self, the future, as well as periodical and unmanageable negative thoughts which frequently linger around the self. Cognitive theories of depression proposed that depressed populations show a greater tendency to have negative interpretations on ambiguous stimuli, situations, and events (1). According to cognitive theories of depression, such a negative interpretation bias is assumed to play a central role for both development and maintenance of depression (1, 2). There is now fairly consistent scientific evidence concerning the interpretative biases in depression. Previous studies have employed various methods to explore this issue, the most prevalent being self-reports of subjects' interpretations of scenarios and stories with ambiguity (3–5). Such methods substantially contributed to the establishment of cognitive theories of depression. Even so, as Lawson and MacLeod (6) put forward, self-reporting methodologies are vulnerable to effects caused by response bias. For instance, depressed individuals probably process the negative and neutral interpretations of ambiguous information in a similar way to non-depressed ones but show a greater inclination to give the more negative interpretations.

In order to circumvent this problem, many studies switched to the usage of performance-based measures, such as priming tasks, but failed to discover interpretation biases in populations with depression (6–8). Some researchers proposed that the failure in finding interpretive biases through priming methods possibly owning to the application of reaction times (RTs) measures to evaluate the cognitive processing of depressed individuals (9). Distinctively, severity of depression is correlated with both the retardation and increased variability of the response latencies to carry out voluntary reactions. Thus, response latencies are not sensitive enough to detect interpretive biases in depressed individuals. To resolve the problems related to response latencies in priming studies, Lawson et al. (9) used physiological indices, like the magnitude of the human startle reflex. They found that depressed people showed a similar eye blink reaction elicited by negative and ambiguous words, but the blink reflexes magnitudes to ambiguous words was much smaller than those to negative words in healthy controls. Previous studies have found that magnitude of the startle reflex was increased after the presentation of negative stimuli (10, 11). Therefore, such findings are consistent with the hypothesis of a negative interpretation bias in depressed individuals.

The heterogeneity of results probably, at least was partially caused by methodological difficulties in evaluating the biased information processing in depression. Given this issue, it is of great necessity to adopt an alternative method, which should not use measurement reflecting speed to execute voluntary responses, and also must avoid the potential impact from response bias effects. As a neurophysiological measure assessing online brain processing mechanisms, event-related brain potentials (ERPs) bear the potential to overcome the limitations mentioned above, providing a unique chance to explore how depressed populations preliminarily process incoming information. Furthermore, evidence from ERPs might be of essential importance to cognitive processing theories of depression (12–14). In addition, featured by high temporal resolution, ERPs can directly measure the neural activity occurred just before the elicitation of behavioral response. A positive ERP component beginning about 300 ms after the stimulus onset has been consistently associated with arousal and emotion (15). Put forward by Kissler et al. (16), this component has been named as the late positive potential (LPP). Studies have demonstrated that the LPP tend to be augmented for emotional stimuli (17, 18). Furthermore, this potential was also found to be correlated with subjective ratings of emotion intensity (19). Amusingly, some researchers have also found that LPP can differentiate negative stimuli from positive ones (20).

The majority of previous studies try to explore the interpretation bias in individuals with depression by using words, sentences, scenarios, and events with ambiguity as experimental stimuli. Such stimuli are loaded with low levels of emotion, thus have poor sensitivity and ecological validity. Recently, considerable empirical researches have used faces with emotional expressions as experimental materials (21, 22). Emotional faces have the following advantages when compared with those used in the majority of previous studies. First, emotional faces are less influenced by different cultural background and people come from different ethnic group incline to interpret basic facial expressions in a similar way (23). Second, facial expressions, as one of the most important message sources in the ongoing stream of various social cues during social interactions, can pass on a wide-spreading of information among social partners (24), about 60% of information (25). Third, interpersonal theories of depression proposed that depressed individuals elicit rejection from others in their social interaction, which in turn exacerbates their future risk of suffering from depression (26). Fourth, faces with emotional expressions are closely allied to the estimations of social approval or disapproval (27) hence it is essential to precisely interpret and react to them for effective social functioning (28). Last but not least, as individuals usually attempt to control their emotional expression in daily interaction, it is quite common to see mild or ambiguous facial expressions. Therefore, it is very difficult to aware and interprets these ambiguous social signals. As a result, it would be more sensitive to use ambiguous facial expressions to explore the interpretive bias in depressed populations. By using facial expressions, some previous studies have detected the interpretation bias in depressed individuals (21, 27, 29).

Individuals with depressive symptoms reside in a stage during which psychometrically identified depression is above the average. However, they do not fulfill the diagnostic criteria of clinical depression overall. Thus, they lie in the middle of a continuum between normal mood and clinical depression. As for preclinical depression, adults with depressive symptoms probably then develop into clinical depression (30). Investigating populations with depressive symptoms allows studying both susceptibility and compensation mechanisms of depression (31). As a consequence, exploration of such mechanisms would enhance our

Abbreviations: ERPs, event-related brain potentials; LPP, late positive potential; NC, normal control; ADs, older adults with depressive symptoms; CES-D, Center for Epidemiologic Studies Depression scale; MMSE, Mini-Mental State Examination; MDD, major depressive disorders; EEG, electroencephalogram; ANOVA, analysis of variance; RTs, reaction times.

comprehension of the underlying processes bring about to clinical relevant depression. Detection of ERPs biomarkers of individuals with depressive symptoms will have important illuminations for early diagnosis of risk populations thus possibly preventing depression onset.

Studies concerning adults and adolescents have revealed that depression and negative interpretation bias is closely correlated, however, its emergence in the elderly still remained unknown due to the discrepancy between young and older adults in depression manifestation and emotion processing (32, 33). First, the elderly with depression showed more sleep disorder and loss of appetite when compared with depressed adults and adolescents [National Institutes of Health (34)]. Second, proposed by the socioemotional selectivity theory, healthy old adults would show a positivity bias in emotion processing compared with the younger ones (33, 35).

In summary, the present study aimed to assess the interpretation bias in the elderly with depressive symptoms when making judgments of facial expressions *via* a priming paradigm. For this purpose, ERPs will be used to evaluate the biased information processing in the elderly. According to the socioemotional selectivity theory proposed by Carstensen (33, 35), we hypothesized that older adult without depressive symptoms would exhibit a positive bias in processing emotional faces. Based on cognitive theories of depression, we hypothesized that the elderly with depressive symptoms would show a negative interpretation bias compared with healthy controls. Measured by RTs, previous studies failed to find interpretation bias in depressed individuals. We hypothesized that the ERP component LPP would reflect an interpretation bias in the elderly with depressive symptoms.

METHOD

Participants

All subjects in the current study were chose from the participants' database of our previous study (36). There are 61 elderly with depressive symptoms and 245 healthy normal controls (NCs) in the database. First, 14 subjects were randomly selected from those 61 elderly with depressive symptoms. A control group was then randomly selected from the 245 normal old adults. The two groups were matched in their demographic variables.

The average age of the healthy NC group was 65.64 years. There are five males and nine females in this group. The mean age of the older adults with depressive symptoms (ADs) was 66.36 years. There are also five males and nine females in this group. The two groups have no difference in their mean age ($p = 0.71$) or education ($p = 0.78$). The Center for Epidemiologic Studies Depression Scale (CES-D) (37) was applied to obtain each participant's depression scores. There are 20 items in the CES-D, and participants are asked to self-rate the presence of their depressive symptoms during the past week on a 4-point Likert-type scale. The total score of the CES-D is 60. Participants with a score of 16 or greater were considered to have depressive symptoms. Studies have shown that the CES-D possess well-established psychometric attributes with older adults (38). The mean CES-D score for the ADs group was 20.21 (SD = 5.65) and that for the NC group was 3.5 (SD = 3.3). The ADs participants had a Mini-Mental State Examination (MMSE) cutoff of ≥24, and they did not meet the DSM-IV clinical criteria for major depressive disorder (MDD). The NC participants had a CES-D cutoff of ≤5 and a MMSE score ≥24.

Written informed consent was obtained from all participants to study participation. They received a compensation for their participation. They all declared that they had no neurological and psychiatric diseases. All participants were right-handed and had normal or corrected-to-normal vision. The clinical and demographic characteristics of these participants are shown in **Table 1**.

Stimuli

Digitalized photographs of affective expressions with both male and female model identities were taken from the Chinese Facial Affective Picture System. The photographs included 870 emotional faces (39). By using the morphing software (Morpheus v. 1.95), affective expressions of each model identity were then blended into each other to create a 50% happy and 50% sad intensity level of ambiguity. Emotional faces of five male and five females with happy and sad expressions, as well as five 50% happy–50% sad ambiguous expressions were applied as primes in the current study. Therefore, there were three kinds of primes, namely happy, sad, and ambiguous facial expressions. Moreover, another series of emotional faces of five male and female with happy and sad expressions were selected from the same Chinese Facial Affective Picture System and used as targets, which resulted in two kinds of targets, happy and sad faces. Hence, the stimulus material for the experiment consisted of 300 distinct images, with 50 happy–happy pairs, 50 happy–sad pairs, 50 sad–happy pairs, 50 sad–sad pairs, 50 ambiguous–happy pairs, and 50 ambiguous–sad pairs. These stimuli were split into five blocks, with 60 trails in each block. A separate set of stimuli was created in the same manner for the practice trials. All pictures were situated within an area of 184 × 198 pixels. Picture size was 7.9 × 7.3 cm^2, and they were shown in the center of the computer screen.

Procedure

Participants with informed consent were given instructions on how to prepare for the ERP recording. In the formal experiment, participants were stayed in a room with dim lighting, sound insulation and electric shield. In each trial, a fixation cross of 400 ms was presented first. Then, a prime face appeared for 200 ms, which was followed by a 100 ms interval. Finally, the target face was presented for 2,000 ms. Following the target face, a blank screen was presented for 1,500 ms, during which the participants were allowed to blink. Participants were required to classify the target face as either "happy" or "sad" as fast and accurately as possible by pushing one of the two horizontally arranged buttons with their index fingers. The face-to-hand assignment was counterbalanced across participants.

TABLE 1 | The clinical and demographic characteristics of the participants.

Characteristics	NC	ADs	*p*-Value
Age (years)	65.64 ± 3.93	66.36 ± 5.20	0.71
Education (years)	12.71 ± 3.29	12.00 ± 3.26	0.78
MMSE	28.64 ± 1.65	27.57 ± 1.91	0.12
CES-D	3.5 ± 3.30	20.21 ± 5.65	<0.01

Electrophysiological Recordings

The electroencephalogram (EEG) was recorded with a 64 Ag/AgCl cap placed in referring to the extended 10–20 positioning system (http://www.neuroscan.com/). EEG signal was recorded with 500 Hz sampling rate and referenced to the right mastoid (M2) online. Impedances were kept below 5 kΩ. During recording, a 30 Hz low-pass filter was used. The eye blinks of participants were corrected mathematically. The remaining artifacts were rejected manually. For the LPP component, segments of 1,000 ms beginning 200 ms pretarget and ending 1,000 ms after target onsets were obtained. A 200 ms pretarget baseline was used to average the segments in order to acquire ERPs. Signals exceeding ±80 μV in any given epoch were discarded automatically.

Behavioral Data Analysis

The judgment RTs were analyzed, while accuracy rates were ignored because of the high accuracy (>95%). The analysis of variance (ANOVA) performed on RTs revealed a significant main effect of prime, $F(1, 26) = 4.48$, $p < 0.05$, $\eta^2 = 0.26$, with judgment latencies of ambiguous primes (617.15 ± 17.91 ms) being faster than that of both happy (633.97 ± 15.98 ms) and sad primes (639.77 ± 18.83 ms), but the happy and sad primes did not differ from each other. Furthermore, no other main effect or interactions approached significance.

ERP Data Analysis

The mean amplitudes in the time range 350–650 ms (LPP) were then exported. According to previous studies and on account of visual inspection of the present data, we focused the analysis of the LPP in this time range over three regions of interest, i.e., frontocentral: FC1, FC3, FCz, FC2, and FC4; centroparietal: CP1, CP3, CPz, CP2, and CP4; parietooccipital: PO3, PO5, POz, PO4, and PO6.

We calculated an ANOVA with the factors prime (happy, sad, and ambiguous), target (happy, sad), and topographical region (frontocentral, centroparietal, and parietooccipital) as a within-subject factor, and group (NC, ADs) as a between-subject factor.

Results showed that there is a significant main effect of group, $F(1, 27) = 16.8$, $p < 0.001$, $\eta^2 = 0.17$; target, $F(1, 82) = 13.66$, $p < 0.001$, $\eta^2 = 0.14$ and topographical region, $F(1, 81) = 39.35$, $p < 0.001$, $\eta^2 = 0.49$. Moreover, the interaction between prime and target also approached significance, $F(1, 81) = 51.59$, $p < 0.001$, $\eta^2 = 0.56$. Simple effect analysis showed that no matter the target was happy or sad faces, there were no significant differences between happy and ambiguous primes, but significant differences were present between happy versus sad and ambiguous versus sad primes, with amplitudes of happy primes larger than that of sad primes ($p < 0.05$), and also larger amplitudes for ambiguous compared to sad primes ($p < 0.05$). ERP waveforms and topographic maps (time range: 350–650 ms) of both sad targets and happy targets for two groups of participants are shown in **Figures 1** and **2**.

In addition, the interaction between prime and group is marginally significant, $F(1, 81) = 2.62$, $p = 0.07$, $\eta^2 = 0.06$. Simple effect analysis showed that ADs have much smaller amplitude than healthy older adults, irrespective of the prime types (all three $ps < 0.01$). For healthy older adults, happy primes did not differ from ambiguous primes ($p > 0.05$), but significant differences were present between happy versus sad and ambiguous versus sad primes, with amplitudes of happy primes larger than that of sad primes ($p < 0.05$), and also larger amplitudes for ambiguous compared to sad primes ($p < 0.05$). For ADs, there were no significant differences between happy versus sad, ambiguous versus sad, and ambiguous versus happy primes (all three $ps > 0.05$). Grand-average ERP waveforms and topographic maps (time range: 350–650 ms) for both groups of participants are shown in **Figures 3** and **4**.

DISCUSSION

By using ERPs, the current study aimed to assess the interpretive bias in the elderly with depressive symptoms when making judgments of facial expressions. We hypothesized that the elderly with depressive symptoms would show a negative interpretation

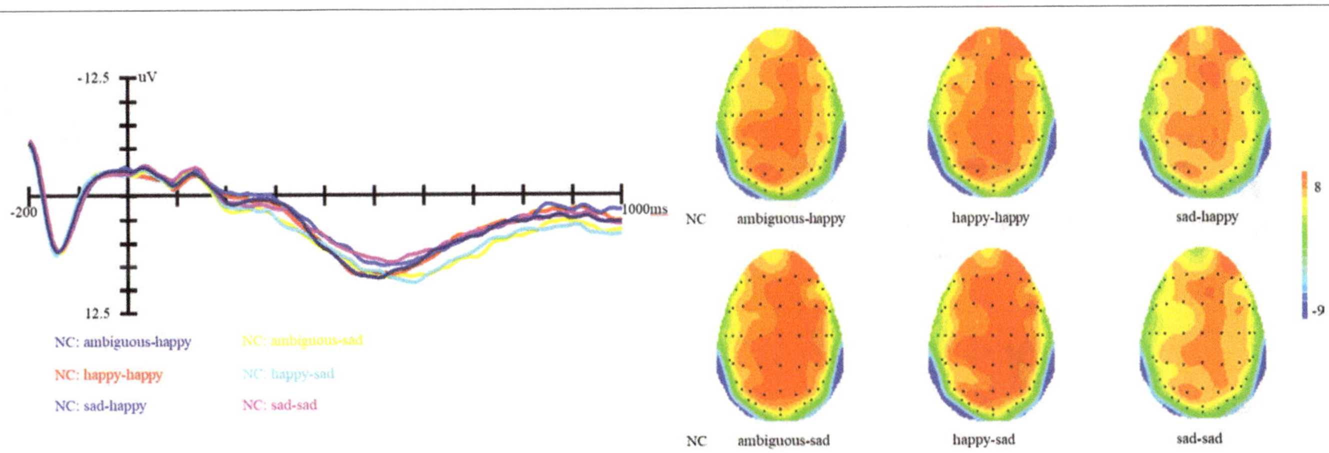

FIGURE 1 | Grand average event-related brain potentials at the electrode CPz of the analyzed topography to ambiguous, happy, and sad facial expressions for both the happy and sad target face for healthy old adults.

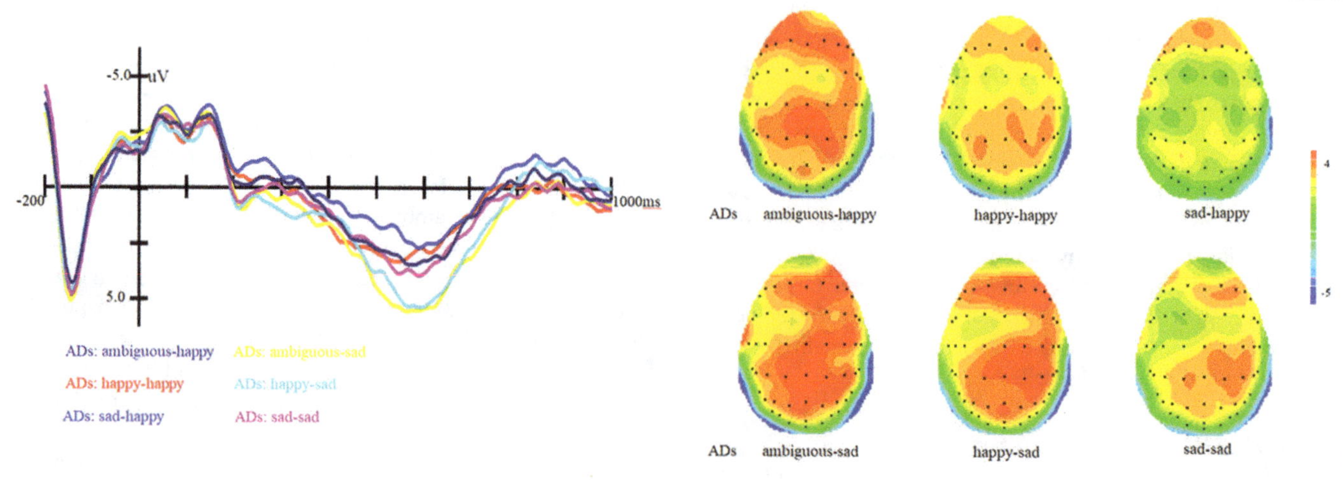

FIGURE 2 | Grand average event-related brain potentials at the electrode CPz of the analyzed topography to ambiguous, happy, and sad facial expressions for both the happy and sad target face for old adults with depressive symptoms.

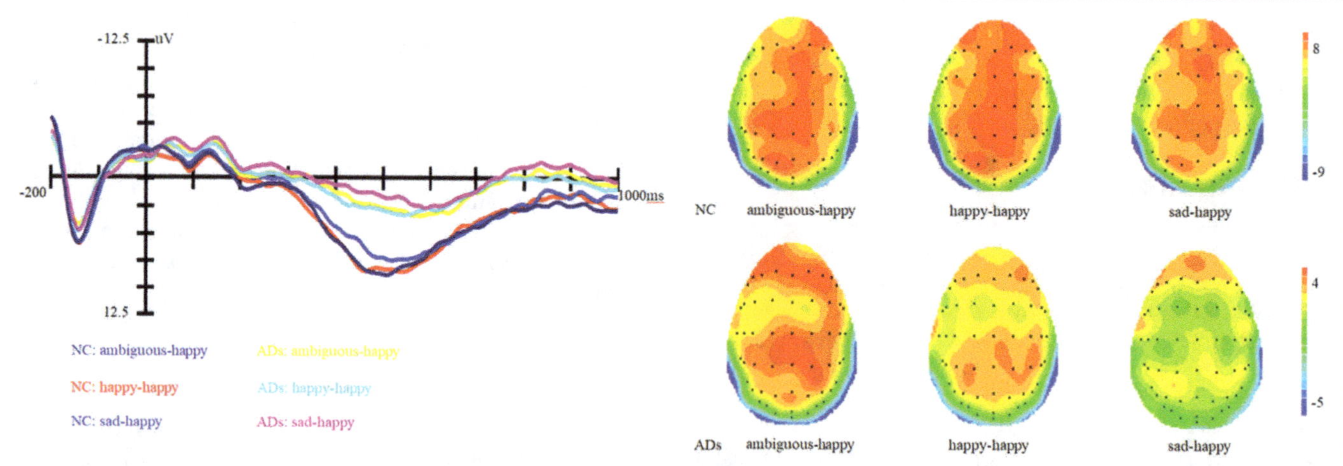

FIGURE 3 | Grand average event-related brain potentials at the electrode CPz of the analyzed topography to ambiguous, happy, and sad facial expressions when the target was a happy face for both the healthy old adults and old adults with depressive symptoms.

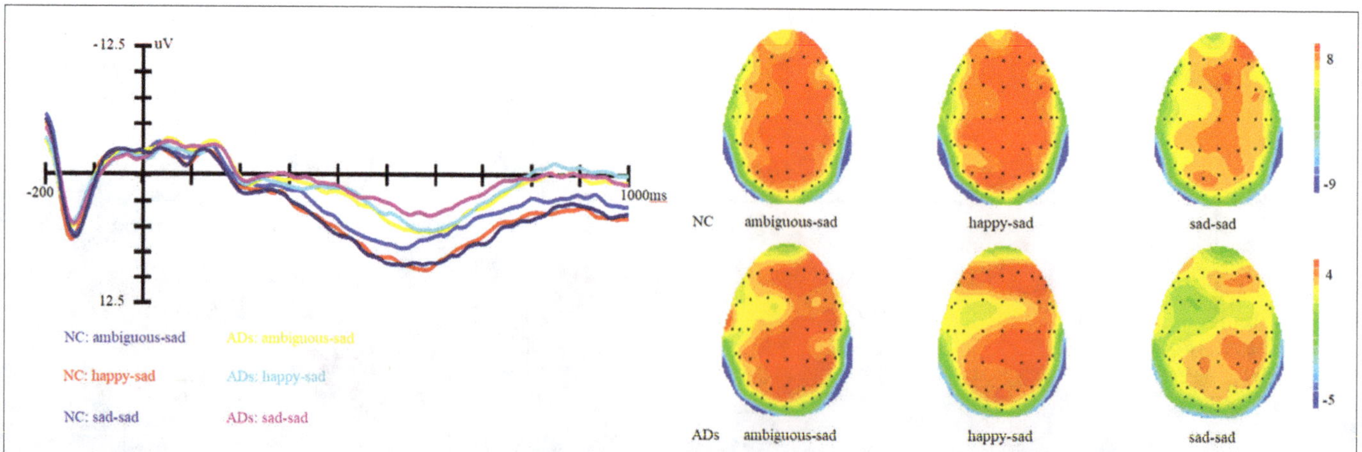

FIGURE 4 | Grand average event-related brain potentials at the electrode CPz of the analyzed topography to ambiguous, happy, and sad facial expressions when the target was a sad face for both the healthy old adults and old adults with depressive symptoms.

bias compared with healthy controls. Results of the current study demonstrated that elderly adults with depressive symptoms have much smaller amplitude than healthy older adults irrespective of the prime types. When processing the targets, the two groups showed different ERP patterns concerning the LPP. The healthy control group revealed no differences between ambiguous and happy primes, irrespective of whether the targets were sad or happy facial expressions. However, significant differences were found between happy and sad and between ambiguous and sad primes. Regarding the elderly with depressive symptoms, there were no significant differences between ambiguous versus happy, ambiguous versus sad primes, and happy versus sad primes. Again, these modulations occurred in a similar strength irrespective of whether a sad or happy target was presented. Concerning reactions times, there was no difference between the two groups.

The LPP reflects a late and controlled attentional evaluation of emotion. Results of the present study with respect to the LPP showed differences between healthy old adults and elderly with depressive symptoms. The LPP findings reveal that normal old adults were more possibly to identify ambiguous facial expressions as happy ones. Such a pattern indicated that there was a positive bias in the normal old adults. This result provided evidence for Carstensen's socioemotional selectivity theory (33, 35), which proposed that normal older adults showed positive preferences for positive over negative emotional information (33, 40). Nevertheless, these characteristics might not apply to the elderly with depressive symptoms. Perhaps, elderly adults with depressive symptoms cannot make a distinction between ambiguous, happy and sad faces, which might suggest an elimination of the positive bias.

Compared to the positive bias observed in healthy controls, the elimination of such a bias in elderly adults with depressive symptoms could also be considered as a kind of negative trend. Therefore, the present study further confirms that there is a depression-linked interpretive bias in depressed individuals and provides further evidence for the cognitive theories of depression (1, 2). However, result of the current study is different from that of Lawson et al. (9). They used the human eye blink reflex to explore the negative interpretation bias in depressed college students and found that depression is associated with a negative interpretation bias. The current study, similar to Lawson et al. (9), used a method which does not depend on subjects' self-reports and can also evade the troubles related to response latency measurement of cognitive processing in individuals with depression, only found an elimination of the positive bias but not a negative bias. It is essential to notice that the difference between our findings and that of Lawson et al. (9) might have been potentially caused by factors such as differences in demographic characteristics of the participants and the kind of depression measures. In Lawson et al. (9), undergraduate students were selected as participants. While in our study, old adults were recruited as participants. Actually, Wood and Kisley (41) had found that old adults and young adults are quite different in processing emotional information. Such differences in participant samples may contribute to the inconsistent findings. Concerning the use of different measurement tools to assess depression, Lawson et al. (9) selected participants with scores on the Beck Depression Inventory. In contrast, we used CES-D to define the depressive symptoms in the elderly. Such differences in measuring depression may also contribute to the inconsistent results. The inconsistency between our study and Lawson et al. (9) also implicated the pressing need for more studies on interpretation bias associated with depression. The current study just catch a glimpse of the neural mechanisms underlying depression, thus future research should explore other related aspects so as to obtain a more integrated understanding of the potential neural underpinnings of the interpretation bias in depression.

The current study demonstrated that the LPP amplitude of elderly adults with depressive symptoms is significantly smaller than that of the healthy older adults. Although the interaction between group and target is marginally significant, simple effect analysis showed that the two groups of participants showed different LPP patterns irrespective of whether a sad or happy target was presented. Concerning such findings, the possible reason is that the sample size of the current study is relatively modest. However, one thing for sure is that depressive symptoms really have some influences on the LPP amplitude of old adults. Therefore, a large sample would be employed in the future to validate the findings of the current study.

CONCLUSION

In summary, the present study found that there exists a positive bias in the healthy elderly. However, depressive symptoms in the elderly not only caused a reduction of LPP amplitude but also an elimination of the positive biases. Such findings highlighted a relation between interpretative biases and depressive symptoms in the elderly by using the neuroscientific method of event-related potentials. The results suggest that ERPs are sensitive to explore the interpretation bias in depressed populations, which enhanced our understanding of the underlying processes bring about to clinical relevant depression and also have important illuminations for early diagnosis of at risk populations. In addition, the present study expanded research concerning interpretation bias to the elderly.

ETHICS APPROVAL AND CONSENT TO PARTICIPATE

The current study was approved by the Ethics Committee of the Institute of Psychology, Chinese Academy of Sciences. Written informed consent of participants was obtained for participation after a detailed explanation of the study procedure.

AVAILABILITY OF DATA AND MATERIALS

The data and materials supporting this study cannot be made publicly available because it will be in conflict with patients' privacy. All interested parties can request the data from lijuan@psych.ac.cn.

AUTHOR CONTRIBUTIONS

JL, HZ, and BD initiated the design for this article together. HZ undertook the statistical analysis and wrote the manuscript. BD participated in the data collection and also made some critical comments on the manuscript. SR made critical comments and revision on the manuscript. As the principal investigator of this project, JL supervised the statistical analysis and the manuscript writing and revision. All authors read and have approved the final manuscript.

ACKNOWLEDGMENTS

We wish to extend our appreciations to all the elderly adults who took part in the current study.

FUNDING

This work was supported by the National Natural Science Foundation of China (31470998, 31271108, and 31671157), Beijing Municipal Science & Technology Commission (Z171100000117006), the Pioneer Initiative of the Chinese Academy of Sciences, Feature Institutes Program (TSS-2015-06), National Key Research and Development Program of China (2016YFC1305904) and the Key Laboratory of Mental Health, Institute of Psychology, Chinese Academy of Sciences (KLMH2014ZK02) granted to JL and also the China Postdoctoral Science Foundation (2015M570164), and the Scientific Foundation of Institute of Psychology, Chinese Academy of Sciences (Y6CX242007) granted to HZ.

REFERENCES

1. Beck AT. Cognitive models of depression. *J Cognit Psychother Int Q* (1987) 1:5–37.
2. Williams JMG, Watts FN, MacLeod CM, Mathews A. *Cognitive Psychology and Emotional Disorders*. 2nd ed. Chichester, England: Wiley (1997).
3. Gupta R, Kar BR. Interpretative bias: indicators of cognitive vulnerability to depression. *Ger J Psychiatry* (2008) 11(3):98–102.
4. Pury CLS. Information-processing predictors of emotional response to stress. *Cognit Emotion* (2002) 16(5):667–83. doi:10.1080/02699930143000400
5. Butler G, Mathews A. Cognitive processes in anxiety. *Adv Behav Res Ther* (1983) 5:51–62. doi:10.1016/0146-6402(83)90015-2
6. Lawson C, MacLeod C. Depression and the interpretation of ambiguity. *Behav Res Ther* (1999) 37(5):463–74. doi:10.1016/S0005-7967(98)00131-4
7. Bisson MAS, Sears CR. The effect of depressed mood on the interpretation of ambiguity, with and without negative mood induction. *Cognit Emotion* (2007) 21(3):614–45. doi:10.1080/02699930600750715
8. Mogg K, Bradbury KE, Bradley BP. Interpretation of ambiguous information in clinical depression. *Behav Res Ther* (2006) 44(10):1411–9. doi:10.1016/j.brat.2005.10.008
9. Lawson C, MacLeod C, Hammond G. Interpretation revealed in the blink of an eye: depressive bias in the resolution of ambiguity. *J Abnorm Psychol* (2002) 111(2):321–8. doi:10.1037/0021-843X.111.2.321
10. Bradley MM, Cuthbert BN, Lang PJ. Startle reflex modulation: emotion or attention? *Psychophysiology* (1990) 27:513–22. doi:10.1111/j.1469-8986.1990.tb01966.x
11. Lang PJ, Bradley MM, Cuthbert BN. Emotion, attention, and the startle reflex. *Psychol Rev* (1990) 97:377–95. doi:10.1037/0033-295X.97.3.377
12. Clark DM, Wells A. A cognitive model of social phobia. In: Heimberg RG, Liebowitz MR, Hope DA, Schneider FR, editors. *Social Phobia: Diagnosis, Assessment, and Treatment*. New York: Guilford Press (1995). p. 69–93.
13. Huppert JD, Foa EB. Maintenance mechanisms in social anxiety: an integration of cognitive biases and emotional processing theory. In: Yiend J, editor. *Cognition, Emotion and Psychopathology: Theoretical, Empirical and Clinical Directions*. New York: Cambridge University Press (2004). p. 213–31.
14. Mathews A, Mackintosh B. A cognitive model of selective processing in anxiety. *Cognit Ther Res* (1998) 22:539–60. doi:10.1023/A:1018738019346
15. Olofsson JK, Nordin S, Sequeira H, Polich J. Affective picture processing: an integrative review of ERP findings. *Biol Psychol* (2008) 77:247–65. doi:10.1016/j.biopsycho.2007.11.006
16. Kissler J, Herbert C, Junghofer M. Emotion and attention in visual word processing – an ERP study. *Biol Psychol* (2009) 80:75–83. doi:10.1016/j.biopsycho.2008.03.004
17. Hajcak G, Macnamara A, Olvet DM. Event-related potentials, emotion, and emotion regulation: an integrative review. *Dev Neuropsychol* (2010) 35:129–55. doi:10.1080/87565640903526504
18. Kaestner EJ, Polich J. Affective recognition memory processing and event-related brain potentials. *Cognit Affect Behav Neurosci* (2011) 11:186–98. doi:10.3758/s13415-011-0023-4
19. Cuthbert BN, Schupp HT, Bradley MM, Birbaumer N, Lang PJ. Brain potentials in affective picture processing: covariation with autonomic arousal and affective report. *Biol Psychol* (2000) 52:95–111. doi:10.1016/S0301-0511(99)00044-7
20. Schacht A, Adler N, Chen PY, Guo TM, Sommer W. Association with positive outcome induces early effects in event-related brain potentials. *Biol Psychol* (2012) 89:130–6. doi:10.1016/j.biopsycho.2011.10.001
21. Beevers CG, Wells TT, Ellis AJ, Fischer K. Identification of emotionally ambiguous interpersonal stimuli among dysphoric and nondysphoric individuals. *Cognit Ther Res* (2009) 33(3):283–90. doi:10.1007/s10608-008-9198-6
22. Jusyte A, Schönenberg M. Threat processing in generalized social phobia: an investigation of interpretation biases in ambiguous facial affect. *Psychiatry Res* (2014) 217(1–2):100–6. doi:10.1016/j.psychres.2013.12.031
23. Ekman P, Friesen WV. Constants across cultures in the face and emotion. *J Pers Soc Psychol* (1971) 17(2):124–9. doi:10.1037/h0030377
24. Mayer JD, DiPaolo M, Salovey P. Perceiving affective content in ambiguous visual stimuli: a component of emotional intelligence. *J Pers Assess* (1990) 54(3–4):772–81. doi:10.1080/00223891.1990.9674037
25. Burgoon JK. Nonverbal signals. In: Knapp ML, Miller GR, editors. *Handbook of Interpersonal Communication*. Beverly Hills, CA: SAGE (1985). p. 344–90.
26. Hames JL, Hagan CR, Joiner TE. Interpersonal processes in depression. *Annu Rev Clin Psychol* (2013) 9:355–77. doi:10.1146/annurev-clinpsy-050212-185553
27. Gilboa-Schechtman E, Foa E, Vaknin Y, Marom S, Hermesh H. Interpersonal sensitivity and response bias in social phobia and depression: labeling emotional expressions. *Cognit Ther Res* (2008) 32(5):605–18. doi:10.1007/s10608-008-9208-8
28. Montagne B, Schutters S, Westenberg HGM, van Honk J, Kessels RPC, de Haan EHF. Reduced sensitivity in the recognition of anger and disgust in social anxiety disorder. *Cogn Neuropsychiatry* (2006) 11:389–401. doi:10.1080/13546800444000254
29. Joormann J, Gotlib IH. Is this happiness I see? Biases in the identification of emotional facial expressions in depression and social phobia? *J Abnorm Psychol* (2006) 115(4):705–14. doi:10.1037/0021-843X.115.4.705
30. Murphy JM, Nierenberg AA, Laird NM, Monson RR, Sobol AM, Leighton AH. Incidence of major depression: prediction from subthreshold categories in the Stirling County study. *J Affect Disord* (2002) 68:251–9. doi:10.1016/S0165-0327(00)00334-7
31. Gruzelier JH. Theory, methods and new directions in the psychophysiology of the schizophrenic process and schizotypy. *Int J Psychophysiol* (2003) 48(3):221–45. doi:10.1016/S0167-8760(03)00055-2
32. Bucks RS, Garner M, Tarrant L, Bradley BP, Mogg K. Interpretation of emotionally ambiguous faces in older adults. *J Gerontol B Psychol Sci Soc Sci* (2008) 63(6):337–43. doi:10.1093/geronb/63.6.P337
33. Carstensen LL, Isaacowitz DM, Charles ST. Taking time seriously: a theory of socioemotional selectivity. *Am Psychol* (1999) 54(3):165–81. doi:10.1037/0003-066X.54.3.165
34. National Institutes of Health. Diagnosis and treatment of depression in late life. *Natl Inst Health Consen Stat* (1991) 9:1–27.
35. Carstensen LL, Mikels JA. At the intersection of emotion and cognition: aging and the positivity effect. *Curr Dir Psychol Sci* (2005) 14(3):117–21. doi:10.1111/j.0963-7214.2005.00348.x

36. Dai BB, Peng YS, Li J. A cross-sectional study of depressive symptom and emotion regulation in older adults. *Chin Ment Health J* (2014) 28(3):192–6. doi:10.3969/j.issn.1000-6729.2014.03.006
37. Radloff LS. The CES-D scale: a self-report depression scale for research in the general population. *Appl Psychol Meas* (1977) 1(3):385–401. doi:10.1177/014662167700100306
38. Lewinsohn PM, Seeley JR, Roberts RE, Allen NB. Center for epidemiologic studies depression scale (CES-D) as a screening instrument for depression among community-residing older adults. *Psychol Aging* (1997) 12(2):277–87. doi:10.1037/0882-7974.12.2.277
39. Gong X, Huang YX, Wang Y, Luo YJ. Revision of the Chinese facial affective picture system. *Chin Ment Health J* (2011) 25(1):40–6. doi:10.3969/j.issn.1000-6729.2011.01.011
40. Murphy NA, Isaacowitz DM. Preferences for emotional information in older and younger adults: a meta-analysis of memory and attention tasks. *Psychol Aging* (2008) 23(2):263–86. doi:10.1037/0882-7974.23.2.263
41. Wood S, Kisley MA. The negativity bias is eliminated in older adults: age-related reduction in event-related brain potentials associated with evaluation categorization. *Psychol Aging* (2006) 21(4):815–20. doi:10.1037/0882-7974.21.4.815

15

Increased Absolute Glutamate Concentrations and Glutamate-to-Creatine Ratios in Patients with Methamphetamine Use Disorders

Wenhan Yang[1], Ru Yang[1], Jing Luo[1], Lei He[1], Jun Liu[1] and Jun Zhang[2*]*

[1] Department of Radiology, Second Xiangya Hospital of Central South University, Changsha, China, [2] Hunan Judicial Police Vocational College, Changsha, China

***Correspondence:**
Jun Liu
junliu123@csu.edu.cn
Jun Zhang
zhangjun888aaa@163.cn*

Introduction: Previous studies have indicated that changes in the concentration of glutamate and related metabolites may mediate the progression of addiction in patients with methamphetamine (MA) use disorders. In the present study, we utilized magnetic resonance spectroscopy (MRS) to investigate absolute glutamate concentrations and metabolite ratios in patients with MA addiction. We further analyzed the association between glutamate concentration and various clinical indicators.

Methods: The present study included 31 unmedicated patients with clinically diagnosed MA dependence (mean age: 30.5 $\pm$ 8.0 years) and 32 age-matched healthy controls (mean age: 32.9 $\pm$ 8.2 years). Patients were evaluated using the Barratt Impulsiveness Scale (BIS-11). We also collected general information regarding the duration and dosage of drug use. Point-resolved spectroscopy was used to quantify the absolute concentrations of metabolites (glutamate, choline, N-acetylaspartate, glutamine, and creatine), as well as the ratio of metabolites to total creatine, using LCModel software. We then compared differences in glutamate levels and psychometric scores between the two groups.

Results: Glutamate-to-creatine ratios in the brainstem were significantly higher in the MA group than in the control group ($t = 2.764$, $p = 0.008$). Glutamate concentrations in the brainstem were also significantly higher in the MA group than in the control group ($t = 2.390$, $p = 0.020$). However, no significant differences in the concentrations or ratios of other metabolites were observed between the two groups (all $p > 0.05$). Glutamate concentration was positively correlated with the duration of drug use ($r = 0.401$, $p = 0.035$) and the total dose of regular addiction (duration of addiction $\times$ regular addiction dose; $r = 0.207$, $p = .040$), but not with BIS-11 scores.

Conclusions: Our findings indicated that glutamate levels in the brainstem are significantly elevated in patients with MA use disorders, and that these levels are significantly associated with the duration and dose of drug use.Such findings suggest that glutamate concentration can be used as an objective biological marker for evaluating/monitoring disease status and treatment efficacy in patients with MA dependence.

Keywords: glutamate, magnetic resonance spectroscopy, substance use disorders, neural circuits, neurotransmitters, methamphetamine, addiction

INTRODUCTION

Methamphetamine (MA) is a highly addictive, widely abused psychostimulant with severe neurotoxic potential (1). Although MA was discovered decades ago, it has recently become one of the most widely used drugs in the world. MA abuse can lead to the emergence and spread of a variety of diseases, increasing the risk of HIV, hepatitis B, hepatitis C, and other diseases due to the sharing of syringes. Additional studies have demonstrated that long-term MA use can lead to elevated blood pressure due to excitation of the sympathetic nervous system, as well as impairments in brain structure, function, and cognition (2). Thus, MA abuse and dependence represent serious public health concerns. However, the diagnosis of MA use disorders has primarily been based on descriptive, symptomatic checklist criteria, and the neural mechanisms underlying the highly addictive nature of the drug remain to be fully elucidated. Further research is required to identify biological markers of MA addiction, and to develop more effective means of monitoring disease status and evaluating the efficacy of therapeutic interventions in patients with MA dependence.

Amphetamine-like psychostimulants are characterized by their ability to bind to dopamine transporters (DATs) (3), which transfer monoamines released into the synapse back into the cytosol, including dopamine. MA binds more rapidly to DAT and is thus more toxic than other amphetamine-like psychostimulants. Although the dopaminergic system is closely related to the formation of addiction, amphetamines are also associated with the adaptation of glutamate signaling (4). Upon entering dopaminergic neurons, amphetamines stimulate endocytosis of the excitatory glutamate transporter EAAT3.

As the main excitatory neurotransmitter in the human central nervous system (CNS), glutamate is involved in a variety of physiological processes. Previous studies have demonstrated that excessive endogenous glutamate is associated with several acute and chronic neurodegenerative diseases (5). Several previous studies have reported that patients with MA addiction exhibit altered levels of glutamate metabolites in the brain. Because glutamate is a key element of the brain's reward system, it may play an intermediate role in the process of addiction. Treatment with N-acetylcysteine (NAC) normalizes glutamate homeostasis and prevents relapse in drug-dependent animals (6). However, the effects of substance addiction on glutamate metabolism in human patients remain unknown. Proton magnetic resonance spectroscopy (1H-MRS) findings regarding brain levels of glutamate in individuals with substance use disorders have been mixed. Some studies have reported that glutamate levels are decreased in patients with alcohol addiction, while others have reported conflicting results. Mon et al. reported that individuals with alcohol dependence exhibited lower baseline concentrations of glutamate in the anterior cingulate cortex than those in the control group (7). Similarly, Bagga et al. reported that glutamate levels were significantly lower in the primary visual cortex in patients with alcohol dependence than in healthy controls (8). However, Frye et al. observed that patients with alcohol dependence exhibited significantly elevated levels of glutamate in the midline anterior cingulate cortex when compared with controls (9). Hermann D et al. found significantly increased glutamate levels during acute alcohol withdrawal in corresponding prefrontal cortex regions of treatment-seeking alcoholic patients and alcohol-dependent rats compared with respective control subjects (10).

When investigating traditional drug dependence, Schmaal et al. observed significant increases in glutamate levels in the anterior cingulate cortex of cocaine users, relative to those observed in healthy controls. Using high-speed amperometry with enzyme-based biosensors, Wakabayashi, and Kiyatkin discovered that an initial intravenous injection of cocaine induces rapid, transient increases in glutamate release in the nucleus accumbens (NAc) of freely moving rats. Moreover, subsequent injections rapidly strengthened this response (11). However, few studies have examined changes in glutamate levels due to the use of synthetic drugs.

White et al. (12) examined the concentration of glutamine metabolites in 26 healthy individuals following oral administration of single, clinically relevant doses of amphetamine (20 mg), MA (20 mg), or placebo. Using MRS, the authors revealed that d-amphetamine administration increased levels of glutamate, glutamine, and creatine in the dorsal anterior cingulate cortex (dACC) 3 days after the peak drug reaction (140–150 min post-ingestion).

In the present study, we aimed to investigate the absolute concentration and ratio of glutamate to other metabolites in patients with MA addiction, in order to aid in the development of a biological marker for evaluating/monitoring disease status as well as the efficacy of therapeutic interventions.

MATERIALS AND METHODS

Participant Characteristics

The present study included 31 unmedicated individuals with MA addiction from Changsha (Hunan Province) undergoing treatment at a drug rehabilitation center in Zhuzhou. All participants provided written informed consent. The experiment was approved by the ethics committee of the Second Xiangya hospital of Central South University. Inclusion criteria were as follows: (1) positive urine test for MA; (2) diagnosis of addiction based on criteria outlined in the fourth edition of the Diagnostic and Statistical Manual of Mental Disorders (DSM-IV), (3) negative urine test for heroin and ketamine; (4) no history of structural brain disease, epilepsy, or head trauma; (5) no contraindications for MRI; (6) no history of mental or psychiatric illness. Patients with a history of serious physical illness, intracranial lesions, mental illness, or MRI contraindications were excluded. Patients meeting the aforementioned criteria underwent MRI examination after 5–30 days of abstinence. We recruited 33 control participants through WeChat, flyers, etc. All participants were right-handed and of Han Chinese descent. Most participants were smokers, while some reported alcohol use as well. Barratt Impulsiveness Scale (BIS-11) scores were obtained for all patients (13) following MRI examination. The demographic characteristics of the experimental and control groups are shown in **Table 1**.

Acquisition/Analysis of MRS Data

All participants underwent imaging in a 3T MRI scanner (MAGNETOM Skyra, Siemens) equipped with a 32-channel phased-array joint head coil. Foam padding and a forehead-restraining strap were utilized to limit head movement during the scanning procedure. To obtain high-quality spectroscopy data, participants were advised regarding the importance of remaining motionless during the procedure. All participants were allowed a moment to relax and move their hands/feet prior to scanning to ensure the quality of MR images. High-resolution, T1-weighted anatomical images of the whole brain were acquired using a three-dimensional fast gradient echo sequence with the following parameters: repetition time (TR) = 1,450 ms, echo time (TE) = 2.0 ms, inversion time (TI) = 900 ms, field-of-view (FOV) = 256 × 256 mm, slice thickness = 1 mm, flip angle = 12°. Slices in the three orthogonal planes were subjected to multiplanar reconstruction in order to localize the volumes of interest (VOI: 10 × 12 × 15 mm = 1.8 cm3). The VOI was positioned to cover the right brainstem in coronal and sagittal slices as a topographic marker (**Figure 1**).

All MRS data were acquired using single-volume localization. Spectral data were acquired via conventional point-resolved spectroscopy (PRESS) using a short TE to ensure optimal selectivity for glutamate. These spectra were also collected with a TR of 1290 ms (average: 240), resulting in a total scan time of over 6.75 min with and without water suppression. Raw data from each acquisition, which consisted of 1,024 points, were collected at a bandwidth of 1,200 Hz. The total examination lasted approximately 10 min for each participant. Spectra were quantified using LCModel software(14, 15).

Cramer–Rao lower bounds (CRLBs) were used to evaluate the accuracy of the amplitude calculation for each component. CRLB estimates represent the %SD of the fit for each metabolite. Only metabolite concentrations with CRLBs below 20% (indicate of high confidence) were accepted and used for the following analyses.

TABLE 1 | Participant characteristics.

	Patients (n = 31) (mean ± *SD*)	Controls (n = 32) (mean ± *SD*)	$\chi t/\chi^2$ /Z value	*p*
Age (years)	30.5 ± 8.0	32.9 ± 8.2	t =-1.139	0.259
GENDER (*N*)				
Male	21	20	$\chi^2 = 0.190$	0.793
Female	10	12		
EDUCATION (*N*)				
Primary school	3	2	Z = -0.377	0.706
Junior high school	20	21		
Senior high school	8	9		
NICOTINE USE (*N*)				
Y	29	26	$\chi^2 = 3.506$	0.257
N	2	6		
FTND	6.1 ± 1.6	5.7 ± 1.5	t = -0.78	0.439
ALCOHOL USE (N)				
Y	12	7	$\chi^2 = 2.119$	0.177
N	19	25		
AUDI	7.6 ± 1.8	6.9 ± 3.4	t = 0.580	0.615

FTND, Fagerstrom Test for Nicotine Dependence; AUDI, Alcohol Use Disorders Identification Test.

Statistical Analysis

Statistical analyses were performed using SPSS 18.0. Demographic characteristics were compared using independent Samples t-tests, chi-square tests, and rank sum tests. Differences in metabolite levels were analyzed using two-sided, independent Samples t-tests and rank sum tests. The data distributions were tested for normality using the Kolmogorov–Smirnov test. Normally distributed data were analyzed using independent Samples t-tests, while non-normally distributed data were analyzed using rank sum tests. Correlations between metabolite levels and clinical characteristics were evaluated using Pearson's correlation coefficients. The level of statistical significance was set at $p < 0.05$.

RESULTS

MRS Relative Metabolite Concentrations

The CRLBs of N-acetylaspartate (NAA), glutamate, creatine, and choline were less than 20% for all participants. Glutamate, **glx (glutamate + glutamine)**, and choline data were excluded for two, two, and three participant of the MA group due to excessive CRLBs. **Glutamine data were not analyzed for the excessive CRLBs of some part of data.** The mean metabolite concentrations in the brainstem are displayed in **Table 2**, **Figures 2**, **Figures 3**. Our findings indicate that glutamate concentrations were higher in the MA group than in the control group [$t_{(57)} = 2.390$, $p = 0.020$]. The ratio of glutamate to creatine was also significantly higher in the MA group than in the control group [$t_{(57)} = 2.764$, $p = 0.008$]. Although the mean **glx (glutamate + glutamine)** concentration was higher in the MA group than in the control group, this difference

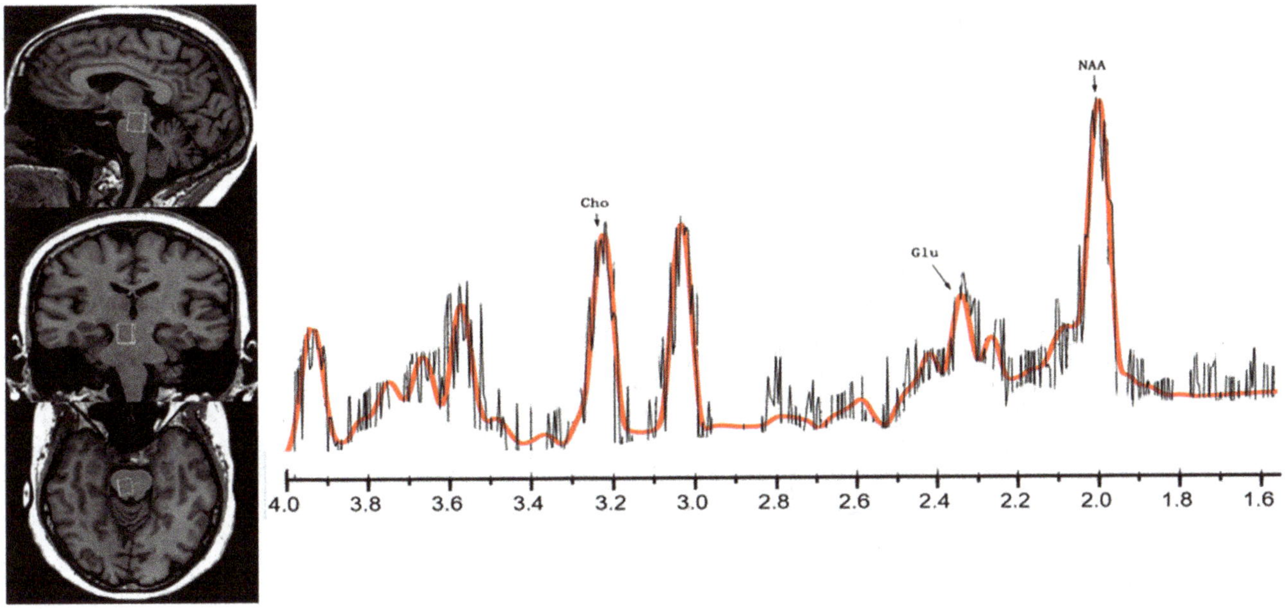

FIGURE 1 | The location and MR spectra of the region of interest in the brainstem on the left side, the localized images of the brainstem from top to bottom are, in order, sagittal, coronal, axial, the interest area located in the midbrain aqueduct in the coronal plane. The result of MR spectra of the right brainstem in the patient (red line) brain is on the other side.

TABLE 2 | Comparison of major metabolites in the brainstem.

Metabolite	Patients (mean ± *SD*)	Controls (mean ± *SD*)	*t*	*p*
NAA	6.25 ± 2.23	6.14 ± 2.13	$t_{(59)}$ = -0.188	0.851
Glu	9.94 ± 2.16	8.48 ± 1.89	$t_{(59)}$ = 2.390	0.020
Glx	11.94 ± 2.73	11.69 ± 3.61	$t_{(59)}$ = -2.98	0.767
tCr	6.56 ± 1.07	6.66 ± 1.37	$t_{(61)}$ = 0.292	0.772
tCho	2.64 ± 0.33	2.87 ± 0.61	$t_{(58)}$ = 1.657	0.103
NAA/tCr	1.13 ± 0.37	1.13 ± 0.48	$t_{(59)}$ = -0.188	0.851
Glu/tCr	1.68 ± 0.73	1.30 ± 0.27	$t_{(59)}$ = 2.764	0.008
Glx/tCr	2.03 ± 0.83	1.77 ± 0.50	$t_{(59)}$ = -0.149	0.143
tCho/tCr	0.43 ± 0.12	0.43 ± 0.16	$t_{(58)}$ = 0.115	0.909

NAA, N-acetyl aspartate; Glu, glutamate; Glx, glutamate+glutamine; tCr, total creatine; tCho, total choline.
Patients: NAA n = 31, Glu n = 29, Glx n = 29, tCr n = 31, tCho n = 29.
Controls: NAA n = 32, Glu n = 32, Glx n = 32, tCr n = 32, tCho n = 31.

was not significant. No significant differences in levels of other metabolites were observed between the two groups (all $p > 0.05$).

Duration of MA Use

Glutamate concentrations and glutamate-to-creatine ratios were significantly higher in patients than controls (**Figures 4**, **5**). In addition, we observed a significant positive correlation between absolute concentrations of glutamate and the duration of MA use (**Figure 6**; $r = 0.401$, $p = 0.035$). Glutamate concentration increased with years of MA use and was also associated with the total dose of regular addiction (duration of addiction × regular addiction dose; $r = 0.207$, $p = 0.040$). Slight negative correlations were also observed between glutamate levels and BIS-11 scores ($r = -0.148$, $p = 0.291$). No significant correlations were observed between levels of other metabolites and clinical characteristics.

DISCUSSION

In the present study, we compared absolute glutamate concentrations and metabolite ratios between patients with MA addiction and healthy controls. Our findings indicated that glutamate concentrations were significantly higher in patients than controls, and that absolute glutamate concentrations were correlated with the duration of MA use.

Glutamate is a vital excitatory neurotransmitter in the brain. The excitatory toxicity of glutamate is related to the pathogenesis of various neurological diseases, such as stroke, amyotrophic lateral sclerosis, and epilepsy (16). Several recent studies have suggested that glutamate is associated with synaptic plasticity in patients with substance addiction (17–20). In addition to its direct influence as an excitatory amino acid, glutamate plays an important role in long-term neuronal enhancement, and is closely related to learning and memory (21, 22). Plasticity of glutamate synapses may be closely related to the long-term process of addiction. Addiction results in long-term alterations to the structure and function of the brain (23, 24), and previous research has indicated that changes in glutamate-mediated neuroplasticity in the reward pathway are critical in the formation of addictive memories, which in turn increase the likelihood of relapse (25). Addictive drugs influence learning

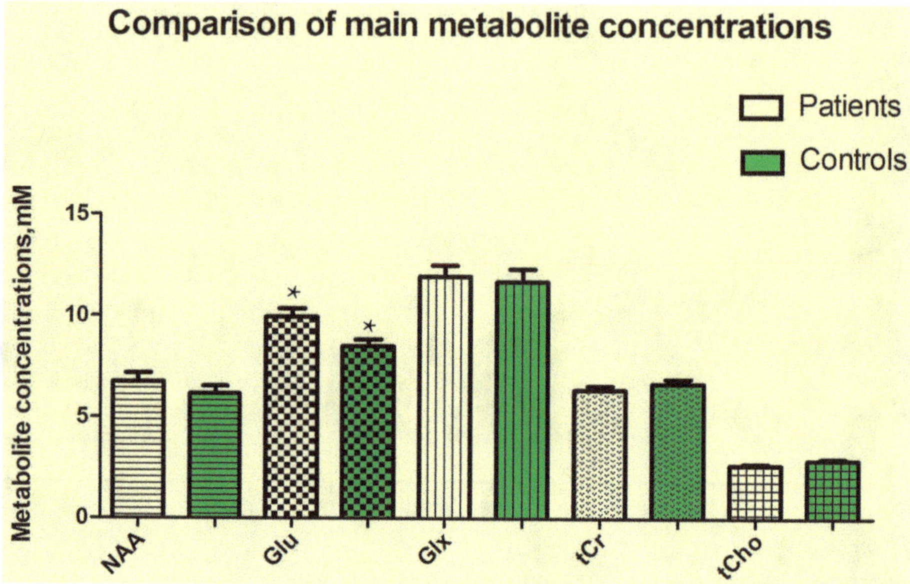

FIGURE 2 | Glutamate concentrations in the brainstem were significantly higher in the MA group than in the control group ($t = 2.390$, $p = 0.020$). No significant differences in the concentrations of other metabolites were observed between the two groups (all $p > 0.05$). *means the existence of statistical differences between the two groups.

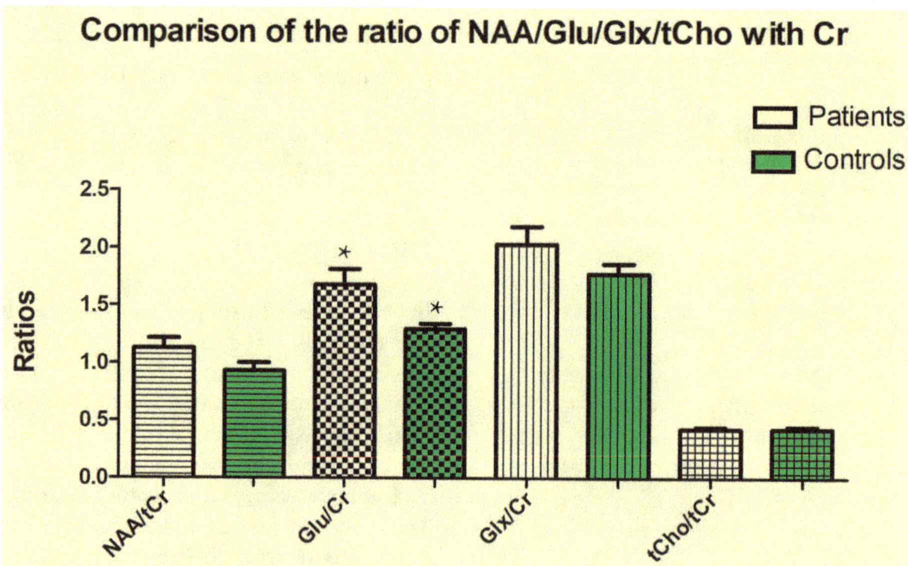

FIGURE 3 | Glutamate-to-creatine ratios in the brainstem were significantly higher in the MA group than in the control group ($t = 2.764$, $p = 0.008$). No significant differences in the ratios of other metabolites were observed between the two groups (all $p > 0.05$). *means the existence of statistical differences between the two groups.

and memory by directly altering dopamine neurotransmission in the midbrain, which leads to subsequent changes in the dorsal and ventral striatum, resulting in increased addiction memory consolidation (26).

The brainstem includes the midbrain, pons, and medulla. The midbrain is an important part of the brain's reward system. The ventral tegmental area (VTA) plays a central role in motivation and reward (27). Addictive drugs are taken up by neurons in the VTA, resulting in adaptation of glutamatergic synapses as well as changes in the dopamine system of the midbrain (28).In addition, the pedunculopontine tegmental nucleus (PPTg) of the brainstem contains neurons that release glutamate, acetylcholine, and GABA, thereby influencing activity in the basal ganglia and limbic region (29–31).Previous studies have indicated that

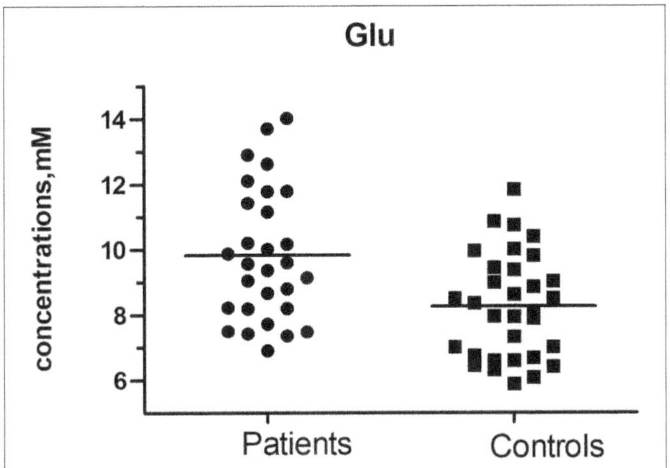

FIGURE 4 | Glu concentration between MA and Control group ($t = 2.390$, $p = 0.020$).

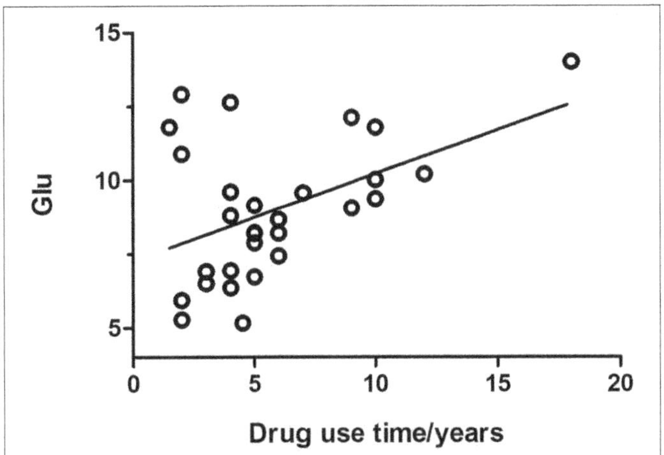

FIGURE 6 | Glutamate concentration was positively correlated with the duration of drug use ($r = 0.401$, $p = 0.035$).

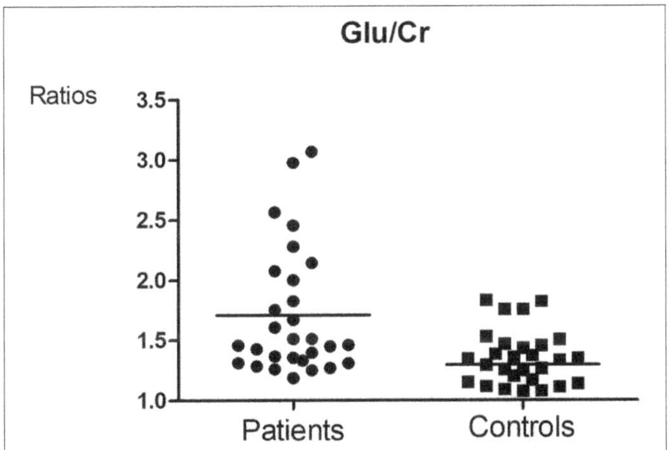

FIGURE 5 | Glutamate-to-creatine ratios between MA and Control group ($t = 2.764$, $p = 0.008$).

glutamate neurons in the ppTg are directly controlled by the VTA, which has been associated with neural regulation in the reward circuit (32).In accordance with previous findings, our results indicated the glutamate levels in the brainstem were higher in the MA group than in the control group. Such findings suggest that elevated glutamate concentrations and glutamate-to-creatine ratios in the brains of patients with MA addiction are associated with changes in synaptic plasticity and the retention of addictive memories. Indeed, it is now widely accepted that increases in extracellular glutamate levels mediate MA-induced neurotoxicity (33). Our results support the hypothesis that glutamate mediates the neuro-modulatory system and reward circuits involved in addiction.

Changes in the neuro-modulatory systems and neural circuits for reward can lead to distinct psychiatric disorders, including addiction (34). Drug addiction is associated with increased dopamine concentrations in the synaptic cleft (35). Neuronal changes in the limbic system can alter behavioral responses to various environmental stimuli associated with reward behavior. Psychostimulants and drug abuse can cause significant synaptic changes in the middle cerebral dopamine system (36). Dopamine is transferred from the ventral tegmental area (VTA) in the midbrain—a process associated with motivation and drug addiction (37).

Drug addiction is a severe mental illness characterized by compulsive drug abuse despite the potential undesirable consequences. Previous studies have indicated that the use of psychoactive stimulants may lead to changes in a wide range of neurological circuits and physiological processes (38). Psychostimulants play a significant role in promoting the structural plasticity of reward circuits in the brain (39). Addiction interacts with the reward system to motivate drug-seeking behavior, inhibit self-control mechanisms, and promote compulsive drug use (40). Such findings may explain the high rate of relapse in patients with drug addiction.

So far, what is known to us is that long-term MA use can lead to structural and functional changes in the brain. The brain's glutamate system plays a key role in long-term plasticity associated with learning and memory. Patients with MA use disorders exhibit persistent cognitive impairments and neurological deficits, which may be related to changes in the prefrontal cortex (PFC) and its glutamatergic projections to the NAc (41). Most previous studies have indicated that the progression of drug addiction is largely due to the adaptive neurobiological response to drug abuse in the corticostriatal glutamatergic and dopaminergic systems in the brain (42, 43). Thus, repeated drug abuse may lead to neurobiological adaptations that promote habitual drug use (44).

Some previous MRS studies have reported that patients with MA use disorders exhibit decreases in NAA/creatine levels, as well as increases in levels of inositol (45, 46). However, in the present study, we observed no significant differences in the concentrations of these metabolites between the MA and control groups. But there are still deficiencies in our experiment. The parameter TE = 33 ms was set, which is a little bit different from the basis data provided for LCModel TE = 30 ms and that is a limitation. To display glx complex (glutamate + glutamine) better, preliminary experiment was designed to detect the optimum echo time (TE). Because of the default setting of TE in LCModel software is 30 ms, 4 TEs around 30 ms (27,30,33, and 36ms) were set. The result shows that the CRLBs (Cramer-Rao) is the lowest and the SNR is the highest when TE = 33 ms. The preliminary experiment also has a limitation that there were only a few subjects in each group. Further studies are required to verify our findings. Another limitation is that there were six matched subjects who could not remember their drug use time accurately, so other six subjects before matched were replaced in **Figure 6**. In addition, changes in the concentrations of glutamate have been implicated in the neuroadaptation processes associated with drug addiction (47). However, such measurements are difficult to obtain due to the overlapping resonance of glutamate and glutamine. We used LCModel software to separate glutamate signals. Our findings indicated that glutamate concentration was higher in the MA group than in the control group, consistent with the findings of Sailasuta et al. (48).

Nonetheless, findings regarding metabolite concentrations in the brains of MA users remain inconsistent. In a 1H-MRS study of 29 patients with MA addiction and 45 healthy controls, Crocker et al. discovered that patients of the MA group exhibited decreased levels of glutamate (49, 50). In contrast to our findings, one previous study involving 44 adolescent MA users and 53 healthy adolescents reported that NAA levels were lower in the anterior cingulate cortex of teenagers in the MA group. Such differences may be due to differences in participant characteristics. Naaijen et al. (51) discovered that glutamate + glutamine (glx) signals were decreased in the anterior cingulate cortex of pediatric patients with autism spectrum disorders (ASD) and attention deficit hyperactivity disorder (ADHD). However, Glx signals were lower in adults with ASD and ADHD, indicating that neurodevelopmental changes in prefrontal glutamate concentration occur throughout the life cycle. Ernst and Chang reported that short-term abstinence from MA use is associated with dynamic abnormalities in glx levels (52), suggesting that normalization of Glx levels may reduce cravings for MA.

Conclusion

Our findings indicated that glutamate concentrations and glutamate-to-creatine ratios were significantly higher in patients with MA use disorders than in controls, and that absolute glutamate concentrations were correlated with the duration of MA use. Such findings may aid in the development of objective biological markers for evaluating/monitor disease status and treatment efficacy in patients with MA dependence.

AUTHOR CONTRIBUTIONS

WY and RY designed the study. JiL and LH conducted the assessments. JZ conducted behavioral and imaging analyses. JuL modified the manuscript and supervised the study. WY wrote the first draft and all authors provided input to the final version of the manuscript.

FUNDING

This study was funded by the National Key Research and Development Program of China, 2016YFC0107104 and the National Natural Science Foundation of China (No. 81671671). This work was partly funded by the National Key Research and Development Program of China (Grant number: 2016YFC0800908).

ACKNOWLEDGMENTS

The authors express their appreciation to their patients and volunteers for participating in this study.

REFERENCES

1. Gibb JW, Kogan FJ. Influence of dopamine synthesis on methamphetamine-induced changes in striatal and adrenal tyrosine hydroxylase activity. *Naunyn Schmiedebergs Arch Pharmacol.* (1979). 310:185–7. doi: 10.1007/BF00500283
2. Chang L, Cloak C, Patterson K, Grob C, Miller EN, Ernst T. Enlarged striatum in abstinent methamphetamine abusers: a possible compensatory response. *Biol Psychiatry* (2005) 57:967–74. doi: 10.1016/j.biopsych.2005.01.039
3. Kalivas PW. Cocaine and amphetamine-like psychostimulants: neurocircuitry and glutamate neuroplasticity. *Dialogues Clin Neurosci.* (2007) 9:389–97.
4. Underhill SM, Wheeler DS, Li M, Watts SD, Ingram SL, Amara. Amphetamine modulates excitatory neurotransmission through endocytosis of the glutamate transporter EAAT3 in dopamine neurons. *Neuron* (2014) 83:404–16. doi: 10.1016/j.neuron.2014.05.043
5. Catarzi,D.,Colotta,V.,Varano,F. Competitive Gly/NMDA receptor antagonists. *Curr Top Med Chem.* (2006) 6:809. doi: 10.2174/156802606777057544
6. Schmaal L, Veltman DJ, Nederveen A, van den Brink W, Goudriaan AE N-acetylcysteine normalizes glutamate levels in cocaine-dependent patients: a randomized crossover magnetic resonance spectroscopy study. *Neuropsychopharmacology* (2012) 37:2143–52. doi: 10.1038/npp.2012.66
7. Mon A, Durazzo TC, Meyerhoff DJ. Glutamate, GABA, and other cortical metabolite concentrations during early abstinence from alcohol and their associations with neurocognitive changes . *Drug Alcohol Depend.* (2012) 125:27–36. doi: 10.1016/j.drugalcdep.2012.03.012
8. Bagga D, Khushu S, Modi S, Kaur P, Bhattacharya D, Garg ML, et al. Impaired visual information processing in alcohol-dependent subjects: a proton magnetic resonance spectroscopy study of the primary visual cortex. *J Stud Alcohol Drugs* (2014) 75:817–26. doi: 10.15288/jsad.2014.75.817

9. Frye MA, Hinton DJ, Karpyak VM, Biernacka JM, Gunderson LJ, Feeder SE, et al. Anterior cingulate glutamate is reduced by acamprosate treatment in patients with alcohol dependence. *J Clin Psychopharmacol.* (2016) 36:669. doi: 10.1097/JCP.0000000000000590
10. Hermann D, Weber-Fahr W, Sartorius A, Hoerst M, Frischknecht U, Tunc-Skarka N, et al. Translational magnetic resonance spectroscopy reveals excessive central glutamate levels during alcohol withdrawal in humans and rats. *Biol Psychiatry* (2012) 71:1015–21. doi: 10.1016/j.biopsych.2011.07.034
11. Wakabayashi KT, Kiyatkin EA. Critical role of peripheral drug actions in experience-dependent changes in nucleus accumbens glutamate release induced by intravenous cocaine. *J Neurochem.* (2014) 128:672–85. doi: 10.1111/jnc.12472
12. White TL, Monnig MA, Walsh EG, Nitenson AZ, Harris AD, Cohen RA, et al. Psychostimulant drug effects on glutamate, Glx, and creatine in the anterior cingulate cortex and subjective response in healthy humans. *Neuropsychopharmacology*(2018) 43:1498–509. doi: 10.1038/s41386-018-0027-7
13. Huang CY, Li CS, Fang SC, Wu CS, Liao DL. The reliability of the Chinese version of the Barratt Impulsiveness Scale version 11, in abstinent, opioid-dependent participants in Taiwan. *J Chin Med Assoc JCMA* (2013) 76:289–95. doi: 10.1016/j.jcma.2013.01.005
14. Provencher SW. Automatic quantitation of localized in vivo 1H spectra with LCModel. *NMR Biomed.* (2001) 14:260–4. doi: 10.1002/nbm.698
15. Provencher SW. Estimation of metabolite concentrations from localized *in vivo* proton NMR spectra. *Magn Reson Med.* (1993) 30:672–9. doi: 10.1002/mrm.1910300604
16. Smith QR, Smith QR. Transport of glutamate and other amino acids at the blood-brain barrier. *J Nutr.* (2000) 130:1016S–22S. doi: 10.1093/jn/130.4.1016S
17. Kalivas PW, Volkow ND. New medications for drug addiction hiding in glutamatergic neuroplasticity. *Mol Psychiatry* (2011) 16:974. doi: 10.1038/mp.2011.46
18. Sugimoto K, Suzuki HI, Fujimura T, Ono A, Kaga N, Isobe Y. A clinically attainable dose of L-asparaginase targets glutamine addiction in lymphoid cell lines. *Cancer Sci.* (2015). 106:1534–43. doi: 10.1111/cas.12807
19. Burnett EJ, Chandler LJ, Trantham-Davidson H. Glutamatergic plasticity and alcohol dependence-induced alterations in reward, affect and cognition. *Prog Neuro Psychopharmacol Biol Psychiatry* (2016) 65:309. doi: 10.1016/j.pnpbp.2015.08.012
20. Borjkhani M, Bahrami F, Janahmadi M. Computational modeling of opioid-induced synaptic plasticity in hippocampus. *PloS ONE* (2018) 13:e0193410. doi: 10.1371/journal.pone.0193410
21. Tzschentke TM. Glutamatergic mechanisms in different disease states: overview and therapeutical implications - an introduction. *Amino Acids* (2002) 23:147–52. doi: 10.1007/s00726-001-0120-8
22. Platt SR. The role of glutamate in central nervous system health and disease - a review. *Vet J.* (2007) 173:278–86. doi: 10.1016/j.tvjl.2005.11.007
23. Zhao M, Fan C, Du J, Jiang H, Chen H, Sun H. Cue-induced craving and physiological reactions in recently and long-abstinent heroin-dependent patients. *Addic Behav.* (2012) 37:393–8. doi: 10.1016/j.addbeh.2011.11.030
24. Kennedy AP, Epstein DH, Phillips KA, Preston KL. Sex differences in cocaine/heroin users: Drug-use triggers and craving in daily life. *Drug Alcohol Depend.* (2013).132:29–37. 10.1016/j.drugalcdep.2012.12.025
25. van Huijstee AN, Mansvelder HD. Glutamatergic synaptic plasticity in the mesocorticolimbic system in addiction. *Front Cell Neurosci.* (2014) 8:466. doi: 10.3389/fncel.2014.00466
26. Schultz W. Dopamine signals for reward value and risk: basic and recent data. *Behav Brain Funct Bbf* (2010) 6:1–9. doi: 10.1186/1744-9081-6-24
27. Lammel S, Lim BK, Malenka RC. Reward and aversion in a heterogeneous midbrain dopamine system. *Neuropharmacology* (2014) 76:351–9. doi: 10.1016/j.neuropharm.2013.03.019
28. Mameli M, Lüscher C. Synaptic plasticity and addiction: learning mechanisms gone awry. *Neuropharmacology* (2011) 61:1052–9. doi: 10.1016/j.neuropharm.2011.01.036
29. Brown RE, Basheer R, McKenna JT, Strecker RE, McCarley RW. et al. Control of sleep and wakefulness. *Physiol Rev.* (2012) 92:1087–187. doi: 10.1152/physrev.00032.2011
30. Yoo JH, Zell V, Wu J, Punta C, Ramajayam N, Shen X, et al. Activation of pedunculopontine glutamate neurons is reinforcing. *J Neurosci.* (2017) 37:38–46. doi: 10.1523/JNEUROSCI.3082-16.2016
31. Gut NK, Winn P. The pedunculopontine tegmental nucleus—A functional hypothesis from the comparative literature. *Movem Disord.* (2016) 31:615–24. doi: 10.1002/mds.26556
32. Koob GF, Volkow ND. Neurobiology of addiction: a neurocircuitry analysis. *Lancet Psychiatry* (2016) 3:760–73. doi: 10.1016/S2215-0366(16)00104-8
33. Tata DA, Yamamoto BK. Chronic stress enhances methamphetamine-induced extracellular glutamate and excitotoxicity in the rat striatum. *Synapse* (2008) 62:325–36. doi: 10.1002/syn.20497
34. Hu H. Reward and aversion. *Ann Rev Neurosci.* (2016) 39:297. doi: 10.1146/annurev-neuro-070815-014106
35. Wilhelm CJ, Johnson RA, Eshleman AJ. Lobeline effects on tonic and methamphetamine-induced dopamine release. *Biochem Pharmacol.* (2008) 75:1411–5. doi: 10.1016/j.bcp.2007.11.019
36. Ja-Hyun B. Dopamine signaling in reward-related behaviors. *Front Neural Circ.* (2013) 7:152. doi: 10.3389/fncir.2013.00152
37. Holly EN, Miczek KA. Ventral tegmental area dopamine revisited: effects of acute and repeated stress. *Psychopharmacology* (2016) 233:163–86. doi: 10.1007/s00213-015-4151-3
38. Kim HJ, Lee JH, Yun K, Kim JH. Alterations in striatal circuits underlying addiction-like behaviors. *Mol Cells* (2017) 40:379–385. doi: 10.14348/molcells.2017.0088
39. Golden SA, Russo SJ. Mechanisms of psychostimulant-induced structural plasticity. *Cold Spring Harbor Perspect Med.* (2012) 2:283–88. doi: 10.1101/cshperspect.a011957
40. Volkow ND, Wang GJ, Tomasi, D, Baler RD.. Unbalanced neuronal circuits in addiction. *Curr Opin Neurobiol.* (2013) 23:639–48. doi: 10.1016/j.conb.2013.01.002
41. Parsegian A, See RE. Dysregulation of dopamine and glutamate release in the prefrontal cortex and nucleus accumbens following methamphetamine self-administration and during reinstatement in rats. *Neuropsychopharmacol Offic Public Am College Neuropsychopharmacol.* (2014) 39:811. doi: 10.1038/npp.2013.231
42. Kalivas PW, Volkow N, Seamans J. unmanageable motivation in addiction: a pathology in prefrontal-accumbens glutamate transmission. *Neuron* (2005) 45:647–50. doi: 10.1016/j.neuron.2005.02.005
43. Gross NB, Duncker PC, Marshall JF. Cortical ionotropic glutamate receptor antagonism protects against methamphetamine-induced striatal neurotoxicity. *Neuroscience* (2011) 199:272. doi: 10.1016/j.neuroscience.2011.09.014
44. George O, Koob GF. Individual differences in prefrontal cortex function and the transition from drug use to drug dependence. *Neurosci Biobehav Rev.* (2010) 35:232. doi: 10.1016/j.neubiorev.2010.05.002
45. Salo R, Nordahl TE, Natsuaki Y, Leamon MH, Galloway GP, Waters C, et al. Attentional control and brain metabolite levels in methamphetamine abusers. *Biol Psychiatry* (2007) 61:1272–80. doi: 10.1016/j.biopsych.2006.07.031
46. Sung YH, Cho SC, Hwang J, Kim SJ, Kim H, Bae S, et al. Relationship between N-acetyl-aspartate in gray and white matter of abstinent methamphetamine abusers and their history of drug abuse: a proton magnetic resonance spectroscopy study. *Drug Alcohol Depend.* (2007) 88:28–35. doi: 10.1016/j.drugalcdep.2006.09.011
47. Reissner KJ, Kalivas PW. Using glutamate homeostasis as a target for treating addictive disorders. *Behav Pharmacol.* (2010) 21:514. doi: 10.1097/FBP.0b013e32833d41b2
48. Sailasuta N, Abulseoud O, Hernandez M, Haghani P, Ross BD, et al. Metabolic abnormalities in abstinent methamphetamine dependent subjects. *Subst Abuse* (2010) 2010:9–20. doi: 10.4137/SART.S4625
49. Crocker CE, Bernier DC, Hanstock CC, Lakusta B, Purdon SE, Seres P. Prefrontal glutamate levels differentiate early phase schizophrenia and methamphetamine addiction: a (1)H MRS study at 3Tesla. *Schizophrenia Res.* (2014) 157:231–7. doi: 10.1016/j.schres.2014.05.004

50. Kim JE, Kim GH, Hwang J, Kim JY, Renshaw PF, Yurgelun-Todd DA, et al. Metabolic alterations in the anterior cingulate cortex and related cognitive deficits in late adolescent methamphetamine users. *Addict Biol.* (2016) 23:327–36. doi: 10.1111/adb.12473
51. Naaijen J, Lythgoe DJ, Amiri H, Buitelaar JK, Glennon JC. Fronto-striatal glutamatergic compounds in compulsive and impulsive syndromes: a review of magnetic resonance spectroscopy studies. *Neurosci Biobehav Rev.* (2015) 52:74–88. doi: 10.1016/j.neubiorev.2015.02.009
52. Ernst T, Chang L. Adaptation of brain glutamate plus glutamine during abstinence from chronic methamphetamine use. *J Neuroimmune Pharmacol.* (2008) 3:165–72. doi: 10.1007/s11481-008-9108-4

16

The Influence of Myelin Oligodendrocyte Glycoprotein on White Matter Abnormalities in Different Onset Age of Drug-Naïve Depression

Feng Wu [1], Lingtao Kong [1], Yue Zhu [1], Qian Zhou [1,2], Xiaowei Jiang [3,4], Miao Chang [3], Yifang Zhou [5], Yang Cao [6], Ke Xu [3], Fei Wang [1,3] and Yanqing Tang [1,5]*

[1] Department of Psychiatry, The First Affiliated Hospital of China Medical University, Shenyang, China, [2] Shanghai Mental Health Center, Shanghai, China, [3] Department of Radiology, The First Affiliated Hospital of China Medical University, Shenyang, China, [4] Brain Function Research Section, The First Affiliated Hospital of China Medical University, Shenyang, China, [5] Department of Gerontology, The First Affiliated Hospital of China Medical University, Shenyang, China, [6] Shenyang Mental Health Center, Shenyang, China

***Correspondence:**
Yanqing Tang
tangyanqing@cmu.edu.cn

Neurophysiological mechanisms of white matter abnormalities in the earlier onset major depressive disorder (eoMDD, onset age ≤25 years old) differ from that in the later onset MDD (loMDD, onset age >25 years old). Myelin oligodendrocyte glycoprotein (MOG) is an important factor influencing white matter development. The influence of MOG on white matter in MDD of different age onset need to be explored. We compared MOG plasma concentrations and diffusion tensor imaging (DTI) data in 35 first-episode medication-naïve MDD patients (23 eoMDD, 12 loMDD), and 32 healthy controls (HC, 17 younger, 15 older). MOG was significantly higher in eoMDD and lower in loMDD compared with HC. Mean diffusivity (MD) values were significantly increased in inferior fronto-occipital fasciculus (IFOF) in eoMDD, and decreased in loMDD. In both younger and older groups, MOG correlated positively with IFOF MD values. Abnormal MOG has different influence in MDD of different age onset, which is linked to MOG's overly active effect on abnormal white matter in eoMDD and markedly weak effect in loMDD cases. Abnormal MOG would be an important factor in white matter damage in MDD; the influence of MOG differs with onset age.

Keywords: major depressive disorder, myelin oligodendrocyte glycoprotein, diffusion tensor imaging, inferior fronto-occipital fasciculus, magnetic resonance imaging, onset age

INTRODUCTION

Previous research (1) has demonstrated that clinical heterogeneity, including the variety of age onsets, is a key factor influencing the treatment of major depressive disorder (MDD). MDD onsets at different ages are assumed to show different clinical symptoms, as well as disease severity and course (2, 3). Convergent evidence suggests that the heritability of MDD onset in the earlier age (eoMDD, onset age ≤25 years old) is influenced by different factors than MDD onset in the later age (loMDD, onset age >25 years old) (4), and that the neurophysiological mechanisms different by age at onset (5–7). Neural development research implied that humans show different neural characteristics at different ages, with brain development rapid, but not totally mature at younger ages, a possible sensitive period (8–14). The brain continues to develop, especially in myelination, until the fourth decade of life, a stable period (9, 15). These principles all imply that age plays an important element of human brain development. Consequently, one might expect neurophysiological differences in the onset of MDD at different ages.

Increasing evidence implicates white matter as an important component of the structural brain changes in MDD (16–18). In the development of the human brain, axon and synaptic pruning would occur quickly, especially in frontal cortex, from adolescence to young adulthood, after which those processes will maintain a stable level (19–23). As one of the myelin associated axon inhibitors (24–29), myelin oligodendrocyte glycoprotein (MOG) is known to limit neurite outgrowth of axon in the maturation of brain, with MOG effects expressed mainly on white matter fibers (30). Although the brain is not mature in adolescence and young adulthood (≤25 years old), because of axon pruning and inadequate myelination, MOG can maintain myelin-axon integrity in normal brain (31). But overexpression of MOG could lead to excessive inhibition of axons (32). In adolescent schizophrenia, errors in pruning localized in frontal cortex has also been demonstrated to be an important element in the pathology of that mental disorder (33). Whether the MOG is also abnormal and leads to axon pruning errors in eoMDD is still unknown.

On the other hand, autopsy studies showed that myelin lesions may exist in adult patients with depression (34), suggesting that myelin lesions may play a key role in the pathology of loMDD (>25 years old). Myelination of human brain gradually increases with age (35) and continues into the fourth decade of life (15, 35–37). The myelin sheaths in the central nervous system (CNS) are produced by oligodendrocytes (38, 39) and also are affected by MOG (36, 40, 41). As a late marker of myelination and oligodendrocyte maturation (31), MOG can concurrently improve the myelination of the CNS (31, 42). This makes information transmission in nerve fibers more rapid and effective, and plays an important role in the maturation of human brain in middle age (15, 37). Lower MOG in more mature adults, accompanied with demyelination, has been found in some nervous system diseases (43–45). Autopsy studies of adult MDD cases also demonstrated decreased MOG gene expression in cortical or subcortical regions of patients' brains (46–48). This suggested that the lower MOG led to a deficit in myelination, which therefore may be a key mechanism in the pathology of loMDD. Based on known differences in the function of MOG at different ages, it seems reasonable to hypothesize that the mechanism of MOG influences MDD differs at different ages of onset. To the best of our knowledge, that age difference has not been explored.

As a factor affecting the development of axons and myelin, MOG may be involved in the white matter abnormalities of MDD; however, the mechanism remains unclear. Diffusion tensor imaging (DTI) is widely used to detect the white matter abnormalities in MDD. Fractional anisotropy (FA) and mean diffusivity (MD) are commonly used to evaluate white matter fiber integrity and microstructure (14, 49–51). We exploited these tools to investigate the effect of MOG on white matter at different ages of MDD onset. Evidence shows that the prefrontal cortex (PFC) is one of the important regions in which MOG is expressed (52). White matter abnormalities of PFC have also been revealed in numerous DTI studies with MDD cases (16, 53–55). Our previous work detected white matter abnormalities in the fornix, which connects the PFC and hippocampus within eoMDD (56). We also found such abnormalities in the superior longitudinal fasciculus (SLF), which connects dorsal lateral prefrontal cortex (DLPFC) and parietal lobe within loMDD (18). These findings suggest that white matter abnormalities in the PFC might be one of the key component of the pathophysiology of MDD. What is not known is what the relationship between white matter abnormalities of PFC and the effect of MOG in eoMDD and loMDD might be; that is an issue we explored in the present research.

In the current study, we recruited the first-episode medication-naïve MDD, and follow up for 6 months to 2 years to exclude the patients turned into bipolar. We measured the concentration of MOG in plasma and FA, MD of white matter of the brain in eoMDD and loMDD, and analyzed the correlation among those measures. We hypothesized that: 1) The concentration of MOG in MDD would differ from those of healthy control participants in different age group; and 2) MOG would be differentially associated with the white matter effects at different ages of MDD onset.

MATERIALS AND METHODS

Participants

We recruited 35 patients (23 eoMDD, 12 loMDD) with diagnosed MDD from outpatients at the Department of Psychiatry, First Affiliated Hospital of China Medical University. All adolescent MDD participants were diagnosed by two trained psychiatrists individually using the Schedule for Affective Disorders and Schizophrenia for School-Age Children (KSADS-PL) and met the following inclusion criteria: fulfilling KSADS-PL criteria; first depressive episode; aged 13–17; no comorbid diagnosis of psychosis, bipolar disorder; and no history of psychotropic medication, electroconvulsive therapy or psychotherapy; severity of depression was assessed through the 17-item Hamilton Depression Rating Scale (HAMD-17) (57) and having a score of at least 17 on HAMD-17. All adult MDD participants were also diagnosed by two trained psychiatrists individually using the Structured Clinical Interview for DSM-IV and met the following inclusion criteria: fulfilling DSM-IV criteria for major depressive disorder; having only a single depressive episode; aged 18–45; exhibiting no comorbid Axis I or II diagnosis; no history of psychotropic medication, electroconvulsive therapy or psychotherapy; having a score of at least 17 on HAMD-17. We followed up for 6 months to 2 years, and excluded the patients who subsequently exhibited a bipolar diagnosis.

By means of advertisements in the same region as the hospital, we also recruited 32 healthy control participants, 17 younger healthy controls (yHC) and 15 older healthy controls (oHC) matched for sex, age and education. The Structured Clinical

Interview for DSM-IV and the KSADS-PL confirmed the absence of DSM-IV Axis I or II disorders. All the participants were assessed HAMD-17.

Exclusion criteria for all participants included the following: any MRI contraindications; history of head injury or neurological disorder; history of substance abuse or dependence; any concomitant medical disorder. We also excluded participants with a history of mood disorders in their first-degree family members. All participants were right-handed and were scanned within 48 h of initial contact. All participants gave written informed consent, and the adolescent participants' parents or legal guardian provided written informed consent after receiving a detailed description of the study. The study was approved by the Ethics Committee of the China Medical University.

Procedure

Plasma Collection

Plasma collection was performed according to standardized protocols. EDTA was used as an anticoagulant. Samples were centrifuged for 10 min at 2,000 × g at 8°C within 30 min of collection and were stored at −80°C until analysis. We used the Bio Trust Specialty Zeal Human MOG ELISA Kit for the determination of MOG concentrations in plasma.

We prepared all standards before starting the assay procedure. All standards and samples were added in duplicate to the Microtiter Plate. We added biotinylated anti-IgG, and combined streptavidin-HRP, TSZ become antibody—antigen—enzyme-antibody complex, after washing completely. We added TMB substrate solution. The intensity of this colored product is directly proportional to the concentration of MOG present in the samples. We measured the optical density (OD) at 450 nm with microtiter plate reader, and calculated MOG concentration by standard curve.

MRI Data Acquisition

Magnetic resonance imaging was performed on a GE Signa HDX 3.0T MRI scanner with a standard head coil at the First Affiliated Hospital of China Medical University, Shenyang, China. DTI was acquired using a spin-echo planar imaging sequence aligned to the anterior commissure-posterior commissure (AC-PC) plane. The diffusion sensitizing gradients were applied along 25 non-collinear directions ($b = 1000$ s/mm^2), together with an axial acquisition without diffusion weighting ($b = 0$). The scan parameters were as follows: TR = 17,000 ms, TE = 85.4 ms, FOV = 24 cm × 24 cm, imaging matrix = 120 × 120, 65 contiguous axial slices of 2 mm without gap. Participants were instructed to rest with their eyes closed but remain awake during scanning. No participant reported falling asleep during the scan when routinely asked immediately after scanning. The high resolution structural image was acquired using a three-dimensional fast spoiled gradient-echo T1-weighted sequence: TR = 7.1 ms, TE = 3.2 ms, FOV = 24 cm × 24 cm, matrix = 240 × 240, slice thickness = 1.0 mm without gap, 176 slices.

MRI Data Processing and Analysis

DTI data were processed by PANDA (Pipeline for Analyzing braiN Diffusion images 1.3.0 http://www.nitrc.org/projects/panda/) software (58), which synthesizes procedures in FSL (http://fsl.fmrib.ox.ac.uk/fsl), diffusion toolkit (http://www.nmr.mgh.harvard.edu/~rpwang/dtk), and MRIcron (http://www.mccauslandcenter.sc.edu/mricro/mricron). Steps are as follows: converting DICOM files into NIfTI images, estimating the brain mask, cropping images, correcting for the eddy-current effect, averaging acquisitions, calculating DTI metrics, and finally, producing diffusion metrics for statistical analysis. The individual images of the diffusion metrics were transformed from native space to a standard Montreal Neurological Institute (MNI) space via spatial normalization (voxel size 2 mm × 2 mm × 2 mm).

Statistical Analysis

We separated the participants into four groups by age and diagnosis: eoMDD (13–25 years of age), loMDD (26–45 years of age), and their paired HC groups. Two-way analysis of variance (ANOVA) with diagnosis (MDD/HC) and age (eo/lo) as between subject factors was used to compare age, education and HAMD scores with SPSS 22.0 software (SPSS Inc., Chicago, Illinois). Two-sample t-test was used to compare illness duration between eoMDD and loMDD groups. MOG concentrations were analyzed using two-way anova tests to detect the age by diagnosis interaction within four groups ($p < 0.05$). Pearson correlations were used to examine the association between MOG and factor score of HAMD.

We also used two-sample t-tests to compare the group differences of FA and MD ($p < 0.005$) within the younger groups and older groups in SPM8, extracted the significantly different ROI values, and used the Pearson's correlation to analyze the correlation between MOG concentration and the ROI values. The contrast map threshold was set at $p < 0.005$ for each voxel, with a cluster size of at least 51 voxels, which was equal to the corrected threshold of $p < 0.05$, as determined by AlphaSim (see program AlphaSim by B.D. Ward in AFNI software. http://afni.nimh.nih.gov/pub/dist/doc/manual/AlphaSim.pdf).

RESULTS

Demographic and Clinical Scales

There were no significant effect of diagnosis or sex in age, education and HAMD scores. MDD and HC groups did not differ significantly in age and education. The effect of diagnosis in HAMD was significant, with significant higher HAMD scores in the MDD group, compared to the HC group ($p = 0.000$). There was no significant effect of age in HAMD. Two-sample t-test showed no difference in the illness duration between eoMDD and loMDD subgroups (**Table 1**).

MOG Results

The interaction result of age by diagnosis of MOG within four groups was significant ($p = 0.026$). In the younger groups, MOG in eoMDD was significantly higher than in yHC ($p = 0.010$). In the older groups, MOG in loMDD was lower than in oHC ($p = 0.049$; **Table 1**).

TABLE 1 | Demographic and clinical data of subjects.

	eoMDD	loMDD	yHC	oHC	Statistic	*P*-values
Number	23	12	17	15	$\chi^2 = 1.101$	0.294
Age (years, mean ± S.D.) [range]	19.44 ± 4.61 [13–25]	33.77 ± 5.86 [26–44]	18.07 ± 3.85 [13–25]	35.28 ± 6.74 [26–45]	$F = 2.782$	0.100
Education (years, mean±S.D.) [range]	11.5 ± 2.57 [7–16]	11.98 ± 3.52 [7–16]	12.68 ± 3.79 [7–18]	13.21 ± 3.42 [9–19]	$F = 0.045$	0.832
HAMD (mean ± S.D.) [range]	22.09 ± 5.01 [17–33]	21.83 ±5.04 [17–32]	0.88 ± 1.58 [0–6]	0.46 ± 0.96 [0–3]	$F = 0.013$	0.908
Duration of illness (month, mean ± S.D.) [range]	5.75 ± 7.11 [0.5–24]	7.85 ± 7.31 [1–24]	N/A	N/A	$t = 0.857$	0.398
MOG (mean ± S.D.)	214.64 ± 71.47	166.19 ± 79.73	178.71 ± 58.69	208.38 ± 63.11	$F = 5.198$	0.026*

*S.D. standard deviation; HAMD, Hamilton Depression Rating Scale; MOG, myelin oligodendrocyte glycoprotein; eoMDD, major depressive disorder onset in the earlier age (onset age ≤25 years old); loMDD, major depressive disorder onset in the later age (onset age >25 years old); yHC, younger healthy controls; oHC, older healthy controls. *P < 0.05.*

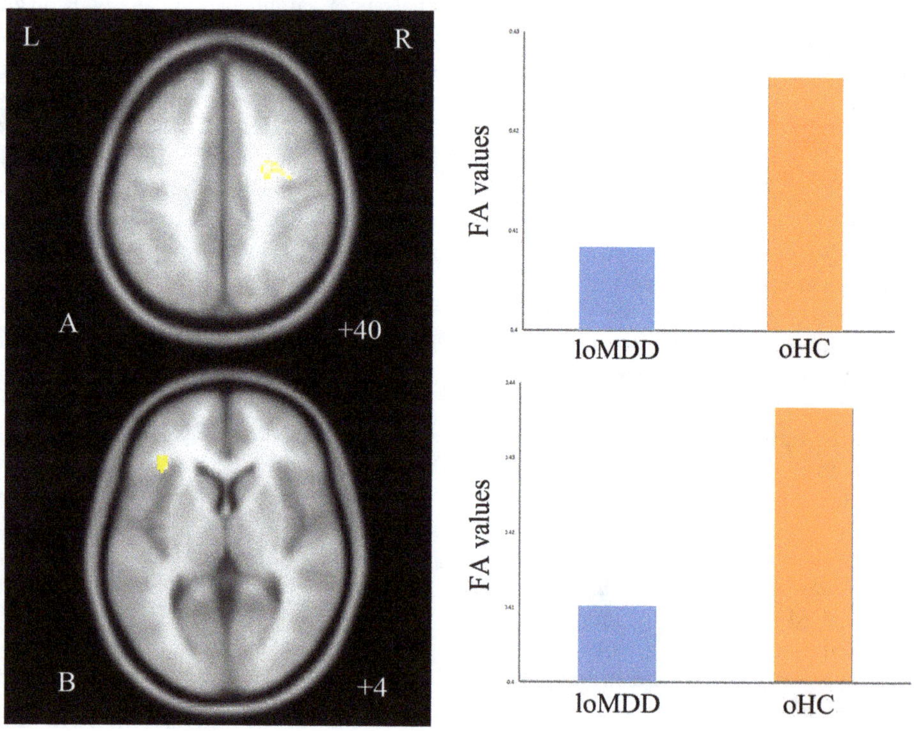

FIGURE 1 | Regions of differences for white matter integrity between medication-naïve patients with major depressive disorder (MDD: eoMDD, onset age ≤25 years old; loMDD, onset age >25 years old) and healthy controls (HC: yHC, younger healthy controls; oHC, older healthy controls). **(A)** The axial image ($z = +40$ mm) shows the significantly decreased fractional anisotropy (FA) values in the right superior longitudinal fasciculus (SLF) with loMDD, compared to oHC. **(B)** The axial image ($z = +4$ mm) shows the significantly decreased FA values in the left inferior fronto-occipital fasciculus (IFOF) with loMDD, compared to oHC. The graph shows FA values for loMDD and oHC.

Correlation Between MOG and FA, MD

We excluded participants who failed to scan or yielded bad quality DTI, leaving 34 MDD (22 eoMDD, 12 loMDD) and 30 HC (17 yHC, 13 oHC) participants for analysis.

With respect to FA values, there were no significantly different regions in the eoMDD group relative to the yHC group, but FA was significantly decreased in the right SLF (cluster size = 81 voxels, maximal point MNI coordinate: $x = 30$ mm, $y = -2$ mm, $z = 40$ mm, $T = 3.07$, $p < 0.05$, corrected) (**Figure 1A**) and left inferior fronto-occipital fasciculus (IFOF) (cluster size = 68 voxels, maximal point MNI coordinate: $x = -38$ mm, $y = 30$ mm, $z = 4$ mm, $T = 3.35$, $p < 0.05$, corrected) (**Figure 1B**) in the loMDD group relative to the oHC group. The correlation between MOG and FA showed no significant association with FA values in the right SLF and left IFOF of loMDD participants.

The MD values were significantly increased in the left IFOF (cluster size = 79 voxels, maximal point MNI coordinate: $x = -18$ mm, $y = -2$ mm, $z = 48$ mm, $T = 3.69$, $p < 0.05$,

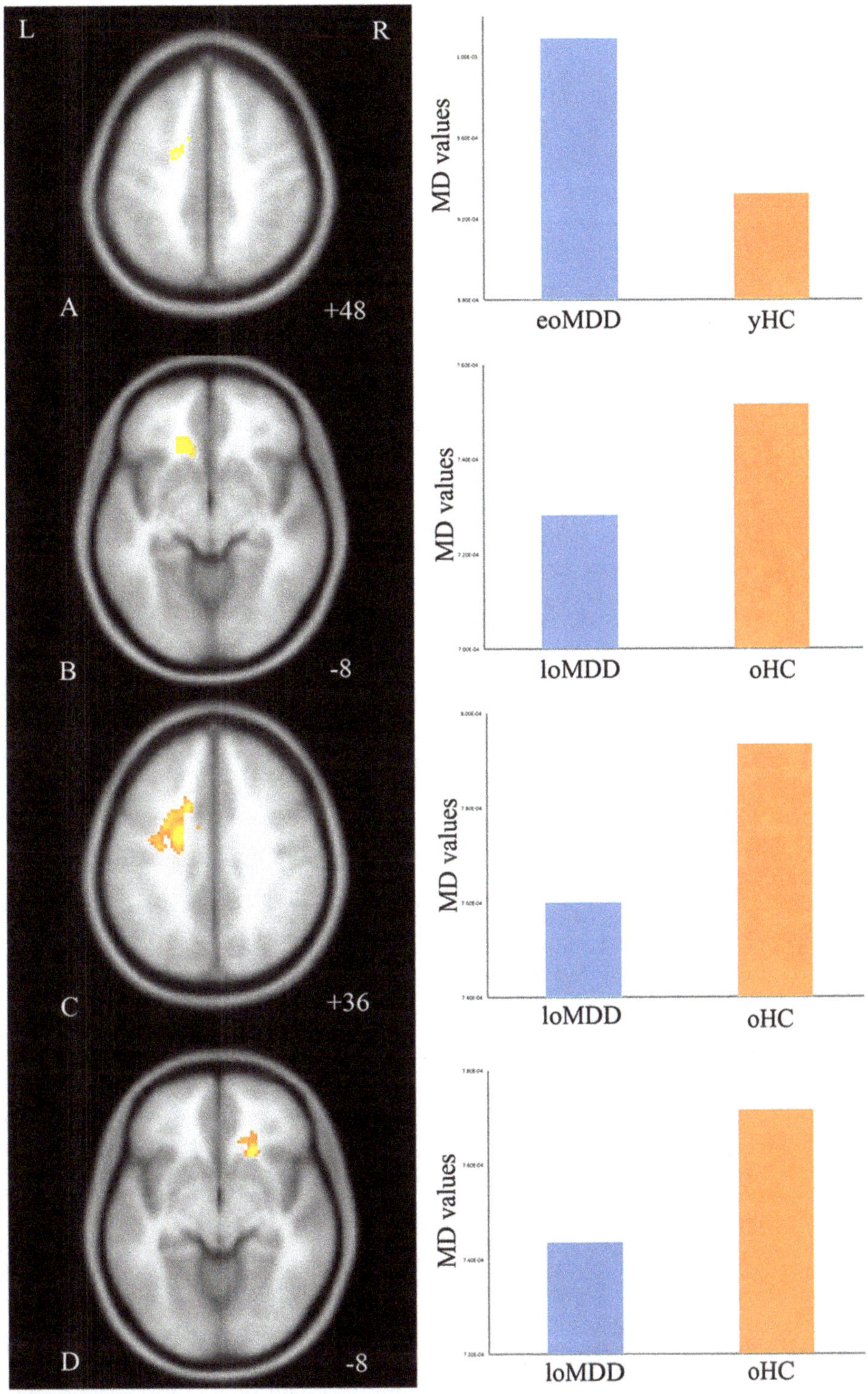

FIGURE 2 | Regions of differences for white matter integrity between medication-naïve patients with major depressive disorder (MDD: eoMDD, onset age ≤25 years old; loMDD, onset age >25 years old) and healthy controls (HC: yHC, younger healthy controls; oHC, older healthy controls). **(A)** The axial image ($z = +48$ mm) shows the significantly increased mean diffusivity (MD) values in the left inferior fronto-occipital fasciculus (IFOF) with eoMDD, compared to yHC. **(B)** The axial image ($z = -8$ mm) shows the significantly decreased MD values in the left IFOF with loMDD, compared to oHC. **(C)** The axial image ($z = +36$ mm) shows the significantly decreased MD values in the left IFOF with loMDD, compared to oHC. **(D)** The axial image ($z = -8$ mm) shows the significantly decreased MD values in the right IFOF with loMDD, compared to oHC. The graph shows MD values for eoMDD, yHC, loMDD, and oHC.

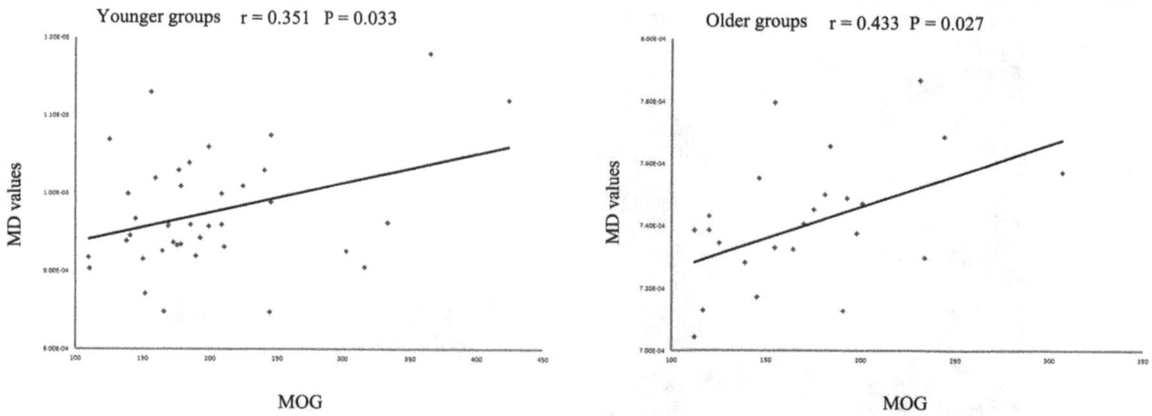

FIGURE 3 | Scatter plots showing significant correlations between myelin oligodendrocyte glycoprotein (MOG) concentration and mean diffusivity (MD) values in the left inferior fronto-occipital fasciculus in different age groups.

corrected) (**Figure 2A**) of the eoMDD group relative to the yHC group. The ROI values of this region were significantly positively correlated with MOG concentration in younger groups ($r = 0.351$, $p = 0.033$; **Figure 3).** In older groups, the MD values were significantly decreased in left IFOF (cluster size = 314 voxels, maximal point MNI coordinate: $x = -18$ mm, $y = 30$ mm, $z = -8$ mm, $T = 4.03$, $p < 0.05$, corrected) (**Figure 2B**), left IFOF (cluster size=1117 voxels, maximal point MNI coordinate: $x = -24$ mm, $y = 0$ mm, $z = 36$ mm, $T = 4.58$, $p < 0.05$, corrected) (**Figure 2C**) and right IFOF (cluster size = 605 voxels, maximal point MNI coordinate: $x = 20$ mm, $y = 28$ mm, $z = -8$ mm, $T = 3.57$, $p < 0.05$, corrected) (**Figure 2D**) in the loMDD group relative to the oHC group. The ROI values of left IFOF (cluster size=314 voxels, maximal point MNI coordinate: $x = -18$ mm, $y = 30$ mm, $z = -8$ mm) is significantly positive correlated with MOG concentration in older groups ($r = 0.443$, $p = 0.027$; **Figure 3**, **Table 2**).

TABLE 2 | Brain regions showing significant differences between major depressive disorder and health control participants.

Brain regions	Cluster size (voxels)	MNI Coordinates			*T*-values
		X	Y	z	
FA					
loMDD < oHC					
Right SLF	81	30	−2	40	3.14
Left IFOF	68	−38	30	4	3.35
MD					
eoMDD > yHC left IFOF	79	−18	−2	48	3.69
loMDD < oHC					
Left IFOF	314	−18	30	−8	4.03
Left IFOF	1117	−24	0	36	4.58
Right IFOF	605	20	28	−8	3.57

eoMDD, major depressive disorder onset in the earlier age (onset age ≤25 years old); loMDD, major depressive disorder onset in the later age (onset age >25 years old); yHC, younger healthy controls; oHC, older healthy controls; FA, fractional anisotropy; MD, mean diffusivity; SLF, superior longitudinal fasciculus; IFOF, inferior fronto-occipital fasciculus.

DISCUSSION

In the current study, we found MOG to be different by age and MDD diagnosis groups. MOG was significantly higher in eoMDD and lower in loMDD compared with HC. The MD increased in IFOF in eoMDD participants, and decreased in IFOF in loMDD cases. We also found that in older and younger groups, MOG showed a positive correlation with MD values in the left IFOF. To our knowledge, this is the first study to detect the MOG plasma concentration *in vivo* MDD patients, and combining MOG and DTI methods *in vivo* to investigate the relationship between MOG and MD in different MDD onset ages. Our findings imply that the abnormality of MOG may have different mechanism influencing white matter at different ages, thereby inducing different symptoms of eoMDD or loMDD.

MOG is highly expressed on some neurons, particularly on large projection neurons, which is a minor component of central culture medium composed of central nervous system (CNS) myelin (30). Other researchers have recognized that MOG limits neurite outgrowth of axons at younger ages (25–27). By contrast, MOG expression increases with age concurrently with CNS myelination (31), and is a late marker of myelination and oligodendrocyte maturation in adults, independent of axonal influence even in absence of axons (59). There is evidence that myelination of human axons is increased with age (36), with the progression of myelination continuing into the fourth decade of life (15). That perspective is consistent with our result of increased MOG by age in HC, reflecting the increasing myelination in normal brain development.

In our study, we found MOG concentration showed a significant age by diagnosis group interaction, which suggested differential change in MOG at different ages of HC and MDD individuals. We found increased MOG in eoMDD. Overexpression of MOG had been proved leading to excessive inhibition of axons (32). Our result of increased MOG in eoMDD may implicate much axon inhibition or pruning, which may lead to an imbalance in young individuals, and result in depressive symptoms in younger age. Our result of decreased MOG in loMDD is same as the autopsy researches. Autopsy studies showed MOG expression down-regulated in BA 21 (47) of MDD patients. According to the function of MOG in myelination, our result suggested that in adulthood, the lower function of myelination may be an important component of the pathology of loMDD, and possibly leading to widely depressive symptoms. Taken together, our study suggested that the mechanism of MOG influence in the CNS of MDD cases depends on the age of onset. Although CNS of MDD individuals is affected by MOG abnormality, the pathophysiology of eoMDD and loMDD are different. Our study has identified for the first time that MOG in plasma is different between MDD and HC, and showed differential influence for different onset ages. The different pathology of eoMDD and loMDD may relate to the MOG's function: on axon pruning too active at younger ages and on myelination too weak at older ages.

Our study also indicated that the abnormal brain region is more focused in IFOF of MDD cases, compared to HC, in both younger groups and older groups. IFOF connects occipital and frontal lobes, which are involved in reading, attention, and visual processing (60, 61) as well as in semantic processing and conceptualizing of visual stimuli (62, 63). Several studies have reported white matter abnormalities of IFOF in MDD (64, 65). Our results of increased MD value of IFOF in eoMDD, consistent with our previous study (56), suggest that white matter abnormalities of IFOF may play an important role in the pathophysiology of MDD in younger age. Furthermore, decreased FA values of SLF and IFOF were detected in loMDD, which is consistent with our previous study (18). In contrast, our results about decreased MD value of IFOF in loMDD was inconsistent with other studies (65). Until now, the essential association of MD with mental disorders has not been fully understood yet. We speculate that age may play a key role in the different change of IFOF between the two age groups of MDD, which need to be further investigated.

MOG showed a positive correlation with MD values in IFOF within both younger and older groups. This suggested that the abnormal MOG may lead to the abnormality of IFOF, which may play an important role in the pathophysiology of MOG-caused MDD. According to our result, we conclude that the increased MOG in eoMDD may implicate much axon pruning in IFOF, possibly leading to depression in younger age. On the other hand, in loMDD, the decreased MOG's function in myelination may lead to more widely damage of white matter in IFOF, resulted in depression in older age. As the first study exploring the correlation between MOG and DTI *in vivo* in MDD patients, the present results may provide a new direction for the study of the pathology of MDD.

Some limitations of this study should be noted. First, as we selected first-episode medication naïve adolescent and adult MDD to minimize the confounds of chronicity, treatment or comorbidity, the relatively small sample size may limit the generalizability of our results as well as our ability to detect relationships between biomarkers and neuroimaging findings in this study. Future studies with larger sample sizes will be important to further understand the neuropathophysiology of MDD. Second, the MOG and white matter development are both continuous processes from early to late life, the age difference between eoMDD and loMDD group may potentially influence the changes in MOG and its effect on white matter integrity. Future studies between eoMDD and loMDD with matched ages are under investigation and longitudinal study would be needed to further explore the changes in MOG and the effect on white matter in MDD patients. Furthermore, the interpretation of results should be cautious because follow-up studies (66) have found that 20–40% of adolescents with MDD develop bipolar disorder within 5 years after the onset of depression. Although we followed our participants for 6 months to 2 years, longer follow-ups should be done. The cross-sectional design of this study did not allow us to distinguish between trait MDD cases and those who later converted to bipolar disorder; longitudinal studies are needed to examine the difference between them.

In summary, our study of first-episode medication-naïve MDD cases demonstrated that MOG abnormality has different effects at different ages of MDD onset. This influence may be the result of MOG's overly active effect on the abnormal white matter in young individuals and comparatively weaker effect at older ages. These findings suggest that abnormal MOG would be an important factor leading to white matter damage in MDD, with the influence different at different onset ages.

AUTHOR CONTRIBUTIONS

FGW, KX, FIW, and YT designed the study. YuZ, QZ, MC, YiZ, and YC acquired the data. FGW, QZ, XJ, and MC analyzed the data. FGW, LK, and FIW wrote the article.

ACKNOWLEDGMENTS

The authors thank Dr. Xuesheng Fan and Dr. Huan Ma of Department of Psychiatry, The First Affiliated Hospital of China Medical University for the help with recruitment of participants. This study was supported by the National Natural Science Foundation of China (81101012 to FGW, 81301166 to LK, 81271499 and 81571331 to YT), the Liaoning Scientific Foundation (2015020532 to FGW and 201602833 to LK), the National Keyresearch and Development Program (2016YFC1306900 to YT), the National Keyresearch and Development Program (2016YFC0904300 to FIW), the National High Tech Development Plan [863] (2015AA020513 to FIW) and the Liaoning Pandeng Scholar (to FIW).

REFERENCES

1. Merikangas KR, Wicki W, Angst J. Heterogeneity of depression. Classification of depressive subtypes by longitudinal course. *Br J Psychiatry* (1994) **164**:342–8. doi: 10.1192/bjp.164.3.342
2. Belmaker RH, Agam G. Major depressive disorder. *N Engl J Med.* (2008) **358**:55–68. doi: 10.1056/NEJMra073096
3. Mondimore FM, Zandi PP, Mackinnon DF, McInnis MG, Miller EB, Crowe RP, et al. Familial aggregation of illness chronicity in recurrent, early-onset major depression pedigrees. *Am J Psychiatry* (2006) **163**:1554–60. doi: 10.1176/ajp.2006.163.9.1554
4. Marazita ML, Neiswanger K, Cooper M, Zubenko GS, Giles DE, Frank E, et al. Genetic segregation analysis of early-onset recurrent unipolar depression. *Am J Hum Genet.* (1997) **61**:1370–8. doi: 10.1086/301627
5. Iorfino F, Hickie IB, Lee RS, Lagopoulos J, Hermens DF. The underlying neurobiology of key functional domains in young people with mood and anxiety disorders: a systematic review. *BMC Psychiatry* (2016) **16**:156. doi: 10.1186/s12888-016-0852-3
6. Scott J, Scott EM, Hermens DF, Naismith SL, Guastella AJ, White D, et al. Functional impairment in adolescents and young adults with emerging mood disorders. *Br J Psychiatry* (2014) **205**:362–8. doi: 10.1192/bjp.bp.113.134262
7. Lee RS, Redoblado-Hodge MA, Naismith SL, Hermens DF, Porter MA, Hickie IB. Cognitive remediation improves memory and psychosocial functioning in first-episode psychiatric out-patients. *Psychol Med.* (2013) **43**:1161–73. doi: 10.1017/S0033291712002127
8. Giorgio A, Watkins KE, Douaud G, James AC, James S, De Stefano N, et al. Changes in white matter microstructure during adolescence. *Neuroimage* (2008) **39**:52–61. doi: 10.1016/j.neuroimage.2007.07.043
9. Yeatman JD, Wandell BA, Mezer AA. Lifespan maturation and degeneration of human brain white matter. *Nat Commun.* (2014) **5**:4932. doi: 10.1038/ncomms5932
10. Fuhrmann D, Knoll LJ, Blakemore SJ. Adolescence as a sensitive period of brain development. *Trends Cogn Sci.* (2015) **19**:558–66. doi: 10.1016/j.tics.2015.07.008
11. Giorgio A, Watkins KE, Chadwick M, James S, Winmill L, Douaud G, et al. Longitudinal changes in grey and white matter during adolescence. *Neuroimage* (2010) **49**:94–103. doi: 10.1016/j.neuroimage.2009.08.003
12. Pfefferbaum A, Sullivan EV. Cross-sectional versus longitudinal estimates of age-related changes in the adult brain: overlaps and discrepancies. *Neurobiol Aging* (2015) **36**:2563–7. doi: 10.1016/j.neurobiolaging.2015.05.005
13. Bava S, Thayer R, Jacobus J, Ward M, Jernigan TL, Tapert SF. Longitudinal characterization of white matter maturation during adolescence. *Brain Res.* (2010) **1327**:38–46. doi: 10.1016/j.brainres.2010.02.066
14. Pohl KM, Sullivan EV, Rohlfing T, Chu W, Kwon D, Nichols BN, et al. Harmonizing DTI measurements across scanners to examine the development of white matter microstructure in 803 adolescents of the NCANDA study. *Neuroimage* (2016) **130**:194–213. doi: 10.1016/j.neuroimage.2016.01.061
15. Arshad M, Stanley JA, Raz N. Adult age differences in subcortical myelin content are consistent with protracted myelination and unrelated to diffusion tensor imaging indices. *Neuroimage* (2016) **143**:26–39. doi: 10.1016/j.neuroimage.2016.08.047
16. Bracht T, Linden D, Keedwell P. A review of white matter microstructure alterations of pathways of the reward circuit in depression. *J Affect Disord.* (2015) **187**:45–53. doi: 10.1016/j.jad.2015.06.041
17. Jiang W, Gong G, Wu F, Kong L, Chen K, Cui W, et al. The papez circuit in first-episode, treatment-naive adults with major depressive disorder: combined atlas-based tract-specific quantification analysis and voxel-based analysis. *PLoS ONE* (2015) **10**:e0126673. doi: 10.1371/journal.pone.0126673
18. Wu F, Tang Y, Xu K, Kong L, Sun W, Wang F, et al. Whiter matter abnormalities in medication-naive subjects with a single short-duration episode of major depressive disorder. *Psychiatry Res.* (2011) **191**:80–3. doi: 10.1016/j.pscychresns.2010.09.002
19. Chugani HT. Biological basis of emotions: brain systems and brain development. *Pediatrics* (1998) **102**:1225–9.
20. Huttenlocher PR. Synaptic density in human frontal cortex - developmental changes and effects of aging. *Brain Res.* (1979) **163**:195–205. doi: 10.1016/0006-8993(79)90349-4
21. Feinberg I, Thode HC Jr, Chugani HT, March JD. Gamma distribution model describes maturational curves for delta wave amplitude, cortical metabolic rate and synaptic density. *J Theor Biol.* (1990) **142**:149–61. doi: 10.1016/S0022-5193(05)80218-8
22. Huttenlocher PR, Dabholkar AS. Regional differences in synaptogenesis in human cerebral cortex. *J Comp Neurol.* (1997) **387**:167–78. doi: 10.1002/(SICI)1096-9861(19971020)387:2<167::AID-CNE1>3.0.CO;2-Z
23. Bourgeois JP, Goldman-Rakic PS, Rakic P. Synaptogenesis in the prefrontal cortex of rhesus monkeys. *Cereb Cortex* (1994) **4**:78–96. doi: 10.1093/cercor/4.1.78
24. McKerracher L, Winton MJ. Nogo on the go. *Neuron* (2002) **36**:345–8. doi: 10.1016/S0896-6273(02)01018-8
25. McKerracher L, David S, Jackson DL, Kottis V, Dunn RJ, Braun PE. Identification of myelin-associated glycoprotein as a major myelin-derived inhibitor of neurite growth. *Neuron* (1994) **13**:805–11. doi: 10.1016/0896-6273(94)90247-X
26. Mukhopadhyay G, Doherty P, Walsh FS, Crocker PR, Filbin MT. A novel role for myelin-associated glycoprotein as an inhibitor of axonal regeneration. *Neuron* (1994) **13**:757–67. doi: 10.1016/0896-6273(94)90042-6
27. Akbik F, Cafferty WB, Strittmatter SM. Myelin associated inhibitors: a link between injury-induced and experience-dependent plasticity. *Exp Neurol.* (2012) **235**:43–52. doi: 10.1016/j.expneurol.2011.06.006
28. Wang KC, Koprivica V, Kim JA, Sivasankaran R, Guo Y, Neve RL, et al. Oligodendrocyte-myelin glycoprotein is a Nogo receptor ligand that inhibits neurite outgrowth. *Nature* (2002) **417**:941–4. doi: 10.1038/nature00867
29. Cafferty WB, McGee AW, Strittmatter SM. Axonal growth therapeutics: regeneration or sprouting or plasticity? *Trends Neurosci.* (2008) **31**:215–20. doi: 10.1016/j.tins.2008.02.004
30. Habib AA, Marton LS, Allwardt B, Gulcher JR, Mikol DD, Hognason T, et al. Expression of the oligodendrocyte-myelin glycoprotein by neurons in the mouse central nervous system. *J Neurochem.* (1998) **70**:1704–11. doi: 10.1046/j.1471-4159.1998.70041704.x
31. Solly SK, Thomas JL, Monge M, Demerens C, Lubetzki C, Gardinier MV, et al. Myelin/oligodendrocyte glycoprotein (MOG) expression is associated with myelin deposition. *Glia* (1996) **18**:39–48.
32. Mishra M, Akatsu H, Heese K. The novel protein MANI modulates neurogenesis and neurite-cone growth. *J Cell Mol Med.* (2011) **15**:1713–25. doi: 10.1111/j.1582-4934.2010.01134.x
33. Selemon LD, Zecevic N. Schizophrenia: a tale of two critical periods for prefrontal cortical development. *Transl Psychiatry* (2015) **5**:e623. doi: 10.1038/tp.2015.115
34. Regenold WT, Phatak P, Marano CM, Gearhart L, Viens CH, Hisley KC. Myelin staining of deep white matter in the dorsolateral prefrontal cortex in schizophrenia, bipolar disorder, and unipolar major depression. *Psychiatry Res.* (2007) **151**:179–88. doi: 10.1016/j.psychres.2006.12.019
35. Wang S, Young KM. White matter plasticity in adulthood. *Neuroscience* (2014) **276**:148–60. doi: 10.1016/j.neuroscience.2013.10.018
36. Flynn SW, Lang DJ, Mackay AL, Goghari V, Vavasour IM, Whittall KP, et al. Abnormalities of myelination in schizophrenia detected *in vivo* with MRI, and post-mortem with analysis of oligodendrocyte proteins. *Mol Psychiatry* (2003) **8**:811–20. doi: 10.1038/sj.mp.4001337
37. O'Rourke M, Gasperini R, Young KM. Adult myelination: wrapping up neuronal plasticity. *Neural Regen Res.* (2014) **9**:1261–4. doi: 10.4103/1673-5374.137571
38. Peters A. The effects of normal aging on myelin and nerve fibers: a review. *J Neurocytol.* (2002) **31**:581–93. doi: 10.1023/A:1025731309829
39. Bercury KK, Macklin WB. Dynamics and mechanisms of CNS myelination. *Dev Cell* (2015) **32**:447–58. doi: 10.1016/j.devcel.2015.01.016
40. Vourc'h P, Andres C. Oligodendrocyte myelin glycoprotein (OMgp): evolution, structure and function. *Brain Res Brain Res Rev.* (2004) **45**:115–24. doi: 10.1016/j.brainresrev.2004.01.003
41. Li G, Crang AJ, Rundle JL, Blakemore WF. Oligodendrocyte progenitor cells in the adult rat CNS express myelin oligodendrocyte glycoprotein (MOG). *Brain Pathol.* (2002) **12**:463–71. doi: 10.1111/j.1750-3639.2002.tb00463.x
42. Mikol DD, Stefansson K. A phosphatidylinositol-linked peanut agglutinin-binding glycoprotein in central nervous system myelin and on oligodendrocytes. *J Cell Biol.* (1988) **106**:1273–9. doi: 10.1083/jcb.106.4.1273

43. Sinmaz N, Nguyen T, Tea F, Dale RC, Brilot F. Mapping autoantigen epitopes: molecular insights into autoantibody-associated disorders of the nervous system. *J Neuroinflammation* (2016) **13**:219. doi: 10.1186/s12974-016-0678-4
44. Maetzler W, Apel A, Langkamp M, Deuschle C, Dilger SS, Stirnkorb JG, et al. Comparable autoantibody serum levels against amyloid- and inflammation-associated proteins in Parkinson's disease patients and controls. *PLoS ONE* (2014) **9**:e88604. doi: 10.1371/journal.pone.0088604
45. Maetzler W, Berg D, Synofzik M, Brockmann K, Godau J, Melms A, et al. Autoantibodies against amyloid and glial-derived antigens are increased in serum and cerebrospinal fluid of Lewy body-associated dementias. *J Alzheimers Dis.* (2011) **26**:171–9. doi: 10.3233/JAD-2011-110221
46. Sokolov BP. Oligodendroglial abnormalities in schizophrenia, mood disorders and substance abuse. Comorbidity, shared traits, or molecular phenocopies? *Int J Neuropsychopharmacol.* (2007) **10**:547–55. doi: 10.1017/S1461145706007322
47. Aston C, Jiang L, Sokolov BP. Transcriptional profiling reveals evidence for signaling and oligodendroglial abnormalities in the temporal cortex from patients with major depressive disorder. *Mol Psychiatry* (2005) **10**:309–22. doi: 10.1038/sj.mp.4001565
48. Barley K, Dracheva S, Byne W. Subcortical oligodendrocyte- and astrocyte-associated gene expression in subjects with schizophrenia, major depression and bipolar disorder. *Schizophr Res.* (2009) **112**:54–64. doi: 10.1016/j.schres.2009.04.019
49. Feldman HM, Yeatman JD, Lee ES, Barde LH, Gaman-Bean S. Diffusion tensor imaging: a review for pediatric researchers and clinicians. *J Dev Behav Pediatr.* (2010) **31**:346–56. doi: 10.1097/DBP.0b013e3181dcaa8b
50. Alexander AL, Hurley SA, Samsonov AA, Adluru N, Hosseinbor AP, Mossahebi P, et al. Characterization of cerebral white matter properties using quantitative magnetic resonance imaging stains. *Brain Connect.* (2011) **1**:423–46. doi: 10.1089/brain.2011.0071
51. Alexander AL, Lee JE, Lazar M, Field AS. Diffusion tensor imaging of the brain. *Neurotherapeutics* (2007) **4**:316–29. doi: 10.1016/j.nurt.2007.05.011
52. Mitkus SN, Hyde TM, Vakkalanka R, Kolachana B, Weinberger DR, Kleinman JE, et al. Expression of oligodendrocyte-associated genes in dorsolateral prefrontal cortex of patients with schizophrenia. *Schizophr Res.* (2008) **98**:129–38. doi: 10.1016/j.schres.2007.09.032
53. Alexopoulos GS, Kiosses DN, Choi SJ, Murphy CF, Lim KO. Frontal white matter microstructure and treatment response of late-life depression: a preliminary study. *Am J Psychiatry* (2002) **159**:1929–32. doi: 10.1176/appi.ajp.159.11.1929
54. Xu K, Jiang W, Ren L, Ouyang X, Jiang Y, Wu F, et al. Impaired interhemispheric connectivity in medication-naive patients with major depressive disorder. *J Psychiatry Neurosci.* (2013) **38**:43–8. doi: 10.1503/jpn.110132
55. Li L, Ma N, Li Z, Tan L, Liu J, Gong G, et al. Prefrontal white matter abnormalities in young adult with major depressive disorder: a diffusion tensor imaging study. *Brain Res.* (2007) **1168**:124–8. doi: 10.1016/j.brainres.2007.06.094
56. Geng H, Wu F, Kong L, Tang Y, Zhou Q, Chang M, et al. Disrupted structural and functional connectivity in prefrontal-hippocampus circuitry in first-episode medication-naive adolescent depression. *PLoS ONE* (2016) **11**:e0148345. doi: 10.1371/journal.pone.0148345
57. Hamilton M. A rating scale for depression. *J Neurol Neurosurg Psychiatry* (1960) **23**:56–62. doi: 10.1136/jnnp.23.1.56
58. Cui Z, Zhong S, Xu P, He Y, Gong G. PANDA: a pipeline toolbox for analyzing brain diffusion images. *Front Hum Neurosci.* (2013) **7**:42. doi: 10.3389/fnhum.2013.00042
59. Rome LH, Bullock PN, Chiappelli F, Cardwell M, Adinolfi AM, Swanson D. Synthesis of a myelin-like membrane by oligodendrocytes in culture. *J Neurosci Res.* (1986) **15**:49–65. doi: 10.1002/jnr.490150106
60. Fox CJ, Iaria G, Barton JJ. Disconnection in prosopagnosia and face processing. *Cortex* (2008) **44**:996–1009. doi: 10.1016/j.cortex.2008.04.003
61. Catani M, Mesulam M. The arcuate fasciculus and the disconnection theme in language and aphasia: history and current state. *Cortex* (2008) **44**:953–61. doi: 10.1016/j.cortex.2008.04.002
62. Indefrey P. The spatial and temporal signatures of word production components: a critical update. *Front Psychol.* (2011) **2**:255. doi: 10.3389/fpsyg.2011.00255
63. Vihla M, Laine M, Salmelin R. Cortical dynamics of visual/semantic vs. phonological analysis in picture confrontation. *Neuroimage* (2006) **33**:732–8. doi: 10.1016/j.neuroimage.2006.06.040
64. Bessette KL, Nave AM, Caprihan A, Stevens MC. White matter abnormalities in adolescents with major depressive disorder. *Brain Imaging Behav.* (2014) **8**:531–41. doi: 10.1007/s11682-013-9274-8
65. Lagopoulos J, Hermens DF, Hatton SN, Battisti RA, Tobias-Webb J, White D, et al. Microstructural white matter changes are correlated with the stage of psychiatric illness. *Transl Psychiatry* (2013) **3**:e248. doi: 10.1038/tp.2013.25
66. Birmaher B, Axelson D, Strober M, Gill MK, Yang M, Ryan N, et al. Comparison of manic and depressive symptoms between children and adolescents with bipolar spectrum disorders. *Bipolar Disord.* (2009) **11**:52–62. doi: 10.1111/j.1399-5618.2008.00659.x

17

Multiple Myeloma, Misdiagnosed as Somatic Symptom Disorder

Jiashu Yao [1†], *Danmei Lv* [2†] *and Wei Chen* [3*]

[1] *Department of Psychiatry, Sir Run Run Shaw Hospital, Hangzhou, China,* [2] *School of Medcine, Zhejiang University, Hangzhou, China,* [3] *Department of Psychiatry, Sir Run Run Shaw Hospital, Hangzhou, China*

***Correspondence:**
Wei Chen
srrcw@zju.edu.cn

These authors have contributed equally to this work

Here we report on a case of a 57-year-old woman with pain and discomfort in multiple sites of upper body who was diagnosed as somatic symptom disorder after completing a partial examinations of relevant parts which turned out to be negative. Finished imageological examinations of all painful parts, she was eventually diagnosed with multiple myeloma after 6-month being misdiagnosed as somatic symptom disorder. This case highlights the importance of completing imageological examinations of all the painful parts of the patient to exclude the possibility of multiple myeloma especially when symptoms are associated with objective signs and treatment has been ineffective; and it is as well as significant to notice characteristics of symptoms and to pay excessive attention directed toward the symptoms in the diagnosis of somatic symptom disorder.

Keywords: misdiagnosis, somatic symptom disorder, somatic symptom and related disorders, multiple myeloma, case report

INTRODUCTION

Multiple myeloma (MM) is characterized by the neoplastic proliferation of immunoglobulin-producing plasma cells. Common presentations include anemia, bone pain, elevated creatinine or serum protein, fatigue, and hypercalcemia. Bone pain, particularly in the back or chest, and less often in the extremities, is present at the time of diagnosis in ~60% of patients (1). Imaging is a key part of the evaluation of all patients with suspected MM. If a patient with multiple myeloma initially presents with only bone pain but is not detected by imaging examination, it is probable to be diagnosed and treated as somatic symptom disorder, then to cause poor prognosis.

Here we report on a case in which a patient with MM was misdiagnosed as somatic symptom disorder (SSD). Written informed consent was obtained from this patient for the publication of this case report.

CASE REPORT

History of Present Illness

On January 4th, 2018, a 57-year-old woman was hospitalized in the department of Psychiatry, Sir Run Run Shaw Hospital because of pain and acid bilge in multiple sites of her upper body for more than 1 year. Over a year ago, the patient started feeling pain and discomfort in the upper left abdomen, and the pain got worse when coughing but with no other discomfort. Two months later, the upper left abdomen pain and acid bilge extended to the front chest, back, abdomen, and upper limbs. The symptoms persisted for months, and aggravated when changing body posture. Test results including cervical MRI, chest CT, abdominal B ultrasound of upper abdomen in a local hospital showed no abnormalities. Treated with Chinese medicine for more than 3 months, there was no significant improvement. About 6 months ago, the patient came to our hospital, expressing the symptoms above and worries about them, with weight loss of about 1–1.5 kg, but denying continuous depression, anxiety, and other symptoms (the score of 24 items of Hamilton Rating Scale for Depression was 12, and Hamilton Anxiety Rating Scale score was 11), and was diagnosed as "somatic symptom disorder." After 4 months of treatment with 60 mg of duloxetine enteric-coated capsules twice daily and hypnotic drugs, the symptoms were obviously alleviated but not completely relieved and there was a significant weight loss of about 5 kg. Therefore, medication was adjusted to escitalopram tablets 20 mg once daily. Two months later, the patient felt no further improvement.

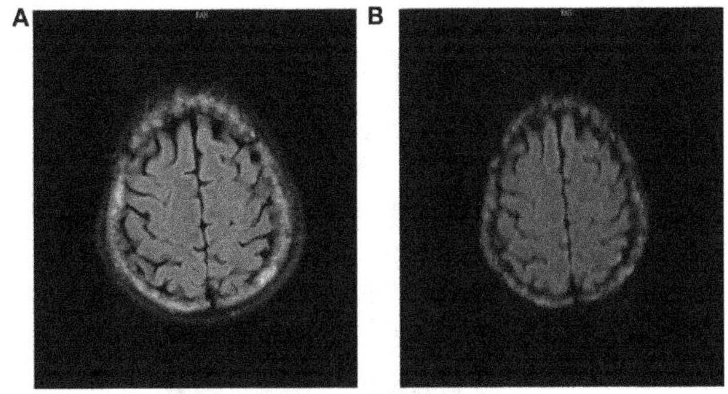

FIGURE 1 | FLAIR **(A)** and DWI **(B)** sequences of cranial MRI showed diffuse thickening of the skull and increasing signal intensity.

Medical History

With hypertension history of more than 10 years, the patient claimed that it's not necessary for her to take any antihypertensive drugs to control blood pressure in recent 1 year. She had bronchitis for 12 years but no medicine was needed. She denied any history of diabetes, heart disease and other diseases and claimed there was no history of surgery and trauma. Also, the patient denied long-term chemical substances, drug or poison exposure history and had no history of smoking and drinking alcohol.

Work-Up and Follow-Up in the Hospital

After admission, due to long-term poor efficacy of the patient, we re-evaluated the patient's physical condition to rule out organic diseases. However, through Blood routine, Blood Biochemistry, Stool Routine, Urine Routine, Chest Film, Electrocardiogram, and so on, no specific abnormality was found. We found that the patient's tumor marker CA-153 was 61.2 U/mL (<25.00 U/mL) and ferritin was 198.70 ug/L (13.00–150.00 ug/L), with no specificity. There was another finding of patient suffering from cholecystitis and gallstones through abdominal ultrasound examination; however, the surgeon suggested that it could not explain the patient's symptoms. When perfecting cranial MRI, we unexpectedly discovered below result: diffuse thickening of the skull and increasing signal intensity. Metastasis? Multiple myeloma? (**Figure 1**).

And lumbar MRI prompted lumbar vertebra, attachment and right iliac bone multiple bone changes, multiple myeloma? Transfer? (**Figure 2**). Skull and pelvis plain radiographs prompted skull, maxillofacial bone, pelvis, and femoral bone changes, multiple myeloma? Transfer? (**Figure 3**).

After perfecting corresponding blood examination, the patient eventually underwent bone marrow aspiration and the results suggested that the patient was suffered from multiple myeloma (**Figure 4**). The patient was finally referred to the hematology department and received appropriate treatment.

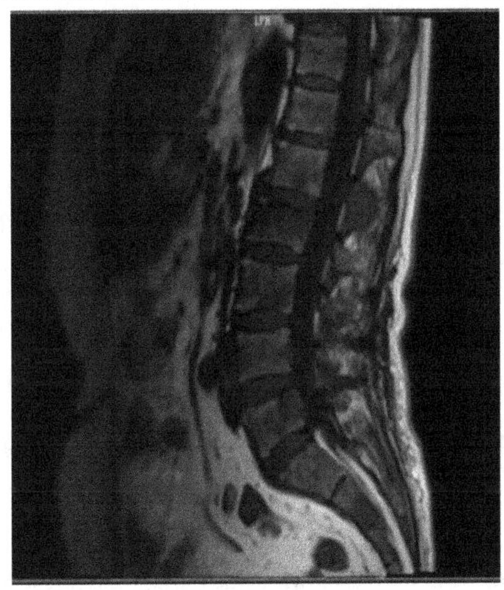

FIGURE 2 | Lumbar MRI prompted lumbar vertebra multiple bone changes.

Discussion

Here we report on a case of a 57-year-old woman with pain and discomfort in multiple sites of upper body who was diagnosed as somatic symptom disorder after completing a partial examinations of relevant parts which turned out to be negative. Finished imageological examinations of all painful parts, she was eventually diagnosed with multiple myeloma after 6-month being misdiagnosed as somatic symptom disorder. This case highlights the importance of completing imageological examinations of all the painful parts of the patient to exclude the possibility of multiple myeloma especially when symptoms are associated with objective signs and treatment has been ineffective; and it is as well as significant to notice characteristics of symptoms and to pay excessive attention directed toward the symptoms in the diagnosis of somatic symptom disorder.

MM is a disease which is characterized by the neoplastic proliferation of immunoglobulin-producing plasma cells. Most patients with MM present with signs or symptoms related to the infiltration of plasma cells into the bone or other organs or to kidney damage from excess light chains. MM accounts for ~1–2% of all cancers and slightly more than 17% of hematologic malignancies (2). Worldwide, there are ~154,000 cases and 101,000 deaths per year attributed to MM (3). MM is also slightly

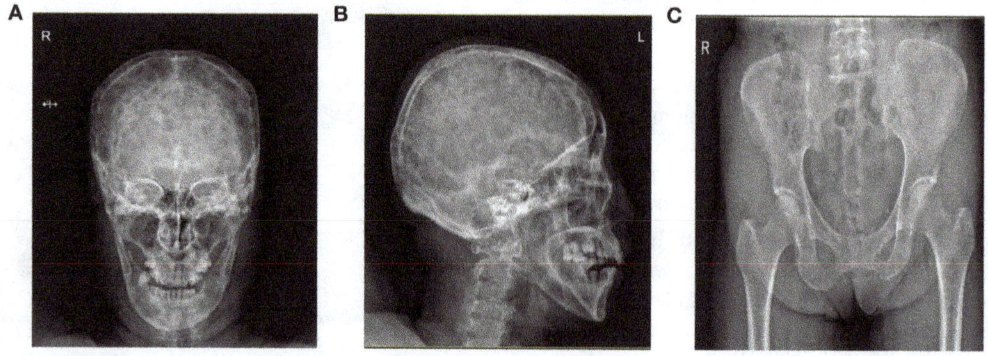

FIGURE 3 | Skull X-ray prompted that the skull and maxillofacial bone **(A,B)** were found to have diffuse worm-like low-density bone destruction and there was no obvious hardening at the edge. **(C)** Pelvis X-ray showed small and low-density bone destruction zone in the pelvis and proximal femur.

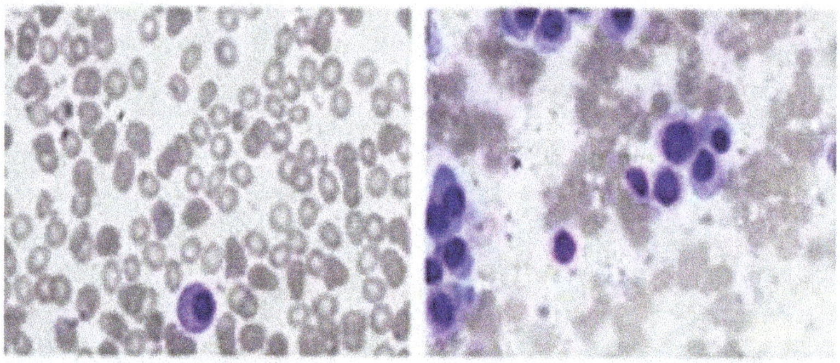

FIGURE 4 | Bone marrow considered multiple myeloma, suggesting a significant increase in the proportion of plasma cells and a small amount of naive plasma cells.

more frequent in men than in women (~1.4:1). The risk of developing MM increases with body mass index (4, 5). MM is a disease of older adults. The median age at diagnosis is 66 years; only 10 and 2% of patients are younger than 50 and 40 years, respectively (1, 6).

Most patients with MM present with signs or symptoms related to the infiltration of plasma cells into the bone or other organs or to kidney damage from excess light chains. As an example, a retrospective analysis of 1,027 sequential patients diagnosed with MM at a single institution found the following symptoms and signs at presentation: Anemia-73%, Bone pain-58%, Elevated creatinine-48%, Fatigue/generalized weakness-32%, Hypercalcemia-28%, Weight loss-24%, one-half of whom had lost ≥9 kg (1).

In American Psychiatric Association's Diagnostic and Statistical Manual, Fifth Edition (DSM-5) (7), SSD is characterized by one or more somatic symptoms that are accompanied by excessive thoughts, feelings, and/or behaviors related to the somatic symptoms. It is estimated the prevalence in the general population is 4% (8, 9) and that among primary care patients is 17% (8, 10). An analysis of individual patient data from nine community studies (total $n > 28{,}000$) found that the most frequent burdensome symptom was pain (11). SSD is not defined by the number of distressful physical symptoms that are present; however, patients who complain about multiple symptoms are more likely to have the disorder. In this case, the patient had a number of pains and acid bilge in multiple locations which are typically present in somatic symptom disorder, with no other symptoms of MM, for instance, anemia, elevated creatinine, fatigue/generalized weakness, hypercalcemia. These enhance the possibilities of misdiagnosing MM as SSD. The percentage of underlying somatic diseases in patients previously diagnosed with SSD is relatively small but unneglectable. A meta-analysis (12) reviewed six diagnostic evaluation studies (total $N = 1{,}804$ patients), 16 follow-up studies (total $N = 2{,}440$ patients), and the percentage of misdiagnosis with SSD was 8.8% (95% CI 1.0–22.2, $p = 0.007$) in diagnostic evaluation studies, 0.5% (95% CI 0.01–1.5, $p = 0.03$) in follow-up studies, while the correct diagnosis shall be diabetes mellitus, duodenal ulcer, Crohn's disease, polymyalgia rheumatica, carcinoma, herniated disc, and so on.

Imaging is a key part of the evaluation of all patients with suspected MM. In this case, we found some related negative imaging test results like cervical MRI, chest CT, abdominal B ultrasound of upper abdomen from another hospital, however, neglected to do examinations of other important parts where the patient reported discomfort, such a lumbar and pelvis imageological examinations. Pain and acid bilge in multiple sites are usually associated with musculoskeletal and nervous system disease, and MRI is the best imaging choice for the early stage of these diseases. In the diagnosis procedure of SSD, thorough physical examination, laboratory tests and imageological examinations are necessary to help clinicians and patients build confidence and ensure that no important diagnosis will be missed (13–15). Moreover, criteria for selective use of tests include objective signs rather than the volume of the concerns expressed by the patient, the presence of complex symptoms, and persistence of symptoms (16). For instance, in our case, the pain of the patient aggravates when the body posture is changed or coughing. This characteristic probably points to a physical disease which is ignored during the early processes of out-patient treatment.

SSD patients always have excessive thoughts, feelings, or behaviors associated with the somatic symptoms. The patient was also anxious because of her symptoms which now we can consider it as healthy anxiety. Clinicians taking a history should determine whether somatic symptoms trigger healthy anxiety or not, in addition, determine whether the patient manifests persistent thoughts and anxiety related to the somatic symptoms, and whether the patient devotes excessive time and energy to the somatic symptoms (17–19). In International Classification of Disease-10 (ICD-10) (20) which is currently widely used in the world, somatoform disorders are defined on the basis of failure to find physical causes rather than the presence of definite psychological and behavioral features. The notion of taking medically unexplained symptoms as the defining feature of ICD-10 somatoform disorders creates a major hindrance to the clinical utility of the diagnosis. There is evidence that the decision about whether symptoms are medically unexplained is unreliable and lacks validity. The inherent dualism in the notion of a lack of medical explanation for somatic symptoms that are cross-sectionally assessed is simplistic and ultimately unhelpful to patent care (21). In ICD-11 (22), excessive attention directed toward the symptoms is highlighted in the diagnosis of Bodily distress disorder.

There is evidence that antidepressants are effective for SSD (23, 24). However, SNRIs could relieve pain by inhibiting reuptake of serotonin and norepinephrine, and suppressing painful sensation uploading regardless of physical disease or psychiatric disorders. Therefore, pain of the patient was obviously alleviated after 4 months of treatment with 60 mg of duloxetine enteric-coated capsules twice daily. This phenomenon also could perplex the revision of the diagnosis.

This case indicates that imageological examinations of all the painful parts of the patient should be completed to exclude the possibility of MM, especially of those whose symptoms are associated with objective signs and treatment has been ineffective. Furthermore, diagnosis of SSD requires not only the elimination of somatic diseases, but also excessive thoughts, feelings, or behaviors associated with the somatic symptoms.

AUTHOR CONTRIBUTIONS

JY wrote the introduction and discussion, DL wrote the case report. WC guided the writing.

REFERENCES

1. Kyle RA, Gertz MA, Witzig TE, Lust JA, Lacy MQ, Dispenzieri A, et al. Review of 1027 patients with newly diagnosed multiple myeloma. *Mayo Clin Proc.* (2003) 78:21–33. doi: 10.4065/78.1.21
2. Siegel RL, Miller KD, Jemal A. Cancer statistics, 2018. *CA Cancer J Clin.* (2018) 68:7–30. doi: 10.3322/caac.21442
3. Fitzmaurice C, Allen C, Barber RM, Barregard L, Bhutta ZA, Brenner H, et al. Global, regional, and national cancer incidence, mortality, years of life lost, years lived with disability, and disability-adjusted life-years for 32 cancer groups, 1990 to 2015: a systematic analysis for the global burden of disease study. *JAMA Oncol.* (2017) 3:524–48. doi: 10.1001/jamaoncol.2016.5688
4. Lauby-Secretan B, Scoccianti C, Loomis D, Grosse Y, Bianchini F, Straif K, et al. Body fatness and cancer–viewpoint of the IARC working group. *N Engl J Med.* (2016) 375:794–8. doi: 10.1056/NEJMsr1606602
5. Kyrgiou M, Kalliala I, Markozannes G, Gunter MJ, Paraskevaidis E, Gabra H, et al. Adiposity and cancer at major anatomical sites: umbrella review of the literature. *BMJ* (2017) 356:j477. doi: 10.1136/bmj.j477
6. Bladé J, Kyle RA. Multiple myeloma in young patients: clinical presentation and treatment approach. *Leuk Lymphoma* (1998) 30:493–501.
7. American Psychiatric Association. *Diagnostic and Statistical Manual of Mental Disorders*. 5th ed. Arlington, VA: American Psychiatric Press [M] (2013).
8. Creed F, Barsky A. A systematic review of the epidemiology of somatisation disorder and hypochondriasis. *J Psychosom Res.* (2004) 56:391–408. doi: 10.1016/S0022-3999(03)00622-6
9. Kirmayer LJ, Robbins JM. Three forms of somatization in primary care: prevalence, co-occurrence, and sociodemographic characteristics. *J Nerv Ment Dis.* (1991) 179:647–55.
10. Escobar JI, Burnam MA, Karno M, Forsythe A, Golding JM. Somatization in the community. *Arch Gen Psychiatry* (1987) 44:713–8. doi: 10.1001/archpsyc.1987.01800200039006
11. Tomenson B, Essau C, Jacobi F, Ladwig KH, Leiknes KA, Lieb R, et al. Total somatic symptom score as a predictor of health outcome in somatic symptom disorders. *Br J Psychiatry* (2013) 203:373–80. doi: 10.1192/bjp.bp.112.114405
12. Eikelboom EM, Tak LM, Roest AM. JGM R: a systematic review and meta-analysis of the percentage of revised diagnoses in functional somatic symptoms. *J Psychosom Res.* (2016) 88:60–7 doi: 10.1016/j.jpsychores.2016.07.001
13. Bensing JM, Verhaak PF. Somatisation: a joint responsibility of doctor and patient. *Lancet* (2006) 367:452–4. doi: 10.1016/S0140-6736(06)68155-5
14. Ring A, Dowrick CF, Humphris GM, Davies J, Salmon P. The somatising effect of clinical consultation: what patients and doctors say and do not say when patients present medically unexplained physical symptoms. *Soc Sci Med.* (2005) 61:1505–15. doi: 10.1016/j.socscimed.2005.03.014
15. Henningsen P, Zipfel S, Herzog W. Management of functional somatic syndromes. *Lancet* (2007) 369:946–55. doi: 10.1016/S0140-6736(07)60159-7
16. Kroenke K. Diagnostic testing and the illusory reassurance of normal results: comment on "Reassurance after diagnostic testing with a low pretest probability of serious disease". *JAMA Intern Med.* (2013) 173:416–7. doi: 10.1001/jamainternmed.2013.11

17. Silverman JJ, Galanter M, Jackson-Triche M, Jacobs DG, Lomax JW, Riba MB, et al. The american psychiatric association practice guidelines for the psychiatric evaluation of adults. *Am J Psychiatry* (2015) 172:798–802. doi: 10.1176/appi.ajp.2015.1720501
18. Bi X, Moos RH, Timko C, Cronkite RC. Family conflict and somatic symptoms over 10 years: a growth mixture model analysis. *J Psychosom Res.* (2015) 78:459–65. doi: 10.1016/j.jpsychores.2015.01.013
19. Croicu C, Chwastiak L, Katon W. Approach to the patient with multiple somatic symptoms. *Med Clin North Am.* (2014) 98:1079–95. doi: 10.1016/j.mcna.2014.06.007
20. World Health Organization. *The ICD-10 Classification of Mental and Behavioural Disorders:Diagnostic Criteria for Research.* Geneva: WHO[M] (1993).
21. Gureje O. Classification of somatic syndromes in ICD-11. *Curr Opin Psychiatry* (2015) 28:345–9. doi: 10.1097/YCO.0000000000000186
22. World Health Organization. *The ICD-11 Classification of Mental and Behavioural Disorders:Diagnostic Criteria for Research.* Geneva: WHO[J] (2018).
23. Kroenke K. Efficacy of treatment for somatoform disorders: a review of randomized controlled trials. *Psychosom Med.* (2007) 69:881–8. doi: 10.1097/PSY.0b013e31815b00c4
24. Sumathipala A. What is the evidence for the efficacy of treatments for somatoform disorders? A critical review of previous intervention studies. *Psychosom Med.* (2007) 69:889–900. doi: 10.1097/PSY.0b013e31815b5cf6

18

Disrupted Cerebellar Connectivity with the Central Executive Network and the Default-Mode Network in Unmedicated Bipolar II Disorder

Xiaomei Luo[1,2†], Guanmao Chen[1,2†], Yanbin Jia[3], JiaYing Gong[2,4], Shaojuan Qiu[1,2], Shuming Zhong[3], Lianping Zhao[1,5], Feng Chen[1,2], Shunkai Lai[3], Zhangzhang Qi[1,2], Li Huang[1,2] and Ying Wang[1,2*]*

[1] Medical Imaging Center, First Affiliated Hospital of Jinan University, Guangzhou, China, [2] Institute of Molecular and Functional Imaging, Jinan University, Guangzhou, China, [3] Department of Psychiatry, First Affiliated Hospital of Jinan University, Guangzhou, China, [4] The Sixth Affiliated Hospital of Sun Yat-sen University, Guangzhou, China, [5] Department of Radiology, Gansu Provincial Hospital, Lanzhou, China

***Correspondence:**
Li Huang
cjr.huangli@vip.163.com
Ying Wang
johneil@vip.sina.com

†These authors have contributed equally to this work

Objective: Bipolar disorder (BD) is a common psychiatric disease. Although structural and functional abnormalities of the cerebellum in BD patients have been reported by recent neuroimaging studies, the cerebellar-cerebral functional connectivity (FC) has not yet been examined. The present study aims to investigate the FC between the cerebellum and cerebrum, particularly the central executive network (CEN) and the default-mode network (DMN) in bipolar II disorder (BD II).

Methods: Ninety-four patients with unmedicated BD II depression and 100 healthy controls (HCs) underwent the resting-state functional magnetic resonance imaging. Seed-based connectivity analyses were performed using cerebellar seeds previously identified as being involved in the CEN (bilateral Crus Ia) and DMN (bilateral Crus Ib).

Results: Compared with HCs, BD II depression patients appeared decreased FC in the right Crus Ia-left dorsal lateral prefrontal cortex (dlPFC) and -left anterior cingulate cortex (ACC), the right Crus Ib-left medial prefrontal cortex (mPFC), -left middle temporal gyrus (MTG), and -left inferior temporal gyrus (ITG). No altered FC between the left Crus Ia or Crus Ib and the cerebral regions was found.

Conclusions: Patients with BD II depression showed disrupted FC between the cerebellum and the CEN (mainly in the left dlPFC and ACC) and DMN (mainly in the left mPFC and temporal lobe), suggesting the significant role of the cerebellum-CEN and -DMN connectivity in the pathogenesis of BD.

Keywords: bipolar disorder, functional magnetic resonance imaging, cerebellar-cerebral functional connectivity, default-mode network, central executive network

INTRODUCTION

Bipolar disorder (BD) is a chronic, severe and fluctuating psychiatric disease and receives widespread attention due to its various clinical manifestation, complicated course, and difficulty in treatment. Though BD consists of recurring episodes of mania and depression, the most common manifestation is the depressive episode, which results in a misdiagnosis as a major depressive disorder (MDD), bringing about mistreatment, huge medical costs, and poor clinical outcome. Despite being a common and important psychiatric illness, the specific pathogenesis of BD remains unclear. The proposal that the cerebellum plays a significant role in the pathophysiological mechanisms of BD was raised these years (1). Some neuroimaging studies have demonstrated structural and functional abnormalities of the cerebellum in BD (2–4).

The cerebellum has traditionally been regarded as an important role in motor control, posture coordination, and linguistic processing. However, recently, some evidence from literatures highlight an association between the cerebellum and higher-order functions, such as non-motor cognition as well as emotion (5–7). Anatomically, the cerebellum of normal human has been divided into ten lobules named I–X, grouped as the anterior lobe (lobules I–V); posterior lobe (lobules VI–IX, including Crus I and Crus II and lobule VIIb); and the flocculonodular lobe (lobule X) (8, 9). And it has been shown to reciprocally connect with many brain regions, like the brainstem reticular nuclei, hypothalamus, periaqueductal gray matter, amygdala, prefrontal cortex, and anterior cingulate cortex (ACC) (10–12). These connections are hypothesized to be the neural substrates for the cerebellar-cerebral functional connectivity (FC). Functionally, several resting-state functional magnetic resonance imaging (rs-fMRI) data have demonstrated FC between the cerebellar subregions and cerebral networks. For instance, using voxel-based analysis, a study has reported strong FC between lobule Crus I, Crus II, and the frontoparietal network; between lobule IX, vermal VIIIb and the default-mode network (DMN); between lobules I–VI, VIII and the sensorimotor networks and so on in 228 normal humans (13). Performing independent component analysis in 15 normal humans, Habas et al. found that cerebellar Crus I and II mainly participated in the bilateral central executive network (CEN), lobule IX participated in the DMN, lobules V–VI participated in the sensorimotor networks, and lobule VI participated in salience network (14). Meanwhile, applying seed-based analysis in 40 normal humans, Krienen and Buckner have also found that subregions in cerebellum had FC with the CEN, DMN, and motor network (15).

The CEN was classically conceptualized as referring to many fields, including working memory, initiation, planning, inhibition, flexibility, and vigilance (16). And the DMN was suggested to subserve ongoing, or default functions of the brain (17). These two networks are recognized as 2 core neurocognitive networks (18), showing dysfunctional connectivity in neuropsychiatric disorders, such as Alzheimer's disease, MDD, and BD (19). Moreover, several rs-fMRI studies have displayed aberrant FC between the cerebellum and the CEN and DMN in MDD (20–22), and schizophrenia (23), suggesting that the cerebellum participated in the pathogenesis of psychiatric diseases. However, only one study paid close attention to the cerebellar FC in BD, which used cerebral seeds to probe the cerebral-cerebellar FC in BD with psychosis, and found cerebral-cerebellar dysconnectivity in selective networks, such as the somatomotor, ventral attention, salience, and frontoparietal networks (24).

BD has two main subtypes, bipolar I disorder (BD I), and bipolar II disorder (BD II), which present different affective states and personality characteristics. According to the Diagnostic and Statistical Manual of Mental Disorders, Fifth Edition (known as DSM-V), BD I have a manic episode while BD II have a hypomanic episode. Though patients with BD II have less severe intensity, several studies suggest that patients with BD II may have a more chronic course, higher frequency of depressive episodes and comorbidity, more suicidal behavior, and rapid cycling than patients with BD I (25–29). There are reports about the genetic (28, 30, 31), metabolic (32), and electrophysiological (25, 33, 34) differences between BD II and BD I. And neuroimaging studies have shown the differences in structure (29, 35–39), and task-based function (40–42) between BD II and BD I. However, most neuroimaging studies, especially rs-fMRI studies, recruited heterogeneous samples of varying BD subtypes that included BD I, BD II. To date, the neurobiology of BD II has been poorly investigated. No prior study has researched the FC between cerebellum and cerebrum in BD II.

In the present study, we collected rs-fMRI data from patients with unmedicated BD II depression and healthy controls (HCs) at relatively large sample scale. To investigate the intrinsic cerebellar-cerebral FC in the CEN and DMN in BD II depression patients and HCs, seed-based correlation analyses were conducted. Cerebellar seeds were used to identify the CEN, and DMN, which were demonstrated to have a cerebral-cerebellar connection by previous studies (7, 15, 21, 22). We hypothesized that BD II depression patients would have aberrant FC in the cerebellum -CEN and -DMN.

METHODS AND MATERIALS

Subjects

A total of 200 individuals ranging in age from 18 to 55 years participated in this study, including 97 currently depressed adults diagnosed with BD II and 103 HCs. The patients were recruited from the psychiatry department, First Affiliated Hospital of Jinan University, Guangzhou, China. All patients met DSM-V criteria for BD II according to the diagnostic assessment by the Structured Clinical Interview for DSM-V Patient Edition (SCID-P). The clinical state was assessed by using the 24-item Hamilton Depression Rating Scale (HDRS) and the Young Mania Rating Scale (YMRS) during the 3-day period prior to the imaging session. To be eligible for the study, all patients should have a total HDRS-24 score of > 21 and total YMRS score of < 7. At the time of testing, all patients were either medication-naïve or were not medicated for at least 6 months. The exclusion criteria included the presence of (a) any other Axis-I psychiatric disorders, (b) a history of electroconvulsive therapy, (c) a history of organic brain disorder, mental retardation, neurological disorders, (d) pregnancy, alcohol/substance abuse or dependence, or any presence of a concurrent and major physical illness, (e) any contraindication to MRI scanning. In addition, 103 right-handed HCs were recruited through local advertisements. To rule out the presence of a current or past history of any psychiatric illness, HCs were carefully screened through a diagnostic interview-the Structured Clinical Interview for DSM-V Non-patient Edition (SCID-NP). Further exclusion criteria for HCs were any history of a current or past significant medical or neurological illness, psychiatric illness in first-degree relatives.

This study was approved by the Ethics Committee of First Affiliated Hospital of Jinan University, Guangzhou, China, and signed a written informed consent for each participant after a full explanation of the study. Two senior clinical psychiatrists confirmed that all subjects had the ability to consent to participate in the examination.

MRI Data Acquisition

Imaging was performed on a GE Discovery MR750 3.0 T System with an 8-channel phased array head coil. Subjects were scanned in a supine, head-first position with symmetrically placed cushions on both sides of the head to decrease motion. Before the scanning, each participant was repeatedly instructed to relax with their eyes closed without falling asleep; after the experiment, only participants who confirmed that they had not fallen asleep were included; otherwise, he/she was excluded.

The rs-fMRI data were acquired using gradient-echo echo-planar imaging sequence with the following parameters: time repetition (TR)/time echo (TE) = 2,000/25 ms, flip angle = 90°, voxel size = 3.75 × 3.75 × 3 mm^3, field of view (FOV) = 240 × 240 mm, matrix = 64 × 64, slice thickness/gap = 3.0/1.0 mm, 35 axial slices covering the whole-brain, and 210 volumes acquired in 7 min. In addition, a three-dimensional brain volume imaging (3D-BRAVO) sequence covering the whole brain was used for structural data acquisition with: TR/TE = 8.2/3.2 ms, flip angle = 12°, bandwidth = 31.25 Hz, slice thickness/gap = 1.0/0 mm matrix=256 × 256, FOV = 240 × 240 mm, NEX = 1, and acquisition time = 3 min 45 s. Routine MRI examination images were also collected for excluding anatomic abnormality. All participants were found by two experienced radiologists to confirm no brain structural abnormalities.

Data Preprocessing

The preprocessing was carried out using Data Processing and Analysis of Brain Imaging (DPABI, http://rfmri.org/DPABI), which is based on Statistical Parametric Mapping (SPM12, http://www.fil.ion.ucl.ac.uk/spm/). For each subject, the first 10 images of the rs-fMRI dataset were excluded to ensure steady-state longitudinal magnetization. The remaining 200 images were first slice-time corrected and then were realigned to the first image for correcting for inter-TR head motion. This realignment correction provided a record of the head motion within the rs-fMRI scan. All subjects should have no more than 2 mm maximum displacement in any plane, 0.2 mm in mean frame-wise displacement (FD) (43), and 2° of angular motion. The individual T1 structural images were segmented (white matter, gray matter, and cerebrospinal fluid) using Segmentation toolbox. Then, the Diffeomorphic Anatomical Registration Through Exponentiated Lie algebra (DARTEL) toolbox was used to create a study specific template for the accurate normalization. Then, resting-state functional images were coregistered to the structural images and transformed into standard Montreal Neurological Institute (MNI) space, resliced to a voxel size of 3 × 3 × 3 mm^3 resolution and smoothed using a 4 mm full width at half maximum (FWHM) Gaussian kernel. Furthermore, the data were removed linear trend and passed through band-pass filtered of 0.01–0.1 Hz. The Friston-24-parameter model of head motion (including the 6 head motion parameters, 6 head motion parameters one time point before, and the 12 corresponding squared items) (44) was chosen based on prior work (45). Several spurious covariates and their temporal derivatives were then regressed out from the time course of each voxel, including the signals of the brain global mean, white matter, and cerebrospinal fluid as well as the Friston-24 parameters of head motion.

FC Analysis

Two previous seed-based rs-fMRI studies have reported that the left cerebellar Crus Ia (MNI coordinates: −12, −78, −28) and right cerebellar Crus Ia (MNI coordinates: 12, −78, −28) participated in the CEN, and the left cerebellar Crus Ib (MNI coordinates: −32, −76, −34) and right cerebellar Crus Ib (MNI coordinates: 34, −80, −36) participated in the DMN in major depressive disorder (21, 22). It was noticed that the bilateral Crus Ib involved in the DMN were asymmetric. These two seeds were defined by Krienen and Buckner in a study that used frontal seeds to investigate the FC between the cerebrum and cerebellum in normal humans (15). They found that the DMN (mPFC) was strongly connected with the bilateral Crus Ib. Thus, we chose these four seeds with a radius of 6 mm to examine the FC between the cerebellum and the CEN and the DMN (**Figure 1**). The seed point reference time series of each seed was extracted by averaging the time series of voxels of each ROI. For each subject, correlation maps were produced by computing the Pearson's correlation coefficients between the time series of the seeds and all the other brain voxels. To improve the normality, the obtained correlation maps were then converted to *z*-values maps using Fisher's *r-to-z* transformation. For all the subjects, four *z*-score maps which represented the intrinsic FC of the four cerebellar seeds were finally obtained.

Statistical Analysis

The two final group of participants included in this study were 94 patients with BD II (mean age, SD, gender ration) and 100 HCs. Independent-sample *t*-tests and χ^2 tests were used to compare the demographic data between the BD II and HCs groups with SPSS 17.0 software (SPSS, Chicago, IL, USA). All tests were two-tailed, and $p < 0.05$ were considered statistically significant.

The one-sample *t*-test was performed on z-score maps to demonstrate the within-group FC spatial distribution of each cerebellar seed for the BD patients and HCs. Then, the two-sample *t*-test was performed to assess the significant differences of the whole brain FC for each cerebellar seed between BD patients and HCs within the union mask of one-sample *t*-test results of both groups. Age, gender, education level, and the mean FD were included as nuisance covariates in the group comparisons. Statistical maps were thresholded using permutation test (PT) as implemented in Permutation Analysis of Linear Models (PALM) (46) and integrated into DPABI. The threshold-free cluster enhancement (TFCE) and voxel-wise

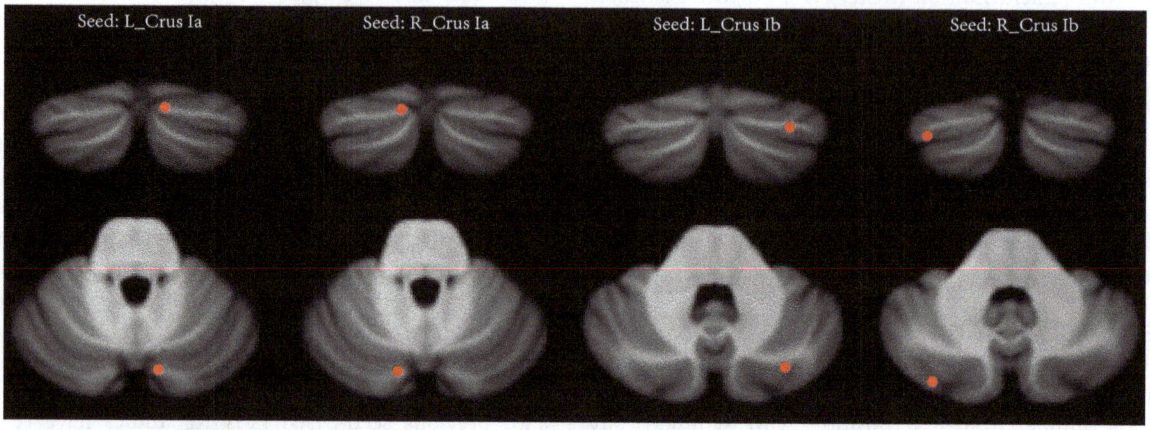

FIGURE 1 | The seeds of the cerebellum. In each hemisphere, two seeds were defined, including the Crus Ia and Crus Ib. L (R), left (right) hemisphere.

correction (VOX) with PT were tested at two-tailed $p < 0.05$ for multiple comparisons. The number of permutations was set at 1,000.

Once statistically significant group differences were observed in any brain FC, we calculated the Pearson correlation coefficients between the clinical variables and FC values in BD II group. These clinical variables included onset age of illness, number of episodes, duration of illness, HDRS score, and YMRS score.

RESULTS

Demographic Information

Table 1 shows the demographic and clinical information of all study participants. Three patients with BD II and three HCs were discarded from further analyses owing to excessive head movement during the image acquisition. Finally, the participants included 94 BD II patients and 100 HCs. The two groups have no significant differences in sex, age, years of education, and FD parameter.

TABLE 1 | Demographic and Clinical Data in BD II patients and HCs.

Variables	BD II	HCs	*P*-Value
No. of participants	94	100	
Gender (M: F)	51:43	45:55	0.198**
Age (years)	27.18 ± 9.15	28.32 ± 8.95	0.383*
Years of education	14.06 ± 2.79	14.72 ± 2.76	0.101*
Age at onset (years)	22.36 ± 8.94	NA	
No. of episodes	3.01 ± 1.45	NA	
Duration of illness (months)	47.11 ± 60.51	NA	
24-item HDRS score (points)	26.02 ± 6.80	NA	
YMRS score (points)	3.98 ± 5.27	NA	
FD values (mm)	0.08 ± 0.04	0.08 ± 0.04	0.497*

*Unless otherwise indicated, data are means ± standard deviation. BD, bipolar disorder; HCs, healthy controls; HDRS, Hamilton Depression Rating Scale; YMRS, Young Mania Rating Scale; FD, framewise displacement for in-scanner head motion; NA, not applicable. **P-value for sex distribution obtained by χ^2 test. *P-values obtained by independent sample tests.*

FC Analysis Within-Group

One-sample *t*-tests displayed the within-group FC patterns in the BD II and HCs group. Within the HCs group, the FC spatial distribution of the bilateral cerebellar Crus Ia is mainly located in the CEN, including the bilateral dlPFC, ACC, and superior parietal cortext. And the FC spatial distribution of the bilateral cerebellar Crus Ib is mainly located in the DMN, including the bilateral mPFC, posterior cingulate cortex, precuneus, inferior parietal lobule, middle temporal gyrus (MTG), and inferior temporal gyrus (ITG). Visual inspection indicated that FC patterns of the bilateral cerebellar Crus Ia and Crus Ib in the BD II group were similar to those of the HCs group.

FC Analysis Between-Group

For the CEN, the patients with BD II displayed decreased FC in the right Crus Ia-left dlPFC, and -left ACC compared with HCs (**Table 2**, **Figure 2**). For the DMN, the patients with BD II displayed decreased FC in the right Crus Ib-left mPFC (ventral mPFC, vmPFC), -left MTG, and -left ITG (fusiform gyrus) compared with HCs (**Table 2**, **Figure 2**). There was no aberrant FC between the left Crus Ia or Crus Ib and the cerebral regions in BD II patients compared to the HCs. In addition, there was no increased FC in the BD II group relative to the HCs group. No significant correlations between the FC values in these regions and any clinical measure (including onset age of illness, number of episodes, duration of illness, HDRS, YMRS scores) in the BD II patients were found.

DISCUSSION

Using well-defined cerebellar seeds, we investigated the alteration of cerebellar-cerebral connectivity in BD II patients and found evidence of abnormalities in selective networks. Particularly, we found decreased cerebellar-cerebral FC in the CEN and DMN, particularly decreased Crus Ia-dlPFC, and ACC connectivity, and Crus Ib-mPFC, MTG, and ITG connectivity in unmedicated

TABLE 2 | Differences of cerebellar-cerebral FC between BD II patients and HCs.

Cerebellar seeds	Significant regions	*t* value	Cluster size (mm^3)	side	MNI			Brodmann area
					x	y	z	
BD<HCs								
R Crus Ia	dlPFC	−4.7902	810	L	−48	27	18	9, 46
	dlPFC	−3.8646	2160	L	−33	6	48	9
	ACC	−4.4720	81	L	−6	33	33	32
R Crus Ib	vmPFC	−3.5598	324	L	−15	57	12	10
	mPFC	−4.4338	1161	L	−24	42	45	8
	MTG	−4.3466	1242	L	−69	−39	−9	21
	ITG (fusiform gyrus)	−3.9390	594	L	−54	−15	−30	20

FC, functional connectivity; BD, bipolar disorder; HCs, healthy controls; MNI, Montreal Neurological Institute; R, right; L, left; dlPFC, dorsal lateral prefrontal cortext; ACC, anterior cingulate cortext; vmPFC, ventral medial prefrontal cortex; mPFC, medial prefrontal cortex; MTG, middle temporal gyrus; ITG, inferior temporal gyrus.

patients with bipolar II depression. This is the first study to report abnormal cerebellar connectivity with the CEN and DMN in patients with bipolar II depression.

The dlPFC and ACC are recognized as important regions within the CEN and are significant roles in maintaining cognition and emotion control (47–49). In this study, we found reduced FC within right Crus Ia-left dlPFC, and right Crus Ia-left ACC in patients with bipolar II depression, suggesting the impaired FC between the cerebellum and the CEN. Using seed-based connectivity analyses, a recent rs-fMRI found reduced cerebro-cerebellar FC in frontoparietal control networks in psychotic BD (24). Another rs-fMRI study reported decreased FC between the cerebellum and the dlPFC in patients with geriatric depression (21). Several studies demonstrated structural and functional abnormality of the dlPFC in BD. For example, several structural MRI studies reported reduced cortical thickness (50, 51) and gray matter volume (52) in the dlPFC in bipolar depression. Additionally, some rs-fMRI studies showed reduced FC between the dlPFC and mPFC (53), right temporal gyrus (54), left insula (55), and amygdala (56) in BD patients using seed-based approach or global brain connectivity method. Furthermore, task-based fMRI studies revealed that BD depressed patients showed decreased activation in the dlPFC and cerebellum during n-back tasks (57, 58). A previous PET study found that decreased dlPFC metabolism was associated with sustained attention deficits in depressed adults with BD (59). The ACC is a key region implicated in mood regulation (60) and might be a possible trait feature of BD (61, 62). An rs-fMRI study revealed decreased FC between the defined cingulo-opercular network (included the dorsal ACC attributed to cognition) and cerebellar network in BD (23). In addition, performing an emotion processing task, BD patients showed decreased activation in the ACC compared to HCs (63, 64). Therefore, disrupt connectivity of the cerebellar Crus Ia-dlPFC and -ACC may be associated with dysfunctional cognition and emotion control in BD II patients.

The DMN was suggested to subserve ongoing, or default functions of the brain such as self-referential mental activity, episodic memory retrieval, inner speech, mental images, emotions, and planning future events (17, 65). In this study, patients with BD II depression showed decreased FC in the cerebellum connected to the mPFC (mainly in the vmPFC). Using seed-based connectivity analyses, Alalade et al. reported that depression patients had reduced FC between the cerebellar seeds and the vmPFC (21). The mPFC is a core hub of the DMN in which abnormalities have been reported in BD (66). Structural MRI found decreased gray matter volume and density predominantly in the vmPFC in BD patients (67–69). And in rs-fMRI studies, Wang et al. found diminished functional connectivity strength (70) and voxel-mirrored homotopic connectivity (71) in the mPFC in non-medicine BD II patients. Using independent component analysis, Öngür et al. reported reduced DMN connectivity in the vmPFC in BD patients (72). Moreover, several studies demonstrated that ruminative self-focus was associated with the aberrant FC/activation in the mPFC in depression (73–76). A task-based fMRI study revealed that BD patients have decreased FC between the vmPFC and the head of the caudate, performing a self-reflection task (77). Taken together, our finding of the aberrant Crus Ib-mPFC connectivity may be involved in the abnormality of self-referential mental activity in BD patients.

The temporal gyrus is suggested to be in involved in several cognitive processing, including visual perception (ITG), language and semantic memory processing (MTG), sensory integration (78). In this study, the depressed BD II patients showed reduced FC between the right Crus Ib and left temporal lobe, including the MTG and ITG. A structural MRI study found reduced cortical thickness in the left MTG, ITG, and vmPFC in BD II patients (79). Two rs-fMRI studies demonstrated that the BD depression patients showed a reduction of functional connectivity strength in the left MTG (80) and reduction of the voxel-mirrored homotopic connectivity in the cerebellum and fusiform (81). Additionally, task-based fMRI studies found reduced activation in the MTG in BD II depression patients during an n-back task (82), and reduced activation in the MTG and ITG in BD I during an attentional task (83) and visuospatial processing task (84). Thus, these studies, united with our findings, suggest that the reduced FC within the Crus Ib-MTG and -ITG may be associated with disruption of cognition in BD.

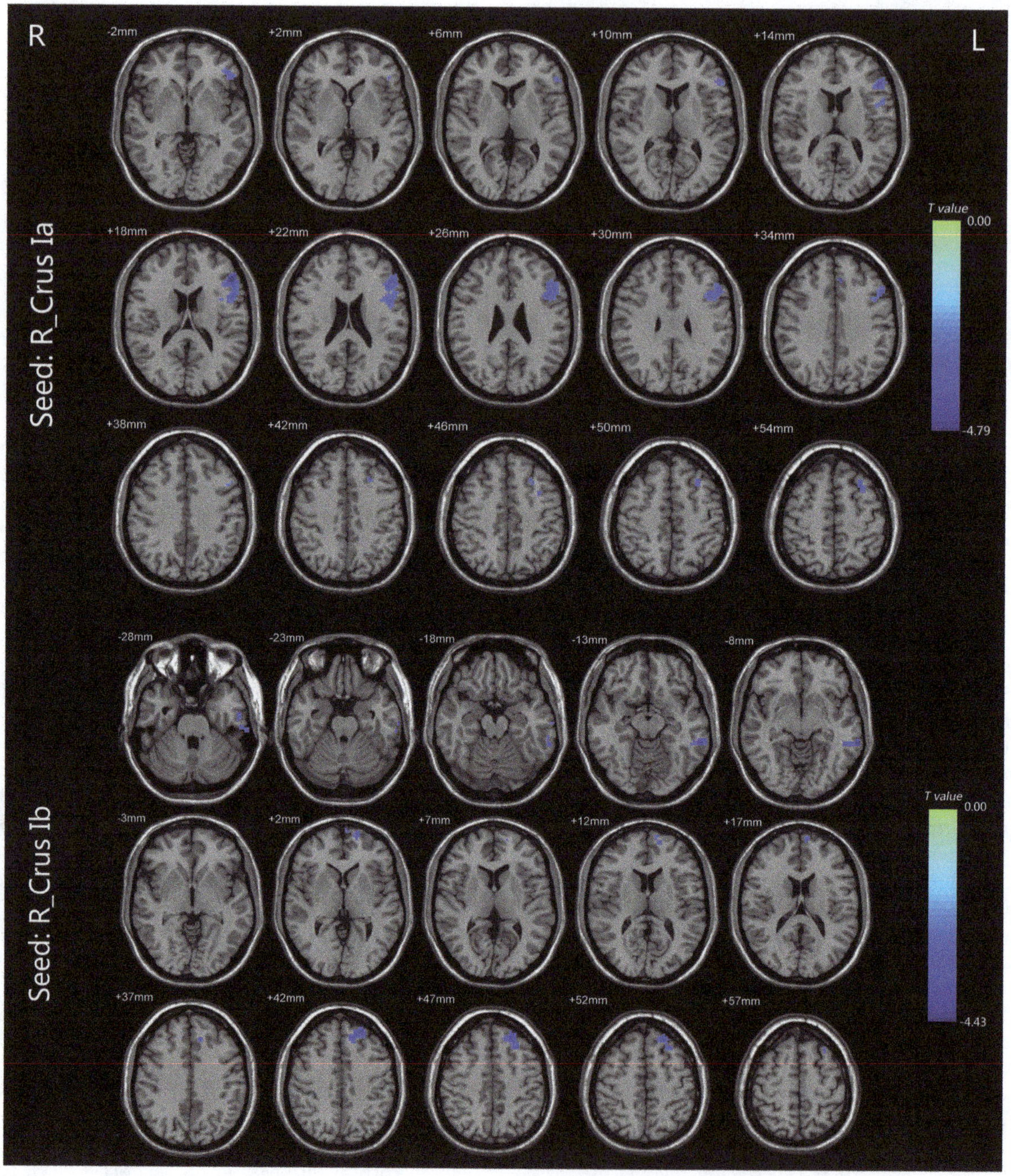

FIGURE 2 | The FC differences between the BD patients and HCs ($p < 0.05$, TFCE corrected). For the CEN, the patients with BD II displayed decreased FC in the right Crus Ia-left dlPFC and left ACC compared with HCs. For the DMN, the patients with BD II displayed decreased FC in the right Crus Ib-left mPFC (vmPFC), left MTG, and left ITG (fusiform gyrus) compared with HCs. Shades of blue denoted decreased FC in the BD group compared with HCs group. The color bars indicate the *t*-values. FC, functional connectivity; BD, bipolar disorder; HCs, healthy controls; TFCE, the threshold-free cluster enhancement; CEN, central executive network; dlPFC, dorsal lateral frontal cortext; ACC, anterior cingulate cortext; DMN, default mode network; mPFC, medial prefrontal cortex; vmPFC, ventral medial prefrontal cortex; MTG, middle temporal gyrus; ITG, inferior temporal gyrus.

What's more, unexpectedly, it's revealed that all the findings of reduced cerebellar-cerebral FC in patients appear between the right cerebellar seeds and the regions in the left cerebral hemisphere. There are pieces of evidence supporting abnormal hemisphere asymmetries in the major psychotic disorders, such as schizophrenia, MDD, and BD. Generally, a predominant left hemisphere disturbance in schizophrenia was reported by psychophysiological, neuropsychological, and neuroimaging studies (85–89). Electrophysiology, rs-fMRI and task-based fMRI studies showed a predominantly left-sided reduction of activity in the PFC in depression (90–94). And several studies found that patients with left hemisphere damage or lesions tended to appear depressive symptoms (95–97), while patients with right hemisphere damage or lesions tended to appear manic symptoms (97, 98). Two studies founded lower activation in the left hemisphere than in the right hemisphere in the BD depression while the opposite in the BD mania (99, 100), which is consistent with our finding of asymmetric left hemisphere disturbance in BD II depression. This phenomenon was reported to be associated with a high percentage of dopaminergic synapses in the left hemisphere, and the dopamine is essential in regulating motor activity, biological substrate of positive emotions and approaching behavior (99). Thus, the hemispheric asymmetry aberrance may be a significant biological substrate in BD.

There were several strengths in our study. First, we recruited a large number of participants of 94 BD II patients and 100 HCs, and the samples of non-medicine patients with BD II depression are homogeneous, while most previous rs-fMRI studies recruited heterogeneous samples of varying BD subtypes including BD I and BD II. Second, we noted permutation test with TFCE for multiple comparison correction in between-group contrast. A recent study demonstrated that the PT with TFCE, which is a strict multiple comparison correction strategy, was best able to reach the balance between family-wise error rate and test-retest reliability/replicability (101). However, there are also some potential limitations that should be taken into consideration. First, without a group of patients with BD in a euthymic episode, it is still not clear whether aberrant cerebellar-cerebral FC is specific to the depression episode of BD or shared by all episodes of the disease. Second, BD patients didn't participate in cognitive test scales, such as the Wisconsin Card Sorting Test, Digit Span Test, and Stroop Color Word Test. Further studies of the correlations between the impaired FC values and cognitive function are needed to support our speculations that the cerebellum-CEN and -DMN FC is involved in the cognition deficits in BD. Third, we didn't analyses the morphology characteristics of the BD patients, which should be considered and combined with our findings to provide more reliable imaging evidence in the pathogenesis of BD. Forth, further studies should be taken to investigate the differences of FC between BD II and BD I. Finally, we confirmed that the participants had not fallen asleep via their self-report, which could not ensure that each participant had not actually fallen asleep during the period of scanning.

CONCLUSION

Patients with BD II depression showed disrupted FC between the cerebellum and the CEN (mainly in the left dlPFC and ACC) and DMN (mainly in the left mPFC, and temporal lobe), suggesting the significant role of the cerebellum-CEN and -DMN connectivity in the pathogenesis of BD.

AUTHOR CONTRIBUTIONS

XL, LH, and YW design the study; GC, YJ, JG, SQ, SZ, LZ, FC, SL, and ZQ contribute to data acquisition; GC contribute to data analysis; XL, GC, LH, and YW write the manuscript. All authors contributed to and have approved the final manuscript.

FUNDING

The study was supported by grants from the National Natural Science Foundation of China (81671670, 81501456, and 81471650); Planned Science and Technology Project of Guangdong Province, China (2014B020212022); Planned Science and Technology Project of Guangzhou, China (1563000653, 201508020004, 201604020007, and 201604020184). The funding organizations played no further role in study design, data collection, analysis and interpretation, and paper writing.

REFERENCES

1. Minichino A, Bersani FS, Trabucchi G, Albano G, Primavera M, Delle Chiaie R, et al. The role of cerebellum in unipolar and bipolar depression: a review of the main neurobiological findings. *Riv Psichiatr.* (2014) 49:124–31. doi: 10.1708/1551.16907
2. Zhao L, Wang Y, Jia Y, Zhong S, Sun Y, Zhou Z, et al. Cerebellar microstructural abnormalities in bipolar depression and unipolar depression: a diffusion kurtosis and perfusion imaging study. *J. Affect. Disord.* (2016) 195:21–31. doi: 10.1016/j.jad.2016.01.042
3. Dolan RJ, Bench CJ, Brown RG, Scott LC, Friston KJ, Frackowiak RS. Regional cerebral blood flow abnormalities in depressed patients with cognitive impairment. *J Neurol Neurosurg Psychiatry* (1992) 55:768–73. doi: 10.1136/jnnp.55.9.768
4. Liu CH, Li F, Li SF, Wang YJ, Tie CL, Wu HY, et al. Abnormal baseline brain activity in bipolar depression: a resting state functional magnetic resonance imaging study. *Psychiatr Res.* (2012) 203:175–9. doi: 10.1016/j.pscychresns.2012.02.007
5. Kirschen MP, Davis-Ratner MS, Milner MW, Chen SHA, Schraedley-Desmond P, Fisher PG, et al. Verbal memory impairments in children after cerebellar tumor resection. *Behav Neurol.* (2008) 20:39–53. doi: 10.1155/2008/817253
6. Laricchiuta D, Petrosini L, Picerni E, Cutuli D, Iorio M, Chiapponi C, et al. The embodied emotion in cerebellum: a neuroimaging study of alexithymia. *Brain Struct Funct.* (2015) 220:2275–87. doi: 10.1007/s00429-014-0790-0
7. Stoodley CJ, Schmahmann JD. Functional topography in the human cerebellum: a meta-analysis of neuroimaging studies. *Neuroimage* (2009) 44:489–501. doi: 10.1016/j.neuroimage.2008.08.039
8. Stoodley CJ, Valera EM, Schmahmann JD. Functional topography of the cerebellum for motor and cognitive tasks: an fMRI study. *Neuroimage* (2012) 59:1560–70. doi: 10.1016/j.neuroimage.2011.08.065
9. Schmahmann JD, Doyon J, McDonald D, Holmes C, Lavoie K, Hurwitz AS, et al. Three-dimensional MRI atlas of the human cerebellum in proportional stereotaxic space. *Neuroimage* (1999) 10:233–60. doi: 10.1006/nimg.1999.0459
10. Vilensky JA, van Hoesen GW. Corticopontine projections from the cingulate cortex in the rhesus monkey. *Brain Res.* (1981) 205:391–5. doi: 10.1016/0006-8993(81)90348-6
11. Haines DE, Dietrichs E, Sowa TE. Hypothalamo-cerebellar and cerebello-hypothalamic pathways: a review and hypothesis concerning cerebellar

circuits which may influence autonomic centers affective behavior. *Brain, Behav Evol.* (1984) 24:198–220. doi: 10.1159/000121317

12. Heath RG, Dempesy CW, Fontana CJ, Myers WA. Cerebellar stimulation: effects on septal region, hippocampus, and amygdala of cats and rats. *Biol Psychiatry* (1978) 13:501–29.
13. Sang L, Qin W, Liu Y, Han W, Zhang YT, Jiang TZ, et al. Resting-state functional connectivity of the vermal and hemispheric subregions of the cerebellum with both the cerebral cortical networks and subcortical structures. *Neuroimage* (2012) 61:1213–25. doi: 10.1016/j.neuroimage.2012.04.011
14. Habas C, Kamdar N, Nguyen D, Prater K, Beckmann CF, Menon V, et al. Distinct cerebellar contributions to intrinsic connectivity networks. *J Neurosci.* (2009) 29:8586–94. doi: 10.1523/JNEUROSCI.1868-09.2009
15. Krienen FM, Buckner RL. Segregated fronto-cerebellar circuits revealed by intrinsic functional connectivity. *Cereb Cortex* (2009) 19:2485–97. doi: 10.1093/cercor/bhp135
16. Smith SM, Fox PT, Miller KL, Glahn DC, Fox PM, Mackay CE, et al. Correspondence of the brain's functional architecture during activation and rest. *Proc Natl Acad Sci USA.* (2009) 106:13040–5. doi: 10.1073/pnas.0905267106
17. Gusnard DA, Raichle ME, Raichle ME. Searching for a baseline: functional imaging and the resting human brain. *Nat Rev Neurosci.* (2001) 2:685–94. doi: 10.1038/35094500
18. Menon V. Large-scale brain networks and psychopathology: a unifying triple network model. *Trends Cogn Sci.* (2011) 15:483–506. doi: 10.1016/j.tics.2011.08.003
19. Sha Z, Xia M, Lin Q, Cao M, Tang Y, Xu K, et al. Meta-connectomic analysis reveals commonly disrupted functional architectures in network modules and connectors across brain disorders. *Cereb Cortex* (2017) 28:4179–94. doi: 10.1093/cercor/bhx273
20. Liu L, Zeng LL, Li YM, Ma QM, Li BJ, Shen H, et al. Altered cerebellar functional connectivity with intrinsic connectivity networks in adults with major depressive disorder. *PLoS ONE* (2012) 7:e39516. doi: 10.1371/journal.pone.0039516
21. Alalade E, Denny K, Potter G, Steffens D, Wang LH. Altered Cerebellar-cerebral functional connectivity in geriatric depression. *PLoS ONE* (2011) 6:e20035. doi: 10.1371/journal.pone.0020035
22. Guo WB, Liu F, Xue ZM, Gao KM, Liu ZN, Xiao CQ, et al. Abnormal resting-state cerebellar-cerebral functional connectivity in treatment-resistant depression and treatment sensitive depression. *Prog Neuropsychopharmacol Biol Psychiatry* (2013) 44:51–7. doi: 10.1016/j.pnpbp.2013.01.010
23. Mamah D, Barch DM, Repovs G. Resting state functional connectivity of five neural networks in bipolar disorder and schizophrenia. *J Affect Dis.* (2013) 150:601–9. doi: 10.1016/j.jad.2013.01.051
24. Shinn AK, Roh YS, Ravichandran CT, Baker JT, Ongur D, Cohen BM. Aberrant cerebellar connectivity in bipolar disorder with psychosis. *Biol Psychiatry Cogn Neurosci Neuroimaging* (2017) 2:438–48. doi: 10.1016/j.bpsc.2016.07.002
25. Ma G, Wang C, Jia Y, Wang J, Zhang B, Shen C, et al. Electrocardiographic and electrooculographic responses to external emotions and their transitions in bipolar i and ii disorders. *Int J Environ Res Public Health* (2018) 15:884. doi: 10.3390/ijerph15050884
26. Baek JH, Park DY, Choi J, Kim JS, Choi JS, Ha K, et al. Differences between bipolar I and bipolar II disorders in clinical features, comorbidity, and family history. *J Affect Disord.* (2011) 131:59–67. doi: 10.1016/j.jad.2010.11.020
27. Dell'Osso B, Shah S, Do D, Yuen LD, Hooshmand F, Wang PW, et al. American tertiary clinic-referred bipolar II disorder versus bipolar I disorder associated with hastened depressive recurrence. *Int J Bipolar Disord.* (2017) 5:2. doi: 10.1186/s40345-017-0072-x
28. Vieta E, Suppes T. Bipolar II disorder: arguments for and against a distinct diagnostic entity. *Bipolar Disord.* (2008) 10:163–78. doi: 10.1111/j.1399-5618.2007.00561.x
29. Ha TH, Her JY, Kim JH, Chang JS, Cho HS, Ha K. Similarities and differences of white matter connectivity and water diffusivity in bipolar I and II disorder. *Neurosci Lett.* (2011) 505:150–4. doi: 10.1016/j.neulet.2011.10.009
30. Lee SY, Chen SL, Chang YH, Chen SH, Chu CH, Huang SY, et al. The ALDH2 and DRD2/ANKK1 genes interacted in bipolar II but not bipolar I disorder. *Pharmacogenet Genomics* (2010) 20:500–6. doi: 10.1097/FPC.0b013e32833caa2b
31. Lee SY, Chen SL, Chen SH, Huang SY, Tzeng NS, Chang YH, et al. The COMT and DRD3 genes interacted in bipolar I but not bipolar II disorder. *World J Biol Psychiatry* (2011) 12:385–91. doi: 10.3109/15622975.2010.505298
32. Chou YH, Wang SJ, Lin CL, Mao WC, Lee SM, Liao MH. Decreased brain serotonin transporter binding in the euthymic state of bipolar I but not bipolar II disorder: a SPECT study. *Bipolar Disord.* (2010) 12:312–8. doi: 10.1111/j.1399-5618.2010.00800.x
33. Zhu QS, Wang JW, Fan HY, Ma GR, Zhang BR, Shen CC, et al. Blink reflex under external emotional-stimuli in bipolar I and II disorders. *Psychiatry Res.* (2018) 259:520–5. doi: 10.1016/j.psychres.2017.11.020
34. Zhu QS, Wang JW, Shen CC, Fan HY, Zhang BR, Ma GR, et al. Inhibitory brainstem reflexes under external emotional-stimuli in bipolar I and II disorders. *BMC Psychiatry* (2017) 17:224. doi: 10.1186/s12888-017-1390-3
35. Abe C, Ekman CJ, Sellgren C, Petrovic P, Ingvar M, Landen M. Cortical thickness, volume and surface area in patients with bipolar disorder types I and II. *J Psychiatr Neurosci.* (2016) 41:240–50. doi: 10.1503/jpn.150093
36. Ha TH, Ha K, Kim JH, Choi JE. Regional brain gray matter abnormalities in patients with bipolar II disorder: a comparison study with bipolar I patients and healthy controls. *Neurosci Lett.* (2009) 456:44–8. doi: 10.1016/j.neulet.2009.03.077
37. Hauser P, Matochik J, Altshuler LL, Denicoff KD, Conrad A, Li X, et al. MRI-based measurements of temporal lobe and ventricular structures in patients with bipolar I and bipolar II disorders. *J Affect Disord.* (2000) 60:25–32. doi: 10.1016/S0165-0327(99)00154-8
38. Liu JX, Chen YS, Hsieh JC, Su TP, Yeh TC, Chen LF. Differences in white matter abnormalities between bipolar I and II disorders. *J Affect Disord.* (2010) 127:309–15. doi: 10.1016/j.jad.2010.05.026
39. Maller JJ, Thaveenthiran P, Thomson RH, McQueen S, Fitzgerald PB. Volumetric, cortical thickness and white matter integrity alterations in bipolar disorder type I and II. *J Affect Disord.* (2014) 169:118–27. doi: 10.1016/j.jad.2014.08.016
40. Caseras X, Murphy K, Lawrence NS, Fuentes-Claramonte P, Watts J, Jones DK, et al. Emotion regulation deficits in euthymic bipolar I versus bipolar II disorder: a functional and diffusion-tensor imaging study. *Bipolar Disord.* (2015) 17:461–70. doi: 10.1111/bdi.12292
41. Dell'Osso B, Cinnante C, Di Giorgio A, Cremaschi L, Palazzo MC, Cristoffanini M, et al. Altered prefrontal cortex activity during working memory task in bipolar disorder: a functional magnetic resonance imaging study in euthymic bipolar I and II patients. *J Affect Disord.* (2015) 184:116–22. doi: 10.1016/j.jad.2015.05.026
42. Caseras X, Lawrence NS, Murphy K, Wise RG, Phillips ML. Ventral striatum activity in response to reward: differences between bipolar i and ii disorders. *Am J Psychiatry* (2013) 170:533–41. doi: 10.1176/appi.ajp.2012.12020169
43. Jenkinson M, Bannister P, Brady M, Smith S. Improved optimization for the robust and accurate linear registration and motion correction of brain images. *Neuroimage* (2002) 17:825–41. doi: 10.1006/nimg.2002.1132
44. Friston KJ, Williams S, Howard R, Frackowiak RS, Turner R. Movement-related effects in fMRI time-series. *Magn Reson Med.* (1996) 35:346–55. doi: 10.1002/mrm.1910350312
45. Satterthwaite TD, Elliott MA, Gerraty RT, Ruparel K, Loughead J, Calkins ME, et al. An improved framework for confound regression and filtering for control of motion artifact in the preprocessing of resting-state functional connectivity data. *Neuroimage* (2013) 64:240–56. doi: 10.1016/j.neuroimage.2012.08.052
46. Winkler AM, Ridgway GR, Douaud G, Nichols TE, Smith SM. Faster permutation inference in brain imaging. *Neuroimage* (2016) 141:502–16. doi: 10.1016/j.neuroimage.2016.05.068
47. Niendam TA, Laird AR, Ray KL, Dean YM, Glahn DC, Carter CS. Meta-analytic evidence for a superordinate cognitive control network subserving diverse executive functions. *Cogn Affect Behav Neurosci.* (2012) 12:241–68. doi: 10.3758/s13415-011-0083-5
48. Breukelaar IA, Antees C, Grieve SM, Foster SL, Gomes L, Williams LM, et al. Cognitive control network anatomy correlates with neurocognitive behavior: a longitudinal study. *Hum Brain Mapp.* (2017) 38:631–43. doi: 10.1002/hbm.23401

49. Brown A, Biederman J, Valera E, Lomedico A, Aleardi M, Makris N, et al. Working memory network alterations and associated symptoms in adults with ADHD and Bipolar Disorder. *J Psychiatr Res.* (2012) 46:476–83. doi: 10.1016/j.jpsychires.2012.01.008
50. Lan MJ, Chhetry BT, Oquendo MA, Sublette ME, Sullivan G, Mann JJ, et al. Cortical thickness differences between bipolar depression and major depressive disorder. *Bipolar Disord.* (2014) 16:378–88. doi: 10.1111/bdi.12175
51. Niu MQ, Wang Y, Jia YB, Wang JJ, Zhong SM, Lin JB, et al. Common and specific abnormalities in cortical thickness in patients with major depressive and bipolar disorders. *Ebiomedicine* (2017) 16:162–71. doi: 10.1016/j.ebiom.2017.01.010
52. Figueroa R, Harenski K, Nicoletti M, Brambilla P, Mallinger AG, Frank E, et al. Dorsolateral prefrontal cortex abnormalities in bipolar disorder - Possible effects of lithium treatment? *Biol Psychiatry* (2000) 47:S103–4. doi: 10.1016/S0006-3223(00)00608-9
53. Favre P, Baciu M, Pichat C, Bougerol T, Polosan M. fMRI evidence for abnormal resting-state functional connectivity in euthymic bipolar patients. *J Affect Disord.* (2014) 165:182–9. doi: 10.1016/j.jad.2014.04.054
54. Dickstein DP, Gorrostieta C, Ombao H, Goldberg LD, Brazel AC, Gable CJ, et al. Fronto-temporal spontaneous resting state functional connectivity in pediatric bipolar disorder. *Biol Psychiatry* (2010) 68:839–46. doi: 10.1016/j.biopsych.2010.06.029
55. Ambrosi E, Arciniegas DB, Madan A, Curtis KN, Patriquin MA, Jorge RE, et al. Insula and amygdala resting-state functional connectivity differentiate bipolar from unipolar depression. *Acta Psychiatr Scand.* (2017) 136:129–39. doi: 10.1111/acps.12724
56. Anticevic A, Brumbaugh MS, Winkler AM, Lombardo LE, Barrett J, Corlett PR, et al. Global prefrontal and fronto-amygdala dysconnectivity in bipolar I disorder with psychosis history. *Biol Psychiatry* (2013) 73:565–73. doi: 10.1016/j.biopsych.2012.07.031
57. Fernandez-Corcuera P, Salvador R, Monte GC, Sarro S, Goikolea JM, Amann B, et al. Bipolar depressed patients show both failure to activate and failure to de-activate during performance of a working memory task. *J Affect Disord.* (2013) 148:170–8. doi: 10.1016/j.jad.2012.04.009
58. Townsend J, Bookheimer SY, Foland-Ross LC, Sugar CA, Altshuler LL. fMRI abnormalities in dorsolateral prefrontal cortex during a working memory task in manic, euthymic and depressed bipolar subjects. *Psychiatr Res.* (2010) 182:22–9. doi: 10.1016/j.pscychresns.2009.11.010
59. Brooks JO, Wang PW, Strong C, Sachs N, Hoblyn JC, Fenn R, et al. Preliminary evidence of differential relations between prefrontal cortex metabolism and sustained attention in depressed adults with bipolar disorder and healthy controls. *Bipolar Disord.* (2006) 8:248–54. doi: 10.1111/j.1399-5618.2006.00310.x
60. Phillips ML, Drevets WC, Rauch SL, Lane R. Neurobiology of emotion perception I: the neural basis of normal emotion perception. *Biol Psychiatry* (2003) 54:504–14. doi: 10.1016/S0006-3223(03)00168-9
61. Liu J, Blond BN, van Dyck LI, Spencer L, Wang F, Blumberg HP. Trait and state corticostriatal dysfunction in bipolar disorder during emotional face processing. *Bipolar Disord.* (2012) 14:432–41. doi: 10.1111/j.1399-5618.2012.01018.x
62. Soeiro-de-Souza MG, Salvadore G, Moreno RA, Otaduy MCG, Chaim KT, Gattaz WF, et al. Bcl-2 rs956572 Polymorphism is associated with increased anterior cingulate cortical glutamate in euthymic bipolar I disorder. *Neuropsychopharmacology* (2013) 38:468–75. doi: 10.1038/npp.2012.203
63. Townsend JD, Torrisi SJ, Lieberman MD, Sugar CA, Bookheimer SY, Altshuler LL. Frontal-amygdala connectivity alterations during emotion downregulation in bipolar i disorder. *Biol Psychiatry* (2013) 73:127–35. doi: 10.1016/j.biopsych.2012.06.030
64. Blumberg HP, Donegan NH, Sanislow CA, Collins S, Lacadie C, Skudlarski P, et al. Preliminary evidence for medication effects on functional abnormalities in the amygdala and anterior cingulate in bipolar disorder. *Psychopharmacology* (2005) 183:308–13. doi: 10.1007/s00213-005-0156-7
65. Greicius MD, Menon V. Default-mode activity during a passive sensory task: uncoupled from deactivation but impacting activation. *J Cogn Neurosci.* (2004) 16:1484–92. doi: 10.1162/0898929042568532
66. Ongur D, Price JL. The organization of networks within the orbital and medial prefrontal cortex of rats, monkeys and humans. *Cereb Cortex* (2000) 10:206–19. doi: 10.1093/cercor/10.3.206
67. Phillips M, Ladouceur C, Drevets W. A neural model of voluntary and automatic emotion regulation: implications for understanding the pathophysiology and neurodevelopment of bipolar disorder. *Mol Psychiatry* (2008) 13:833–57. doi: 10.1038/mp.2008.65
68. Narita K, Suda M, Takei Y, Aoyama Y, Majima T, Kameyama M, et al. Volume reduction of ventromedial prefrontal cortex in bipolar II patients with rapid cycling: a voxel-based morphometric study. *Prog Neuropsychopharmacol Biol Psychiatry* (2011) 35:439–45. doi: 10.1016/j.pnpbp.2010.11.030
69. Wise T, Radua J, Via E, Cardoner N, Abe O, Adams TM, et al. Common and distinct patterns of grey-matter volume alteration in major depression and bipolar disorder: evidence from voxel-based meta-analysis. *Mol Psychiatry* (2017) 22:1455–63. doi: 10.1038/mp.2016.72
70. Wang Y, Zhong SM, Jia YB, Sun Y, Wang B, Liu T, et al. Disrupted resting-state functional connectivity in nonmedicated bipolar disorder. *Radiology* (2016) 280:529–36. doi: 10.1148/radiol.2016151641
71. Wang Y, Zhong S, Jia Y, Zhou Z, Zhou Q, Huang L. Reduced interhemispheric resting-state functional connectivity in unmedicated bipolar II disorder. *Acta Psychiatr Scand.* (2015) 132:400–7. doi: 10.1111/acps.12429
72. Ongur D, Lundy M, Greenhouse I, Shinn AK, Menon V, Cohen BM, et al. Default mode network abnormalities in bipolar disorder and schizophrenia. *Psychiatry Res.* (2010) 183:59–68. doi: 10.1016/j.pscychresns.2010.04.008
73. Zhu XL, Wang X, Xiao J, Liao J, Zhong MT, Wang W, et al. Evidence of a dissociation pattern in resting-state default mode network connectivity in first-episode, treatment-naive major depression patients. *Biol Psychiatry* (2012) 71:611–7. doi: 10.1016/j.biopsych.2011.10.035
74. Cooney RE, Joormann J, Eugene F, Dennis EL, Gotlib IH. Neural correlates of rumination in depression. *Cogn Affect Behav Neurosci.* (2010) 10:470–8. doi: 10.3758/CABN.10.4.470
75. Farb NAS, Anderson AK, Bloch RT, Segal ZV. Mood-linked responses in medial prefrontal cortex predict relapse in patients with recurrent unipolar depression. *Biol. Psychiatry* (2011) 70:366–72. doi: 10.1016/j.biopsych.2011.03.009
76. Bartova L, Meyer BM, Diers K, Rabl U, Scharinger C, Popovic A, et al. Reduced default mode network suppression during a working memory task in remitted major depression. *J Psychiatr Res.* (2015) 64:9–18. doi: 10.1016/j.jpsychires.2015.02.025
77. Zhang L, Vander Meer L, Opmeer EM, Marsman JC, Ruhe HG, Aleman A. Altered functional connectivity during self- and close other-reflection in patients with bipolar disorder with past psychosis and patients with schizophrenia. *Neuropsychologia* (2016) 93:97–105. doi: 10.1016/j.neuropsychologia.2016.09.020
78. Onitsuka T, Shenton ME, Salisbury DF, Dickey CC, Kasai K, Toner SK, et al. Middle and inferior temporal gyrus gray matter volume abnormalities in chronic schizophrenia: an MRI study. *Am J Psychiatry* (2004) 161:1603–11. doi: 10.1176/appi.ajp.161.9.1603
79. Elvsashagen T, Westlye LT, Boen E, Hol PK, Andreassen OA, Boye B, et al. Bipolar II disorder is associated with thinning of prefrontal and temporal cortices involved in affect regulation. *Bipolar Disord.* (2013) 15:855–64. doi: 10.1111/bdi.12117
80. Lv D, Lin W, Xue Z, Pu W, Yang Q, Huang X, et al. Decreased functional connectivity in the language regions in bipolar patients during depressive episodes but not remission. *J Affect Disord.* (2016) 197:116–24. doi: 10.1016/j.jad.2016.03.026
81. Wang Y, Zhong SM, Jia YB, Zhou ZF, Wang B, Pan JY, et al. Interhemispheric resting state functional connectivity abnormalities in unipolar depression and bipolar depression. *Bipolar Disord.* (2015) 17:486–95. doi: 10.1111/bdi.12315
82. Brooks JO, Vizueta N, Penfold C, Townsend JD, Bookheimer SY, Altshuler LL. Prefrontal hypoactivation during working memory in bipolar II depression. *Psychol Med.* (2015) 45:1731–40. doi: 10.1017/S0033291714002852
83. Cerullo MA, Eliassen JC, Smith CT, Fleck DE, Nelson EB, Strawn JR, et al. Bipolar I disorder and major depressive disorder show similar

brain activation during depression. *Bipolar Disord.* (2014) 16:703–12. doi: 10.1111/bdi.12225
84. Singh MK, Chang KD, Kelley RG, Cui X, Sherdell L, Howe ME, et al. Reward processing in adolescents with bipolar I disorder. *J Am Acad Child Adolesc Psychiatry* (2013) 52:68–83. doi: 10.1016/j.jaac.2012.10.004
85. McCarley RW, Shenton ME, O'Donnell BF, Faux SF, Kikinis R, Nestor PG, et al. Auditory P300 abnormalities and left posterior superior temporal gyrus volume reduction in schizophrenia. *Arch Gene Psychiatry* (1993) 50:190–7. doi: 10.1001/archpsyc.1993.01820150036003
86. Heidrich A, Strik WK. Auditory P300 topography and neuropsychological test performance: evidence for left hemispheric dysfunction in schizophrenia. *Biol Psychiatry* (1997) 41:327–35. doi: 10.1016/S0006-3223(96)00030-3
87. Kalb R, Raydt G, Reulbach U, Kornhuber J. Symmetry reversal in schizophrenia. *Psychiatry Clin Neurosci.* (2003) 57:353–60. doi: 10.1046/j.1440-1819.2003.01131.x
88. Schroder J, Wenz F, Schad LR, Baudendistel K, Knopp MV. Sensorimotor cortex and supplementary motor area changes in schizophrenia. a study with functional magnetic resonance imaging. *Br J Psychiatry* (1995) 167:197–201. doi: 10.1192/bjp.167.2.197
89. Yurgelun-Todd DA, Waternaux CM, Cohen BM, Gruber SA, English CD, Renshaw PF. Functional magnetic resonance imaging of schizophrenic patients and comparison subjects during word production. *Am J Psychiatry* (1996) 153:200–5. doi: 10.1176/ajp.153.2.200
90. Bruder GE, Stewart JW, McGrath PJ. Right brain, left brain in depressive disorders: clinical and theoretical implications of behavioral, electrophysiological and neuroimaging findings. *Neurosci Biobehav Rev.* (2017) 78:178–91. doi: 10.1016/j.neubiorev.2017.04.021
91. Kemp AH, Griffiths K, Felmingham KL, Shankman SA, Drinkenburg W, Arns M, et al. Disorder specificity despite comorbidity: resting EEG alpha asymmetry in major depressive disorder and post-traumatic stress disorder. *Biol Psychol.* (2010) 85:350–4. doi: 10.1016/j.biopsycho.2010.08.001
92. Stewart JL, Coan JA, Towers DN, Allen JJB. Resting and task-elicited prefrontal EEG alpha asymmetry in depression: support for the capability model. *Psychophysiology* (2014) 51:446–55. doi: 10.1111/psyp.12191
93. Fitzgerald PB, Laird AR, Maller J, Daskalakis ZJ. A meta-analytic study of changes in brain activation in depression. *Hum Brain Mapp.* (2008) 29:683–95. doi: 10.1002/hbm.20613
94. Harmon-Jones E, Gable PA, Peterson CK. The role of asymmetric frontal cortical activity in emotion-related phenomena: a review and update. *Biol Psychol.* (2010) 84:451–62. doi: 10.1016/j.biopsycho.2009.08.010
95. Black FW. Unilateral brain lesions and MMPI performance: a preliminary study. *Percept Mot Skills* (1975) 40:87–93. doi: 10.2466/pms.1975.40.1.87
96. Gasparrini WG, Satz P, Heilman K, Coolidge FL. Hemispheric asymmetries of affective processing as determined by the minnesota multiphasic personality inventory. *J Neurol Neurosurg Psychiatry* (1978) 41:470–3. doi: 10.1136/jnnp.41.5.470
97. Robinson RG, Price TR. Post-stroke depressive disorders: a follow-up study of 103 patients. *Stroke* (1982) 13:635–41. doi: 10.1161/01.STR.13.5.635
98. Sackeim HA, Greenberg MS, Weiman AL, Gur RC, Hungerbuhler JP, Geschwind N. Hemispheric asymmetry in the expression of positive and negative emotions. Neurologic evidence. *Arch Neurol.* (1982) 39:210–8. doi: 10.1001/archneur.1982.00510160016003
99. Garcia-Toro M, Montes JM, Talavera JA. Functional cerebral asymmetry in affective disorders: new facts contributed by transcranial magnetic stimulation. *J Affect Disord.* (2001) 66:103–9. doi: 10.1016/S0165-0327(00)00276-7
100. Koek RJ, Yerevanian BI, Tachiki KH, Smith JC, Alcock J, Kopelowicz A. Hemispheric asymmetry in depression and mania. a longitudinal QEEG study in bipolar disorder. *J Affect Disord.* (1999) 53:109–22. doi: 10.1016/S0165-0327(98)00171-2
101. Chen X, Lu B, Yan CG. Reproducibility of R-fMRI metrics on the impact of different strategies for multiple comparison correction and sample sizes. *Hum Brain Mapp.* (2018) 39:300–18. doi: 10.1002/hbm.23843

19

Insomnia Really Hurts: Effect of a Bad Night's Sleep on Pain Increases with Insomnia Severity

Yishul Wei[1], *Tessa F. Blanken*[1,2] *and Eus J. W. Van Someren*[1,2,3*]

[1] Department of Sleep and Cognition, Netherlands Institute for Neuroscience, An Institute of the Royal Netherlands Academy of Arts and Sciences, Amsterdam, Netherlands, [2] Department of Integrative Neurophysiology, Center for Neurogenomics and Cognitive Research, Amsterdam Neuroscience, Vrije Universiteit Amsterdam, Amsterdam, Netherlands, [3] Department of Psychiatry, Amsterdam UMC, Vrije Universiteit Amsterdam, Amsterdam, Netherlands

***Correspondence:**
Eus J. W. Van Someren
e.j.w.someren@vu.nl

Insomnia and chronic pain are highly prevalent conditions and are often comorbid. Somatic complaints other than pain are also often observed in insomnia. Poor sleep and pain are known to mutually reinforce each other. However, it is unknown whether the habitual severity of insomnia modulates the acute effect of a particularly bad night's sleep on the next day's pain severity, and whether it modulates the acute effect of pain on the following night's sleep quality. Using data from 3,508 volunteers (2,684 female, mean age 50.09 y), we addressed these questions in addition to the associations between the habitual severity of insomnia, somatic complaints, and pain. Results indicated that people suffering from more severe habitual insomnia showed stronger mutual acute within-day reactivity of pain and poor sleep quality. The same increased reactivity was found in people with more severe habitual pain. Interestingly, the acute within-day mutual reactivity of pain and sleep quality showed consistent asymmetry. Pain worsened more after a particularly bad night's sleep than it improved after a particularly good night's sleep. Likewise, sleep worsened more after a day with more-than-usual pain than it improved after a day with less-than-usual pain. Future interventions may profit from addressing this asymmetric mutual reactivity especially in people with severe comorbid insomnia and chronic pain.

Keywords: sleep quality, pain, insomnia disorder, somatic complaints, symptom dynamics, reactivity, sensitization

INTRODUCTION

Insomnia is the most prevalent sleep disorder and the second most prevalent mental disorder in Western countries (1). The prevalence of insomnia estimated by epidemiological studies ranges from 6% to one third, depending on the definition of insomnia and the source population (2). Furthermore, insomnia represents an important risk factor for the development of various medical conditions, including cardiovascular diseases (3, 4), diabetes (5), and other mental disorders (6).

Insomnia is often observed to accompany somatic complaints, including pain. Between 50 and 88% of people with chronic pain who seek medical help also complain about insomnia (7, 8) and, vice versa, at least 40% of people with insomnia have chronic pain (9, 10). Disrupted sleep further predicts the frequency (11), extent (12), and intensity (13) of pain in the general population. Other somatic complaints besides pain have also been linked to insomnia, although such associations have been studied less extensively (14–16).

It is generally accepted that the relationship between pain and insomnia is reciprocal (17, 18). Recent large-scale longitudinal population-based studies have convincingly shown that insomnia predicts new incidence of chronic pain (19, 20) and vice versa (21, 22). Among patients with chronic pain, insomnia symptoms not only are associated with greater pain intensity, pain-related disability, and depression (23, 24), but also have impacts on prognosis (25–28). A limitation of these studies on the consequences of insomnia on pain, already acknowledged by some authors, is that insomnia is almost always assessed with self-reports on sleep problems, while daytime impairments which are part of the defining characteristics of insomnia (29, 30) have typically not been taken into account.

Although the above-mentioned observational studies provide compelling evidence for the impacts of disrupted sleep on pain, interventional studies often find that treatments targeting insomnia only contribute to small reduction of pain in patients with comorbid insomnia and chronic pain (31, 32). The reasons for this discrepancy between observational and interventional studies are at present insufficiently understood. It could be that improved sleep quality alleviates pain to a less extent than insomnia aggravates pain in general. Alternatively, the observed associations between pain and sleep quality may be confounded or modulated by other factors. Systematically studying individual differences in the reactivity profile with respect to pain and sleep quality may provide clues about the factors involved.

The current study aims at depicting a clearer picture of the relationship between sleep quality and pain along these lines. Using data from a psychometric database contributed by volunteers in the community, we first answer the question, "Do painful conditions improve after a particularly good night's sleep to the same degree as they worsen after a particularly bad night's sleep?" and the corresponding question regarding the reverse effect of pain on sleep. We next explore the possibility that a person's reactivity to poor sleep in terms of pain severity might depend on the baseline insomnia severity. In other words: Does a bad night's sleep increase the next day's pain to the same degree in people with habitual poor sleep as it does in people with habitual good sleep? Likewise, one might ask whether painful experience affects subsequent sleep to the same degree in people with habitual poor sleep as it does in people with habitual good sleep. The same two questions can be asked for people with less vs. more habitual pain. We complement the investigation with assessments of associations of habitual insomnia severity with the overall severity of habitual pain and somatic complaints. To our knowledge, this is the first study to investigate how mutual vulnerabilities between acute pain and disturbed sleep may be modulated by habitual pain and disturbed sleep.

MATERIALS AND METHODS

Participants

Questionnaire data were obtained through the Netherlands Sleep Registry (NSR), an online platform for psychometric data collection across the general population. Volunteers for the NSR include good and poor sleepers recruited through advertisement on the internet, television, radio, magazines, and newspapers as well as through flyers distributed in health care institutions and conventions. Each participant registered for an account on the NSR website (www.sleepregistry.nl) and could then complete a wide array of survey modules online concerning demographics, personality, psychosocial well-being, life events, and medical history. Each of the online survey modules contains one or more questionnaires, as detailed previously (33). Because the sheer number of surveys precluded the possibility of completing all modules in one sitting, participants were allowed to fill them out bit by bit at self-chosen times and places. As a result, a different number of participants had completed each individual survey module at the time of analysis. The current analyses utilized data entered between January 2011 and October 2017 by a total number of 3508 participants. No exclusion criteria other than missing of questionnaire data necessary for the subsequent analyses was imposed. The ethics committee of the Academic Medical Center, University of Amsterdam, Amsterdam, The Netherlands, and the Central Committee on Research Involving Human Subjects, The Hague, The Netherlands, approved of unsigned informed consent because volunteers participated anonymously without revealing their full names and addresses and were not exposed to any intervention or behavioral constraint.

Measures

Insomnia Severity Index (ISI)

The Insomnia Severity Index (34) is a seven-item Likert scale measuring the severity of nighttime and daytime symptoms of insomnia. Each item is a 5-point rating (0–4) concerning a distinct aspect of insomnia over a 2-week period, denoted hereafter as "habitual." The total sum score, ranging from 0 to 28, provides an overall index of insomnia severity. The ISI has been shown to have good psychometric properties, including high diagnostic accuracy (34–36).

Four-Dimensional Symptom Questionnaire (4-DSQ)

The Four-Dimensional Symptom Questionnaire (37) comprises 4 subscales: distress, somatization, anxiety, and depression. Each subscale measures the severity of a suite of psychological symptoms over a 1-week period, denoted hereafter as "habitual." The questionnaire has been designed so that the overlap between subscales is minimal. That is, symptoms specific to depression, anxiety, and somatic complaints are captured by the corresponding subscales, while the distress subscale assesses non-specific symptoms reflecting the general level of mental distress. The ranges of the subscales are, respectively, 0–32 for distress, 0–32 for somatization, 0–24 for anxiety, and 0–12 for depression. The 4-DSQ has been shown to have good psychometric properties, including high diagnostic accuracy (37–40).

Chronic Pain Grade (CPG)

The Chronic Pain Grade (41) assesses pain severity across a period up to 6 months, denoted hereafter as "habitual". It provides 3 quantitative scores, i.e. pain intensity, pain-related disability, and days with pain-related disability. For clinical purposes the scores can be combined to determine a final categorical grade (5 levels from pain-free to high disability–severely limiting). Given the aim of the current study, only the pain intensity score (range: 0–100) was used.

The pain assessment module of the NSR also contains 4 items about the perceived acute relationship between sleep and pain, similar to those used in a previous study (42). The perceived acute effect of sleep on pain is addressed by 2 items, "If I sleep worse/better than usual on one night, the next day the chance of feeling pain is ..." and the answer options are "much smaller," "smaller," "somewhat smaller," "as usual," "somewhat bigger," "bigger," and "much bigger" (coded as −3, −2, −1, 0, 1, 2, and 3, respectively). The perceived acute effect of pain on sleep is addressed by 2 items, "If I have a day with more/less pain than usual, the following night I usually sleep ..." and the answer options are "much worse," "worse," "somewhat worse," "as usual," "somewhat better," "better," and "much better" (coded as −3, −2, −1, 0, 1, 2, and 3, respectively).

Statistical Analyses

We first calculated Spearman correlation coefficients to examine the associations of habitual insomnia severity with the habitual severity of somatic complaints and habitual pain intensity. Next, linear regression was employed to control for possible effects of age, sex, and the other 4-DSQ subscales.

Data on perceived acute within-day sleep–pain relationship were analyzed in 3 steps. First, Wilcoxon signed-rank tests were performed to evaluate whether the central tendency of each rating significantly deviated from the 0 rating that indicates "as usual," i.e., no effect. Second, two Wilcoxon signed-rank tests ensued to compare (1) the absolute acute effect of worse-than-usual sleep with that of better-than-usual sleep on subsequent pain, and (2) the absolute acute effect of more-than-usual pain with that of less-than-usual pain on subsequent sleep. Finally, Spearman correlation coefficients were used to investigate whether habitual insomnia severity and habitual pain intensity modulated the strength of the within-day mutual reactivity of pain and sleep quality. In addition to statistical significance, the robustness of the correlations was further verified by their 95% bootstrap confidence intervals (computed over 10,000 resampling iterations).

RESULTS

The distributions of age, sex, ISI, 4-DSQ subscales, CPG pain intensity score, and ratings on perceived acute sleep–pain relationship are presented in **Table 1**. Of all participants, 2497 completed the 4-DSQ, 2873 completed the CPG together with ratings on perceived acute sleep–pain relationship, and 1862 completed all of the questionnaires. People who completed only the CPG did not differ from those who also completed the 4-DSQ in terms of habitual pain or insomnia severity (**Table 2**). People who completed only the 4-DSQ had less severe habitual insomnia and somatic complaints as compared to those who also completed the CPG. The difference in habitual insomnia severity was secondary to the difference in sex distribution as the ISI within each sex did not differ between the subsamples (results not shown). In contrasts, the differences in somatic complaints between subsamples remained significant even when comparisons were performed separately for each sex (results not shown).

TABLE 1 | Characteristics of participants (mean ± standard deviation).

Age (y)	50.09 ± 15.24
Sex (female/male)	2684/824
ISI	10.12 ± 7.17
4-DSQ (N = 2,497)	
Distress	10.08 ± 8.12
Somatization	7.11 ± 5.62
Anxiety	2.25 ± 3.65
Depression	1.50 ± 2.84
CPG pain intensity (N = 2,873)	40.42 ± 20.08
Perceived sleep–pain relationship (N = 2,873)	
Pain after worse sleep[a]	0.52 ± 0.82
Pain after better sleep[a]	−0.38 ± 0.76
Sleep after more pain[b]	−0.50 ± 0.97
Sleep after less pain[b]	0.18 ± 0.63

4-DSQ, Four-Dimensional Symptom Questionnaire; CPG, Chronic Pain Grade; ISI, Insomnia Severity Index.
[a]*Responses to the items "If I sleep worse/better than usual on one night, the next day the chance of feeling pain is ..." with ratings ranging from −3 (much smaller) to 3 (much bigger).*
[b]*Responses to the items "If I have a day with more/less pain than usual, the following night I usually sleep ..." with ratings ranging from −3 (much worse) to 3 (much better).*

Habitual insomnia severity (ISI) correlated with the somatization subscale of the 4-DSQ (Spearman correlation coefficient = 0.47, $p < 0.001$), and with the pain intensity score from the CPG (Spearman correlation coefficient = 0.33, $p < 0.001$). Regression coefficients are presented in **Tables 3**, **4**, for models with the somatization subscale of the 4-DSQ as outcome and with the pain intensity score from the CPG as outcome, respectively. In **Table 3** one sees that habitual insomnia severity was robustly positively associated with the habitual severity of somatic complaints, even after controlling for the effects of the other 4-DSQ subscales (depression, anxiety, and general distress). Similarly, in **Table 4** one sees that habitual insomnia severity was robustly positively associated with habitual pain intensity, even after controlling for the effects of all 4-DSQ subscales (depression, anxiety, somatization, and general distress).

Table 1 also shows that, as expected, people reported to have more pain than usual after they experienced a particularly bad night's sleep and less pain than usual after they experienced a particularly good night's sleep. Wilcoxon signed-rank tests confirmed that these ratings significantly differed from 0 (both $p < 0.001$). Interestingly, the acute impact of changes in sleep quality on pain was not symmetric. A particularly bad night's sleep increased the next day's pain significantly more than a particularly good night's sleep ameliorated the next day's pain (mean difference ± standard deviation = 0.13 ± 0.63, $p < 0.001$).

Similarly, people reported to have significantly worse sleep than usual following a day during which they experienced more pain than usual ($p < 0.001$). They also reported to have significantly better sleep than usual following a day during

TABLE 2 | Characteristics of participants (mean ± standard deviation) within subsamples according to questionnaires completed.

	CPG + 4-DSQ (N = 1,862)	CPG only (N = 1,011)	4-DSQ only (N = 635)
Age (y)	50.83 ± 14.46	48.81 ± 16.67*	49.96 ± 14.97
Sex (female/male)	1459/403	782/229	443/192***
ISI	10.17 ± 7.10	10.36 ± 7.16	9.61 ± 7.41*
4-DSQ			
Distress	10.34 ± 8.06	–	9.33 ± 8.23***
Somatization	7.59 ± 5.59	–	5.72 ± 5.49***
Anxiety	2.35 ± 3.72	–	1.95 ± 3.44**
Depression	1.53 ± 2.87	–	1.43 ± 2.73
CPG pain intensity	40.81 ± 19.86	39.70 ± 20.47	–
Perceived sleep–pain relationship			
Pain after worse sleep[a]	0.52 ± 0.82	0.51 ± 0.82	–
Pain after better sleep[a]	−0.38 ± 0.75	−0.40 ± 0.76	–
Sleep after more pain[b]	−0.50 ± 0.97	−0.49 ± 0.97	–
Sleep after less pain[b]	0.19 ± 0.64	0.18 ± 0.62	–

4-DSQ, Four-Dimensional Symptom Questionnaire; CPG, Chronic Pain Grade; ISI, Insomnia Severity Index.

, **, * Significance of difference from the "CPG + 4-DSQ" subsample (*p < 0.05, **p < 0.01, ***p < 0.001) as determined by Fisher exact test for sex and by Wilcoxon rank-sum tests for the other variables.*

[a]Responses to the items "If I sleep worse/better than usual on one night, the next day the chance of feeling pain is ..." with ratings ranging from −3 (much smaller) to 3 (much bigger).

[b]Responses to the items "If I have a day with more/less pain than usual, the following night I usually sleep ..." with ratings ranging from −3 (much worse) to 3 (much better).

which they experienced less pain than usual ($p < 0.001$). The acute impact of changes in pain on sleep quality was again not symmetric. A day with more pain than usual worsened the night's sleep quality more than a day with less pain than usual improved the night's sleep quality (mean difference ± standard deviation = $0.31 \pm 1.01, p < 0.001$).

Remarkably, all of the 4 ratings on perceived acute sleep–pain relationship significantly correlated with the pain intensity score from the CPG, and 3 out from 4 significantly correlated with the ISI (**Table 5**). **Figure 1** visualizes how the mutual acute within-day reactivity of pain and sleep quality was modulated by habitual insomnia severity. Participants are grouped according to clinical cutoffs of the ISI (34). The left panel of **Figure 1** shows that the acute effect of sleep quality on the next day's pain increased in both directions with increasing habitual insomnia severity. The blue bars in the right panel of **Figure 1** illustrate that the improvement in sleep quality after a day with less pain than usual was independent of habitual insomnia severity within the subclinical range (the two groups with ISI < 15), while in the clinical insomnia groups (ISI ≥ 15), the benefit for sleep due to a day with less pain than usual disappeared with increasing habitual insomnia severity. In strong contrast, the red bars in the right panel of **Figure 1** illustrate that acute worsening of sleep after a day with more pain than usual continued to increase with more severe habitual insomnia.

TABLE 3 | Regression model with habitual severity of somatization / somatic complaints as outcome variable (N = 2,497).

	Regression coefficient	Standard error	t	p
(Intercept)	2.074	0.390	5.31	<0.001
Age (y)	−0.005	0.006	−0.79	0.43
Female	0.656	0.202	3.25	0.001
ISI	0.115	0.015	7.85	<0.001
4-DSQ Distress	0.302	0.020	15.46	<0.001
4-DSQ Anxiety	0.387	0.032	12.02	<0.001
4-DSQ Depression	−0.191	0.044	−4.34	<0.001

4-DSQ, Four-Dimensional Symptom Questionnaire; ISI, Insomnia Severity Index.

DISCUSSION

The current study delineates the perceived acute within-day sleep–pain relationship in a community-based sample on top of the associations between habitual insomnia and habitual somatic complaints (including pain). We show, in addition to robust associations of habitual insomnia severity with the habitual severity of somatic complaints and pain, that people in general perceive reciprocal, but asymmetric, acute effects of incidental changes in sleep quality and pain severity on each other—with the effects of worse sleep and more pain than usual larger than those of better sleep and less pain than usual, respectively. Importantly, the strength of the perceived acute reciprocal effects is generally stronger in people with more severe habitual insomnia and pain, with the notable exception being that the benefit for sleep due to a day with less pain than usual is gradually lost with increasing habitual insomnia severity.

The associations of the perceived acute sleep–pain relationship with habitual insomnia severity and habitual pain intensity reported here are novel and may have clinical implications. It is known that people with insomnia exhibit larger night-to-night sleep variability than people without (43).

This larger variability may be in part driven by larger fluctuations in the severity of physical symptoms, in line with a recent study showing that self-reported nocturnal wake time is associated with the fluctuation in pain over a week (44). Our results further refine this association by highlighting an asymmetric effect of the fluctuation in pain on sleep quality, especially for people with severe habitual insomnia or pain. In fact, in people with severe habitual insomnia, transient reduction of pain has virtually no effect on subsequent sleep quality (**Figure 1**). When it comes to treatment programs for patients with chronic pain, especially for those with severe comorbid insomnia, it therefore cannot be assumed that sleep problems would automatically be resolved upon alleviation of pain—a point already emphasized by other authors (45, 46). The acute effect of the fluctuation in sleep quality on pain is also asymmetric, and increases with habitual insomnia or pain severity in both directions. The increase is larger for worse-than-usual sleep than for better-than-usual sleep, resulting in even more exaggerated asymmetry in people with severe habitual insomnia or chronic pain (cf. **Figure 1**). This could possibly explain why previous interventional studies have reported only weak and inconsistent effects of treatments targeting insomnia on pain in patients with clinically comorbid insomnia and chronic pain (31, 32). Possible reactivity differences between people may therefore need to be carefully considered in future intervention development to achieve more efficient management of comorbid insomnia and chronic pain.

To our knowledge, the perceived acute sleep–pain relationship has only been investigated within a specific clinical sample in a smaller-scale study (42). Our results about the asymmetric perceived acute sleep–pain relationship agree with that study, thereby demonstrating generalizability. A handful of previous community-based studies investigated the relationship between habitual insomnia severity and habitual somatic complaints (14–16) and more specifically between habitual insomnia severity and habitual pain intensity (13, 47). However, the definitions of insomnia adopted by most of these studies referred only to night-time symptoms (difficulty initiating sleep, difficulty maintaining sleep, early morning awakening, nonrestorative sleep and/or poor sleep quality) whereas we here evaluated insomnia severity using the ISI which also assesses daytime impairments. Furthermore, different sets of psychological symptoms (or none at all) were controlled for in different studies, making comparisons somewhat difficult. The most similar study to the current one, but of a smaller scale, was conducted by Zhang et al. (15). That study reported robust associations of the ISI with the severity of pain and non-pain somatic complaints over the prior week, after controlling for the Hospital Anxiety and Depression Scale scores (48) which overlap in content with the distress, anxiety and depression subscales of the 4-DSQ. In conclusion, our result with respect to somatic complaints within 1 week can be regarded as corroborating the finding of Zhang et al. (15), whereas the result on pain intensity generalizes their finding to a longer reference period (up to 6 months).

The mechanisms underlying the relationship between insomnia and pain (or somatic complaints in general) are still not well understood (18, 49). It is known that short or disrupted sleep can acutely induce low pain threshold (50, 51). Chronic insomnia, in particular, is associated with hypersensitivity to interoceptive input which may involve heightened brain excitability, attentional bias, or deficient salience filtering (52, 53). The caudate nucleus, a subcortical structure known to be involved in pain suppression (54), has also been shown to be affected in insomnia (55). Thus, insomnia may trigger a cascade of neuronal changes leading to central sensitization—which has long been considered a major contributor to chronic pain (56). The reverse influence of chronic pain on sleep is equally

TABLE 4 | Regression model with habitual pain intensity as outcome variable ($N = 1,862$).

	Regression coefficient	Standard error	t	p
(Intercept)	15.56	1.97	7.90	<0.001
Age (y)	0.18	0.03	6.01	<0.001
Female	3.25	1.02	3.20	0.001
ISI	0.50	0.07	6.91	<0.001
4-DSQ Distress	−0.12	0.10	−1.26	0.21
4-DSQ Somatization	1.29	0.10	13.41	<0.001
4-DSQ Anxiety	−0.21	0.16	−1.33	0.18
4-DSQ Depression	0.44	0.21	2.08	0.04

4-DSQ, Four-Dimensional Symptom Questionnaire; ISI, Insomnia Severity Index.

TABLE 5 | Spearman correlation coefficients between perceived acute sleep–pain relationship and habitual insomnia/pain severity ($N = 2,873$; brackets indicate 95% bootstrap confidence intervals).

	Sleep → Pain		Pain → Sleep	
	Pain after worse sleep[a]	Pain after better sleep[a]	Sleep after more pain[b]	Sleep after less pain[b]
ISI	0.19*** [0.16, 0.23]	−0.13*** [−0.17, −0.10]	−0.20*** [−0.23, −0.16]	−0.02 [−0.05, 0.02]
CPG pain intensity	0.19*** [0.15, 0.22]	−0.06** [−0.10, −0.02]	−0.26*** [−0.30, −0.22]	0.10*** [0.06, 0.14]

CPG, Chronic Pain Grade; ISI, Insomnia Severity Index.

$^{**}p < 0.01$, $^{***}p < 0.001$.

[a]*Responses to the items "If I sleep worse/better than usual on one night, the next day the chance of feeling pain is ..." with ratings ranging from −3 (much smaller) to 3 (much bigger).*

[b]*Responses to the items "If I have a day with more/less pain than usual, the following night I usually sleep ..." with ratings ranging from −3 (much worse) to 3 (much better).*

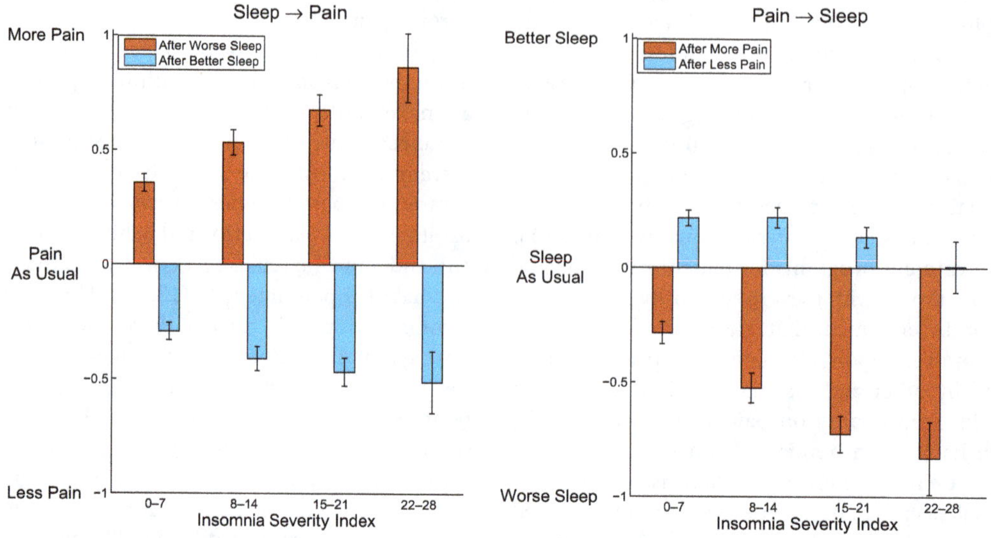

FIGURE 1 | Average perceived pain after a better night and worse night of sleep than usual **(Left)**, and average perceived sleep quality after a day with more pain and less pain than usual **(Right)**, within subgroups of participants defined by clinical cutoffs of the Insomnia Severity Index. Error bars indicate 95% confidence intervals.

if not even more elusive (57) and might involve dysregulation of the hypothalamic-pituitary-adrenal axis (58). In addition, various behavioral and cognitive factors have been proposed to mediate the mutual influences of pain and poor sleep, including medication (59), catastrophizing (60), pre-sleep arousal (61), negative mood (62, 63) and attention (64). Clearly, more research is needed to better understand the interactions between insomnia and chronic pain, two highly prevalent conditions for which comorbidity is not unusual.

Some limitations of our study can be mentioned. First, we investigated the acute bidirectional effects of sleep quality and pain by means of subjective ratings. The real effects, as would be observed with repeated measurements of present pain and sleep quality, might differ from the perceived ones. On the other hand, subjective experience and conception about sleep and pain are not at all trivial as compared to objective indicators of their relationship. Even if the measured acute effects were purely subjective, the results reported here would still be of clinical relevance as they would in this case signify that dysfunctional beliefs about the consequences of poor sleep and pain were most exaggerated in people with severe symptomology and thus might represent an especially effective venue for interventions (46). Second, data were taken from a psychometric database which received input from volunteers. As a consequence, the sample might not precisely represent the general population. Third, participants could fill out different questionnaires at different times, possibly resulting in weaker observed associations than could be found with simultaneous completion. In light of these limitations and our novel results, future longitudinal studies with population-based samples are warranted so as to obtain more accurate symptom dynamics in the general population. Such insights may in turn facilitate future research on intervention strategies in line with the emerging "systems" approaches to psychopathology and psychotherapy.

AUTHOR CONTRIBUTIONS

YW and TB collected and analyzed data. EV supervised the project. YW wrote the manuscript. All authors participated in the revision of the manuscript.

FUNDING

Research leading to these results has received funding from the Netherlands Organization of Scientific Research (NWO) grant VICI-453.07.001, the European Research Council Advanced Grant 671084 INSOMNIA, and the Bial Foundation grant 190/16.

REFERENCES

1. Wittchen HU, Jacobi F, Rehm J, Gustavsson A, Svensson M, Jönsson B, et al. The size and burden of mental disorders and other disorders of the brain in Europe 2010. *Eur Neuropsychopharmacol.* (2011) 21:655–79. doi: 10.1016/j.euroneuro.2011.07.018
2. Ohayon MM. Epidemiology of insomnia: what we know and what we still need to learn. *Sleep Med Rev.* (2002) 6:97–111. doi: 10.1053/smrv.2002.0186
3. Sofi F, Cesari F, Casini A, Macchi C, Abbate R, Gensini GF. Insomnia and risk of cardiovascular disease: a meta-analysis. *Eur J Prev Cardiol.* (2014) 21:57–64. doi: 10.1177/2047487312460020
4. He Q, Zhang P, Li G, Dai H, Shi J. The association between insomnia symptoms and risk of cardio-cerebral vascular events: a meta-analysis of prospective cohort studies. *Eur J Prev Cardiol.* (2017) 24:1071–82. doi: 10.1177/2047487317702043

5. Cappuccio FP, D'Elia L, Strazzullo P, Miller MA. Quantity and quality of sleep and incidence of type 2 diabetes: a systematic review and meta-analysis. *Diabetes Care* (2010) 33:414–20. doi: 10.2337/dc09-1124
6. Alvaro PK, Roberts RM, Harris JK. A systematic review assessing bidirectionality between sleep disturbances, anxiety, and depression. *Sleep* (2013) 36:1059–68. doi: 10.5665/sleep.2810
7. Tang NKY. Insomnia co-occurring with chronic pain: clinical features, interaction, assessments and possible interventions. *Rev Pain* (2008) 2:2–7. doi: 10.1177/204946370800200102
8. Alföldi P, Wiklund T, Gerdle B. Comorbid insomnia in patients with chronic pain: a study based on the Swedish quality registry for pain rehabilitation (SQRP). *Disabil Rehabil.* (2014) 36:1661–9. doi: 10.3109/09638288.2013.864712
9. Ohayon MM. Relationship between chronic painful physical condition and insomnia. *J Psychiatr Res.* (2005) 39:151–9. doi: 10.1016/j.jpsychires.2004.07.001
10. Taylor DJ, Mallory LJ, Lichstein KL, Durrence HH, Riedel BW, Bush AJ. Comorbidity of chronic insomnia with medical problems. *Sleep* (2007) 30:213–8. doi: 10.1093/sleep/30.2.213
11. Edwards RR, Almeida DM, Klick B, Haythornthwaite JA, Smith MT. Duration of sleep contributes to next-day pain report in the general population. *Pain* (2008) 137:202–7. doi: 10.1016/j.pain.2008.01.025
12. Mundal I, Bjørngaard JH, Nilsen TIL, Nicholl BI, Gråwe RW, Fors EA. Long-term changes in musculoskeletal pain sites in the general population: the HUNT study. *J Pain* (2016) 17:1246–56. doi: 10.1016/j.jpain.2016.08.006
13. Liu X, Xiao S, Zhou L, Hu M, Zhou W, Liu H. Sleep quality and covariates as predictors of pain intensity among the general population in rural China. *J Pain Res.* (2018) 11:857–66. doi: 10.2147/JPR.S156731
14. Kim K, Uchiyama M, Liu X, Shibui K, Ohida T, Ogihara R, et al. Somatic and psychological complaints and their correlates with insomnia in the Japanese general population. *Psychosom Med.* (2001) 63:441–6. doi: 10.1097/00006842-200105000-00013
15. Zhang J, Lam S-P, Li SX, Tang NL, Yu MWM, Li AM, et al. Insomnia, sleep quality, pain, and somatic symptoms: sex differences and shared genetic components. *Pain* (2012) 153:666–73. doi: 10.1016/j.pain.2011.12.003
16. Wong JY-H, Fong DY-T, Chan KK-W. Anxiety and insomnia as modifiable risk factors for somatic symptoms in Chinese: a general population-based study. *Qual Life Res.* (2015) 24:2493–8. doi: 10.1007/s11136-015-0984-9
17. Smith MT, Haythornthwaite JA. How do sleep disturbance and chronic pain inter-relate? Insights from the longitudinal and cognitive-behavioral clinical trials literature. *Sleep Med Rev.* (2004) 8:119–32. doi: 10.1016/S1087-0792(03)00044-3
18. Finan PH, Goodin BR, Smith MT. The association of sleep and pain: an update and a path forward. *J Pain* (2013) 14:1539–52. doi: 10.1016/j.jpain.2013.08.007
19. Mork PJ, Vik KL, Moe B, Lier R, Bardal EM, Nilsen TIL. Sleep problems, exercise and obesity and risk of chronic musculoskeletal pain: the Norwegian HUNT study. *Eur J Public Health* (2014) 24:924–9. doi: 10.1093/eurpub/ckt198
20. Uhlig BL, Sand T, Nilsen TI, Mork PJ, Hagen K. Insomnia and risk of chronic musculoskeletal complaints: longitudinal data from the HUNT study, Norway. *BMC Musculoskelet Disord.* (2018) 19:128. doi: 10.1186/s12891-018-2035-5
21. Ødegård SS, Sand T, Engstrøm M, Zwart J-A, Hagen K. The impact of headache and chronic musculoskeletal complaints on the risk of insomnia: longitudinal data from the Nord-Trøndelag health study. *J Headache Pain* (2013) 14:24. doi: 10.1186/1129-2377-14-24
22. Skarpsno ES, Nilsen TIL, Sand T, Hagen K, Mork PJ. Do physical activity and body mass index modify the association between chronic musculoskeletal pain and insomnia? Longitudinal data from the HUNT study, Norway. *J Sleep Res.* (2018) 27:32–9. doi: 10.1111/jsr.12580
23. McCracken LM, Iverson GL. Disrupted sleep patterns and daily functioning in patients with chronic pain. *Pain Res Manag.* (2002) 7:75–9. doi: 10.1155/2002/579425
24. Ashworth PCH, Davidson KM, Espie CA. Cognitive–behavioral factors associated with sleep quality in chronic pain patients. *Behav Sleep Med.* (2010) 8:28–39. doi: 10.1080/15402000903425587
25. Davies KA, Macfarlane GJ, Nicholl BI, Dickens C, Morriss R, Ray D, et al. Restorative sleep predicts the resolution of chronic widespread pain: results from the EPIFUND study. *Rheumatology* (2008) 47:1809–13. doi: 10.1093/rheumatology/ken389
26. Mundal I, Gråwe RW, Bjørngaard JH, Linaker OM, Fors EA. Prevalence and long-term predictors of persistent chronic widespread pain in the general population in an 11-year prospective study: the HUNT study. *BMC Musculoskelet Disord.* (2014) 15:213. doi: 10.1186/1471-2474-15-213
27. Aili K, Nyman T, Svartengren M, Hillert L. Sleep as a predictive factor for the onset and resolution of multi-site pain: a 5-year prospective study. *Eur J Pain* (2015) 19:341–9. doi: 10.1002/ejp.552
28. Alföldi P, Dragioti E, Wiklund T, Gerdle B. Spreading of pain and insomnia in patients with chronic pain: results from a national quality registry (SQRP). *J Rehabil Med.* (2017) 49:63–70. doi: 10.2340/16501977-2162
29. American Psychiatric Association. *Diagnostic and Statistical Manual of Mental Disorders.* 5th ed. Washington, DC: American Psychiatric Publishing (2013).
30. American Academy of Sleep Medicine. *International Classification of Sleep Disorders.* 3rd ed. Darien, IL: American Academy of Sleep Medicine (2014).
31. Finan PH, Buenaver LF, Runko VT, Smith MT. Cognitive-behavioral therapy for comorbid insomnia and chronic pain. *Sleep Med Clin.* (2014) 9:261–74. doi: 10.1016/j.jsmc.2014.02.007
32. Tang NKY, Lereya ST, Boulton H, Miller MA, Wolke D, Cappuccio FP. Nonpharmacological treatments of insomnia for long-term painful conditions: a systematic review and meta-analysis of patient-reported outcomes in randomized controlled trials. *Sleep* (2015) 38:1751–64. doi: 10.5665/sleep.5158
33. Benjamins JS, Migliorati F, Dekker K, Wassing R, Moens S, Blanken TF, et al. Insomnia heterogeneity: characteristics to consider for data-driven multivariate subtyping. *Sleep Med Rev.* (2017) 36:71–81. doi: 10.1016/j.smrv.2016.10.005
34. Bastien CH, Vallières A, Morin CM. Validation of the insomnia severity index as an outcome measure for insomnia research. *Sleep Med.* (2001) 2:297–307. doi: 10.1016/S1389-9457(00)00065-4
35. Morin CM, Belleville G, Bélanger L, Ivers H. The insomnia severity index: psychometric indicators to detect insomnia cases and evaluate treatment response. *Sleep* (2011) 34:601–8. doi: 10.1093/sleep/34.5.601
36. Wong ML, Lau KNT, Espie CA, Luik AI, Kyle SD, Lau EYY. Psychometric properties of the sleep condition indicator and insomnia severity index in the evaluation of insomnia disorder. *Sleep Med.* (2017) 33:76–81. doi: 10.1016/j.sleep.2016.05.019
37. Terluin B, van Marwijk HWJ, Adèr HJ, de Vet HCW, Penninx BWJH, Hermens MLM, et al. The four-dimensional symptom questionnaire (4DSQ): a validation study of a multidimensional self-report questionnaire to assess distress, depression, anxiety and somatization. *BMC Psychiatry* (2006) 6:34. doi: 10.1186/1471-244X-6-34
38. Terluin B, Brouwers EPM, van Marwijk HWJ, Verhaak PFM, van der Horst HE. Detecting depressive and anxiety disorders in distressed patients in primary care; comparative diagnostic accuracy of the four-dimensional symptom questionnaire (4DSQ) and the hospital anxiety and depression scale (HADS). *BMC Fam Pract.* (2009) 10:58. doi: 10.1186/1471-2296-10-58
39. Terluin B, Smits N, Brouwers EPM, de Vet HCW. The four-dimensional symptom questionnaire (4DSQ) in the general population: scale structure, reliability, measurement invariance and normative data: a cross-sectional survey. *Health Qual Life Outcomes* (2016) 14:130. doi: 10.1186/s12955-016-0533-4
40. Sitnikova K, Dijkstra-Kersten SMA, Mokkink LB, Terluin B, van Marwijk HWJ, Leone SS, et al. Systematic review of measurement properties of questionnaires measuring somatization in primary care patients. *J Psychosom Res.* (2017) 103:42–62. doi: 10.1016/j.jpsychores.2017.10.005
41. Von Korff M, Ormel J, Keefe FJ, Dworkin SF. Grading the severity of chronic pain. *Pain* (1992) 50:133–49. doi: 10.1016/0304-3959(92)90154-4
42. Blågestad T, Pallesen S, Grønli J, Tang NKY, Nordhus IH. How perceived pain influence sleep and mood more than the reverse: a novel, exploratory study with patients awaiting total hip arthroplasty. *Front Psychol.* (2016) 7:1689. doi: 10.3389/fpsyg.2016.01689
43. Buysse DJ, Cheng Y, Germain A, Moul DE, Franzen PL, Fletcher M, et al. Night-to-night sleep variability in older adults with and without chronic insomnia. *Sleep Med.* (2010) 11:56–64. doi: 10.1016/j.sleep.2009.02.010
44. Ravyts SG, Dzierzewski JM, Grah SC, Buman MP, Aiken-Morgan AT, Giacobb PR jr, et al. Sleep and pain in mid- to late-life: an exploration

of day-to-day pain inconsistency. *Clin Gerontol.* (2018) 41:123–9. doi: 10.1080/07317115.2017.1345818
45. Wilson KG, Kowal J, Ferguson EJ. Clinically important change in insomnia severity after chronic pain rehabilitation. *Clin J Pain* (2016) 32:784–91. doi: 10.1097/AJP.0000000000000325
46. Tang NKY. Cognitive behavioural therapy in pain and psychological disorders: towards a hybrid future. *Prog Neuro-Psychopharmacol Biol Psychiatry* (2018). doi: 10.1016/j.pnpbp.2017.02.023. [Epub ahead of print].
47. Sutton DA, Moldofsky H, Badley EM. Insomnia and health problems in Canadians. *Sleep* (2001) 24:665–70. doi: 10.1093/sleep/24.6.665
48. Zigmond AS, Snaith RP. The hospital anxiety and depression scale. *Acta Psychiatr Scand.* (1983) 67:361–70. doi: 10.1111/j.1600-0447.1983.tb09716.x
49. Boakye PA, Olechowski C, Rashiq S, Verrier MJ, Kerr B, Witmans M, et al. A critical review of neurobiological factors involved in the interactions between chronic pain, depression, and sleep disruption. *Clin J Pain* (2016) 32:327–36. doi: 10.1097/AJP.0000000000000260
50. Lautenbacher S, Kundermann B, Krieg J-C. Sleep deprivation and pain perception. *Sleep Med Rev.* (2006) 10:357–69. doi: 10.1016/j.smrv.2005.08.001
51. Schrimpf M, Liegl G, Boeckle M, Leitner A, Geisler P, Pieh C. The effect of sleep deprivation on pain perception in healthy subjects: a meta-analysis. *Sleep Med.* (2015) 16:1313–20. doi: 10.1016/j.sleep.2015.07.022
52. van der Werf YD, Altena E, van Dijk KD, Strijers RLM, De Rijke W, Stam CJ, et al. Is disturbed intracortical excitability a stable trait of chronic insomnia? A study using transcranial magnetic stimulation before and after multimodal sleep therapy. *Biol Psychiatry* (2010) 68:950–5. doi: 10.1016/j.biopsych.2010.06.028
53. Wei Y, Ramautar JR, Colombo MA, Stoffers D, Gómez-Herrero G, van der Meijden WP, et al. I keep a close watch on this heart of mine: increased interoception in insomnia. *Sleep* (2016) 39:2113–24. doi: 10.5665/sleep.6308
54. Wunderlich AP, Klug R, Stuber G, Landwehrmeyer B, Weber F, Freund W. Caudate nucleus and insular activation during a pain suppression paradigm comparing thermal and electrical stimulation. *Open Neuroimag J.* (2011) 5:1–8. doi: 10.2174/1874440001105010001
55. Stoffers D, Altena E, van der Werf YD, Sanz-Arigita EJ, Voorn TA, Astill RG, et al. The caudate: a key node in the neuronal network imbalance of insomnia? *Brain* (2014) 137:610–20. doi: 10.1093/brain/awt329
56. Latremoliere A, Woolf CJ. Central sensitization: a generator of pain hypersensitivity by central neural plasticity. *J Pain* (2010) 10:895–926. doi: 10.1016/j.jpain.2009.06.012
57. Foo H, Mason P. Brainstem modulation of pain during sleep and waking. *Sleep Med Rev.* (2003) 7:145–54. doi: 10.1053/smrv.2002.0224
58. Roehrs T, Roth T. Sleep and pain: interaction of two vital functions. *Semin Neurol.* (2005) 25:106–16. doi: 10.1055/s-2005-867079
59. Bohra MH, Kaushik C, Temple D, Chung SA, Shapiro CM. Weighing the balance: how analgesics used in chronic pain influence sleep? *Br J Pain* (2014) 8:107–18. doi: 10.1177/2049463714525355
60. MacDonald S, Linton SJ, Jansson-Fröjmark M. Avoidant safety behaviors and catastrophizing: shared cognitive-behavioral processes and consequences in co-morbid pain and sleep disorders. *Int J Behav Med.* (2008) 15:201–10. doi: 10.1080/10705500802222675
61. Byers HD, Lichstein KL, Thorn BE. Cognitive processes in comorbid poor sleep and chronic pain. *J Behav Med.* (2016) 39:233–40. doi: 10.1007/s10865-015-9687-5
62. O'Brien EM, Waxenberg LB, Atchison JW, Gremillion HA, Staud RM, McCrae CS, et al. Negative mood mediates the effect of poor sleep on pain among chronic pain patients. *Clin J Pain* (2010) 26:310–9. doi: 10.1097/AJP.0b013e3181c328e9
63. Generaal E, Vogelzangs N, Penninx BWJH, Dekker J. Insomnia, sleep duration, depressive symptoms, and the onset of chronic multisite musculoskeletal pain. *Sleep* (2017) 40:zsw030. doi: 10.1093/sleep/zsw030
64. Harrison L, Wilson S, Heron J, Stannard C, Munafò MR. Exploring the associations shared by mood, pain-related attention and pain outcomes related to sleep disturbance in a chronic pain sample. *Psychol Health* (2016) 31:565–77. doi: 10.1080/08870446.2015.1124106

20

Increased Salience Network Activity in Patients with Insomnia Complaints in Major Depressive Disorder

Chun-Hong Liu[1,2]*, Jing Guo[3], Shun-Li Lu[2], Li-Rong Tang[2], Jin Fan[4], Chuan-Yue Wang[2], Lihong Wang[5]*, Qing-Quan Liu[1] and Cun-Zhi Liu[3]

[1] Beijing Hospital of Traditional Chinese Medicine, Beijing Institute of Traditional Chinese Medicine, Capital Medical University, Beijing, China, [2] Beijing Key Laboratory of Mental Disorders, Department of Radiology, Beijing Anding Hospital, Capital Medical University, Beijing, China, [3] Acupuncture and Moxibustion Department, Beijing Hospital of Traditional Chinese Medicine, Capital Medical University, Beijing, China, [4] Department of Psychiatry, Icahn School of Medicine at Mount Sinai, New York, NY, United States, [5] Department of Psychiatry, University of Connecticut Health Center, Farmington, CT, United States

***Correspondence:**
Chun-Hong Liu
chunhongliu11@163.com;
Lihong Wang
lwang@uchc.edu

Background: Insomnia is one of the main symptom correlates of major depressive disorder (MDD), but the neural mechanisms underlying the multifaceted interplay between insomnia and depression are not fully understood.

Materials and methods: Patients with MDD and high insomnia (MDD-HI, $n = 24$), patients with MDD and low insomnia (MDD-LI, $n = 37$), and healthy controls (HCs, $n = 51$) were recruited to participate in the present study. The amplitude of low-frequency fluctuations (ALFF) during the resting state were compared among the three groups.

Results: We observed ALFF differences between the three groups in the right inferior frontal gyrus/anterior insula (IFG/AI), right middle temporal gyrus, left calcarine, and bilateral dorsolateral prefrontal cortex (dlPFC). Further region of interest (ROI) comparisons showed that the increases in the right IFG/AI reflected an abnormality specific to insomnia in MDD, while increases in the bilateral dlPFC reflected an abnormality specific to MDD generally. Increased ALFF in the right IFG/AI was also found to be correlated with sleep disturbance scores when regressing out the influence of the severity of anxiety and depression.

Conclusion: Our findings suggest that increased resting state ALLF in IFG/AI may be specifically related to hyperarousal state of insomnia in patients with MDD, independently of the effects of anxiety and depression.

Keywords: insomnia, depression, resting-state, low-frequency fluctuation, salience networks

INTRODUCTION

Major depressive disorder (MDD) is characterized by a sustained depressive mood, anhedonia, and sleep abnormalities, alongside a number of motivational and social behaviors (1). Globally, it is a major cause of disability (2). Epidemiological studies have shown that MDD frequently co-occurs with insomnia and insomnia can persist into the remission or recovery stage (3–6). Importantly, the relationship between insomnia and depression is bidirectional with the severity of sleep disturbances positively correlated to the overall severity of depression and to a poor quality of life

(7). Insomnia may also increase the severity of depression and the risk of suicidality (8). Indeed, insomnia, which is a disorder that is independent of depression (9), has a prognostic value as a risk factor for subsequent depressive episodes (3, 10). In longitudinal studies of adults with MDD, insomnia has been shown to increase the risk of recurrence of new depressive episodes twofold to fourfold (11, 12). Additionally, the re-emergence of insomnia can predict the recurrence of a new depressive episode (13). Insomnia can also lead to poor responses to various forms of treatment for depression (3). Treatments for insomnia might help with treatments of depressive symptoms (14). Likewise, insomnia significantly affects the symptoms that are correlated with MDD (15). So, as there appears to be an interplay between insomnia and depression that is multifaceted, examining the specific underlying brain abnormalities associated with insomnia in patients with MDD, could produce data that may lead to the availability of individualized therapies for patients with MDD. However, the neural mechanisms underlying insomnia and MDD comorbidity are currently unclear.

Intrinsic functional connectivity (FC) studies show that several large-scale brain networks have been considered as potential neural substrates in MDD, including the default mode network, the frontoparietal and dorsal attention network, and the salience networks [for a review, see Ref. (16, 17)]. The majority of the above studies have focused on the relationship between three core intrinsic connectivity networks, suggesting that psychiatric disorders, including MDD, could be explained in part by the triple network model (18). However, there is as yet no systematic evidence for the specific abnormalities that may be associated with MDD where symptoms of insomnia coexist. Within the triple network, the salience network, which mainly involves the amygdala, the anterior insula (AI) and the dorsal anterior cingulate cortex (dACC) has recently been identified as playing an essential role in both insomnia and MDD (18, 19). The right AI within the salience network is predominantly responsible for the integration of autonomic, visceromotor, emotional and interoceptive responses (18). As a result, the salience network is postulated to mediate the emotional, vegetative and somatic aspects of depression, including sleep disturbances (20). Using simultaneous resting-state functional magnetic resonance imaging (rsfMRI) and electroencephalogram (EEG) recordings, Chen et al. (21) observed that patients with insomnia who were not depressed had increased ventral insula co-activation within the salience system when they were compared with healthy controls (HCs) at rest. Interestingly, the subjects with insomnia in Chen et al.'s study (21) had higher anxiety and depression scores than the HC group, although the scores were below clinical thresholds. The increased co-activation of the insula/salience network observed in patients with insomnia could be indicative of unconscious anxiety/depression, or of insufficient gating of sensory stimuli (22). Using an interoceptive attention task, Avery et al. (23) demonstrated a decrease in the insular activation in MDD patients, but the anxiety level in this particular MDD group was not examined. Interestingly, one of our previous studies on depressed patients with anxiety also revealed increased resting-state activity in the AI (close to the middle insula region) (24). However, Guo et al. found that there was a decrease in the short-range strength of FC in the right insula in drug-naïve MDD patients and no regional activity was observed in the insula (25, 26). So, whether increased co-activity of the AI within the salience system is related to anxiety, depression, or insomnia remains unclear; it was anticipated that analyzing regional spontaneous brain activity in MDD patients with insomnia should assist in clarifying this.

A number of techniques have been developed for the analysis of the data generated by rsfMRI, including FC, regional homogeneity (ReHo), the amplitude of low-frequency fluctuations (ALFF), and the fractional amplitude of low-frequency fluctuations (fALFF). ReHo depicts the local coherency of a given voxel to those of neighboring voxels and is limited in its usefulness between spatially distant brain domains (27). Traditional seed-based FC was initially used to measure correlations based on low-frequency fluctuating signals (28). ALFF measures the absolute strength or intensity of low-frequency oscillations and has a higher test–retest reliability in gray matter than white matter (29). ALFF has repeatedly been reported to reflect concurrent local neuronal activity (24, 30), and is an effective technique for examining the fluctuations in disease-related regional spontaneous activity strength during the resting state. It has been demonstrated to be abnormal in a number of psychiatric disorders, including MDD and bipolar disorder (27, 31).

To validate the above hypothesis, it is essential to assess whether the regional spontaneous brain activity in the salience network prevails when a comorbidity of insomnia and depression exists. Interestingly, a reduction in γ-aminobutyric acid in dACC within the salience network has been identified in both primary insomnia and MDD using single-voxel proton magnetic spectroscopy (1H-MRS) (32). As strong links between insomnia and MDD have already been established, we hypothesized that patients with comorbid insomnia and MDD would display abnormal ALFF in regional spontaneous activity, especially in the salience network. Confirmation of this will provide important information for furthering understanding of the mechanisms underlying MDD and high insomnia (MDD-HI). As individuals with MDD-HI may not necessarily be in a highly aroused or ruminative state, but would be expected to be lethargic or mindless, we hypothesized that increased right insular activity would be observed during the resting state in MDD-HI patients. We hypothesized further that these alterations may be an essential biomarker for insomnia with MDD after adjusting for anxiety and depression as a covariate. The aim of the current study was to clarify these issues and so enhance understanding of the neural mechanisms in the high-insomnia subtype of MDD.

MATERIALS AND METHODS

Participants

The present study was approved by the Research Ethics Review Board of Beijing Anding Hospital, Capital Medical University and State Key Laboratory of Cognitive Neuroscience and Learning, Beijing Normal University. After study procedures were fully explained to participants, they gave written consent before experiments were initiated.

Subsets of the data used here have been used in previous studies (24). The participants included 24 MDD-HI and 37 patients with MDD and low insomnia (MDD-LI) who were outpatients and inpatients at Beijing Anding Hospital, Capital Medical University. Also, 51 age-, gender-, education-matched, and right-handed HCs were included in the present study. All 61 participants with MDD were diagnosed by two experienced psychiatrists using the Structured Clinical Interview (SCID) for the Diagnostic and Statistical Manual for Mental Disorders, Fourth Edition (DSM-IV) (33). Sleep disturbances (consisting of inability to fall asleep, night waking, and waking too early) were evaluated using the 17-item Hamilton Depression Rating Scale (HAMD) (34, 35) and the sleep disturbance factor of the HAMD insomnia subscale, including items 4 (insomnia-early), 5 (insomnia-middle), and 6 (insomnia-late) (36–38). According to Park et al. (37), the cutoff point for MDD patients with "low insomnia" was an insomnia level ≤3 on the HAMD subscale and for "high insomnia" was an insomnia level ≥4. The baseline depressive symptoms were derived from the adjusted HAMD scores in which the scores for the sleep items (questions 4–6) were removed to measure severity of depression and to minimize any effects of sleep disturbances on severity of depression (37–40). The severity of anxiety was evaluated based on the Hamilton Anxiety Rating Scale (HAMA) (34). Participants' details are presented in **Table 1**. Inclusion criteria have been previously reported (31), with all participants: (1) 18–60 years old; (2) right handed; (3) meeting the DSM-IV diagnostic criteria for MDD; (4) no history of current serious medical or neurological illness; (5) no history of other psychiatric disorders (e.g., schizophrenia and obsessive-compulsive disorder) or an anxiety disorder (e.g., panic disorder, generalized anxiety disorder or a specific phobia); (6) no history of trauma resulting in loss of consciousness; (7) no diagnosis of dementia or developmental disorder; and (8) no history of alcohol and substance abuse or dependence. The HCs were interviewed with the non-patient edition of SCID. Exclusion criteria included the presence of any DSM-IV axis-I diagnosis, any current serious medical or neurological illness, a history of neurological or neuropsychiatric illness, a history of head trauma with loss of consciousness, and a positive history of a major psychiatric disorder, dementia, or mental retardation.

Image Acquisition

Images were acquired using a Siemens Trio 3-Tesla MRI scanner at the National Key Laboratory for Cognitive Neuroscience and Learning, Beijing Normal University, Beijing. All rsfMRI data were acquired using an echo-planar imaging (EPI) sequence with the following parameters: 33 axial slices, repetition time (TR) = 2,000 ms, echo time (TE) = 30 ms, flip angle (FA) = 90°, thickness/gap = 3.5/0.6 mm, field of view (FOV) = 220 mm^2 × 220 mm, and matrix size = 64 mm × 64 mm with 240 volumes. A resting state was defined as when subjects performed no specific cognitive tasks during scanning. All participants were instructed to be still, shut their eyes, clear their minds and not to fall asleep.

TABLE 1 | Group demographics and clinical measures.

Measure (mean ± SD)	MDD-LI (*n* = 37)	MDD-HI (*n* = 24)	HC (*n* = 51)	Statistical value	*p*-Value
Age, years	34.27 ± 11.23	41.33 ± 12.51	35.53 ± 12.53	2.69	0.07[#]
Years of education	15.11 ± 2.99	14.17 ± 2.93	15.76 ± 2.36	2.88	0.06[#]
Gender (male/female)	9/28	12/12	23/28	5.35	0.07[Δ]
Illness duration (years)	5.58 ± 6.21	9.94 ± 11.15		1.96	0.06[*]
Number of depressive episodes	2.24 ± 1.34	2.46 ± 2.06		0.49	0.62[*]
HAMD	13.57 ± 7.00	26.17 ± 6.93		6.89	<0.001[#]
Adjusted HAMD	9.24 ± 6.21	16.08 ± 5.93		4.28	<0.001[#]
HAMA	11.70 ± 7.75	20.04 ± 8.85		3.88	<0.001[#]
Sleep disturbance	2.19 ± 0.74	5.04 ± 0.91		13.45	<0.001[#]
Antidepressants	42	19			
SSRI	26	12			
SNRI	7	5			
Mirtazapine	1	0			
Trazodone	1	2			
TCA	3	0			
Flupentixol and melitracen tetracyclic	4	1			
Antipsychotics	10	2			
Quetiapine	6	2			
Resperidone	2	0			
Aripiprazole	2	0			
Benzodiazepines	3	3			
Lonazepan	1	3			
Oxazepam	2	0			
Medication-free	0	4			

Adjusted Hamilton Depression Rating Scale (HAMD) score means HAMD scores after omission of sleep questions. MDD-HI, MDD patients with high insomnia; MDD-LI, MDD patients with low insomnia; HC, healthy controls; HAMD, Hamilton Depression Rating Scale; HAMA, Hamilton Anxiety Rating Scale; SSRI, selective serotonin reuptake inhibitor; SNRI, selective serotonin and noradrenalin reuptake inhibitor; TCA, tricyclic antidepressant.

[#]p-Values for one-way ANOVA, [*]p-values for two-sample t-tests, and [Δ]p-values for chi-square test.

Image PreProcessing

Image preprocessing was performed using Data Processing Assistant and Resting-State fMRI (DPARSF) Advanced Edition[1] (41) and the Statistical Parametric Mapping software package (SPM8)[2] MATLAB (MathWorks) toolboxes. The first 10 volumes of each participant's functional time points were removed for signal stabilization to allow them to adapt to scanner noise. Slice timing and head motion correction were conducted first. Head motion was evaluated by the realigning parameters that were estimated by SPM and reported in "ExcludeSubjects.txt" in the "RealignParameter" directory. In addition the mean frame-wise displacement was calculated to measure the scrubbing-related microhead motion of each subject. The largest mean frame-wise displacement (FD, Jenkinson) of all the subjects was <0.2 mm (42). No participant was excluded from additional analysis by excessive motion criterion (>2 mm of translation or >2° of rotation in any direction) and frame-wise displacement values. Then, the structural image of each participant was coregistered to the head motion-corrected EPI image. The coregistered structural images were segmented using a unified segmentation algorithm, which significantly improved the accuracy of spatial normalization, and were then transformed into standard Montreal Neurological Institute (MNI) space. The EPI images were also spatially normalized to MNI space by applying the parameters of structural image normalization and were resampled to a voxel size of 3 mm × 3 mm × 3 mm. Finally, EPI images were spatially smoothed with a Gaussian kernel of 4-mm full width at half maximum (FWHM). In addition, linear trend removal and temporal band-pass filtering (0.01–0.08 Hz) were performed. At last, nuisance covariates, e.g., head motion parameters, global mean time courses, white matter time courses, and cerebrospinal fluid time courses were regressed out.

ALFF Map Calculation

The filtered time series of each voxel was transformed into the frequency domain using a fast Fourier transformation, and the power spectrum was obtained. The square root was calculated at each frequency of the power spectrum because the power of a given frequency is proportional to the square of the amplitude of this frequency. The averaged square root across 0.01–0.08 Hz at each voxel was taken as the ALFF. The ALFF value of each voxel was also divided by the raw mean ALFF value for standardization purposes in order to reduce the effects of variability across participants (43). The mean individual ALFF maps were analyzed statistically.

Statistical Analyses

The most updated bug-fixed version of the Resting State functional magnetic resonance imaging (fMRI) Data Analysis Toolkit AlphaSim program in AFNI for multiple comparisons (RESTplus 1.1_20160113) was used for statistical analyses. We performed one-way analysis of variance (ANOVA) across the ALFF among the three groups with sex, age, education level, adjusted HAMD, and HAMA scores as covariates. The statistically corrected threshold of $p < 0.05$ within the whole-brain mask (size, 276,133 mm^3) was determined with Monte Carlo simulations [parameters: single voxel $p = 0.01$, FWHMx = 4.575 mm, FWHMy = 4.564 mm, FWHMz = 4.508 mm, cluster size = 486 mm^3 and 1,000 iterations (44)]. For the regions showing significant differences among the three groups, we conducted further region of interest (ROI) analysis across the MDD-HI, MDD-LI and HC groups to investigate whether these regions showed abnormalities specific to insomnia or MDD. Additionally, voxel-wise Pearson's correlation analyses were performed to indicate the relationships between the ALFFs with sleep disturbance scores with age, gender, educational level, HAMA, and adjusted HAMD scores as covariates in pooled MDD patients (including both the MDD-HI and MDD-LI groups).

RESULTS

Demographic and Clinical Characteristics

In **Table 1**, the demographic details and clinical characteristics of the participants in the study are summarized. The individuals in the MDD-HI, MDD-LI, and HC groups were well matched for age, sex distribution and years in education. The adjusted HAMD, sleep disturbance, and HAMA scores were highly correlated ($r = 0.803$ and $p < 0.001$ for adjusted HAMD and sleep disturbance scores; $r = 0.842$ and $p < 0.001$ for adjusted HAMD and HAMA scores, and $r = 0.567$ and $p < 0.001$ for HAMA and sleep disturbance scores) in pooled MDD patients. Mean FD did not differ among individuals in the MDD-HI (0.080 ± 0.032), MDD-LI (0.077 ± 0.033), and HC (0.077 ± 0.033) groups in the final sample ($F[2, 110] = 0.328$, $p = 0.744$).

Differences in ALFF Values Between Groups

One-way ANOVA demonstrated that there were significant differences among the three groups ($p < 0.05$, corrected) in the right inferior frontal gyrus/anterior insula (IFG/AI), the right middle temporal gyrus, the left calcarine, and the bilateral dorsolateral prefrontal cortex (dlPFC) (**Figure 1A**; **Table 2**).

ROI-Wise ALFF Comparisons

We conducted ROI analyses within the ALFF differences among the three groups. The ALFF values of the five brain regions with significant difference in Section "Differences in ALFF Values Between Groups" were averaged, yielding an ROI-wise mean ALFF value. The MDD-HI group had significantly increased ALFF values in the right IFG/AI region ($p < 0.001$) when they were compared with the ALFF values in the MDD-LI group. The MDD-HI group had significantly increased ALFF values in the right IFG/AI ($p < 0.001$), the left dlPFC ($p < 0.001$), and the right dlPFC ($p < 0.041$) when compared with the HC group. In contrast, the MDD-LI group exhibited significantly increased ALFF values in the right middle temporal gyrus ($p < 0.001$) and the bilateral dlPFC ($p < 0.001$), as well as decreased ALFF values

[1]http://rfmri.org/DPARSF.
[2]http://www.fil.ion.ucl.ac.uk/spm.

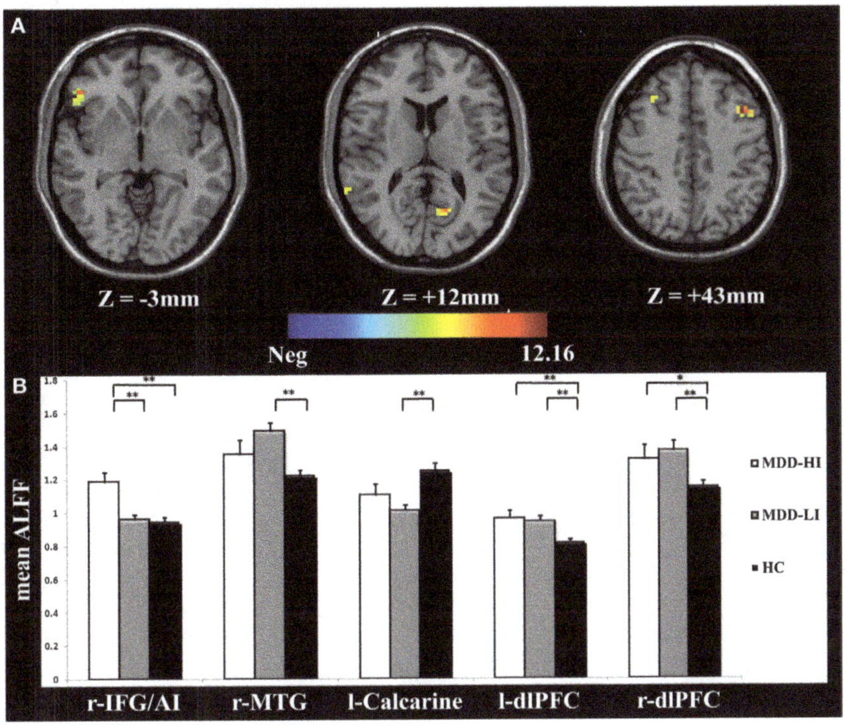

FIGURE 1 | (A) Analysis of variance (ANOVA) of the amplitude of low-frequency fluctuation (ALFF) values of the three groups with the covariates of age, gender, educational level, and adjusted Hamilton Depression Rating Scale (HAMD) scores. The color bar represents the *F*-value from ANOVA. The numbers below the images refer to the *z*-coordinates according to the Montreal Neurological Institute (MNI) atlas. The statistical threshold was set at $|F| = 4.83$ ($p = 0.01$) with a cluster size of 486 mm^3, which corresponded to an AlphaSim corrected $p < 0.05$. **(B)** The bar graphs represent mean ALFF values in each region of interest (ROI) for r-IFG/AI, r-MTG, l-Calcarine, l-dlPFC, and r-dlPFC, respectively. r-IFG/AI, right inferior frontal gyrus/anterior insula; r-MTG, right middle temporal gyrus; l-Calcarine, left calcarine; l- dlPFC, left dorsolateral prefrontal cortex; r-dlPFC, right dorsolateral prefrontal cortex.

TABLE 2 | Brain areas with significant differences in the ALFF values among three groups.

Brain regions	Side	Brodmann areas	Talairach coordinates			*K*	*F*-value
			x	*y*	*z*		
IFG/AI	R	47	51	33	−3	29	10.08
Middle temporal gyrus	R	22	63	−51	9	36	8.28
Calcarine	L		−15	−66	12	18	9.05
dlPFC	R		21	30	33	26	9.03
dlPFC	L		−39	15	42	22	12.16

ALFF, amplitude of low-frequency fluctuation; K, cluster number; IFG, inferior frontal gyrus; AI, anterior insula; dlPFC, dorsolateral prefrontal cortex.

in the left calcarine ($p < 0.001$) relative to the HC group. These results are illustrated in **Figure 1B**. More significantly, it was determined that the right IFG/AI displayed alterations that were more specific to insomnia in MDD and increased ALFF values in the bilateral dlPFC were related more in general to MDD. The mean Cohen's *d* in the right IFG/AI for MDD-HI vs. MDD-LI groups, MDD-HI vs. HC groups and MDD-LI vs. HC groups were 1.12, 1.05, and −0.03, respectively. The effect-size correlation, *ry*, in the right IFG/AI for MDD-HI vs. MDD-LI groups, MDD-HI vs. HC groups, and MDD-LI vs. HC groups were 1.12, 0.47, and −0.02, respectively.

Correlation Analyses

Voxel-wise regression analyses indicated that the increased ALFF values in the right IFG/AI (peak coordinate: 48, 33, 0) and in the right dACC (peak coordinate: 12, 30, 33) were significantly correlated with the sleep disturbance scores of pooled MDD patients (after controlling for the anxiety and adjusted depression scores; **Figure 2A**). ROI analysis confirmed that this correlation was not due to outliers (**Figure 2B**). The detailed correlation results between the ALFF measurements and the severity of sleep disturbance scores at the whole-brain level are presented in **Table 3**.

DISCUSSION

In the present study, the alterations in resting-state activity specific to insomnia in MDD were examined by comparing the changes in ALFF among subjects with MDD-HI, MDD-LI, and HC. MDD-HI patients had significantly increased ALFF values in the right IFG/AI when compared with MDD-LI patients. Furthermore, increased IFG/AI activity was correlated with the severity of insomnia symptoms after controlling for anxiety and

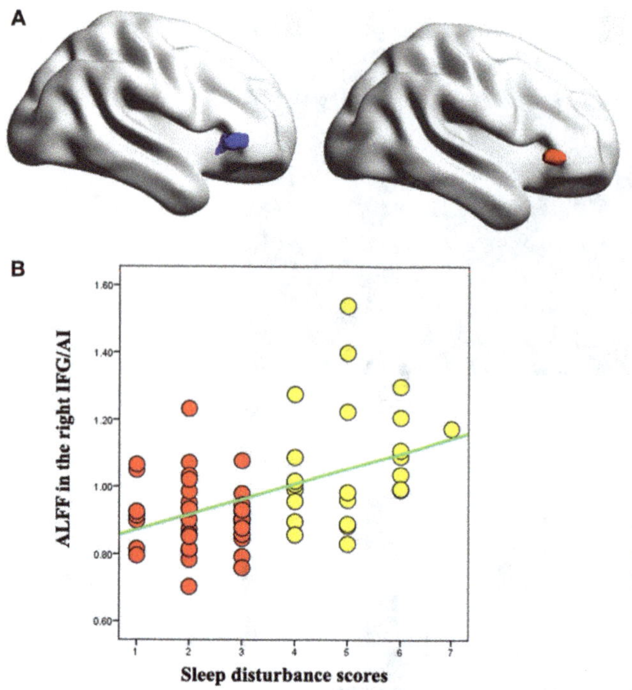

FIGURE 2 | (A) Left: voxel-wise correlation analysis between the amplitude of low-frequency fluctuation (ALFF) values and sleep disturbance scores revealed positive correlation in the right inferior frontal gyrus/anterior insula (IFG/AI) in pooled major depressive disorder (MDD) patients with high and low insomnia (peak coordinate: 48, 33, 0) with age, gender, educational level, anxiety, and adjusted depression scores as covariates (navy blue). Right: the right IFG/AI region from analysis of variance (ANOVA) of the three groups with the covariates of age, gender, educational level, and adjusted depression scores (red). The two right IFG/AI clusters obviously overlapped. **(B)** Region of interest (ROI) analysis of the correlation analysis between the right IFG/AI ALFF values and the sleep disturbance scores confirmed that the results from the whole-brain analysis were not driven by outliers. Yellow dots represent MDD patients with high insomnia, and red dots represent MDD patients with low insomnia.

TABLE 3 | Voxel-wise correlation analysis between the ALFF values and the sleep disturbance scores in pooled MDD patients including both low and high insomnia.

Brain region		Side	Talairach coordinates			Voxels	*r*	*p*
			x	*y*	*z*			
ALFF	**Positive correlation**							
	IFG/AI	Right	48	33	0	47	0.49	<0.01
	Middle cingulum	Right	12	30	33	18	0.54	<0.01

ALFF, amplitude of low-frequency fluctuation; IFG/AI, inferior frontal gyrus/anterior insula.

adjusted depression scores. More importantly, it was found that the right IFG/AI is the key node of the salience network. Taken together, the results presented here suggest that abnormalities in the salience network are profoundly involved in the sleep disturbances associated with MDD. In addition, increased ALFF values in the bilateral dlPFC were consistently demonstrated to exist in both the MDD-HI and MDD-LI groups when compared with the HC group. This suggests that increased ALFF values in the dlPFC represent the characteristic physiological change associated with MDD.

The salient network is thought to be responsible for the dynamic switching between the default mode network and the interactions of the central executive network (45), hence, the central role and relevance of the salience network in MDD has been previously described (46, 47). The salience network can be further subdivided into the dorsal and ventral salience networks (48, 49). The dorsal salience network is related to attention and the switching between cognitive resources, while the ventral system is related to emotional processing (48, 49). Likewise, the insula has been parcellated into the dorsal AI, ventral AI and posterior insula by Deen et al. (50), as in a report by Cauda et al. (51). The dorsoanterior insula is associated with cognitive processes including monitoring the interoceptive state and the ventroanterior insula is related to emotional processing (52). In the present study, MDD-HI patients had significantly increased ALFF values in the right IFG/AI relative to MDD-LI patients. The increased IFG/AI and dACC activity was correlated with the severity of the symptoms of insomnia after controlling for anxiety and the adjusted depression scores. The increased dorso-AI activity and its correlation with the severity of insomnia might indicate that the salience network may be specifically related to hyperarousal state of insomnia in patients with MDD, independently of the effects of anxiety and depression.

When combining the findings for the MDD-HI group and the MDD-LI group and comparing them to the HC group, significantly increased ALFF values in the right middle temporal gyrus and bilateral dlPFC were noted, but decreased ALFF values in the left calcarine. These results are largely consistent with the findings of Liu et al. (53), where ALFF values were investigated in 30 treatment-naïve MDD subjects. It was found that MDD patients had significantly increased ALFF values in the bilateral ventral/dorsal ACC, the left dlPFC, the left superior frontal cortex, and the left inferior parietal cortex, as well as decreased ALFF values in the bilateral occipital cortex, the cerebellum and the right superior temporal cortex. The regions affected are largely located in the cortico-limbic circuits, as demonstrated by previous authors (18, 54). Interestingly, analysis of ROI demonstrated that an increased right dlPFC ALFF value is a consistent finding across MDD groups with HI and LI. The involvement of the dlPFC in major depression has been a primary focus of previous studies. Our research group and others have demonstrated that subjects with MDD have attenuated activation or low metabolism in the dlPFC while performing cognitive tasks (55, 56). The data on the dlPFC reported here are in accordance with the general finding that dlPFC activity may be related to a depressive state and might, therefore, serve as a neuroimaging marker of MDD (57).

The HAMD sleep items evaluate three sleep periods, while the Pittsburgh Insomnia Rating Scale evaluates day time sleepiness/dysfunction. The HAMD sleep items may simplify insomnia and place less emphasis on patients with only a single dimension of insomnia, which may be the case in a quarter of MDD patients (58). Moreover, HAMD sleep items are widely recognized to be well correlated with sleep diaries (36). The Pittsburgh Insomnia Rating Scale is a more subjective rating of sleep quality including insomnia, which takes into account subjective ratings of sleep, sleep timings, and sleep duration, as well as daytime dysfunction (38). Our definition of insomnia using the three sleep questions in the HAMD has also been adopted as the main objective measure of insomnia in MDD (36). So, the definition of insomnia based on questions from the HAMD subscales can be considered to be the main objective measure of insomnia in MDD.

The present study has several limitations. First, almost none of the patients were medication-free at the time of the scans due to serious practical and ethical issues, so possible confounding effects of medication could be not ruled out. Also, as detailed lifetime data were not collected (e.g., duration of medication and dose), we could not rule out the potential impact of medication by including it as a covariate in the analyses. Given the fact that the current findings concerning depression are consistent with previous work in treatment-naïve MDD patients (59), it could be argued that the major findings of this study are valid, regardless of the medication issue. Clearly, further studies in treatment-naïve patients with and without symptoms of insomnia are necessary to confirm the current findings. A second limitation of the present study is that it did not include insomnia patients not suffering with MDD. To best clarify the underlying neural mechanisms specifically related to MDD with insomnia and to MDD without insomnia, future studies should involve a larger number of MDD patients as well as insomniacs without MDD. Third, follow-up of MDD patients is necessary to determine which are likely to develop HI. Fourth, the mean ages of the MDD-LI, MDD-HI and HC groups were 34.27 (SD = 14.6), 41.33 (SD = 12.51), and 35.53 (SD = 12.53), respectively. Although the mean age of the MDD-HI group was above that of the MDD-LI group, they were both representative of the adult population with MDD (60). Fifthly, we performed family wise error (FWE) corrected using threshold-free cluster enhancement (TFCE) in FSL (61) and multiple comparisons using false discovery rate (FDR) correction. However, the results were negative. The final limitation of the present study is that insomnia was only measured using the insomnia factor in the HAMD. Further investigations should now be conducted employing additional tools to assess insomnia and sleep, such as the Pittsburgh Insomnia Rating Scale, polysomnography, or sleep diaries to improve the accuracy of the insomnia measurements.

In summary, the key findings of the present study were increased intrinsic neural oscillation within the right IFG/AI in MDD patients with HI, which was independent of symptoms of anxiety or depression. Although we cannot rule out the influence of medication on intrinsic neural oscillations, consistent findings in the IFG/AI between the present study and previous reports in the literature suggest that there is a high possibility of the involvement of the salience network in insomnia, rather than a medication effect. Confirmation of the findings presented here will help to establish whether there is an insomnia subtype of MDD patient. The present results also extend those of previous studies and demonstrate that increased intrinsic neural oscillations in the right dlPFC during the resting state is a characteristic change in the depressive state that merits further investigation as a potential imaging marker for MDD.

AUTHOR CONTRIBUTIONS

C-HL and JG designed the study, along with S-LL, L-RT, JF, C-YW, LW, and Q-QL. C-HL, JG, S-LL, L- T, and C-YW collected the original imaging data. C-HL, JF, and LW managed and analyzed the imaging data. C-HL, L-RT, JF, C-YW, LW, and Q-QL wrote the manuscript. All authors contributed to and have approved the final manuscript.

ACKNOWLEDGMENTS

The authors gratefully acknowledge the Beijing Normal University Imaging Center for Brain Research and Prof. Yu-Feng Zang for their contributions to MRI data acquisition, Prof. Franco Cauda and Dr. Bin Jing for their assistance with the insular subregion mask.

REFERENCES

1. Whiteford HA, Degenhardt L, Rehm J, Baxter AJ, Ferrari AJ, Erskine HE, et al. Global burden of disease attributable to mental and substance use disorders: findings from the Global Burden of Disease study 2010. *Lancet* (2013) 382:1575–786. doi:10.1016/S0140-6736(13)61611-6
2. Paulus MP, Stein MB. An insular view of anxiety. *Biol Psychiatry* (2006) 60:383–7. doi:10.1016/j.biopsych.2006.03.042
3. Baglioni C, Battagliese G, Feige B, Spiegelhalder K, Nissen C, Voderholzer U, et al. Insomnia as a predictor of depression. A meta-analytic evaluation of longitudinal epidemiological studies. *J Affect Disord* (2011) 135:10–9. doi:10.1016/j.jad.2011.01.011
4. Riemann D, Voderholzer U. Primary insomnia: a risk factor to develop depression? *J Affect Disord* (2003) 76:255–9. doi:10.1016/S0165-0327(02)00072-1
5. Riemann D. Insomnia and comorbid psychiatric disorders. *Sleep Med* (2007) 8(Suppl 4):S15–20. doi:10.1016/S1389-9457(08)70004-2
6. Tsuno N, Besset A, Ritchie K. Sleep and depression. *J Clin Psychiatry* (2005) 66:1254–69. doi:10.4088/JCP.v66n1008
7. McCall WV, Reboussin BA, Cohen W. Subjective measurement of insomnia and quality of life in depressed inpatients. *J Sleep Res* (2000) 9:43–8. doi:10.1046/j.1365-2869.2000.00186.x
8. Walker MP. The role of sleep in cognition and emotion. *Ann N Y Acad Sci* (2009) 1156:168–97. doi:10.1111/j.1749-6632.2009.04416.x
9. Harvey AG. Insomnia: symptom or diagnosis? *Clin Psychol Rev* (2001) 21:1037–59. doi:10.1016/S0272-7358(00)00083-0
10. Jindal RD, Thase ME. Treatment of insomnia associated with clinical depression. *Sleep Med Rev* (2004) 8:19–30. doi:10.1016/S1087-0792(03)00025-X
11. Breslau N, Roth T, Rosenthal L, Andreski P. Sleep disturbance and psychiatric disorders: a longitudinal epidemiological study of young adults. *Biol Psychiatry* (1996) 39:411–8. doi:10.1016/0006-3223(95)00188-3
12. Chang PP, Ford DE, Mead LA, Cooper-Patrick L, Klag MJ. Insomnia in young men and subsequent depression. The Johns Hopkins Precursors study. *Am J Epidemiol* (1997) 146:105–14. doi:10.1093/oxfordjournals.aje.a009241
13. Manber R, Chambers AS. Insomnia and depression: a multifaceted interplay. *Curr Psychiatry Rep* (2009) 11:437–42. doi:10.1007/s11920-009-0066-1
14. Howland RH. Sleep interventions for the treatment of depression. *J Psychosoc Nurs Ment Health Serv* (2011) 49:17–20. doi:10.3928/02793695-20101208-01

15. Yao Z, Wang L, Lu Q, Liu H, Teng G. Regional homogeneity in depression and its relationship with separate depressive symptom clusters: a resting-state fMRI study. *J Affect Disord* (2009) 115:430–8. doi:10.1016/j.jad.2008.10.013
16. Kaiser RH, Andrews-Hanna JR, Wager TD, Pizzagalli DA. Large-scale network dysfunction in major depressive disorder: a meta-analysis of resting-state functional connectivity. *JAMA Psychiatry* (2015) 72:603–11. doi:10.1001/jamapsychiatry.2015.0071
17. Mulders PC, van Eijndhoven PF, Schene AH, Beckmann CF, Tendolkar I. Resting-state functional connectivity in major depressive disorder: a review. *Neurosci Biobehav Rev* (2015) 56:330–44. doi:10.1016/j.neubiorev.2015.07.014
18. Menon V. Large-scale brain networks and psychopathology: a unifying triple network model. *Trends Cogn Sci* (2011) 15:483–506. doi:10.1016/j.tics.2011.08.003
19. Spiegelhalder K, Regen W, Baglioni C, Nissen C, Riemann D, Kyle SD. Neuroimaging insights into insomnia. *Curr Neurol Neurosci Rep* (2015) 15:9. doi:10.1007/s11910-015-0527-3
20. Groenewold NA, Opmeer EM, de Jonge P, Aleman A, Costafreda SG. Emotional valence modulates brain functional abnormalities in depression: evidence from a meta-analysis of fMRI studies. *Neurosci Biobehav Rev* (2013) 37:152–63. doi:10.1016/j.neubiorev.2012.11.015
21. Chen MC, Chang C, Glover GH, Gotlib IH. Increased insula coactivation with salience networks in insomnia. *Biol Psychol* (2014) 97:1–8. doi:10.1016/j.biopsycho.2013.12.016
22. Hairston IS, Talbot LS, Eidelman P, Gruber J, Harvey AG. Sensory gating in primary insomnia. *Eur J Neurosci* (2010) 31:2112–21. doi:10.1111/j.1460-9568.2010.07237.x
23. Avery JA, Drevets WC, Moseman SE, Bodurka J, Barcalow JC, Simmons WK. Major depressive disorder is associated with abnormal interoceptive activity and functional connectivity in the insula. *Biol Psychiatry* (2014) 76:258–66. doi:10.1016/j.biopsych.2013.11.027
24. Liu CH, Ma X, Song LP, Fan J, Wang WD, Lv XY, et al. Abnormal spontaneous neural activity in the anterior insular and anterior cingulate cortices in anxious depression. *Behav Brain Res* (2015) 281:339–47. doi:10.1016/j.bbr.2014.11.047
25. Guo W, Liu F, Chen J, Wu R, Zhang Z, Yu M, et al. Decreased long-and short-range functional connectivity at rest in drug-naive major depressive disorder. *Aust N Z J Psychiatry* (2016) 50:763–9. doi:10.1177/0004867415617835
26. Guo W, Liu F, Yu M, Zhang J, Zhang Z, Liu J, et al. Decreased regional activity and network homogeneity of the fronto-limbic network at rest in drug-naive major depressive disorder. *Aust N Z J Psychiatry* (2015) 49:550–6. doi:10.1177/0004867415577978
27. Liu CH, Li F, Li SF, Wang YJ, Tie CL, Wu HY, et al. Abnormal baseline brain activity in bipolar depression: a resting state functional magnetic resonance imaging study. *Psychiatry Res* (2012) 203:175–9. doi:10.1016/j.pscychresns.2012.02.007
28. Guo W, Cui X, Liu F, Chen J, Xie G, Wu R, et al. Increased anterior default-mode network homogeneity in first-episode, drug-naive major depressive disorder: a replication study. *J Affect Disord* (2018) 225:767–72. doi:10.1016/j.jad.2017.08.089
29. Fox MD, Raichle ME. Spontaneous fluctuations in brain activity observed with functional magnetic resonance imaging. *Nat Rev Neurosci* (2007) 8:700–11. doi:10.1038/nrn2201
30. Zuo XN, Di Martino A, Kelly C, Shehzad ZE, Gee DG, Klein DF, et al. The oscillating brain: complex and reliable. *Neuroimage* (2010) 49:1432–45. doi:10.1016/j.neuroimage.2009.09.037
31. Liu CH, Ma X, Wu X, Fan TT, Zhang Y, Zhou FC, et al. Resting-state brain activity in major depressive disorder patients and their siblings. *J Affect Disord* (2013) 149:299–306. doi:10.1016/j.jad.2013.02.002
32. Plante DT, Jensen JE, Schoerning L, Winkelman JW. Reduced γ-aminobutyric acid in occipital and anterior cingulate cortices in primary insomnia: a link to major depressive disorder? *Neuropsychopharmacology* (2012) 37:1548–57. doi:10.1038/npp.2012.4
33. First M, Spitzer R, Gibbon M, Williams J. *Structured Clinical Interview for DSM-IV Axis I Disorders*. American Psychiatric Pub (1997).
34. Hamilton M. A rating scale for depression. *J Neurol Neurosurg Psychiatry* (1960) 23:56–62. doi:10.1136/jnnp.23.1.56
35. Kennedy SH. Core symptoms of major depressive disorder: relevance to diagnosis and treatment. *Dialogues Clin Neurosci* (2008) 10:271–7.
36. Manber R, Blasey C, Arnow B, Markowitz JC, Thase ME, Rush AJ, et al. Assessing insomnia severity in depression: comparison of depression rating scales and sleep diaries. *J Psychiatr Res* (2005) 39:481–8. doi:10.1016/j.jpsychires.2004.12.003
37. Park SC, Kim JM, Jun TY, Lee MS, Kim JB, Jeong SH, et al. Prevalence and clinical correlates of insomnia in depressive disorders: the CRESCEND study. *Psychiatry Investig* (2013) 10:373–81. doi:10.4306/pi.2013.10.4.373
38. Troxel WM, Kupfer DJ, Reynolds CF III, Frank E, Thase ME, Miewald JM, et al. Insomnia and objectively measured sleep disturbances predict treatment outcome in depressed patients treated with psychotherapy or psychotherapy-pharmacotherapy combinations. *J Clin Psychiatry* (2012) 73:478–85. doi:10.4088/JCP.11m07184
39. Trivedi MH, Bandelow B, Demyttenaere K, Papakostas GI, Szamosi J, Earley W, et al. Evaluation of the effects of extended release quetiapine fumarate monotherapy on sleep disturbance in patients with major depressive disorder: a pooled analysis of four randomized acute studies. *Int J Neuropsychopharmacol* (2013) 16:1733–44. doi:10.1017/S146114571300028X
40. Lowe A, Rajaratnam SM, Hoy K, Taffe J, Fitzgerald PB. Can sleep disturbance in depression predict repetitive transcranial magnetic stimulation (rTMS) treatment response? *Psychiatry Res* (2013) 210:121–6. doi:10.1016/j.psychres.2013.04.028
41. Chao-Gan Y, Yu-Feng Z. DPARSF. A MATLAB toolbox for "pipeline" data analysis of resting-state fMRI. *Front Syst Neurosci* (2010) 4:13. doi:10.3389/fnsys.2010.00013
42. Jenkinson M, Bannister P, Brady M, Smith S. Improved optimization for the robust and accurate linear registration and motion correction of brain images. *Neuroimage* (2002) 17:825–41. doi:10.1006/nimg.2002.1132
43. Zang YF, He Y, Zhu CZ, Cao QJ, Sui MQ, Liang M, et al. Altered baseline brain activity in children with ADHD revealed by resting-state functional MRI. *Brain Dev* (2007) 29:83–91. doi:10.1016/j.braindev.2006.07.002
44. Stein MB, Simmons AN, Feinstein JS, Paulus MP. Increased amygdala and insula activation during emotion processing in anxiety-prone subjects. *Am J Psychiatry* (2007) 164:318–27. doi:10.1176/ajp.2007.164.2.318
45. Chand GB, Dhamala M. The salience network dynamics in perceptual decision-making. *Neuroimage* (2016) 134:85–93. doi:10.1016/j.neuroimage.2016.04.018
46. Bressler SL, Menon V. Large-scale brain networks in cognition: emerging methods and principles. *Trends Cogn Sci* (2010) 14:277–90. doi:10.1016/j.tics.2010.04.004
47. Uddin LQ. Salience processing and insular cortical function and dysfunction. *Nat Rev Neurosci* (2015) 16:55–61. doi:10.1038/nrn3857
48. Touroutoglou A, Bliss-Moreau E, Zhang J, Mantini D, Vanduffel W, Dickerson BC, et al. A ventral salience network in the macaque brain. *Neuroimage* (2016) 132:190–7. doi:10.1016/j.neuroimage.2016.02.029
49. Touroutoglou A, Hollenbeck M, Dickerson BC, Feldman Barrett L. Dissociable large-scale networks anchored in the right anterior insula subserve affective experience and attention. *Neuroimage* (2012) 60:1947–58. doi:10.1016/j.neuroimage.2012.02.012
50. Deen B, Pitskel NB, Pelphrey KA. Three systems of insular functional connectivity identified with cluster analysis. *Cereb Cortex* (2011) 21:1498–506. doi:10.1093/cercor/bhq186
51. Cauda F, Costa T, Torta DM, Sacco K, D'Agata F, Duca S, et al. Meta-analytic clustering of the insular cortex: characterizing the meta-analytic connectivity of the insula when involved in active tasks. *Neuroimage* (2012) 62:343–55. doi:10.1016/j.neuroimage.2012.04.012
52. Liu CH, Jing B, Ma X, Xu PF, Zhang Y, Li F, et al. Voxel-based morphometry study of the insular cortex in female patients with current and remitted depression. *Neuroscience* (2014) 262:190–9. doi:10.1016/j.neuroscience.2013.12.058
53. Liu J, Ren L, Womer FY, Wang J, Fan G, Jiang W, et al. Alterations in amplitude of low frequency fluctuation in treatment-naïve major depressive disorder measured with resting-state fMRI. *Hum Brain Mapp* (2014) 35:4979–88. doi:10.1002/hbm.22526
54. Fitzgerald PB, Laird AR, Maller J, Daskalakis ZJ. A meta-analytic study of changes in brain activation in depression. *Hum Brain Mapp* (2008) 29:683–95. doi:10.1002/hbm.20426
55. Halari R, Simic M, Pariante CM, Papadopoulos A, Cleare A, Brammer M, et al. Reduced activation in lateral prefrontal cortex and anterior cingulate during attention and cognitive control functions in medication-naïve adolescents with depression compared to controls. *J Child Psychol Psychiatry* (2009) 50:307–16. doi:10.1111/j.1469-7610.2008.01972.x

56. Wagner G, Sinsel E, Sobanski T, Köhler S, Marinou V, Mentzel HJ, et al. Cortical inefficiency in patients with unipolar depression: an event-related FMRI study with the Stroop task. *Biol Psychiatry* (2006) 59:958–65. doi:10.1016/j.biopsych.2005.10.025
57. Wang L, Krishnan KR, Steffens DC, Potter GG, Dolcos F, McCarthy G. Depressive state- and disease-related alterations in neural responses to affective and executive challenges in geriatric depression. *Am J Psychiatry* (2008) 165:863–71. doi:10.1176/appi.ajp.2008.07101590
58. Sunderajan P, Gaynes BN, Wisniewski SR, Miyahara S, Fava M, Akingbala F, et al. Insomnia in patients with depression: a STAR*D report. *CNS Spectr* (2010) 15:394–404. doi:10.1017/S1092852900029266
59. Adamo D, Ruoppo E, Leuci S, Aria M, Amato M, Mignogna MD. Sleep disturbances, anxiety and depression in patients with oral lichen planus: a case-control study. *J Eur Acad Dermatol Venereol* (2005) 29:291–7. doi:10.1111/jdv.12525
60. Kok RM, Reynolds CF III. Management of depression in older adults: a review. *JAMA* (2017) 317:2114–22. doi:10.1001/jama.2017.5706
61. Smith SM, Nichols TE. Threshold-free cluster enhancement: addressing problems of smoothing, threshold dependence and localisation in cluster inference. *Neuroimage* (2009) 44:83–98. doi:10.1016/j.neuroimage.2008.03.061

21

Weighted Random Support Vector Machine Clusters Analysis of Resting-State fMRI in Mild Cognitive Impairment

Xia-an Bi[1*], *Qian Xu*[1], *Xianhao Luo*[2], *Qi Sun*[1] *and Zhigang Wang*[1]

[1] *College of Information Science and Engineering, Hunan Normal University, Changsha, China,* [2] *College of Mathematics and Statistics, Hunan Normal University, Changsha, China*

Correspondence:
Xia-an Bi
bixiaan@hnu.edu.cn

The identification of abnormal cognitive decline at an early stage becomes an increasingly significant conundrum to physicians and is of major interest in the studies of mild cognitive impairment (MCI). Support vector machine (SVM) as a high-dimensional pattern classification technique is widely employed in neuroimaging research. However, the application of a single SVM classifier may be difficult to achieve the excellent classification performance because of the small-sample size and noise of imaging data. To address this issue, we propose a novel method of the weighted random support vector machine cluster (WRSVMC) in which multiple SVMs were built and different weights were given to corresponding SVMs with different classification performances. We evaluated our algorithm on resting state functional magnetic resonance imaging (RS-fMRI) data of 93 MCI patients and 105 healthy controls (HC) from the Alzheimer's Disease Neuroimaging Initiative (ADNI) cohort. The maximum accuracy given by the WRSVMC is 87.67%, demonstrating excellent diagnostic power. Furthermore, the most discriminative brain areas have been found out as follows: gyrus rectus (REC.L), precentral gyrus (PreCG.R), olfactory cortex (OLF.L), and middle occipital gyrus (MOG.R). These findings of the paper provide a new perspective for the clinical diagnosis of MCI.

Keywords: mild cognitive impairment, weighted random support vector machine cluster, classification, abnormal brain areas, resting-state fMRI

INTRODUCTION

Mild cognitive impairment (MCI) is a clinical entity which represents a state of slightly cognitive deficits for age and education, but does not markedly affect activities of daily life (1, 2). Studies show that healthy controls (HC) convert to Alzheimer's disease (AD) at an annual rate of 1–2% (3). Nevertheless, the rate of MCI patients who progress to AD is between 10 and 15% per year (4), implying that MCI may be a high-risk state for developing AD dementia. At present, there is no exact therapy which could completely stop or reverse the progression of AD (5). It is hence crucial to identify MCI patients and explore pathological changes in their brains, in order to offer timely treatment and slow down the transition from MCI to AD.

Neuroimaging techniques play increasingly important roles in the investigation of brain dysfunctions of MCI patients (6). In particular, the resting-state functional magnetic resonance imaging (RS-fMRI) may be one of the most popular brain imaging techniques due to its numerous advantages (7). On the one hand, RS-fMRI has higher spatial resolution than electroencephalogram (EEG) (8). On the other hand, RS-fMRI is noninvasive compared to position emission tomography (PET) and computed tomography (CT) (9). In addition, RS-fMRI is easier to implement without requiring specific tasks when compared to task-state fMRI (10). The application of RS-fMRI could help to enhance the understanding of spontaneous brain activities of MCI patients.

Graph theory is a reliable approach which offers a suitable framework for the study of brain neural network at a whole-brain connectivity level (11, 12). The literature on graph theory reports that MCI patients compared to HC show the altered functional connectivity (FC) and a clear disrupted topological pattern in the brain network (13, 14). Therefore, the graph theory metrics may possess predictive information that helps to classify MCI patients from HC. It is a promising approach that the discriminative graph theory metrics are considered as predictor features to build a classifier for excellent classification performance (15, 16).

Support vector machine (SVM) has been widely utilized for analysis of neuroimaging data to assist the identification of MCI (17). Zhang et al. (18) employed a linear SVM and achieved a classification accuracy of 79.02% for 346 MCI vs. 207 HC. Yu et al. (19) achieved an accuracy of 79.65% when using the SVM with leave-one-out cross validation to classify 170 patients with MCI from 169 HC. Zhang and Shen (20) reported an accuracy of 83.2% using the multi-modal SVM to discriminate between 91 MCI patients and 50 HC. Beheshti et al. (21) used the SVM classifier to yield a classification accuracy of 70.38% when distinguishing 87 MCI patients and 61 HC. Li et al. (22) achieved an accuracy of 77.4% for 99 MCI vs. 52 HC using the SVM. Because these MCI studies above usually considered a single SVM which may not be robust enough in dealing with neuroimaging data, the classification accuracies reported by the studies were universally lower than 85%.

To improve the accuracy and robustness of the classification algorithm, a novel approach of weighted random support vector machine cluster (WRSVMC) was put forward in this paper. Compared to a single SVM classifier, the WRSVMC has the following advantages: (1) The WRSVMC is robust because it consists of a great deal of SVM classifiers; (2) The classification accuracy of the WRSVMC is improved because the influences of strong SVM base classifiers are enhanced by a weighted method; (3) The abnormal brain areas could be found out using the WRSVMC based on the optimal subset of features; (4) The WRSVMC achieves an high accuracy of 87.67%, indicating that the abnormal brain areas which we have found were considerably convincing. In the process of exploring the abnormal brain areas, brain areas are ranked in accordance with the amount of discriminative information. We mainly discussed the first four brain areas as follows: gyrus rectus (REC.L), precentral gyrus (PreCG.R), olfactory cortex (OLF.L) and middle occipital gyrus (MOG.R). The gyrus rectus is considered to be a newly discovered abnormal brain area in patients with MCI because it is rarely studied in neuroimaging literature on MCI. The remaining three abnormal brain areas are consistent with the claims in existing literature involving MCI (23–25). In a word, these findings help us to understand the underlying pathologic mechanisms of MCI.

MATERIALS AND METHODS

Demographic Information

The publicly available RS-fMRI data was obtained from Alzheimer's Disease Neuroimaging Initiative (ADNI) cohort (http://adni.loni.usc.edu/) (26) whose primary goal was to study the pathogenesis and treatment of MCI and AD by exploring multifarious imaging data (27). We initially collected 231 subjects' RS-fMRI data, including 93 MCI patients and 138 HC. 33 HC were excluded due to excessive head movements during the preprocessing, leaving 93 MCI patients (48 males and 45 females) and 105 HC (42 males and 63 females) for further analysis. We used Chi-squared test and found no significant discrepancy between the MCI patients and HC with respect to sex ($\chi^2 = 2.683$, $p = 0.101$). All data was anonymized according to the Health Insurance Portability and Accountability (HIPAA) guidelines, and followed the research procedures and ethical guidelines determined by the Institutional Review Boards (IRB) of the participating agencies.

Data Acquisition

All participants were imaged on a Siemens TRIO 3 Tesla machine. Resting state functional images were acquired using the scanning parameters as bellow: repetition time (TR) = 3,000 ms, echo time (TE) = 30 ms, pixel spacing X/pixel spacing Y = 3.3/3.3 mm, acquisition matrix = 64×64, flip angle = 80, axial slices = 48, slice thickness = 3.313 mm, without slice gap, 140 time points. During the RS-fMRI scanning, all subjects should lie still and close their eyes without thinking of anything systematically.

Data Preprocessing

Image preprocessing was carried out by employing the Data Processing Assistant for Resting State fMRI (DPARSF) (www.restfmri.net) software. Briefly, the preprocessing steps were as bellow: converting data from DICOM to NIFTI format; discarding the first 10 volumes due to magnetization instability; correcting for time offset between slices; correcting for head motion between volumes; normalizing data with the echo-planar imaging (EPI) template; spatial smoothing using a Gaussian kernel with the full width-half maximum (FWHM) = 6 mm; linear de-trending; performing band-pass filtering (0.01–0.08 Hz); regressing out several spurious variables.

The Application of Graph Theory

Graph theory is an ideal approach to investigate the characteristics of the complex brain functional connectivity (FC) network. The application of graph theory is likely to help to improve the understanding of neural activities in the diseased and healthy human brain. In our experiment, we utilized the internationally common anatomical automatic labeling (AAL) atlases (28) to define the regions of interest (ROIs). Both the left and right brains could be divided into 45 ROIs, resulting in 90 ROIs. Each ROI is defined as a node in brain FC network. The time series of all voxels within each of ROIs are averaged to obtain the mean time series of each ROI, and the Pearson correlation coefficients are computed between each pair of mean time series. Therefore, a 90×90 FC network is constructed. Then a cut-off value in the range of $[0, 1]$ is applied to FC

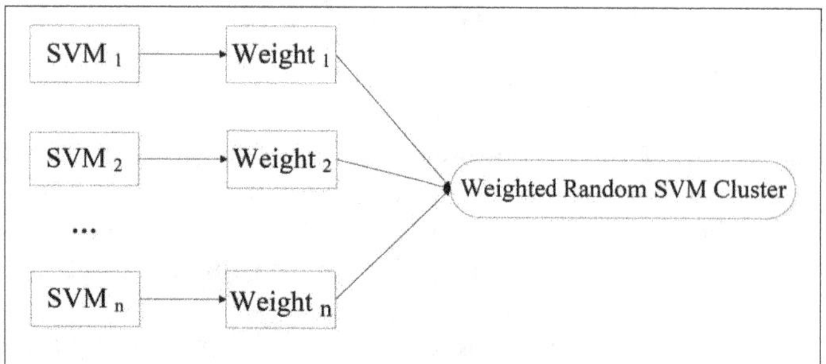

FIGURE 1 | The idea of WRSVMC.

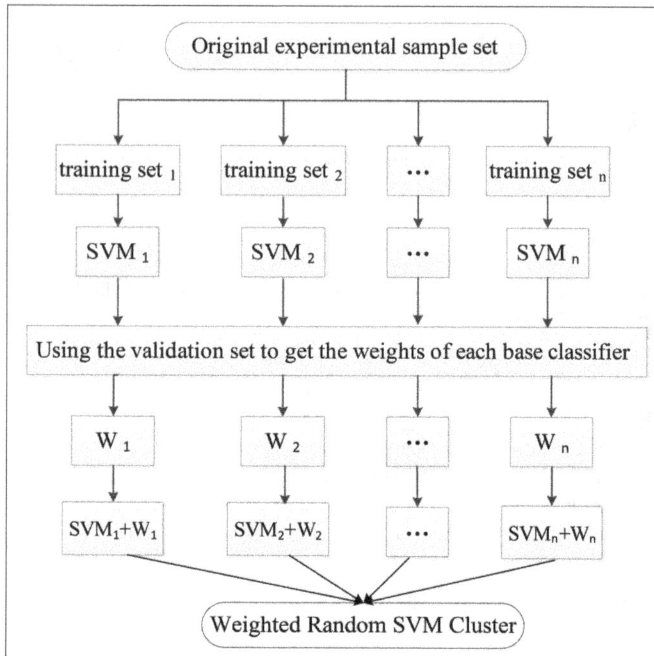

FIGURE 2 | The training process of the WRSVMC.

network to get binary undirected graph. Specifically, the weight of the edge is 1 if there is an edge between two nodes, otherwise the weight is 0.

In this paper, the following graph theory metrics in the binary undirected graph are considered: degree, local efficiency, shortest path and clustering coefficient. These graph metrics are supported to be significantly different between the brain connectivity networks of HC and MCI patients (29–31). For each subject, 90 degrees, 4,005 shortest paths, 90 local efficiencies and 90 clustering coefficients are obtained and they are then utilized as classification features for subsequent experiments.

The Weighted Random SVM Cluster

The Design of the WRSVMC

Machine learning techniques are widely utilized for pattern recognition, among which the SVM model shows excellent performance in classifying high-dimensional neuroimaging data (32). However, only a single SVM is not stable and there is a general problem of low classification accuracy for it. Bi et al. (33) proposed the random SVM cluster (RSVMC) which showed better generalization performance compared to a single SVM classifier. However, it is noteworthy that the performance of a single SVM classifier built in RSVMC may be considerably different. The RSVMC adopts a simple voting rule that the same weights are assigned to different SVMs, ignoring the differences between strong classifiers and weak classifiers. Therefore, there is still room for the improvement of the RSVMC algorithm.

We put forward a novel approach of WRSVMC in this paper. Different weights are calculated for different SVM classifiers. The higher the SVM's accuracy is, the greater weight the SVM gets. As a result, the influences of the base classifiers with excellent classification performances are enhanced during the voting process, promoting the discriminative ability of the WRSVMC. **Figure 1** exhibits the idea of our proposed WRSVMC.

In the first stage, the experimental sample set is split into the "training and validation" set and the test set. Then, the training process is followed. Specifically, a part of the samples are randomly selected from the "training and validation" set as the training set, and some features are randomly chosen from all features to construct a SVM classifier. The remaining validation set is used to calculate the single SVM's classification accuracy which is used as its weight. The training process is repeated for n times to obtain n SVM classifiers with weights, resulting in a WRSVMC which is more robust and accurate. **Figure 2** describes the training process of the WRSVMC.

The WRSVMC could be used to forecast the class label of each test sample. Firstly, each test sample is fed into a WRSVMC classifier, and the amount of votes for each sample's label is weighted. The total amount of votes belonging to class a is denoted as S_a

$$S_a = \sum_{i=1}^{n} \mathrm{I}(f_i(x) = a) \times W_i \tag{1}$$

where x represents a sample in the test set; $f_i(x)$ is the class label predicted by i-th SVM based on the test sample; $(\cdot)$ is the indicator function which takes values 0 and 1. If the test sample is predicted to be class a, the value equals to 1; otherwise, the value equals to 0.

Then the final predicted label A of the test sample is represented by the label with the maximum total amount of votes.

$$A = \mathrm{Arg\ max}(S_a) \tag{2}$$

By comparing the predicted label with the actual label, we could get the number of test samples that were correctly classified, denoted as T_{true}. The classification accuracy P_{true} of the WRSVMC is given by:

$$P_{true} = \frac{T_{true}}{T} \tag{3}$$

where T is the number of samples in the test set.

The Classification of the WRSVMC

It is assumed that there are a total of N samples collected, of which N_1 is the number of HC and N_2 is that of MCI patients, where $N = N_1 + N_2$. Each sample has $4,275$ $(90 + 4,005 + 90 + 90)$ dimensional features, then marking the label of MCI patients as $+1$ and that of HC as -1. One of our tasks is to discriminate between MCI patients and HC based on 4,275 features.

First, 198 samples from ADNI cohort are split into 125 samples as the "training and validation" set and 73 samples as the test set. Next, 65 training samples are chosen from the "training and validation" set, and 65 features are picked out from 4,275 dimensional features to train a single SVM classifier. The cost parameter c for each SVM classifier is set to Inf, and the radial basis function (RBF) kernel is selected with a bandwidth σ of 3. Then, the remaining validation set is used to calculate the SVM's classification accuracy, which represents the weight of corresponding SVM. This training process is repeated for 500 times in the experiment.

The 73 test samples are put into the WRSVMC and each of 500 SVMs votes at the same time. The amount of votes for each SVM should be its weight, thus avoiding the disadvantages of voting with equal rights. The results of 500 SVMs are calculated and the class with the maximum total amount of votes is considered as the predicted class of the new sample. The number of the new samples that are correctly classified is divided by 73, which represents the classification performance of the WRSVMC.

The amount of base classifiers in the WRSVMC is initially set to 500. In general, with expansion of the amount of SVM classifiers, the WRSVMC could converge to lower generalization errors. But excessive SVM classifiers also increase experimental training time and even lead to overfitting. Therefore, the different amounts of SVM classifiers need to be tested. We use the classification accuracy of the WRSVMC as a guideline to decide the optimal amount of SVM classifiers in the WRSVMC.

Feature Selection of the WRSVMC

Each SVM randomly selects features, resulting in different classification performances. However, the SVMs with high performances make more contributions to the performance of the WRSVMC. We extract the features of the above-mentioned SVMs and thus obtain the important features of the WRSVMC. Details are as follows.

Firstly, the 73 unseen samples are utilized to evaluate the performance of each of 500 weighted SVM classifiers. The SVMs with classification accuracies above 50% are considered to be effective classifiers and these SVMs would be retained in the WRSVMC. Then the value of each feature of the selected SVMs is multiplied by the corresponding weight as the score of the feature, denoted as $Score_{i,j}$:

$$Score_{i,j} = \sum_{k=1}^{T} H_{k,j} \times W_i \quad (4)$$

where $H_{k,j}$ represents the j-th feature value of the k-th test sample.

The scores of the same feature are accumulated and the features ranking in the top 400 in terms of total scores are considered as important features (as shown in **Figure 3**).

$$\text{Score}_j = \sum_{i=1}^{n} \text{Score}_{i,j} \quad (5)$$

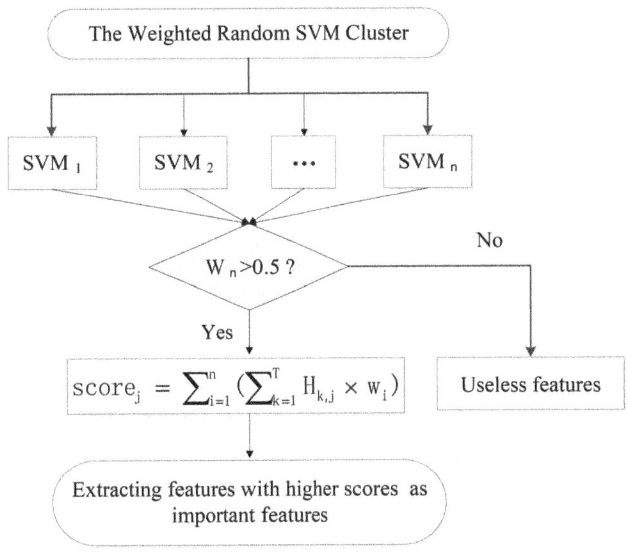

FIGURE 3 | The extraction of important features.

Feature selection is conducted because of the fact that some input features are redundant and less relevant for the WRSVMC. Specifically, the 65 dimensional features are randomly chosen from the top p features of the 400 important features to perform the WRSVMC. We select a value for p from the set $\{70, 72, \cdots, 400\}$. The classification performance of the WRSVMC is regarded as a guideline to find the optimal p in the experiment. The feature set of the top p features extracted from the 400 important features of the WRSVMC with the highest performance is considered as the optimal subset of features. As a result, the most discriminative features are chosen and meanwhile the redundant features are excluded.

In this study, we utilize the optimal subset of features to explore the most discriminative brain areas. Firstly, we detect the brain areas corresponding to each optimal feature. Then the brain areas are ranked in accordance with the frequencies of brain areas. The higher the frequency is, the more abnormal the brain area becomes.

RESULTS

The Performances of WRSVMC

Figure 4 shows three boxplots comparing the generalization performances of the WRSVMC, RSVMC (33) and a non-SVM classifier, i.e., random forest (RF) which is an ensemble learner and has considerably wide applications in neuroimaging data. The box plots refer to the results of 50 experiments which perform these three classification algorithm respectively. It can be seen from the **Figure 4** that the WRSVMC reports the comparatively higher classification accuracies in the range of 75–85% compared to the RSVMC with the range of 70–80% and the RF with the range of 70–78%. The maximum accuracy of the WRSVMC that we put forward is higher, and the overall performance is better.

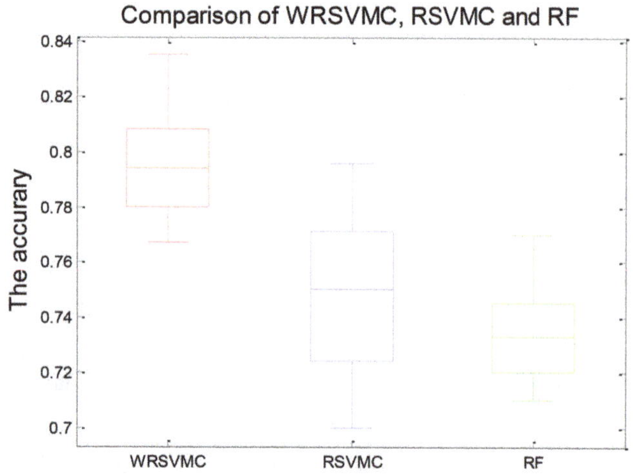

FIGURE 4 | The generalization performance of the WRSVMC, RSVMC, and RF.

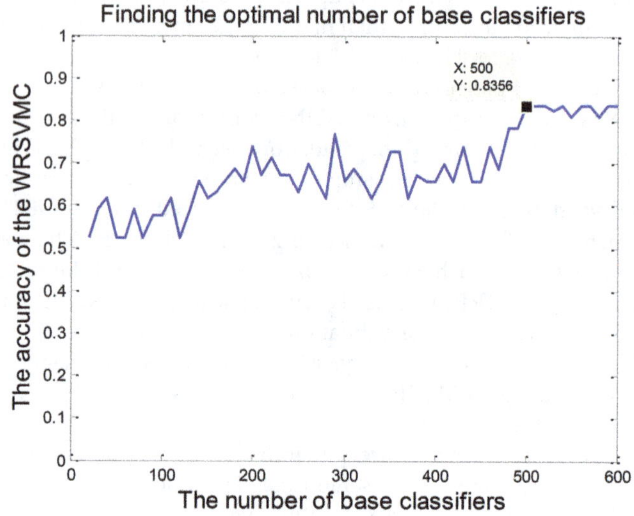

FIGURE 5 | The optimal amount of SVM classifiers.

TABLE 1 | The statistical significance of results between the algorithms.

Classifiers (Mean ± SD)	WRSVMC	RSVMC	RF	*P*-value
Accuracy (%)	0.80 ± 0.02	0.75 ± 0.03	0.73 ± 0.02	0.000[a]/0.000[b]

[a] *The P-value of the two-sample t-test between the WRSVMC and RSVMC.*
[b] *The P-value of the two-sample t-test between the WRSVMC and RF.*

TABLE 2 | The features with higher scores.

Score (rounded)	Feature
13	ORBinf.L-IOGL
12	IFGoperc.L-PCL.R PHG.L- LING.L PAL.L- MTG.L HIP.L -PCL.R SMG.R- TPOsup.L
11	REC.L- PHG.L SPG.R- MTG.R LING.L- HES.L SMG.L- ITG.L SMA.R- CAL.L ORBinf.L- ROL.R

Table 1 exhibits the statistical significance of results between the WRSVMC and other two methods. The two-sample *t*-test is conducted to examine the differences of the WRSVMC/RSVMC and WRSVMC/RF respectively and the *P*-values are close to 0.00 and 0.00, which indicates that the differences between the WRSVMC and other two classification methods are statistical significance. In addition, the complexities of these three ensemble classifiers depend on the number n of the base classifiers. Accordingly, all the complexities of the three algorithms are $O(n)$. In a word, the experimental results show that our new WRSVMC is highly effective and stable.

The Optimal Amount of Base Classifiers

The amount of SVM classifiers in the WRSVMC with the minimum classification error is regarded as the optimal amount of SVM classifiers. In the first place, we gradually adjust the amount of SVMs from 20 to 600, with a step size of 10. Then, the classification performances of the WRSVMC with different amounts of SVMs are calculated. It can be seen from **Figure 5** that our proposed WRSVMC based on all the original features achieves a maximum accuracy of 83.56%, and it becomes stable at the stage where the amount of the SVM classifier is 500. Therefore, 500 is selected to be the optimal amount of the SVM base classifiers.

The Important Features

The important features should make important influences on the WRSVMC. We employ the score to measure the influence of each feature, and finally extract the features ranking in the top 400 in terms of scores as important features. **Table 2** shows the features whose scores are rounded to 13, 12, and 11 sequentially. All of the features listed are the shortest paths between two ROIs, indicating that shortest path makes greater contribution to classification compared to other graph theory metrics. The features with the scores rounded to 13 or 12 are the shortest paths between ORBinf.L and IOG.L, IFGoperc.L and PCL.R, ORBinf.L and IOG.L, PHG.L and LING.L, PAL.L and MTG.L, HIP.L and PCL.R, SMG.R, and TPOsup.L respectively.

The Optimal Subset of Features

Feature selection is performed for exploring the optimal subset of features from 400 "important features" to further enhance the final performance. The optimal p ($70 \leq p \leq 400$) could be found when the WRSVMC using the features set which consists of the top p features achieves the highest performance. As shown in **Figure 6**, the WRSVMC reports the highest accuracy of 87.67% when p is 270. Hence, the optimal subset of features comprises the top 270 dimensional features. At the same time, the WRSVMC achieves a sensitivity of 91.67% and specificity of 83.78% based on the most discriminative features. These features are used to explore the corresponding brain areas in the next experiment.

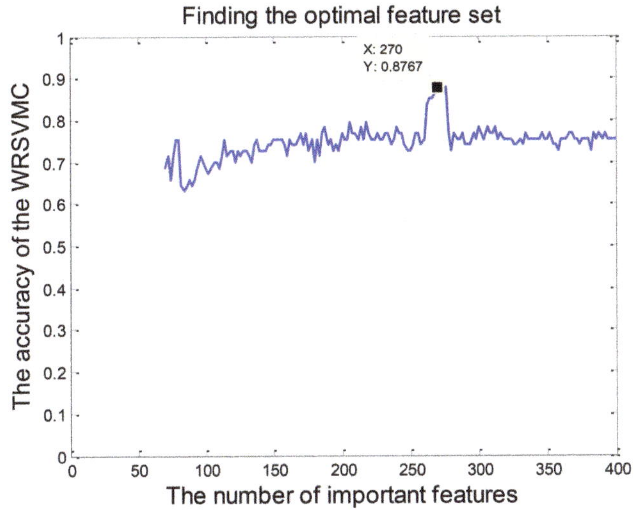

FIGURE 6 | The number of optimal features.

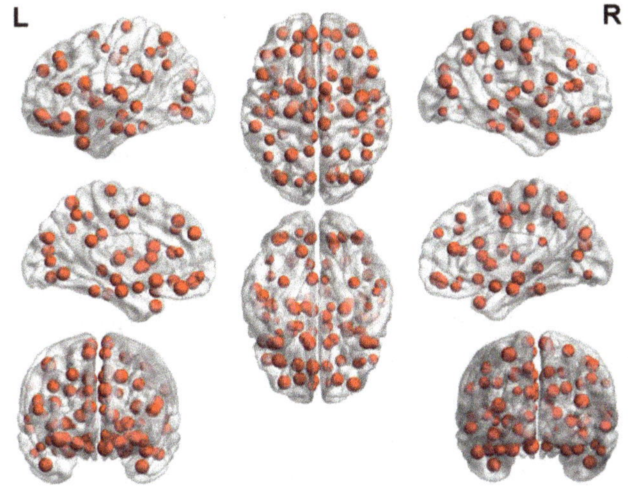

FIGURE 7 | The frequency of each brain area.

The Abnormal Brain Areas

Figure 7 depicts the locations of ROIs. Each node in the graph represents a ROI. The higher the frequency is, the larger the node becomes. The specific frequencies for some discriminative ROIs are shown in **Table 3**. The brain areas corresponding to the optimal subset of features with relatively higher frequecnies (11, 10 and 9) are as bellow: gyrus rectus (REC.L), precentral gyrus (PreCG.R), olfactory cortex (OLF.L), middle occipital gyrus (MOG.R), median cingulate and paracingulate gyri (DCG.L), superior parietal gyrus (SPG.L), inferior frontal gyrus (IFGoperc.L) and middle frontal gyrus (ORBmid.R).

DISCUSSION

Classification Effect

In this paper, we combine RS-fMRI with the graph theory, and put forward a novel approach of WRSVMC to accurately distinguish MCI patients and HC. RS-fMRI is a reliable tool in mapping the brain FC networks due to its high-spatial resolution and noninvasive. Graph theory represents a powerful framework for the study of complex brain network properties. Furthermore, to the best of our knowledge, the WRSVMC is first applied to the neuroimaging data, which may be of great impact on neuroimaging research. The WRSVMC not only achieves a high accuracy of 87.67% (as shown in **Figure 6**), but also is employed to facilitate the detection of abnormal brain areas, which provides valuable insight into the diagnosis of MCI.

The SVM as a high-dimensional pattern classification technique has attracted more and more attention recently and has been showed to be an effective approach for the identification of MCI patients using medical imaging data. Zhang et al. (34) employed a multi-kernel SVM (MK-SVM) method for 91 MCI vs. 50 HC classifications and achieved an accuracy of 76.4%. Granziera et al. (35) used the SVM classifier to reach an accuracy of 75% when separating 42 MCI and 77 HC. Ye et al. (36) adopted the MK-SVM method fusing multi-modality data and achieved an accuracy of 82.13% discriminating between 52 HC and 99 MCI patients. Long et al. (37) reported an accuracy of 82.8% using the SVM based identification algorithm to classify 64 MCI patients from 60 HC. The performance metrics, e.g., accuracy, sensitivity and specificity of these SVM algorithms are listed in **Table 4**.

Most of the single SVM algorithms dealing with neuroimaging data possess the low classification accuracy because of the small number of samples and image noise. In addition, plenty of researches only focus on classification and rarely study abnormal brain regions associated with MCI. To address these problems, we innovatively propose the WRSVMC which represents the weighted ensemble of individual SVM, and produces better classification performance compared to a single SVM classifier. Feature selection is a crucial stage to deal with large-size feature vectors based on the graph theory metrics in our proposed WRSVMC algorithm. Specifically, we utilize the score to assess the influence of each input feature, and extract the top 400 features as the important features. Then, the classification performance of the WRSVMC is considered as a criterion to explore the optimal subset of features from the 400 important features. Finally, we utilize the optimal subset of features to search the corresponding brain areas which are mapped in **Figure 7**. The high accuracy of 87.67% (as shown in **Figure 6**) given by the WRSVMC suggests that the abnormal brain areas that we have found are considerably convincing.

In the process of building a WRSVMC, the training set is randomly selected from all the data and the features are randomly chosen from all the features, reflecting the randomness of the WRSVMC. As a result, each SVM classifier is considerably differentiated due to the random samples and random features, which could ensure that there is no overfitting issue during the training procedure of the proposed WRSVMC method to some extent. In addition, the WRSVMC works well on the test

TABLE 3 | The brain areas with higher frequency.

Frequency	Brain area
11	REC.L
10	PreCG.R OLF.L
9	MOG.R DCG.L SPG.L IFGoperc.L ORBmid.R
8	SFGdor.L ORBmid.L SMA.R SFGmed.L INS.R ACG.R DCG.R HIP.R PHG.L PHG.R PCL.R PUT.L HES.L TPOsup.L

TABLE 4 | The performance of our WRSVMC and existing SVM algorithm.

Author	Method	Accuracy(%)	Sensitivity(%)	Specificity(%)
(34)	MK-SVM	76.4	81.8	66
(35)	SVM	75	60	83
(36)	MK-SVM	82.13	87.68	71.54
(37)	SVM	83.1	82.8	83.3
This paper	WRSVMC	87.67	91.67	83.78

set, which demonstrates an excellent generalization performance, implying a very low possibility of overfitting.

In the experiment, some initial parameter values are set to build the WRSVMC. We now discuss whether these parameter values are appropriate. On the one hand, the cost parameter c for each SVM is set to *Inf* and the RBF kernel with a bandwidth σ of 3 is chosen. Although we artificially select these specific parameter values, we test other parameter values and find no considerable differences with respect to the classification accuracy of the WRSVMC, which indicates that the WRSVMC is stable and universal. On the other, a cut-off value of 0.25 is employed for the brain FC network. When a larger cut-off value is given, the network turns into more granular and fragmented. We conduct a grid search of different cut-off values and find that the optimal cut-off value is still 0.25.

Analysis of the Brain Areas With Higher Frequencies

Our findings suggest that abnormal brain areas associated with MCI mainly involve in gyrus rectus, olfactory cortex, precentral gyrus, and middle occipital gyrus. Next, detailed analysis of these brain areas was discussed.

Gyrus Rectus

The gyrus rectus possesses the highest frequency compared to other ROIs, which indicates that the gyrus rectus makes a great contribution to our WRSVMC algorithm.

The gyrus rectus is located in the frontal lobe's basal surface (38). The frontal lobe plays an important part in executive function, memory, decision-making and so on Fang et al. (39). Hence, the gyrus rectus may associate with cognitive and memory functions. Joo et al. (40) reported that the gyrus rectus resection had a temporary negative influence on memory recall and language. Qiu et al. (41) showed that the gyrus rectus played a vital role in efficient communications. Kristine et al. (42) found that the gyrus rectus was crucial to inhibit improper behavior. Georgiopoulos et al. (43) reported that the gyrus rectus may be relevant to executive function.

A great deal of previous literature showed that Alzheimer's disease (AD) was linked to abnormal gyrus rectus (44, 45). However, little was known about the relationship between MCI and abnormal gyrus rectus. Neuroimaging literature has shown that MCI is a precursor to AD (46, 47), indicating that MCI patients may have the certain gyrus rectus abnormality which is found in patients with AD. In this paper, we considered gurus rectus to be a newly discovered abnormal brain area in patients with MCI due to the highest frequency. Bahar-Fuchs et al. (48) found out considerable amyloid-β burden in gyrus rectus region of amnestic MCI patients compared to HC, which supported our findings to some extents.

The abnormal gyrus rectus is likely to bring about deficits in executive and cognitive functions and lead to memory loss in patients with MCI. The discovery of this new abnormal brain area provides a new perspective for the clinical diagnosis and intervention of MCI.

Olfactory Cortex

The olfactory cortex obtains a relatively high frequency which suggests that the olfactory cortex plays a decisive role in our WRSVMC method.

The olfactory cortex refers to the classical cellular structure of nervous cortex, which is primarily involved in associative learning and memory (49). Yaniv et al. (50) observed the changes in the olfactory (piriform) cortex in the odor memory task. Daniels et al. (51) found out the crucial role of the olfactory cortex in emotional memory processing. Stone et al. (52) reported that the stimulation of olfactory cortex led to enhanced spatial memory. Goto et al. (53) showed that the verbal memory function had a positive correlation with the olfactory cortex volume.

The abnormal olfactory cortex was observed in numerous MCI studies. Zhang et al. (54) found out the disrupted connectivity between the right olfactory cortex and other hub areas in patients with amnestic MCI. Kirova et al. (55) mentioned that MCI patients showed neurofibrillary tau tangles and amyloid plaques in the olfactory cortex. Risacher et al. (24) found that olfactory cortex's *in vivo* activation was lessened in MCI patients. Vasavada et al. (56) observed the alterations of olfactory cortex activity in patients with MCI. Guzman et al. (57) discovered that olfactory cortex and hippocampus volume play the important roles in affecting memory impairment in patients with amnestic MCI.

The abnormal olfactory cortex may refer to a decline in higher-order memory processing and spatial cognitive function in MCI patients. The discovery of olfactory cortex provides assistance for clinical diagnosis of MCI.

Precentral Gyrus

The precentral gyrus gets a comparatively high frequency which make clears that the precentral gyrus is a crucial part in our WRSVMC algorithm.

The precentral gyrus is a major motor cortex which is parallel to the central sulcus. Qiu et al. (41) mentioned that the precentral gyrus is involved in language, memory and motor functions, and have a large impact on efficient communications. Sakurai et al. (58) discoverd that the damage of the precentral gyrus led to acalculia with decreased verbal short-term memory. Sakreida et al. (59) found that the core regions of the precentral gyrus were activated when understanding the language content. Chang (60) reported that the 6-year-old children learning instrumental musical for more than a year showed alterations in the precentral gyrus.

Several studies of MCI reported the correlations between MCI and abnormal precentral gyrus. Chirles et al. (23) found that bilateral precentral gyrus showed increased correlations with other brain areas after an exercise intervention in the MCI group. Han et al. (61) pointed out significantly increased connectivity between the posterior cingulate cortex and the precentral gyrus in MCI patients. Rose et al. (62) observed considerably increased mean diffusivity measurements in the right precentral gyrus in MCI patients. Lin et al. (63) mentioned that the right precentral gyrus was identified with significantly interaction effects by employing the analysis of covariance in patients with MCI.

The abnormal precentral gyrus may lead to challenges in learning knowledge, sluggish behavior, and reduced executive functions in MCI patients. The discovery of precentral gyrus provides new insights into the identification of MCI.

Middle Occipital Gyrus

The middle occipital gyrus gains the relatively high frequency which means that the middle occipital gyrus has a significant influence on our WRSVMC method.

The middle occipital gyrus is the largest gyrus in the occipital lobe, which is the visual processing center of brain. Mickley Steinmetz et al. (64) observed that the amygdala activation was associated with modulation of the middle occipital gyrus when processing emotional stimuli. van Dam et al. (65) reported that the fractional amplitude of low frequency fluctuations (fALFF) had a significant correlation with short-term memory within left middle occipital gyrus. Lauer et al. (66) found that patients with abnormal middle occipital gurus had a poor performance on visual memory. Arsalidou et al. (67) found that static faces showed less activity than dynamic faces in left middle occipital gyrus.

The middle occipital gyrus abnormality was found in a mass of MCI studies. Jacobs et al. (68) found out the significantly increased connectivity from the right middle occipital/angular gyrus to the inferior parietal lobule in amnestic MCI patients. Alexopoulos et al. (69) observed the lower perfusion in the left middle occipital lobe in MCI patients. Makizako et al. (70) found that poor performance in the 6-min walking distance (6MWD) was linked to the decreased cerebral gray matter volume in middle occipital gyrus in MCI patients. Wang et al. (25) found out the significantly decreased FC between the middle occipital lobe and the left thalamus in MCI patients.

The abnormal middle occipital gyrus may result in visual memory impairment and cognitive loss in MCI patients. The discovery of middle occipital gyrus offers assistance for clinical diagnosis and discrimination of MCI.

LIMITATIONS

The current study still has some limitations. First of all, the internationally accepted AAL template is employed to define the brain areas and the whole brain is divided into 90 ROIs, which leads to the fact that the division scale of the complex brain is still not small enough. The template for dividing the brain can be selected at a smaller scale to offer more informative and precise description for brain neural network. Then, the choice of graph theory metrics in this paper is based on the existing literature. However, there is no unified conclusion on how to select the most discriminative input features. With the deepening of research, more significant and meaningful predictor features can be considered to build the WRSVMC algorithm. Finally, the neuroimaging data we have obtained is the fMRI data of all subjects. Other modality of data could be utilized at the same time such as structural magnetic resonance imaging (sMRI), which could provide complementary information.

AUTHOR CONTRIBUTIONS

XB proposed the design of the work and revised it critically for important intellectual content. QX and QS carried out the experiment for the work and drafted part of the work. XL and ZW collected, interpreted the data and drafted part of the work. All the authors approved the final version to be published and agreed to be accountable for all aspects of the work in ensuring that questions related to the accuracy or integrity of any part of the work are appropriately investigated and resolved.

ACKNOWLEDGMENTS

This work is supported by the National Science Foundation of China (No. 61502167).

REFERENCES

1. Andrei C, Manuela P, Alin C, Daniel T, Cristinel S, Ziad N. General issues encountered while diagnosing mild cognitive impairment in Romanian patients. *Int J Geriatr Psychiatry* (2017) 32:116–7. doi: 10.1002/gps.4531
2. Hampstead BM, Sathian K, Bikson M, Stringer AY. Combined mnemonic strategy training and high-definition transcranial direct current stimulation for memory deficits in mild cognitive impairment. *Alzheimers Dement Transl Res Clin Interv.* (2017) 3:459–70. doi: 10.1016/j.trci.2017.04.008

3. Liu D, Zhang L, Li Z, Zhang X, Wu Y, Yang H, et al. Thinner changes of the retinal nerve fiber layer in patients with mild cognitive impairment and Alzheimer's disease. *BMC Neurol.* (2015) 15:14. doi: 10.1186/s12883-015-0268-6
4. Ramírez J, Górriz JM, Ortiz A, Martínez-Murcia FJ, Segovia F, Salas-Gonzalez D, et al. Ensemble of random forests one vs. rest classifiers for MCI and AD prediction using ANOVA cortical and subcortical feature selection and partial least squares. *J Neurosci Methods* (2018) 302:47–57. doi: 10.1016/j.jneumeth.2017.12.005
5. Kunneman M, Smets EMA, Bouwman FH, Schoonenboom NSM, Zwan MD, Pel-Littel R, et al. Clinicians' views on conversations and shared decision making in diagnostic testing for Alzheimer's disease: the ABIDE project. *Alzheimers Dement Transl Res Clin Interv.* (2017) 3:305–13. doi: 10.1016/j.trci.2017.03.009
6. Gruber O, F142. The use of neuroimaging markers in stratified diagnosis and therapy of schizophrenic and affective disorders. *Schizophr Bull.* (2018) 44:S275–5. doi: 10.1093/schbul/sby017.673
7. Caceda R, Bush K, James GA, Stowe Z, Knight B, Kilts C. 471. Resting brain connectivity differentiates suicidal ideation from acute suicidal behavior. *Biol Psychiatry* (2017) 81:S192. doi: 10.1016/j.biopsych.2017.02.955
8. Turner J, Damaraju E, Van Erp T, Mathalon D, Ford J, Voyvodic J, et al. A multi-site resting state fMRI study on the amplitude of low frequency fluctuations in schizophrenia. *Front Neurosci.* (2013) 7:137. doi: 10.3389/fnins.2013.00137
9. Sechi G, Demurtas R, Boadu W, Ortu E. Letter re: alterations of functional connectivity of the motor cortex in Fabry disease: an RS-fMRI study. *Neurology* (2017) 89:1842. doi: 10.1212/WNL.0000000000004566
10. Wang J-B, Zheng L-J, Cao Q-J, Wang Y-F, Sun L, Zang Y-F, et al. Inconsistency in abnormal brain activity across cohorts of ADHD-200 in children with attention deficit hyperactivity disorder. *Front Neurosci.* (2017) 11:320. doi: 10.3389/fnins.2017.00320
11. Keown CL, Datko MC, Chen CP, Maximo JO, Jahedi A, Müller R-A. Network organization is globally atypical in autism: a graph theory study of intrinsic functional connectivity. *Biol Psychiatry Cogn Neurosci Neuroimag.* (2017) 2:66–75. doi: 10.1016/j.bpsc.2016.07.008
12. Vecchio F, Miraglia F, Piludu F, Granata G, Romanello R, Caulo M, et al. "Small World" architecture in brain connectivity and hippocampal volume in Alzheimer's disease: a study via graph theory from EEG data. *Brain Imag Behav.* (2017) 11:473–85. doi: 10.1007/s11682-016-9528-3
13. López ME, Engels MMA, van Straaten ECW, Bajo R, Delgado ML, Scheltens P, et al. MEG beamformer-based reconstructions of functional networks in mild cognitive impairment. *Front Aging Neurosci.* (2017) 9:107. doi: 10.3389/fnagi.2017.00107
14. Song J, Birn RM, Boly M, Meier TB, Nair VA, Meyerand ME, et al. Age-related reorganizational changes in modularity and functional connectivity of human brain networks. *Brain Connect.* (2014) 4:662–76. doi: 10.1089/brain.2014.0286
15. Hojjati SH, Ebrahimzadeh A, Khazaee A, Babajani-Feremi A, Alzheimer's Disease Neuroimaging I. Predicting conversion from MCI to AD using resting-state fMRI, graph theoretical approach and SVM. *J Neurosci Methods* (2017) 282:69–80. doi: 10.1016/j.jneumeth.2017.03.006
16. Khazaee A, Ebrahimzadeh A, Babajani-Feremi A, Alzheimer's Disease Neuroimaging I. Classification of patients with MCI and AD from healthy controls using directed graph measures of resting-state fMRI. *Behav Brain Res.* (2017) 322:339–50. doi: 10.1016/j.bbr.2016.06.043
17. Asgari M, Kaye J, Dodge H. Predicting mild cognitive impairment from spontaneous spoken utterances. *Alzheimers Dement Transl Res Clin Interv.* (2017) 3:219–28. doi: 10.1016/j.trci.2017.01.006
18. Zhang J, Liu M, Le A, Gao Y, Shen D. Alzheimer's disease diagnosis using landmark-based features from longitudinal structural MR images. *IEEE J Biomed Health Inform.* (2017) 21:1607–16. doi: 10.1109/JBHI.2017.2704614
19. Yu K, Wang X, Li Q, Zhang X, Li X, Li S. Individual morphological brain network construction based on multivariate euclidean distances between brain regions. *Front Hum Neurosci.* (2018) 12:204. doi: 10.3389/fnhum.2018.00204
20. Zhang D, Shen D. Multi-modal multi-task learning for joint prediction of multiple regression and classification variables in Alzheimer's disease. *NeuroImage* (2012) 59:895–907. doi: 10.1016/j.neuroimage.2011.09.069
21. Beheshti I, Maikusa N, Daneshmand M, Matsuda H, Demirel H, Anbarjafari G, Japanese-Alzheimer's Disease Neuroimaging I. Classification of Alzheimer's disease and prediction of mild cognitive impairment conversion using histogram-based analysis of patient-specific anatomical brain connectivity networks. *J Alzheimers Dis.* (2017) 60:295–304. doi: 10.3233/JAD-161080
22. Li F, Tran L, Thung KH, Ji S, Shen D, Li J. A robust deep model for improved classification of AD/MCI patients. *IEEE J Biomed Health Inform.* (2015) 19:1610–6. doi: 10.1109/JBHI.2015.2429556
23. Chirles TJ, Reiter K, Weiss LR, Alfini AJ, Nielson KA, Smith JC. Exercise training and functional connectivity changes in mild cognitive impairment and healthy elders. *J Alzheimers Dis.* (2017) 57:845–56. doi: 10.3233/JAD-161151
24. Risacher SL, Tallman EF, West JD, Yoder KK, Hutchins GD, Fletcher JW, et al. Olfactory identification in subjective cognitive decline and mild cognitive impairment: Association with tau but not amyloid positron emission tomography. *Alzheimers Dement Diagn Assess Dis Monitor.* (2017) 9:57–66. doi: 10.1016/j.dadm.2017.09.001
25. Wang Z, Jia X, Liang P, Qi Z, Yang Y, Zhou W, et al. Changes in thalamus connectivity in mild cognitive impairment: evidence from resting state fMRI. *Eur J Radiol.* (2012) 81:277–85. doi: 10.1016/j.ejrad.2010.12.044
26. Liu M, Zhang D, Shen D. Relationship induced multi-template learning for diagnosis of Alzheimer's disease and mild cognitive impairment. *IEEE Trans Med Imag.* (2016) 35:1463–74. doi: 10.1109/TMI.2016.2515021
27. Wang B, Niu Y, Miao L, Cao R, Yan P, Guo H, et al. Decreased complexity in Alzheimer's disease: resting-state fMRI evidence of brain entropy mapping. *Front Aging Neurosci.* (2017) 9:378. doi: 10.3389/fnagi.2017.00378
28. Jin C, Chao Y-P, Lin L, Fu Z, Zhang B, Wu S. The study of graph measurements for hub identification in multiple parcellated brain networks of healthy older adult. *J Med Biol Eng.* (2017) 37:653–65. doi: 10.1007/s40846-017-0259-8
29. Bujnoskova E, Marecek R, Mikl M, Fousek J, Selnes P, Hessen E, et al. ID 326-Functional connectivity alterations and their relation to pathophysiological changes in mild cognitive impairment. *Clin Neurophysiol.* (2016) 127:e126–7. doi: 10.1016/j.clinph.2015.11.429
30. Pereira JB, Mijalkov M, Kakaei E, Mecocci P, Vellas B, Tsolaki M, et al. Abnormal network organization in patients with mild cognitive impairment and Alzheimer's disease. *Alzheimers Dement* (2016) 12:P34. doi: 10.1016/j.jalz.2016.06.048
31. Mathotaarachchi SS, Pascoal TA, Shin M, Benedet AL, Kang M-S, Struyfs H, et al. Graph-theory analysis shows a highly efficient but redundant network in mci tau propagation. *Alzheimers Dement.* (2017) 13:P1275–6. doi: 10.1016/j.jalz.2017.06.1914
32. Song S, Zhan Z, Long Z, Zhang J, Yao L. Comparative study of SVM methods combined with voxel selection for object category classification on fMRI data. *PLoS ONE* (2011) 6:e17191. doi: 10.1371/journal.pone.0017191
33. Bi X-A, Shu Q, Sun Q, Xu Q. Random support vector machine cluster analysis of resting-state fMRI in Alzheimer's disease. *PLoS ONE* (2018) 13:e0194479. doi: 10.1371/journal.pone.0194479
34. Zhang D, Wang Y, Zhou L, Yuan H, Shen D. Multimodal classification of Alzheimer's disease and mild cognitive impairment. *NeuroImage* (2011) 55:856–67. doi: 10.1016/j.neuroimage.2011.01.008
35. Granziera C, Daducci A, Donati A, Bonnier G, Romascano D, Roche A, et al. A multi-contrast MRI study of microstructural brain damage in patients with mild cognitive impairment. *NeuroImage Clin.* (2015) 8:631–9. doi: 10.1016/j.nicl.2015.06.003
36. Ye T, Zu C, Jie B, Shen D, Zhang D. Discriminative multi-task feature selection for multi-modality classification of Alzheimer's disease. *Brain Imag Behav.* (2016) 10:739–49. doi: 10.1007/s11682-015-9437-x
37. Long Z, Jing B, Guo R, Li B, Cui F, Wang T, et al. A Brainnetome Atlas based mild cognitive impairment identification using hurst exponent. *Front Aging Neurosci.* (2018) 10:103. doi: 10.3389/fnagi.2018.00103
38. Destrieux C, Terrier LM, Andersson F, Love SA, Cottier J-P, Duvernoy H, et al. A practical guide for the identification of major sulcogyral structures of the human cortex. *Brain Struct Func.* (2017) 222:2001–15. doi: 10.1007/s00429-016-1320-z
39. Fang S, Wang Y, Jiang T. The influence of frontal lobe tumors and surgical treatment on advanced cognitive functions. *World Neurosurg.* (2016) 91:340–6. doi: 10.1016/j.wneu.2016.04.006

40. Joo MS, Park DS, Moon CT, Chun YI, Song SW, Roh HG. Relationship between gyrus rectus resection and cognitive impairment after surgery for ruptured anterior communicating artery aneurysms. *J Cerebrovasc Endovasc Neurosurg.* (2016) 18:223–8. doi: 10.7461/jcen.2016.18.3.223
41. Qiu A, Mori S, Miller MI. Diffusion tensor imaging for understanding brain development in early life. *Ann Rev Psychol.* (2015) 66:853–76. doi: 10.1146/annurev-psych-010814-015340
42. Kristine MK, Olga Dal M, Selene S, Eric MW, Vanessa R, Jordan G, et al. Areas of brain damage underlying increased reports of behavioral disinhibition. *J Neuropsychiatry Clin Neurosci.* (2015) 27:193–8. doi: 10.1176/appi.neuropsych.14060126
43. Georgiopoulos C, Warntjes M, Dizdar N, Zachrisson H, Engstrom M, Haller S, et al. Olfactory impairment in Parkinson's disease studied with diffusion tensor and magnetization transfer imaging. *J Parkinsons Dis.* (2017) 7:301–11. doi: 10.3233/JPD-161060
44. Frings L, Yew B, Flanagan E, Lam BYK, Hüll M, Huppertz H-J, et al. Longitudinal gray and white matter changes in frontotemporal dementia and Alzheimer's disease. *PLoS ONE* (2014) 9:e90814. doi: 10.1371/journal.pone.0090814
45. Xie Y, Cui Z, Zhang Z, Sun Y, Sheng C, Li K, et al. Identification of amnestic mild cognitive impairment using multi-modal brain features: a combined structural MRI and diffusion tensor imaging study. *J Alzheimers Dis.* (2015) 47:509–22. doi: 10.3233/JAD-150184
46. Carr VA, Bernstein JD, Favila SE, Rutt BK, Kerchner GA, Wagner AD. Individual differences in associative memory among older adults explained by hippocampal subfield structure and function. *Proc Natl Acad Sci USA.* (2017) 114:12075. doi: 10.1073/pnas.1713308114
47. Lao Y, Nguyen B, Tsao S, Gajawelli N, Law M, Chui H, et al. A T1 and DTI fused 3D corpus callosum analysis in MCI subjects with high and low cardiovascular risk profile. *NeuroImage Clin.* (2017) 14:298–307. doi: 10.1016/j.nicl.2016.12.027
48. Bahar-Fuchs A, Chetelat G, Villemagne VL, Moss S, Pike K, Masters CL, et al. Olfactory deficits and amyloid-beta burden in Alzheimer's disease, mild cognitive impairment, and healthy aging: a PiB PET study. *J Alzheimers Dis.* (2010) 22:1081–7. doi: 10.3233/JAD-2010-100696
49. You Y, Novak L, Clancy K, Li W. Human olfactory cortex contributes to emotional and perceptual aspects of aversive associative learning and memory. *bioRxiv* (2017). doi: 10.1101/193748
50. Yaniv C, David P, Wilson DA. Dynamic cortical lateralization during olfactory discrimination learning. *J Physiol.* (2015) 593:1701–14. doi: 10.1113/jphysiol.2014.288381
51. Daniels JK, Vermetten E. Odor-induced recall of emotional memories in PTSD–review and new paradigm for research. *Exp Neurol.* (2016) 284:168–80. doi: 10.1016/j.expneurol.2016.08.001
52. Stone SSD, Teixeira CM, DeVito LM, Zaslavsky K, Josselyn SA, Lozano AM, et al. Stimulation of entorhinal cortex promotes adult neurogenesis and facilitates spatial memory. *J Neurosci.* (2011) 31:13469. doi: 10.1523/JNEUROSCI.3100-11.2011
53. Goto M, Abe O, Miyati T, Yoshikawa T, Hayashi N, Takao H, et al. Entorhinal cortex volume measured with 3T MRI is positively correlated with the Wechsler memory scale-revised logical/verbal memory score for healthy subjects. *Neuroradiology* (2011) 53:617–22. doi: 10.1007/s00234-011-0863-1
54. Zhang B, Zhang X, Zhang F, Li M, Schwarz CG, Zhang J, et al. Characterizing topological patterns in amnestic mild cognitive impairment by quantitative water diffusivity. *J Alzheimers Dis.* (2015) 43:687–97. doi: 10.3233/JAD-140882
55. Kirova A-M, Bays RB, Lagalwar S. Working memory and executive function decline across normal aging, mild cognitive impairment, and Alzheimer's diease. *BioMed Res Int.* (2015) 2015:9. doi: 10.1155/2015/748212
56. Vasavada MM, Wang J, Eslinger PJ, Gill DJ, Sun X, Karunanayaka P, et al. Olfactory cortex degeneration in Alzheimer's disease and mild cognitive impairment. *J Alzheimers Dis.* (2015) 45:947–58. doi: 10.3233/JAD-141947
57. Guzman VA, Carmichael OT, Schwarz C, Tosto G, Zimmerman ME, Brickman AM. White matter hyperintensities and amyloid are independently associated with entorhinal cortex volume among individuals with mild cognitive impairment. *Alzheimers Dement J Alzheimers Assoc.* (2013) 9:S124–31. doi: 10.1016/j.jalz.2012.11.009
58. Sakurai Y, Furukawa E, Kurihara M, Sugimoto I. Frontal phonological agraphia and acalculia with impaired verbal short-term memory due to left inferior precentral gyrus lesion. *Case Rep Neurol.* (2018) 10:72–82. doi: 10.1159/000487849
59. Sakreida K, Scorolli C, Menz M, Heim S, Borghi A, Binkofski F. Are abstract action words embodied? An fMRI investigation at the interface between language and motor cognition. *Front Hum Neurosci.* (2013) 7:125. doi: 10.3389/fnhum.2013.00125
60. Chang Y. Reorganization and plastic changes of the human brain associated with skill learning and expertise. *Front Hum Neurosci.* (2014) 8:35. doi: 10.3389/fnhum.2014.00035
61. Han SD, Arfanakis K, Fleischman DA, Leurgans SE, Tuminello ER, Edmonds EC, et al. Functional connectivity variations in mild cognitive impairment: associations with cognitive function. *J Int Neuropsychol Soc.* (2011) 18:39–48. doi: 10.1017/S1355617711001299
62. Rose SE, McMahon KL, Janke AL, O'Dowd B, de Zubicaray G, Strudwick MW, et al. Diffusion indices on magnetic resonance imaging and neuropsychological performance in amnestic mild cognitive impairment. *J Neurol Neurosurg Psychiatry* (2006) 77:1122–8. doi: 10.1136/jnnp.2005.074336
63. Lin F, Ren P, Lo RY, Chapman BP, Jacobs A, Baran TM, et al. Insula and inferior frontal gyrus' activities protect memory performance against Alzheimer's disease pathology in old age. *J Alzheimers Dis.* (2017) 55:669–78. doi: 10.3233/JAD-160715
64. Mickley Steinmetz KR, Addis DR, Kensinger EA. The effect of arousal on the emotional memory network depends on valence. *NeuroImage* (2010) 53:318–24. doi: 10.1016/j.neuroimage.2010.06.015
65. van Dam WO, Decker SL, Durbin JS, Vendemia JMC, Desai RH. Resting state signatures of domain and demand-specific working memory performance. *NeuroImage* (2015) 118:174–182. doi: 10.1016/j.neuroimage.2015.05.017
66. Lauer J, Moreno-López L, Manktelow A, Carroll EL, Outtrim JG, Coles JP, et al. Neural correlates of visual memory in patients with diffuse axonal injury. *Brain Inj.* (2017) 31:1513–20. doi: 10.1080/02699052.2017.1341998
67. Arsalidou M, Morris D, Taylor MJ. Converging evidence for the advantage of dynamic facial expressions. *Brain Topogr.* (2011) 24:149–63. doi: 10.1007/s10548-011-0171-4
68. Jacobs HIL, Van Boxtel MPJ, Heinecke A, Gronenschild EHBM, Backes WH, Ramakers IHGB, et al. Functional integration of parietal lobe activity in early Alzheimer disease. *Neurology* (2012) 78:352. doi: 10.1212/WNL.0b013e318245287d
69. Alexopoulos P, Sorg C, Förschler A, Grimmer T, Skokou M, Wohlschläger A, et al. Perfusion abnormalities in mild cognitive impairment and mild dementia in Alzheimer's disease measured by pulsed arterial spin labeling MRI. *Eur Arch Psychiatry Clin Neurosci.* (2012) 262:69–77. doi: 10.1007/s00406-011-0226-2
70. Makizako H, Shimada H, Doi T, Park H, Yoshida D, Suzuki T. Six-minute walking distance correlated with memory and brain volume in older adults with mild cognitive impairment: a voxel-based morphometry study. *Dement Geriatr Cogn Dis Extra* (2013) 3:223–32. doi: 10.1159/000354189

22

Effects of DISC1 Polymorphisms on Resting-State Spontaneous Neuronal Activity in the Early-Stage of Schizophrenia

Ningzhi Gou[1,2], Zhening Liu[1,2], Lena Palaniyappan[3], Mingding Li[4], Yunzhi Pan[1,2], Xudong Chen[1,2], Haojuan Tao[1,2], Guowei Wu[1,2], Xuan Ouyang[1,2], Zheng Wang[1,2], Taotao Dou[5], Zhimin Xue[1,2] and Weidan Pu[6,7]**

[1] Mental Health Institute, Second Xiangya Hospital, Central South University, Changsha, China, [2] Key Laboratory of Psychiatry and Mental Health of Hunan Province, The China National Clinical Research Center for Mental Health Disorders, National Technology Institute of Psychiatry, Changsha, China, [3] Departments of Psychiatry and Medical Biophysics & Robarts and Lawson Research Institutes, University of Western Ontario, London, ON, Canada, [4] Zhejiang University School of Medicine, Zhejiang University, Hangzhou, China, [5] Department of Neurosurgery, The First affiliated Hospital of Xinjiang Medical University, Urumqi, China, [6] Medical Psychological Center, Second Xiangya Hospital, Central South University, Changsha, China, [7] Medical Psychological Institute of Central South University, Changsha, China

***Correspondence:**
Zhimin Xue
x.zhimin@csu.edu.cn
Weidan Pu
weidanpu@csu.edu.cn

Background: Localized abnormalities in the synchrony of spontaneous neuronal activity, measured with regional homogeneity (ReHo), has been consistently reported in patients with schizophrenia (SCZ) and their unaffected siblings. To date, little is known about the genetic influences affecting the spontaneous neuronal activity in SCZ. *DISC1*, a strong susceptible gene for SCZ, has been implicated in neuronal excitability and synaptic function possibly associated with regional spontaneous neuronal activity. This study aimed to examine the effects of *DISC1* variations on the regional spontaneous neuronal activity in SCZ.

Methods: Resting-state fMRI data were obtained from 28 SCZ patients and 21 healthy controls (HC) for ReHo analysis. Six single nucleotide polymorphisms (SNPs) of *DISC1* gene were genotyped using the PCR and direct sequencing.

Results: Significant diagnosis × genotype interactions were noted for three SNPs (rs821616, rs821617, and rs2738880). For rs821617, the interactions were localized to the precuneus, basal ganglia and pre-/post-central regions. Significant interactive effects were identified at the temporal and post-central gyri for rs821616 (Ser704Cys) and the inferior temporal gyrus for rs2738880. Furthermore, *post-hoc* analysis revealed that the *DISC1* variations on these SNPs exerted different influences on ReHo between SCZ patients and HC.

Conclusion: To our knowledge this is the first study to unpick the influence of *DISC1* variations on spontaneous neuronal activity in SCZ; Given the emerging evidence that ReHo is a stable inheritable phenotype for schizophrenia, our findings suggest the DISC1 variations are possibly an inheritable source for the altered ReHo in this disorder.

Keywords: schizophrenia, *DISC1*, regional homogeneity, resting-state neuronal activity, genotype

INTRODUCTION

Schizophrenia (SCZ) is a severe and devastating neurodevelopmental disorder with a wide range of clinical clusters and fits a complex mode of inheritance with thousands of genetic variations with small effects (1, 2). It is proposed that distinct schizophrenia-related single nucleotide polymorphisms (SNPs) may be associated with subsets of heritable phenotypes or endo-phenotypes. Recent studies have applied genetic-imaging approach to assess the association of genetic variations with brain morphology and function as such endo-phenotypes in SCZ (3–6). The Regional Homogeneity (ReHo) (7), measuring the local synchronization of neuronal activity at rest, has been successfully applied to fMRI studies in SCZ, majority of which documented decreased ReHo in wide-spread areas including prefrontal, temporal, cingulate, precuneus, and occipital gyri (8–15). Notably, researches using the ReHo have consistently showed that the incoherent neuronal activity was shared by SCZ patients and their healthy siblings (11, 16, 17), implying the incoherence of spontaneous neuronal activity in SCZ is highly associated with inheritable factors. However, owing to the current literatures that few studies, up to date, have examined these inheritable factors for ReHo, the neural mechanism by which the genetic mutants contribute to the altered spontaneous neuronal activity in SCZ remains unknown.

Disrupted-in-Schizophrenia-1 (*DISC1*), a strong susceptible gene for SCZ (18–20), has been shown to be involved in multiple neural processes such as the neurite extension, neuronal proliferation, migration (21–24), and synaptic plasticity within various brain areas (25–27), independently or interactively with other genes such as *NUDEL*, *YWHAE* (rs28365859), and et al (28–31). Particularly, recent studies have established robust evidence for the involvement of the *DISC1* in neuronal excitability and synaptic functioning (32, 33). For example, knockdown of *DISC1* in rats has been shown to regulate surface levels of the AMPA-type glutamate receptor subunit GLUR1, and the frequency of miniature excitatory postsynaptic currents in cortical neuron (34); Another study reveals that knockdown of *DISC1* in mice leads to accelerated formation of dendritic spines in newborn neurons that have both glutamatergic and GABAergic synapses in the dentate gyrus (35); Moreover, the influence of *DISC1* on synapse function has also been evidenced by one postmortem study using light and electron microscopic approach, which demonstrates that *DISC1* localizes at postsynaptic structures highly associated with synapse functioning in both symmetric and asymmetric synapses (36). Taken together, these studies are suggestive of a regulatory role of the *DISC1* in synaptic functioning (especially for the glutamatergic neuron) which is highly associated with the spontaneous neuronal activity in local brain areas. Combining the evidence of the abnormal spontaneous neuronal activity (measured with ReHo) in SCZ patients and their siblings, it is possible that *DISC1* may be involved in the genetic mechanism of SCZ through its effect on the spontaneous neuronal activity.

Previous studies have indicated the involvement of *DISC1* variations in the brain morphological alteration (4, 37–39) and dysfunction during cognitive tasks associated with SCZ (6, 40, 41). Notably, a prior work by our group found that six *DISC1* SNPs were significantly and consistently associated with the morphological and functional abnormalities of precuneus, and that the precuneus gray matter loss was related to the symptom severity in SCZ patients (42). What should be noted is that our prior work recruited a patient sample with a relatively chronic illness duration (18.1 ± 15.9 years). Given the evidence that long hospitalization, medication and environmental stimulus such as stigma and living place may influence the gene expression through epigenetic processes (43, 44), the present study only recruited a patient sample in the early-stage of SCZ (illness duration < 5 years) (45, 46), although which somewhat overlaps with the prior work. The present study, according to our knowledge, is the first study aiming to investigate the genetic influences of *DISC1* polymorphisms on the resting-state spontaneous neuronal activity (measured with ReHo) in SCZ.

MATERIALS AND METHODS

Participants

A total of 28 patients at the early-stage (45, 46) of SCZ were recruited through the Institute of Mental Health, Second Xiangya hospital of Central South University, Changsha, China. Twenty-one healthy controls (HC) were recruited from Changsha city area. All participants were right-handed and no other contraindications to fMRI scanning (e.g., no cardiovascular and metallic implants). All patients were diagnosed with SCZ according to the Structural Clinical Interview for DSM-IV, Patient version (SCID-I/P). The Positive and Negative Syndrome Scale (PANSS) (47) was used as instruments of clinical assessment. Exclusion criteria for participants were neurological or comorbid psychiatric disorders (Axis I or Axis II), history of head injury, other serious illness, alcohol or substance dependence, exposure to electroconvulsive therapy, pregnant or breastfeeding (HC with a history of SCZ or a family history of psychosis were also excluded). All HC were well matched with the SCZ in terms of gender ($\chi^2 = 0.458$, $P = 0.498$) and years of education ($t = 0.000$, $P = 1.000$), except for age ($t = -2.939$, $P = 0.005$). Differences in demographic details (age, gender, education) were also examined across the genotype groups. Informed consent was given by all participants and the study was approved by the Ethics Committee of the Second Xiangya Hospital, Central South University.

Genotyping

DNA was extracted from whole venous blood samples. Since our prior work by Gong et al has identified 6 DISC1 SNPs (rs3738401, rs2738880, rs1535530, rs821616, rs821617, and rs12133766) that are consistently associated with resting-state functional alterations in schizophrenia patients, this study focused on the contribution of these SNPs to the abnormality of regional homogeneity at rest in this severe mental disorder. We genotyped *DISC1* SNPs using the PCR and direct sequencing (42). After sequencing, these six SNPs were identified with minor allele frequency > 5% in our sample. Based on our prior work (42), the genotypic groups were divided based on the dominant model: T-allele carriers vs. A homozygotes for rs821616; G-allele carries vs. A homozygotes for rs821617; G-allele carriers vs. A homozygotes for rs2738880; A-allele carriers vs. G homozygotes for rs3738401; C-allele carriers vs. T homozygotes for rs1535530; A-allele carriers vs. G homozygotes for rs12133766. The number of subjects of each genotype for each given SNP was listed in the Table S1.

MRI Data Acquisition and Image Preprocessing

All subjects underwent functional MRI scanning using 1.5-T GE Signa Twinspeed MR scanner (General Electric Medical System, Milwaukee, USA). The participants were informed to lay supine in the scanner with their heads fixed with foam pads and a belt and remain motionless with eyes closed. Gradient-echo echo planar imaging (EPI) was used to acquire resting-state functional images with the following parameters: repetition time/echo time (TR/TE) = 2,000/40 ms, 33 axial slices, 24 × 24 matrix, 90° flip angle, 5 mm section thickness, 1 mm slice gap. For each subject, fMRI scanning lasted for 6 min and 180 volumes were obtained. The fMRI data preprocessing was conducted by SPM8 (University College London, UK; http://www.fil.ion.ucl.ac.uk/spm) and DPARSF (http://restfmri.net/forum/DPARSF). The first 10 volumes of each functional time series were discarded for signal equilibrium and participants' adaptation to the scanning noise. The remaining 170 volumes were analyzed. The steps included slice timing, head-motion correction, spatial normalization in Montreal Neurological Institute (MNI) space and resampling with 3 × 3 × 3 mm^3 resolution. The head motion of all subjects was <2.0 mm maximum displacement in any direction of x, y, and z and 2.0° in any angular dimension, then band-pass filter (0.01–0.08 Hz) were conducted to reduce low-frequency drift and high-frequency noise; finally, nuisance covariates, including the global mean signal, white matter, and cerebrospinal fluid signals were regressed out.

ReHo Analysis

ReHo maps were calculated using the Kendall's coefficient of concordance (KCC) of the time series within a 27-voxel cubic neighborhood (7), KCC was computed using a cubic cluster size of 27 voxels based on the assumption that a voxel was temporally similar to those of its neighbors, a high ReHo value implies that the resting-state time series have high synchronization with those of its nearest neighbors (26 voxels). To reduce the influence of individual variations in the KCC value, normalizations of ReHo maps were done by dividing the KCC among each voxel by the averaged KCC of the whole brain. Finally smoothed with a Gaussian kernel of 4 × 4 × 4 mm full-width at half maximum (FWHM), we obtained a ReHo map of each subject for statistical analysis.

Statistical Analysis

Demographic and clinical data were analyzed using SPSS, version 19.0 (SPSS, Inc., Chicago, IL), fMRI data analysis was performed using Statistic Parameter Mapping 8 software (SPM8; www.fil.ion.ucl.ac.uk/spm). Deviation of the genotype counts from the Hardy–Weinberg equilibrium (HWE) was tested using a chi-square goodness-of-fit test. Statistical differences in genotypic between SCZ and HC were evaluated by the Chi-square test at significance level of $P < 0.05$. The linkage disequilibrium (LD) analysis was applied to detect the internal relationship of SNPs. In this study, demographic data (age, gender, and education) across diagnosis and genotypes were compared by either two sample *T*-test or χ^2 test. A 2 × 2 full-factorial model was performed using SPM8 (http://www.fil.ion.ucl.ac.uk/spm), with diagnosis and genotype as between-subject factors by including age and gender as covariates. This full-factorial model allowed us to characterize the main effect of diagnosis, genotype, and diagnosis × genotype interactive effect on the spontaneous neuronal activity. AlphaSim correction (as provided in the REST toolbox) (48) based on the Monte Carlo simulation, was conducted with a combined threshold of $P < 0.005$ at voxel level and $P < 0.001$ at cluster level (at least 30 voxels), which were applied to statistical maps derived from the full factorial model (48–50). We have listed the number of voxels and the smoothness sizes corresponding to the main effect and interactive effect of each given SNP after AlphaSim correction in the Table S2. The ReHo values were automatically calculated and extracted from the regions of interests, and then *post-hoc* analysis was performed to investigate the simple effects of these factors (disease status and genotypes). For further verifying our findings, a permutation-based nonparametric test using the Randomize tool in FSL (http://fsl.fmrib.ox.ac.uk/fsl/fslwiki/Randomize) was performed with family-wise error (FWE) correction ($P < 0.05$) for multiple comparisons corrections. A two-way ANCOVA within general linear model (GLM) framework was performed to calculate the main effect of disease and genotypes as well as the interactive effects between the two factors. All GLM designs included age and sex as covariates. For each GLM, *P*-values were calculated employing permutation-based statistics (10,000 permutations) (51, 52) for multiple comparisons correction. Pearson correlations were calculated between ReHo values and behavioral data including PANSS scores, illness duration and medication dosage in SCZ. Significance was set at $P < 0.05$.

RESULTS

Demographic and Genotypic Characteristics in Our Sample

Demographic and clinical data were summarized in **Table 1**. No significant differences were found between SCH and HC group in terms of gender, education, except for the age ($P < 0.05$) which was entered as the covariate into further fMRI data analysis. The genotypes allele distribution did not deviate from Hardy–Weinberg equilibrium (HWE) within the group (SCZ or HC) and with the groups combined ($P > 0.05$) for four SNPs (except for the SNPs rs3738401 and rs12133766 due to their being unsatisfactory with HWE). The genotype groups did not significantly differ with respect to age, gender, and education for the survived four SNPs ($P > 0.05$). Linkage disequilibrium (LD) analysis of SNPs was tested using Haploview software. R^2 for each pair of SNPs were calculated. No other pairwise SNPs showed a high level of LD except the pair of rs821616 and rs821617 ($R^2 = 0.8$, $P < 0.001$).

TABLE 1 | Demographic and clinical characteristics of SCZ and HC.

Variables	SCZ	HC	*P*-value
Number	28	21	
Age(years)	23.9 (5.4)	28.8 (6.1)	0.005*
Gender (M/F)	16/12	14/7	0.498
Education (years)	12.9(2.0)	12.9 (3.8)	1.000
Illness Duration (months)	15.1 (14.2)	–	–
MD (clz eq[a]) (mg/d)	384.9 (243.8)	–	–
SNPs			
Rs821617 (G+/AA)	6/22	7/14	0.350
Rs821616 (Cys+/SerSer)	9/19	6/15	0.788
Rs2738880 (G+/AA)	18/10	10/11	0.243
Rs1535530 (C+/TT)	14/14	11/10	0.869
PANSS total score	85.7 (19.9)	–	–
PANSS positive score	17.8 (6.5)	–	
PANSS negative score	21.0 (6.2)	–	
PANSS general score	38.9 (9.4)	–	

*Data are given as mean (standard deviation) *$P < 0.05$.*
[a]clz eq, chlorpromazine equivalents; MD, medication dose; SCH, schizophrenia; HC, healthy controls; PANSS, positive and negative syndrome scale.

Interactions and Simple Effects Between Diagnosis and Genotype Groups

As shown in the **Table 2**, significant group × genotype interactive effects on the ReHo were found for three SNPs (rs821617, rs821616, rs2738880). For rs821617, a significant interaction was found in the right precuneus (PCUN), middle occipital gyrus (MOG), basal ganglia (BG), post-central gyrus (PostCG), and left pre-central gyrus (PreCG), calcarine (CAL) (**Figures 1A1–F1**). Further *post-hoc* analysis indicated that for G allele carriers, SCZ showed lower ReHo in the right PCUN (**Figure 1A2**), MOG (**Figure 1B2**), and left CAL (**Figure 1C2**) comparing to HC, while no significance of ReHo was observed between A homozygous SCZ and HC group; Meanwhile, the G-allele carriers showed lower ReHo in the right PCUN, MOG, and higher ReHo in the right BG (**Figure 1D2**), PostCG (**Figure 1E2**), and left PreCG (**Figure 1F2**) than the AA carriers in SCZ group, whereas the HC group showed the opposite findings in the above regions.

For Ser704Cys, the genotype × diagnosis interactions were found in the left middle temporal gyrus (MTG), extending to superior temporal gyrus (STG) (**Figure 2A1**) and PostCG (**Figure 2B1**). Further *post-hoc* analysis showed that for Cys allele carriers (**Figures 2A2,B2**), SCZ group showed lower ReHo in the left MTG and PostCG compared to HC group, while for Ser homozygous SCZ group showed higher ReHo in the left MTG than HC group; Meanwhile, in the HC group, the Ser homozygotes showed lower ReHo than the Cys-allele carriers in the left MTG and PostCG, which was not observed in the SCZ group.

For rs2738880, the genotype × diagnosis interaction was found in the left inferior temporal gyrus (ITG) (**Figure 3A1**). Further *post-hoc* analysis (**Figure 3A2**) showed that for the G-allele carriers, SCZ group showed lower ReHo in the left ITG compared to HC, whereas an opposite finding was observed in the A homozygotes; Meanwhile, G-allele carriers showed lower ReHo compared to A homozygotes in SCZ group, while in HC group an opposite pattern was revealed.

Main Effect of *DISC1* Genotypes on ReHo Across All Subjects

For rs821617, the G carriers showed lower ReHo in the right middle frontal gyrus (MFG) compared with the A homozygous group (**Figure 4A**); For Ser704Cys, Ser homozygotes showed higher ReHo in the left MFG than Cys-allele carriers (**Figure 4B**); For rs2738880 and rs1535530, no significant genotype main effects were found.

Main Effect of Diagnosis on ReHo

Patients with SCZ showed lower ReHo compared to healthy controls in the bilateral thalamus (THA) (**Figures 5A,B**).

The findings using non-parametric test ($P < 0.001$, uncorrected) were quite similar with our original results (see Table S3). Rs821616 and rs821617 were found to have significant interactive effects of genotypes with diagnosis on the ReHo in distributed brain regions, which located at the temporal gyrus for the rs821616 and the PCUN, MOG, PUTA, PostCG, and PreCG for the rs821617. In addition, a main effect of *DISC1* genotypes was observed in the MFG in all subjects. However, only the interactive effects between rs821617 and diagnosis on the PCUN and visual cortex were survived after FWE correction.

Correlation

There were no significant correlations of ReHo with severity of symptoms, illness duration, or medicine dosage in SCZ ($P > 0.05$).

DISCUSSION

This study, according to our knowledge, is the first to document the genetic effect of *DISC1* variations on the resting-state regional neuronal activity in SCZ. Of six *DISC1* SNPs, three (Ser704Cys, rs821617, rs2738880) were found to have significant interactive effects of genotypes with diagnosis on the ReHo in distributed brain regions, which located at the temporal and PostCG for the rs821616, the ITG for the rs2738880, and the PCUN, BG, MOG, CAL, PostCG, and PreCG for the rs821617. Previous studies have reported that the altered spontaneous neuronal activity (measured with ReHo) in those regions above was shared between SCZ patients and their unaffected siblings (11, 16). Our findings provide the novel evidence that variations of *DISC1* gene may potentially underlie these shared abnormalities associated with SCZ. Further simple genotypic effects revealed in the current study suggest a complicated pattern of genetic influence of *DISC1* variations on the resting-state neuronal activity. In addition, a main effect of *DISC1* genotypes was observed in the MFG in all subjects. No significant correlations of ReHo with severity of symptoms in SCZ.

The *DISC1* Ser704Cys SNP has been widely studied in human beings, identifying a close relationship of this allele with brain morphology and functioning which are impaired in SCZ (37, 38, 40, 41, 53, 54). Notably, one volumetric study has identified

TABLE 2 | Main effect and interactive effects across diagnosis and genotypes.

Contrast	Cluster size	*P*-value	Effect size (partial η^2)	MNI coordinates			Region
				x	y	z	
MAIN EFFECT OF DIAGNOSIS							
	112	1.00*E*−06	0.40	−15	−15	12	THA (VLN)
	55	1.40*E*−05	0.34	12	−12	9	THA (VLN)
MAIN EFFECT OF GENOTYPES							
rs821617	31	1.80*E*−05	0.33	42	15	54	MFG
rs821616	69	2.00*E*−06	0.39	−30	36	48	MFG
INTERACTION: GENOTYPE × DIAGNOSIS							
rs821617	101	3.00*E*−05	0.33	3	−75	51	PCUN
	53	4.40*E*−05	0.32	42	−81	0	MOG
	115	2.60*E*−04	0.26	−3	−93	6	CAL
	41	2.90*E*−05	0.33	24	−9	9	PUTA
	38	2.90*E*−05	0.33	21	−3	−6	PALL
	91	8.10*E*−05	0.30	−33	−18	45	PreCG
	116	2.45*E*−04	0.27	33	−33	45	PostCG
rs821616	35	2.60*E*−05	0.33	−60	−51	9	MTG (extending to STG)
	40	2.30*E*−05	0.34	−39	−42	63	PostCG
rs2738880	63	1.80*E*−05	0.35	−51	−54	−6	ITG

AlphaSim correction with a combined statistical thresholds of $P < 0.005$ at voxel level and $P < 0.001$ at cluster level. THA, thalamus; MFG, middle frontal gyrus; PCUN, precuneus; MOG, middle occipital gyrus; CAL, calcarine; PUTA, putamen; PALL, pallidum; ITG, inferior temporal gyrus; STG, MTG, superior/middle temporal gyrus; PreCG, Pre-central gyrus; PostCG, Post-central gyrus; VLN, Ventral Lateral Nucleus.

significant diagnosis (SCZ vs. HC) × genotype (Cys+ vs. SerSer) interaction on the gray matter volumes in the frontal and temporal cortices (54); another task-induced fMRI study also showed diagnosis × genotype interaction on brain activation in the frontal cortex during a verbal fluency task (6). The evidence together indicates that genetic variation of the *DISC1* Ser704Cys may relate to the risk of SCZ and interplay with the disease for abnormal brain morphology and task-oriented functions. The present study found the interactive effects of Ser704Cys with diagnosis on the ReHo in the MTG (extending to the STG) and PostCG, further demonstrating the involvement of this SNP in the abnormal resting-state neuronal activity associated with SCZ.

In particular, the MTG and STG, responsible for comprehension and conceptual or semantic processing (55), have been consistently documented to be critical in the neuropathology of psychotic symptoms (especially for hallucinations) in SCZ (56). One fMRI study showed that the altered activation in the temporal gyrus in the siblings of SCZ during the N-back task (57). Most importantly, abnormal ReHo in these regions has been observed to be shared by SCZ patients and their unaffected siblings (11), suggesting the inheritable influence on the functional activity of the MTG and STG in SCZ. Our findings provide the first evidence that *DISC1* Ser704Cys mutations may be the genetic source for this inheritable influence.

Rs821617, has a tight linkage with rs821616 leading to the change of amino acid (K800R) in *DISC1* protein isoform b (NM001164538; http://www.ncbi.nlm.nih.gov/protein/NP_001158010.1). A prior study by our group in chronic patients reported the involvement of this locus in the development of SCZ, documenting that a significant association between rs821617 and abnormal functional connectivity of the PCUN with frontal cortex in SCZ (42). Consistently, this study found a significant interaction of this SNP with diagnosis on the resting-state PCUN activity. This consistent finding across chronic and early-stage patients may suggest that the influence of DISC1 variation (especially for the rs821617) may be not modulated by the long hospitalization, medication and other environmental factors such as stigma, living place (43, 44). Future neuroimaging-genetic studies using longitudinal design will be verify this notion.

The PCUN, broadly known as the key node in the so-called "default mode network" (DMN) (58), is associated with episodic memory, self-referential processing, and visuo-spatial imagery (59–61), which are all consistently observed to be impaired in SCZ, such as the self-processing (62) and insight (63). Functional alteration in this region has been repeatedly found in unaffected siblings of SCZ across cognition-related state (57, 64, 65) and resting-state (66). Notably, by applying the ReHo, a recent fMRI study reported altered resting-state neuronal activity in the PCUN in healthy siblings of SCZ (16), which supports that the PCUN dysfunction may be a potential neuroimaging endophenotype for SCZ. Our finding may further reveal that genetic underpinning of this endophenotype is associated with the *DISC1* rs821617 polymorphisms. Most interestingly, our further simple effects showed that in G-carriers, but not in A homozygotes, SCZ patients exhibited reduced ReHo relative to HC in the PCUN, suggesting the G allele of this SNP may be engaged in the neuropathology of SCZ through its specific influence on the resting-state PCUN activity.

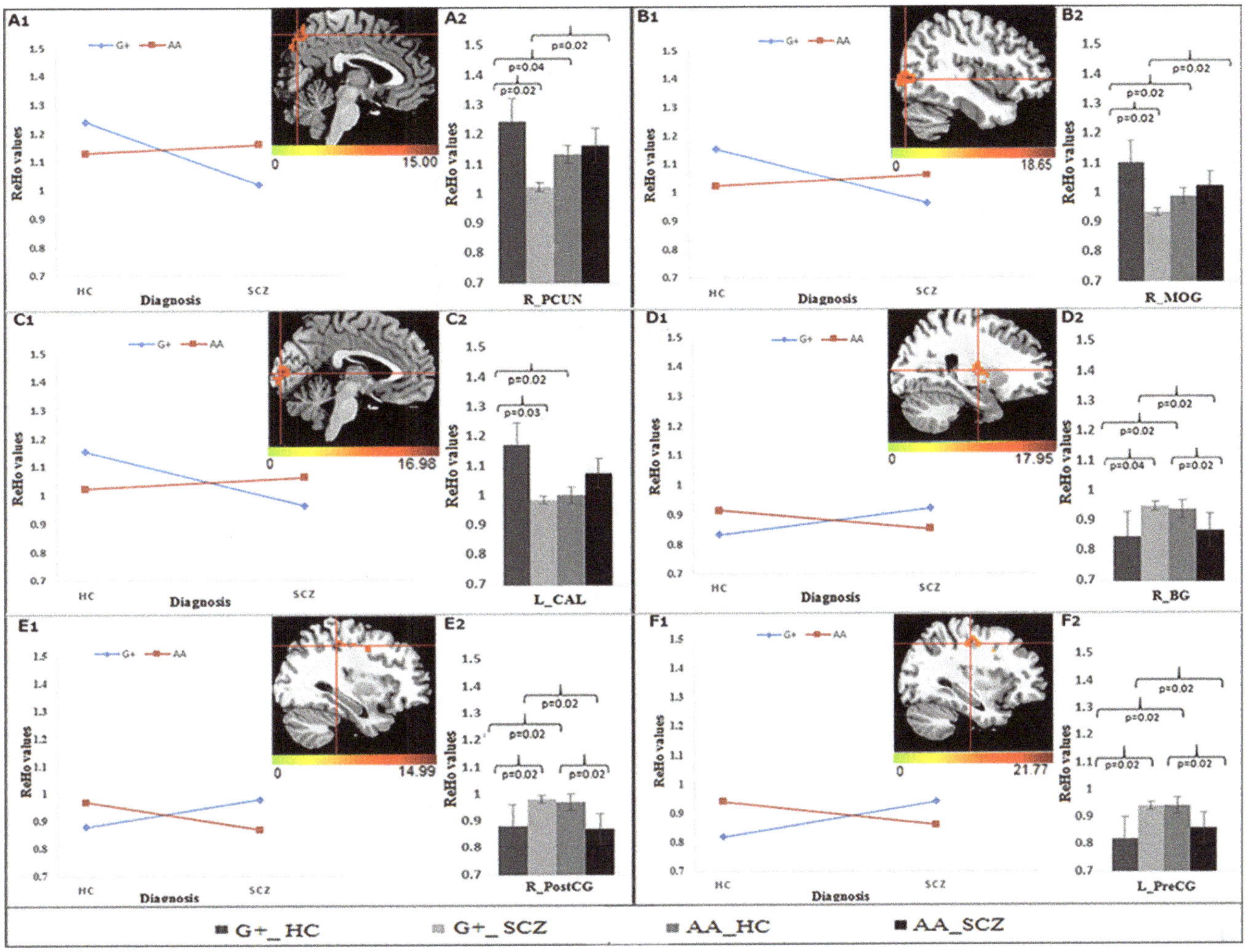

FIGURE 1 | The interaction and simple effect between rs821617 genotypes and diagnosis on ReHo. **(A1–F1)** Clusters of significance for the interaction. **(A1)** R-PCUN, **(B1)** R-MOG, **(C1)** L-CAL, **(D1)** R-BG, **(E1)** R-PostCG, **(F1)** L-PreCG. **(A2–F2)** Plots show the simple effect resulted from the genotype G+ vs. AA across diagnosis.

Another key region identified as related with the rs821617 is the BG (putamen and pallidum), which is well-known for its dopaminergic hyperfunction associated with the biological mechanism of SCZ. Inheritable contributions to the BG functional and structural abnormalities have been also revealed in previous studies involving SCZ patients and their unaffected siblings (67–71), which may be originated from the *DISC1* rs821617 mutations observed in this study. The role of the *DISC1* gene in regulating dopaminergic function (72) may partly explain the *DISC1* rs821617 mutations affect the BG resting-state neuronal activity in SCZ.

Additionally, we also found a significant interaction between rs2738880 genotype and diagnosis on the ReHo in the ITG, which is a key region responsible for language processing, working memory, social cognition and emotional visual processes. The morphological and functional alterations have been consistently found in SCZ patients (73–76) and their healthy siblings (76), as well as the subjects with psychosis risk syndrome (PRS) (12). As a rare variation in intron region upstream the exon 9 of DSC1 gene, the rs2738880 was examined in only one study (42) and its exact mechanism on brain activity still remains unclear.

Despite the interactions between diagnosis and *DISC1* genotypes on the resting-state neuronal activity, our findings also showed informative simple effects. These complicated simple effects may be characterized by two features. Firstly, the *DISC1* mutations may exert different genetic effects on ReHo between SCZ and HC. For rs821617 and rs2738880, the genotype effects on ReHo in SCZ are completely opposite to that in the HC, while the significant rs821616 genotype effects are observed in HC, but not in SCZ. These findings echo with previous studies (6, 77) and comply with the notion that SCZ fits a complex mode of inheritance with numerous genetic variations (19, 78), where the effects of numbers of alleles combine to form a continuum of internal phenotypic variation in brain function in SCZ. However, how *DISC1* interacts with other genes or environmental factors to influence the resting-state neuronal activity in SCZ still calls for future studies. Secondly, we observed that in rs821616 T-allele carriers, but not in A homozygotes, SCZ exhibited reduced

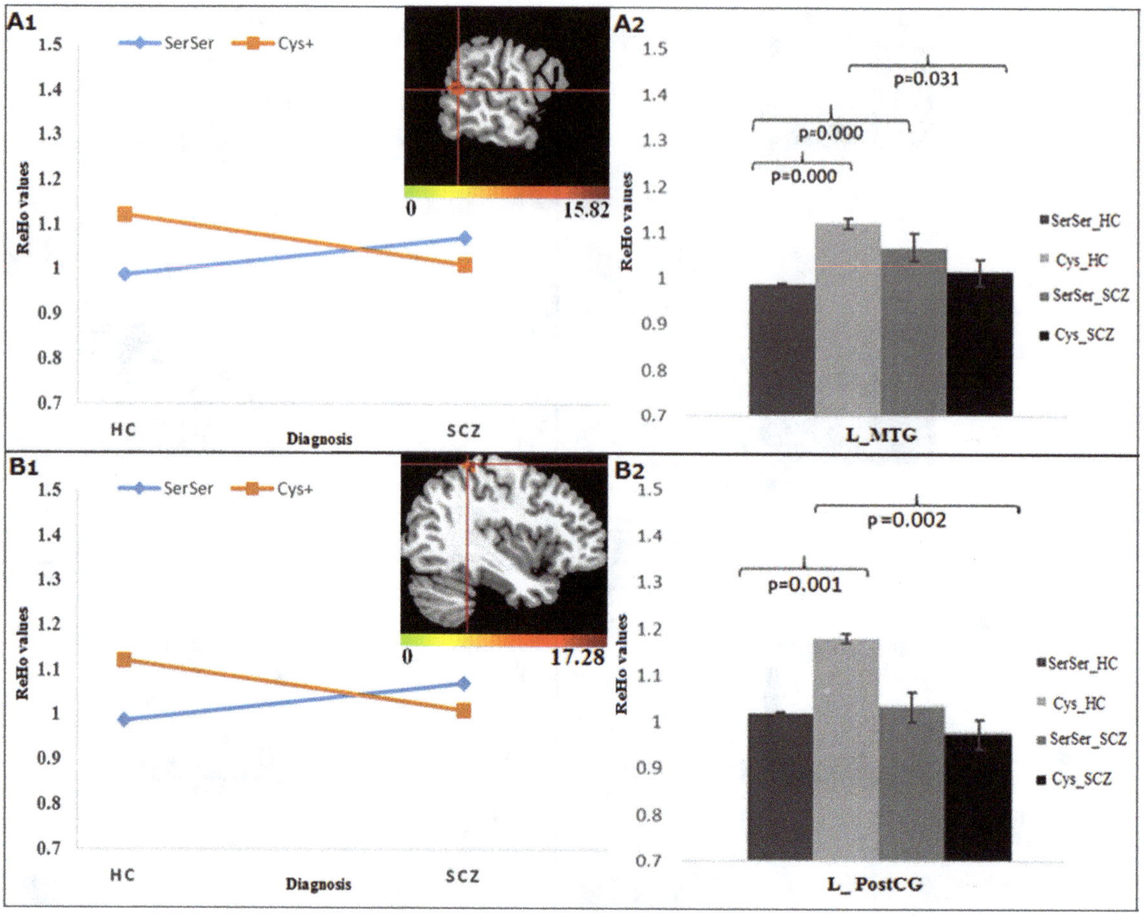

FIGURE 2 | The interaction and simple effect between Ser704Cys genotypes and diagnosis. **(A1,B1)** Clusters of significance in the L-MTG, STG, and PostCG. **(A2,B2)** The simple effect of Ser704Cys in these clusters.

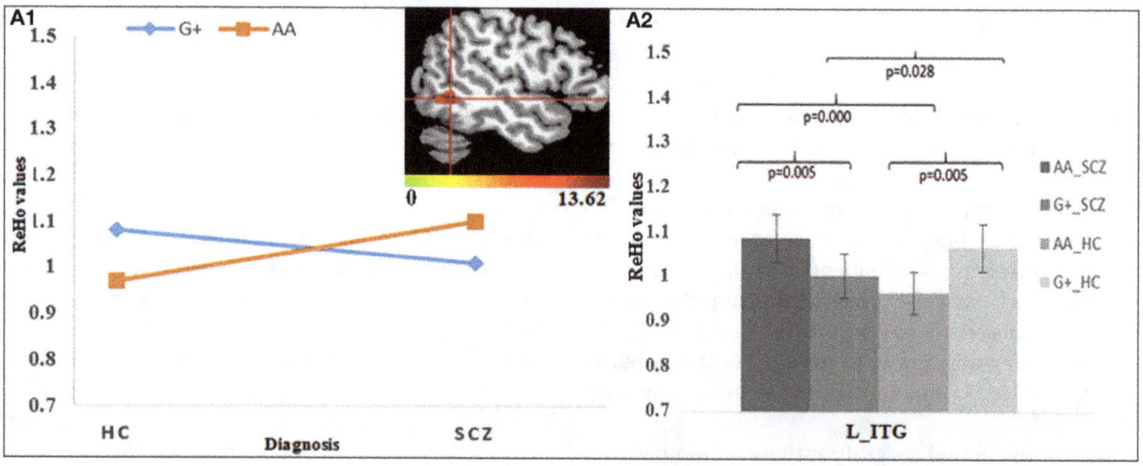

FIGURE 3 | The interaction and simple effect between rs2738880 genotypes and diagnosis. **(A1)** Cluster of significance for the interaction effect in the L-ITG. **(A2)** The simple effect in the L-ITG.

ReHo in the PostCG relative to HC, interestingly, the same pattern was also observed in rs821617 G-allele carriers. These findings imply that the T allele of rs821616 and the G allele of rs821617 may be engaged in the neuropathology of SCZ through their specific influences on the resting-state neuronal activity.

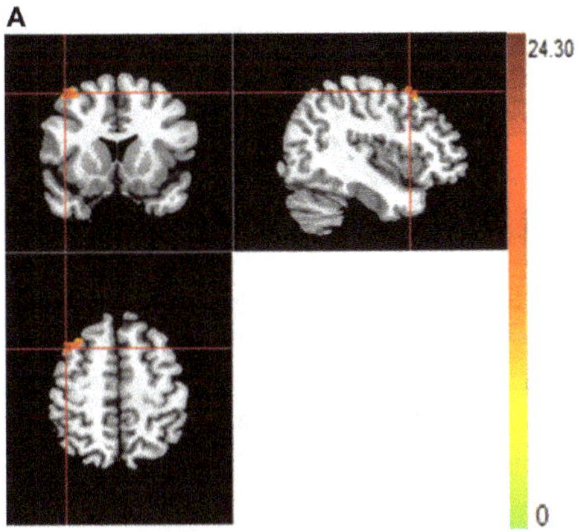

FIGURE 4 | (A,B) The images show the main effect of genotypes. The hot color indicate that ReHo is lower when carrying the G-allele of rs821617, T-allele of rs821616 than homozygotes group for all subjects. **(A)** R-MFG for rs821617 **(B)** L-MFG for rs821616.

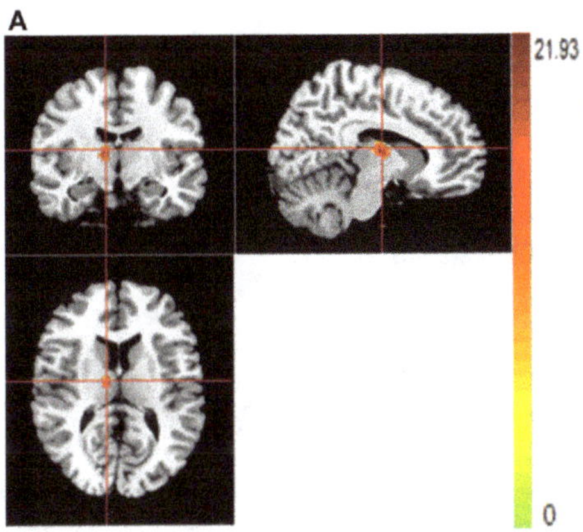

FIGURE 5 | (A,B) The images show the main effect of diagnosis. The hot color indicate that ReHo is higher in HC than SCZ for all SNPs. **(A)** R-THA **(B)** L-THA.

Robust biological evidence has supported the critical role of *DISC1* gene in the brain morphology and functioning. Traditionally, *DISC1* protein is suggested to be essential in neurite outgrowth and neuronal migration (21–24, 36), recent evidence implicates that mutations of *DISC1* disrupt synapse formation, regression and function, finally leading to the dysfunctional neurotransmission and altered neuronal activity (32, 33), such as the glutamatergic and the dopaminergic pathways, eventually inducing schizophrenia-like symptoms including positive, negative, and cognitive symptoms (34, 72). The present study, using a genetic-neuroimaging approach *in vivo*, extends previous evidence to show a significant influence of *DISC1* mutations on the regional spontaneous neuronal activity in SCZ patients.

Several limitations should be noted in this study. First of all, our sample is relatively small. For the purpose of further verifying our results, we did a non-parametric test using 10,000 permutations on our neuroimaging-genetic data and showed similar findings with our prior results. Most importantly, the interactive effects between rs821617 and diagnosis on the precuneus and visual cortex still survived after FWE correction, increasing the reliability of our findings. However, these findings in the present study need to be verified and replicated in future studies with a relatively large sample; Secondly, no correlations between ReHo and symptom severity were observed in this study. The study by Gong et al. also did not find associations between functional alterations and symptoms, but found a correlation of gray matter loss of precuneus with negative symptoms. The null finding of correlation analysis may be accounted for by our relatively small sample. However, since previous studies never found the correlations of clinical symptoms with ReHo, another possible explanation is that the synchrony of spontaneous neuronal activity could be used qualitatively to help locate functional alterations, but not as a quantitative marker for evaluating SCZ symptoms. Thirdly, this study recruited the patients in the early stage of SCZ to control the effects of medication and hospitalization on the resting-state neuronal activity, which along with the methodological distinctions (ReHo vs. functional connectivity) may account for the differences between our findings and the prior work by Gong et al. However, the effect of antipsychotic medications and illness duration could not be completely ruled out. Future studies on first-episode drug-naïve patients may put further insight on the relationship of *DISC1* mutants with SCZ brain functional abnormalities. Fourthly, environmental factors including stress and childhood trauma have been proven to interact with genetic variants to contribute to the development of SCZ (79, 80). Interestingly, a recent study found that the mutant *DISC1* mice exposed to a diet containing neurotoxicant (Pb2+) produced the brain and behavior abnormalities consistent with SCZ (81), suggesting *DISC1* variations related to SCZ may be relevant to the environmental xenobiotics. However, this study did not obtain such environmental information in our samples. It still calls for future study to examine how *DISC1* variants interact with risky environmental factors to influence the neurodevelopment of SCZ.

In summary, this study highlights the importance of the *DISC1* polymorphisms in the modulation of resting-state neuronal activity in SCZ. Our findings support that the *DISC1* variations are highly associated with the abnormal resting-state neuronal activity repeatedly observed in SCZ, and potentially, extend the evidence to show the genetic underpinning of the shared alterations of resting-state spontaneous neuronal activity (endo-phenotype) between SCZ and their unaffected siblings. The complicated simple effects suggest that the *DISC1* gene possibly interact with other genes or environmental factors to contribute to the altered resting-state neuronal activity in SCZ, and thus, future studies in the framework of gene-gene or gene-environment interaction are called for to provide further insight into the genetic mechanism of resting-state brain dysfunction in SCZ. Moreover, recent evidence demonstrates that reduced ReHo benefits from 13 weeks paliperidone treatment mainly targeting at the dopaminergic pathways in SCZ patients (82), suggesting that alterations of ReHo may be a potential pharmacological target for SCZ treatment. Our findings possibly provide a means to target specific regions with highest degree of localized connectivity abnormalities for therapeutic purposes in this severe mental disorder.

AUTHOR CONTRIBUTIONS

WP: designed the study; NG and WP: analyzed, interpreted the data, and wrote the first draft of the manuscript; ZX, ZL, ML, and LP: provided fMRI technical support and revised it critically for important intellectual content. Other authors collected the data and provided assistance for statistical analysis. All authors contributed to and have approved the final manuscript.

FUNDING

The work was supported by grants from the National Natural Science Foundations of China (81671335 and 81171287 to ZX, 81561168021, 2016YFSF090142, 81271485, and 81471362 to ZL, 81401125 to WP, 81301161 to HT, 81701325 to GW) and the Graduates' innovation Projects of Central South University (2016zzts548 to NG).

ACKNOWLEDGMENTS

We would like to thank Zhong He from the Department of Radiology of Second Xiangya hospital, Central South University, for his assistance in fMRI data; Meanwhile, we would like to thank Yicheng Long for his contributions to the further analysis of data.

REFERENCES

1. Zheng F, Yan H, Liu B, Yue W, Fan L, Liao J, et al. ALDH2 Glu504Lys confers susceptibility to schizophrenia and impacts hippocampal-prefrontal functional connectivity. *Cereb Cortex* (2017) **27**:2034–40. doi: 10.1093/cercor/bhw056
2. Burdick KE, Kamiya A, Hodgkinson CA, Lencz T, DeRosse P, Ishizuka K, et al. Elucidating the relationship between DISC1, NDEL1 and NDE1 and the risk for schizophrenia: evidence of epistasis and competitive binding. *Hum Mol Genet.* (2008) **17**:2462–73. doi: 10.1093/hmg/ddn146
3. Prata DP, Mechelli A, Picchioni MM, Fu CH, Toulopoulou T, Bramon E, et al. Altered effect of dopamine transporter 3'UTR VNTR genotype on prefrontal and striatal function in schizophrenia. *Arch Gen Psychiatry* (2009) **66**:1162–72. doi: 10.1001/archgenpsychiatry.2009.147
4. Trost S, Platz B, Usher J, Scherk H, Wobrock T, Ekawardhani S, et al. DISC1 (disrupted-in-schizophrenia 1) is associated with cortical grey matter volumes in the human brain: a voxel-based morphometry (VBM) study. *J Psychiatr Res.* (2013) **47**:188–96. doi: 10.1016/j.jpsychires.2012.10.006
5. Chakirova G, Whalley HC, Thomson PA, Hennah W, Moorhead TW, Welch KA, et al. The effects of DISC1 risk variants on brain activation in controls, patients with bipolar disorder and patients with schizophrenia. *Psychiatry Res.* (2011) **192**:20–8. doi: 10.1016/j.pscychresns.2011.01.015
6. Prata DP, Mechelli A, Picchioni M, Fu CH, Kane F, Kalidindi S, et al. No association of Disrupted-in-Schizophrenia-1 variation with prefrontal function in patients with schizophrenia and bipolar disorder. *Genes Brain Behav.* (2011) **10**:276–85. doi: 10.1111/j.1601-183X.2010.00665.x
7. Zang Y, Jiang T, Lu Y, He Y, and Tian L. Regional homogeneity approach to fMRI data analysis. *Neuroimage* (2004) **22**:394–400. doi: 10.1016/j.neuroimage.2003.12.030
8. Zhuo CJ, Zhu JJ, Wang CL, Wang LN, Li J, and Qin W. Increased local spontaneous neural activity in the left precuneus specific to auditory verbal hallucinations of schizophrenia. *Chin Med J.* (2016) **129**:809–13. doi: 10.4103/0366-6999.178974
9. Gao B, Wang Y, Liu W, Chen Z, Zhou H, Yang J, et al. Spontaneous activity associated with delusions of schizophrenia in the left medial superior frontal gyrus: a resting-state fMRI study. *PLoS ONE* (2015) **10**:e0133766. doi: 10.1371/journal.pone.0133766
10. Liu H, Liu Z, Liang M, Hao Y, Tan L, Kuang F, et al. Decreased regional homogeneity in schizophrenia: a resting state functional magnetic resonance imaging study. *Neuroreport* (2006) **17**:19–22. doi: 10.1097/01.wnr.0000195666.22714.35

11. Liu C, Xue Z, Palaniyappan L, Zhou L, Liu H, Qi C, et al. Abnormally increased and incoherent resting-state activity is shared between patients with schizophrenia and their unaffected siblings. *Schizophr Res.* (2016) **171**:158–65. doi: 10.1016/j.schres.2016.01.022
12. Wang S, Wang G, Lv H, Wu R, Zhao J, Guo W. Abnormal regional homogeneity as potential imaging biomarker for psychosis risk syndrome: a resting-state fMRI study and support vector machine analysis. *Sci Rep.* (2016) **6**:27619. doi: 10.1038/srep27619
13. Jiang S, Zhou B, Liao Y, Liu W, Tan C, Chen X, et al. [Primary study of resting state functional magnetic resonance imaging in early onset schizophrenia using ReHo]. *Zhong Nan Da Xue Xue Bao Yi Xue Ban* (2010) **35**:947–51. doi: 10.3969/j.issn.1672-7347.2010.09.008
14. Yu R, Hsieh MH, Wang HL, Liu CM, Liu CC, Hwang TJ, et al. Frequency dependent alterations in regional homogeneity of baseline brain activity in schizophrenia. *PLoS ONE* (2013) **8**:e57516. doi: 10.1371/journal.pone.0057516
15. Liu Y, Zhang Y, Lv L, Wu R, Zhao J, Guo W. Abnormal neural activity as a potential biomarker for drug-naive first-episode adolescent-onset schizophrenia with coherence regional homogeneity and support vector machine analyses. *Schizophr Res.* (2017) **192**:408–15. doi: 10.1016/j.schres.2017.04.028
16. Liao H, Wang L, Zhou B, Tang J, Tan L, Zhu X, et al. A resting-state functional magnetic resonance imaging study on the first-degree relatives of persons with schizophrenia. *Brain Imaging Behav.* (2012) **6**:397–403. doi: 10.1007/s11682-012-9154-7
17. Xiao B, Wang S, Liu J, Meng T, He Y, Luo X. Abnormalities of localized connectivity in schizophrenia patients and their unaffected relatives: a meta-analysis of resting-state functional magnetic resonance imaging studies. *Neuropsychiatr Dis Treat.* (2017) **13**:467–75. doi: 10.2147/NDT.S126678
18. Baron M. Genetics of schizophrenia and the new millennium: progress and pitfalls. *Am J Hum Genet.* (2001) **68**:299–312. doi: 10.1086/318212
19. Sawa A, Snyder SH. Schizophrenia: diverse approaches to a complex disease. *Science* (2002) **296**:692–5. doi: 10.1126/science.1070532
20. Millar JK, Wilsonannan JC, Anderson S, Christie S, Taylor MS, Semple CA, et al. Disruption of two novel genes by a translocation co-segregating with schizophrenia. *Hum Mol Genet.* (2000) **9**:1415. doi: 10.1093/hmg/9.9.1415
21. Kamiya A, Kubo K, Tomoda T, Takaki M, Youn R, Ozeki Y, et al. A schizophrenia-associated mutation of DISC1 perturbs cerebral cortex development. *Nat Cell Biol.* (2005) **7**:1167–78. doi: 10.1038/ncb1328
22. Miyoshi K, Honda A, Baba K, Taniguchi M, Oono K, Fujita T, et al. Disrupted-In-Schizophrenia 1, a candidate gene for schizophrenia, participates in neurite outgrowth. *Mol Psychiatry* (2003) **8**:685–94. doi: 10.1038/sj.mp.4001352
23. Ozeki Y, Tomoda T, Kleiderlein J, Kamiya A, Bord L, Fujii K, et al. Disrupted-in-Schizophrenia-1 (DISC-1): mutant truncation prevents binding to NudE-like (NUDEL) and inhibits neurite outgrowth. *Proc Natl Acad Sci USA* (2002) **100**:289–94. doi: 10.1073/pnas.0136913100
24. Brandon NJ, Handford EJ, Schurov I, Rain JC, Pelling M, Duran-Jimeniz B, et al. Disrupted in Schizophrenia 1 and Nudel form a neurodevelopmentally regulated protein complex: implications for schizophrenia and other major neurological disorders. *Mol Cell Neurosci.* (2004) **25**:42–55. doi: 10.1016/j.mcn.2003.09.009
25. Austin CP, Ma L, Ky B, Morris JA, Shughrue PJ. DISC1 (Disrupted in Schizophrenia-1) is expressed in limbic regions of the primate brain. *Neuroreport* (2003) **14**:951–4. doi: 10.1097/01.wnr.0000074342.81633.63
26. Meyer KD, Morris JA. Immunohistochemical analysis of Disc1 expression in the developing and adult hippocampus. *Gene Expr Patterns* (2008) **8**:494–501. doi: 10.1016/j.gep.2008.06.005
27. Schurov IL, Handford EJ, Brandon NJ, Whiting PJ. Expression of disrupted in schizophrenia 1 (DISC1) protein in the adult and developing mouse brain indicates its role in neurodevelopment. *Mol Psychiatry* (2004) **9**:1100–10. doi: 10.1038/sj.mp.4001574
28. Hayashi MA, Portaro FC, Bastos MF, Guerreiro JR, Oliveira V, Gorrao SS, et al. Inhibition of NUDEL (nuclear distribution element-like)-oligopeptidase activity by disrupted-in-schizophrenia 1. *Proc Natl Acad Sci USA* (2005) **102**:3828–33. doi: 10.1073/pnas.0500330102
29. Takahashi T, Nakamura Y, Nakamura Y, Aleksic B, Takayanagi Y, Furuichi A, et al. The polymorphism of YWHAE, a gene encoding 14-3-3epsilon, and orbitofrontal sulcogyral pattern in patients with schizophrenia and healthy subjects. *Prog Neuropsychopharmacol Biol Psychiatry* (2014) **51**:166–71. doi: 10.1016/j.pnpbp.2014.02.005
30. Mata I, Perez-Iglesias R, Roiz-Santianez R, Tordesillas-Gutierrez D, Gonzalez-Mandly A, Berja A, et al. Additive effect of NRG1 and DISC1 genes on lateral ventricle enlargement in first episode schizophrenia. *Neuroimage* (2010) **53**:1016–22. doi: 10.1016/j.neuroimage.2009.11.010
31. Nicodemus KK, Kolachana BS, Vakkalanka R, Straub RE, Giegling I, Egan MF, et al. Evidence for statistical epistasis between catechol-O-methyltransferase (COMT) and polymorphisms in RGS4, G72 (DAOA), GRM3, and DISC1: influence on risk of schizophrenia. *Hum Genet.* (2007) **120**:889–906. doi: 10.1007/s00439-006-0257-3
32. Bennett MR. Schizophrenia: susceptibility genes, dendritic-spine pathology and gray matter loss. *Prog Neurobiol.* (2011) **95**:275–300. doi: 10.1016/j.pneurobio.2011.08.003
33. Ma TM, Abazyan S, Abazyan B, Nomura J, Yang C, Seshadri S, et al. Pathogenic disruption of DISC1-serine racemase binding elicits schizophrenia-like behavior via D-serine depletion. *Mol Psychiatry* (2013) **18**:557–67. doi: 10.1038/mp.2012.97
34. Hayashi-Takagi A, Takaki M, Graziane N, Seshadri S, Murdoch H, Dunlop AJ, et al. Disrupted-in-Schizophrenia 1 (DISC1) regulates spines of the glutamate synapse via Rac1. *Nat Neurosci.* (2010) **13**:327–32. doi: 10.1038/nn.2487
35. Duan X, Chang JH, Ge S, Faulkner RL, Kim JY, Kitabatake Y, et al. Disrupted-In-Schizophrenia 1 regulates integration of newly generated neurons in the adult brain. *Cell* (2007) **130**:1146–58. doi: 10.1016/j.cell.2007.07.010
36. Kirkpatrick B, Xu L, Cascella N, Ozeki Y, Sawa A, Roberts RC. DISC1 immunoreactivity at the light and ultrastructural level in the human neocortex. *J Compar Neurol.* (2006) **497**:436–50. doi: 10.1002/cne.21007
37. Li Y, Liu B, Hou B, Qin W, Wang D, Yu C, et al. Less efficient information transfer in Cys-allele carriers of DISC1: a brain network study based on diffusion MRI. *Cereb Cortex* (2013) **23**:1715–23. doi: 10.1093/cercor/bhs167
38. Sprooten E, Sussmann JE, Moorhead TW, Whalley HC, ffrench-Constant C, Blumberg HP, et al. Association of white matter integrity with genetic variation in an exonic DISC1 SNP. *Mol Psychiatry* (2011) **16**:688–9. doi: 10.1038/mp.2011.15
39. Duff BJ, Macritchie KAN, Moorhead TWJ, Lawrie SM, Blackwood DHR. Human brain imaging studies of DISC1 in schizophrenia, bipolar disorder and depression: a systematic review. *Schizophr Res.* (2013) **147**:1–13. doi: 10.1016/j.schres.2013.03.015
40. Prata DP, Mechelli A, Fu CH, Picchioni M, Kane F, Kalidindi S, et al. Effect of disrupted-in-schizophrenia-1 on pre-frontal cortical function. *Mol Psychiatry* (2008) **13**:915–7. doi: 10.1038/mp.2008.76
41. Di Giorgio A, Blasi G, Sambataro F, Rampino A, Papazacharias A, Gambi F, et al. Association of the SerCys DISC1 polymorphism with human hippocampal formation gray matter and function during memory encoding. *Eur J Neurosci.* (2008) **28**:2129–36. doi: 10.1111/j.1460-9568.2008.06482.x
42. Gong X, Lu W, Kendrick KM, Pu W, Wang C, Jin L, et al. A brain-wide association study of DISC1 genetic variants reveals a relationship with the structure and functional connectivity of the precuneus in schizophrenia. *Hum Brain Mapp.* (2014) **35**:5414–30. doi: 10.1002/hbm.22560
43. Aguilera O, Fernandez AF, Munoz A, Fraga MF. Epigenetics and environment: a complex relationship. *J Appl Physiol.* (2010) **109**:243–51. doi: 10.1152/japplphysiol.00068.2010
44. Copoglu US, Igci M, Bozgeyik E, Kokacya MH, Igci YZ, Dokuyucu R, et al. DNA methylation of BDNF gene in Schizophrenia. *Med Sci Monit.* (2016) **22**:397–402. doi: 10.12659/MSM.895896
45. Guo X, Zhai J, Liu Z, Fang M, Wang B, Wang C, et al. Effect of antipsychotic medication alone vs combined with psychosocial intervention on outcomes of early-stage schizophrenia: a randomized, 1-year study. *Arch Gen Psychiatry* (2010) **67**:895–904. doi: 10.1001/archgenpsychiatry.2010.105
46. Pu W, Li L, Zhang H, Ouyang X, Liu H, Zhao J, et al. Morphological and functional abnormalities of salience network in the early-stage of paranoid schizophrenia. *Schizophr Res.* (2012) **141**:15–21. doi: 10.1016/j.schres.2012.07.017
47. Kay SR, Fiszbein A, Opler LA. The Positive and Negative Syndrome Scale (PANSS) for schizophrenia. *Schizophr Bull.* (1987) **13**:261–276.
48. Song XW, Dong ZY, Long XY, Li SF, Zuo XN, Zhu CZ, et al. REST: a toolkit for resting-state functional magnetic resonance imaging data processing. *PLoS ONE* (2011) **6**:e25031. doi: 10.1371/journal.pone.0025031

49. Lorenz RC, Kruger JK, Neumann B, Schott BH, Kaufmann C, Heinz A, et al. Cue reactivity and its inhibition in pathological computer game players. *Addict Biol.* (2013) **18**:134–46. doi: 10.1111/j.1369-1600.2012.00491.x
50. Song X, Qian S, Liu K, Zhou S, Zhu H, Zou Q, et al. Resting-state BOLD oscillation frequency predicts vigilance task performance at both normal and high environmental temperatures. *Brain Struct Funct.* (2017) **222**:4065–77. doi: 10.1007/s00429-017-1449-4
51. Holmes AP, Blair RC, Watson JD, Ford I. Nonparametric analysis of statistic images from functional mapping experiments. *J Cereb Blood Flow Metab.* (1996) **16**:7–22. doi: 10.1097/00004647-199601000-00002
52. Winkler AM, Ridgway GR, Webster MA, Smith SM, Nichols TE. Permutation inference for the general linear model. *Neuroimage* (2014) **92**:381–97. doi: 10.1016/j.neuroimage.2014.01.060
53. Callicott JH, Straub RE, Pezawas L, Egan MF, Mattay VS, Hariri AR, et al. Variation in DISC1 affects hippocampal structure and function and increases risk for schizophrenia. *Proc Natl Acad Sci USA* (2005) **102**:8627–32. doi: 10.1073/pnas.0500515102
54. Takahashi T, Suzuki M, Tsunoda M, Maeno N, Kawasaki Y, Zhou SY, et al. The Disrupted-in-Schizophrenia-1 Ser704Cys polymorphism and brain morphology in schizophrenia. *Psychiatry Res.* (2009) **172**:128–35. doi: 10.1016/j.pscychresns.2009.01.005
55. Wei T, Liang X, He Y, Zang Y, Han Z, Caramazza A, et al. Predicting conceptual processing capacity from spontaneous neuronal activity of the left middle temporal gyrus. *J Neurosci.* (2012) **32**:481–9. doi: 10.1523/JNEUROSCI.1953-11.2012
56. Hickok G, Poeppel D. Dorsal and ventral streams: a framework for understanding aspects of the functional anatomy of language. *Cognition* (2004) **92**:67–99. doi: 10.1016/j.cognition.2003.10.011
57. Callicott JH, Egan MF, Mattay VS, Bertolino A, Bone AD, Verchinksi B, et al. Abnormal fMRI response of the dorsolateral prefrontal cortex in cognitively intact siblings of patients with schizophrenia. *Am J Psychiatry* (2003) **160**:709–19. doi: 10.1176/appi.ajp.160.4.709
58. Buckner RL, Andrews-Hanna JR, Schacter DL. The brain's default network: anatomy, function, and relevance to disease. *Ann NY Acad Sci.* (2008) **1124**:1–38. doi: 10.1196/annals.1440.011
59. Chen C, Xiu D, Chen C, Moyzis R, Xia M, He Y, et al. Regional homogeneity of resting-state brain activity suppresses the effect of dopamine-related genes on sensory processing sensitivity. *PLoS ONE* (2015) **10**:e0133143. doi: 10.1371/journal.pone.0133143
60. Cavanna AE, Trimble MR. The precuneus: a review of its functional anatomy and behavioural correlates. *Brain* (2006) **129**(Pt 3):564–83. doi: 10.1093/brain/awl004
61. Pu W, Rolls ET, Guo S, Liu H, Yu Y, Xue Z, et al. Altered functional connectivity links in neuroleptic-naive and neuroleptic-treated patients with schizophrenia, and their relation to symptoms including volition. *Neuroimage Clin.* (2014) **6**:463–74. doi: 10.1016/j.nicl.2014.10.004
62. Zhao W, Luo L, Li Q, Kendrick KM. What can psychiatric disorders tell us about neural processing of the self. *Front Hum Neurosci.* (2013) **7**:485. doi: 10.3389/fnhum.2013.00485
63. Fagetagius C, Boyer L, Padovani R, Richieri R, Mundler O, Lancon C, et al. Schizophrenia with preserved insight is associated with increased perfusion of the precuneus. *J Psychiatry Neurosci.* (2012) **37**:297–304. doi: 10.1503/jpn.110125
64. de Achaval D, Villarreal MF, Costanzo EY, Douer J, Castro MN, Mora MC, et al. Decreased activity in right-hemisphere structures involved in social cognition in siblings discordant for schizophrenia. *Schizophr Res.* (2012) **134**:171–9. doi: 10.1016/j.schres.2011.11.010
65. Hanssen E, van der Velde J, Gromann PM, Shergill SS, de Haan L, Bruggeman R, et al. Neural correlates of reward processing in healthy siblings of patients with schizophrenia. *Front Hum Neurosci.* (2015) **9**:504. doi: 10.3389/fnhum.2015.00504
66. Chang X, Shen H, Wang L, Liu Z, Xin W, Hu D, et al. Altered default mode and fronto-parietal network subsystems in patients with schizophrenia and their unaffected siblings. *Brain Res.* (2014) **1562**:87–99. doi: 10.1016/j.brainres.2014.03.024
67. Brahmbhatt SB, Haut K, Csernansky JG, Barch DM. Neural correlates of verbal and nonverbal working memory deficits in individuals with schizophrenia and their high-risk siblings. *Schizophr Res.* (2006) **87**:191–204. doi: 10.1016/j.schres.2006.05.019
68. Vink M, Ramsey NF, Raemaekers M, Kahn RS. Striatal dysfunction in schizophrenia and unaffected relatives. *Biol Psychiatry* (2006) **60**:32–9. doi: 10.1016/j.biopsych.2005.11.026
69. Woodward ND, Tibbo P, Purdon SE. An fMRI investigation of procedural learning in unaffected siblings of individuals with schizophrenia. *Schizophr Res.* (2007) **94**:306–16. doi: 10.1016/j.schres.2007.04.026
70. Mamah D, Harms MP, Wang L, Barch D, Thompson P, Kim J, et al. Basal ganglia shape abnormalities in the unaffected siblings of schizophrenia patients. *Biol Psychiatry* (2008) **64**:111–20. doi: 10.1016/j.biopsych.2008.01.004
71. Seidman LJ, Faraone SV, Goldstein JM, Goodman JM, Kremen WS, Matsuda G, et al. Reduced subcortical brain volumes in nonpsychotic siblings of schizophrenic patients: a pilot magnetic resonance imaging study. *Am J Med Genet.* (1997) **74**:507–14.
72. Dahoun T, Trossbach SV, Brandon NJ, Korth C, Howes OD. The impact of Disrupted-in-Schizophrenia 1 (DISC1) on the dopaminergic system: a systematic review. *Transl Psychiatry* (2017) **7**:e1015. doi: 10.1038/tp.2016.282
73. Onitsuka T, Shenton ME, Salisbury DF, Dickey CC, Kasai K, Toner SK, et al. Middle and inferior temporal gyrus gray matter volume abnormalities in chronic schizophrenia: an MRI study. *Am J Psychiatry* (2004) **161**:1603–11. doi: 10.1176/appi.ajp.161.9.1603
74. Tang J, Liao Y, Zhou B, Tan C, Liu W, Wang D, et al. Decrease in temporal gyrus gray matter volume in first-episode, early onset schizophrenia: an MRI study. *PLoS ONE* (2012) **7**:e40247. doi: 10.1371/journal.pone.0040247
75. Kuroki N. Middle and inferior temporal gyrus gray matter volume abnormalities in first-episode schizophrenia: an MRI study. *Am J Psychiatry* (2006) **163**:2103. doi: 10.1176/appi.ajp.163.12.2103
76. Liu H, Kaneko Y, Ouyang X, Li L, Hao Y, Chen EY, et al. Schizophrenic patients and their unaffected siblings share increased resting-state connectivity in the task-negative network but not its anticorrelated task-positive network. *Schizophr Bull.* (2012) **38**:285–94. doi: 10.1093/schbul/sbq074
77. Wei Q, Diao F, Kang Z, Gan Z, Han Z, Zheng L, et al. The effect of DISC1 on regional gray matter density of schizophrenia in Han Chinese population. *Neurosci Lett.* (2012) **517**:21–4. doi: 10.1016/j.neulet.2012.03.098
78. Harrison PJ, Weinberger DR. Schizophrenia genes, gene expression, and neuropathology: on the matter of their convergence. *Mol Psychiatry* (2005) **10**:40–68. doi: 10.1038/sj.mp.4001558
79. Ballinger MD, Saito A, Abazyan B, Taniguchi Y, Huang CH, Ito K, et al. Adolescent cannabis exposure interacts with mutant DISC1 to produce impaired adult emotional memory. *Neurobiol Dis.* (2015) **82**:176–84. doi: 10.1016/j.nbd.2015.06.006
80. Wang HG, Jeffries JJ, Wang TF. Genetic and developmental perspective of language abnormality in autism and schizophrenia: one disease occurring at different ages in humans? *Neuroscientist* (2016) **22**:119–31. doi: 10.1177/1073858415572078
81. Abazyan B, Dziedzic J, Hua KG, Abazyan S, Yang CX, Mori S, et al. Chronic exposure of mutant DISC1 mice to lead produces sex-dependent abnormalities consistent with schizophrenia and related mental disorders: a gene-environment interaction study. *Schizophr Bull.* (2014) **40**:575–84. doi: 10.1093/schbul/sbt071
82. Bai Y, Wang W, Xu J, Zhang F, Yu H, Luo C, et al. Altered resting-state regional homogeneity after 13 weeks of paliperidone injection treatment in schizophrenia patients. *Psychiatry Res.* (2016) **258**:37–43. doi: 10.1016/j.pscychresns.2016.10.008

23

Neuroimaging Studies of Suicidal Behavior and Non-Suicidal Self-Injury in Psychiatric Patients

Carmen Domínguez-Baleón [1†], Luis F. Gutiérrez-Mondragón [1†], Adrián I. Campos-González [2,3†] and Miguel E. Rentería [2,3]*

[1] *Licenciatura en Ciencias Genómicas, Centro de Ciencias Genómicas, Universidad Nacional Autónoma de México, Cuernavaca, Mexico,* [2] *Department of Genetics & Computational Biology, QIMR Berghofer Medical Research Institute, Brisbane, QLD, Australia,* [3] *Faculty of Medicine, The University of Queensland, Herston, QLD, Australia*

***Correspondence:**
Miguel E. Rentería
miguel.renteria@qimrberghofer.edu.au

[†] *These authors have contributed equally to this work*

Background: With around 800,000 people taking their own lives every year, suicide is a growing health concern. Understanding the factors that underlie suicidality and identifying specific variables associated with increased risk is paramount for increasing our understanding of suicide etiology. Neuroimaging methods that enable the investigation of structural and functional brain markers *in vivo* are a promising tool in suicide research. Although a number of studies in clinical samples have been published to date, evidence about neuroimaging correlates for suicidality remains controversial.

Objective: Patients with mental disorders have an increased risk for both suicidal behavior and non-suicidal self-injury. This manuscript aims to present an up-to-date overview of the literature on potential neuroimaging markers associated with SB and NSSI in clinical samples. We sought to identify consistently reported structural changes associated with suicidal symptoms within and across psychiatric disorders.

Methods: A systematic literature search across four databases was performed to identify all English-language neuroimaging articles involving patients with at least one psychiatric diagnosis and at least one variable assessing SB or NSSI. We evaluated and screened evidence in these articles against a set of inclusion/exclusion criteria and categorized them by disease, adhering to the PRISMA guidelines.

Results: Thirty-three original scientific articles investigating neuroimaging correlates of SB in psychiatric samples were found, but no single article focusing on NSSI alone. Associations between suicidality and regions in frontal and temporal cortex were reported by 15 and 9 studies across four disorders, respectively. Furthermore, differences in hippocampus were reported by four studies across three disorders. However, we found a significant lack of replicability (consistency in size and direction) of results across studies.

Conclusions: Our systematic review revealed a lack of neuroimaging studies focusing on NSSI in clinical samples. We highlight several potential sources of bias in published studies, and conclude that future studies should implement more rigorous study designs to minimize bias risk. Despite several studies reporting associations between SB and anatomical differences in the frontal cortex, there was a lack of consistency across them. We conclude that better-powered samples, standardized neuroimaging and analytical protocols are needed to continue advancing knowledge in this field.

Keywords: neuroimaging, psychiatric patients, self-harm, suicide attempt, depression, schizophrenia, bipolar disorder

INTRODUCTION

Intentional self-harm defies the human intrinsic drive of self-preservation. However, both suicidal behavior (SB) and non-suicidal self-injury (NSSI) are surprisingly common in the population (1). Every year, more than 800,000 people around the world die by suicide (2). In fact, suicide is the second leading cause of death in people aged between 15 and 29 (2), plus it is increasingly recognized as a concerning public health issue in both developed and developing nations alike. Therefore, better prediction, prevention and intervention strategies are urgently needed.

It is estimated that for every completed suicide, there are between 10 and 20 attempts (3). Lifetime prevalence of SB is 9.2% for suicidal ideation, 3.1% for suicidal planning, and 2.7% for suicide attempts (4). Notably, lifetime prevalence of NSSI is estimated between 4 and 6% (including self-cutting, biting, or burning) in adult community samples (5, 6), but it is substantially higher in adolescents (14–47%) (7–9) and clinical samples (21–61%) (5).

The etiology of SB and NSSI is complex and knowledge about their underlying neurobiological mechanisms is limited (10). Several biological pathways have been implicated in the development and progression of NSSI and SB. Specifically, endogenous opioid deficiencies and altered levels of endocannabinoids in the brain have been associated with depression, anxiety, and suicide-related disorders (11, 12). Historically, the study of NSSI and SB has been hindered due to their behavioral nature, and by the common assumption that these behaviors are symptoms or consequences of other underlying mental disorders (13). Hence, despite their preventable nature, it is difficult to detect suicidal tendencies in time to prevent a fatal outcome, as the most common method for risk assessment consists of asking the patient whether he or she has experienced any type of suicidal thoughts. However, given that the topic is considered "taboo" and carries a big stigma in many societies, it is not uncommon for individuals to restrain from communicating their true intentions (14).

SB and NSSI show a strong relationship with mental health disorders (15). In fact, suicide is the most common cause of premature death in patients with major psychotic and mood disorders and up to 90% of individuals who commit suicide present at least one (often undiagnosed or untreated) axis I major psychiatric disorder (16–18). Some psychiatric conditions known for having increased suicide risk include major depressive disorder (MDD), bipolar disorder (BIP), schizophrenia (SCZ), and schizoaffective disorders and borderline personality disorder (BPD), among others (15). A recent meta-review concluded that these conditions are also associated with an increased risk of all-cause mortality and self-harm (15). Although NSSI and SB are routinely assessed as secondary items for some mental disorders, there is considerable variation in how that assessment is made. For instance, the timescale, degree of severity and specific constructs (e.g., ideation, attempt, or intent) vary widely even within single disorders such as MDD (13).

While knowledge about the underlying mechanisms of SB and NSSI remains elusive (19), it is acknowledged that individual genetic factors in combination with environmental stressors influence suicidal outcomes (20). A twin study showed that genetic factors explain a significant part of the variance in NSSI (37% for males and 59% for females) and SB (41 and 55%, respectively) (20). Furthermore, these behaviors are strongly correlated ($r = 0.49-0.61$), and the correlation is largely explained by shared genes (62 and 76% for males and females, respectively) (20). Notably, it is still unknown to what extent the genetic and neural mechanisms that lead to a suicidal attempt are common or distinct across different psychiatric disorders.

Neuroimaging methods, such as magnetic resonance imaging (MRI), allow for the non-invasive interrogation of brain structure and function *in vivo* (21). By comparing groups of patients and healthy controls and applying statistical methods that control for possible confounding covariates such as age, sex, ethnicity, or treatment, it is possible to explore the neural correlates of suicide vulnerability with unprecedented detail. Nonetheless, as with any other scientific approaches, a set of study design principles should be implemented to avoid possible confounding factors and sources of bias to affect study outcomes.

Here we present a systematic review of the literature on neuroimaging studies of SB and NSSI in patients with mental disorders. In addition to summarizing the results of published studies, we assessed potential sources of bias following the PRISMA guidelines. We hypothesized that neuroanatomical differences associated with SB and NSSI would be consistent within disorders. Furthermore, given that affective mental disorders are genetically correlated (22), we also expected some commonalities across disorders to emerge. Overall, we hope to be able to provide a valuable collection of information that can enable more powerful, better-designed analyses of SB and NSSI; also to allow a deeper understanding of these conditions that can ultimately lead to more effective prevention and intervention strategies.

MATERIALS AND METHODS

Literature Search

Two reviewers conducted literature searches in Google Scholar, PsycINFO, EMBASE, and PubMed for neuroimaging articles investigating SB (ideation, planning, or attempt) and NSSI in patients with psychiatric disorders. We defined three sets of keywords, comprising (i) self-harm and suicide terms, (ii) neuroimaging terms, and (iii) psychiatric disorder terms (**Table 1** and **Supplementary Material**). For each list, we included synonyms or equivalent terms for each of the terms. Subsequently, we used combinations of keywords (one from each category) to systematically query the databases (**Figure 1**).

Inclusion Criteria

In this review, we focused only on structural MRI studies, and not those involving computed tomography or functional MRI techniques. We included only original articles written in English. Therefore, unpublished studies, non-peer-reviewed articles, articles published in a language other than English, case reports, conference abstracts, meta-analyses, review articles, editorials, and articles not assessing neuroimaging phenotypes relative to suicidal symptoms were excluded. The inclusion or exclusion of an article was assessed independently by three of the authors, and in cases of disagreement it was discussed case by case until an agreement was reached.

Data Collection Process

All published articles relating suicidality with neuroanatomical phenotypes were thoroughly read by at least three authors. Information on cortical or subcortical phenotype comparisons between patients with suicidal symptoms (as reported by the study) and healthy controls or non-suicidal patients was extracted from tables, figures and the main text of the results section of each article reviewed. Each author contributed to creating and corroborating **Tables 2–7**. Measurements were collected as standardized values or statistical differences (*Z*-scores, Cohen's d, *F*-score, etc.) in volumetric, thickness, or surface area measurements, and stored as a simplified outcome variable assessing differences between suicidal cases vs. non-suicidal cases and/or healthy controls (**Tables 2–7**).

TABLE 1 | Keywords used to query the bibliographic databases.

Suicidal behavior/NSSI	Neuroimaging	Psychiatric disorders
Self-harm, suicide, suicide attempt, suicidal behavior, suicidal ideation, self-mutilation, self-injury, self-poisoning.	Magnetic-resonance imaging, MRI, brain imaging, neuroimaging.	Psychiatry, psychiatric patients, mental disorder, mental health, psychiatric diagnosis, depression, mdd, major depressive disorder, schizophrenia, bipolar disorder, anorexia nervosa, bulimia nervosa, post-traumatic stress disorder, ptsd, alcohol use disorder, substance use disorder, cannabis, alcoholism, borderline personality disorder, anxiety, alcohol abuse, anxiety disorders, eating disorders.

Bias Risk Assessment

Typical bias risk assessment instruments (e.g., Cochrane) are intended for interventional studies such as randomized controlled trials. For case-control studies searching for neurobiological associations, there is, to the best of our knowledge, no gold standard instrument for performing bias risk assessment. Nonetheless, we acknowledge the importance of finding possible sources of bias in the reviewed literature. Thus, we devised a table including possible sources of confounding or bias in structural neuroimaging association studies, including key design, and statistical aspects such as matching suitable controls and cases, assessing absence of mental disorders in the control group, assessing MRI scans for artifacts and pathological findings, etc. Three authors independently filled this table indicating whether a study had a low, medium or high risk of bias for all constructs. As an example, for the construct "controls matched to subjects," a study that perfectly matched demographics between controls and cases would receive a score of low risk, while a study with only partially matching controls

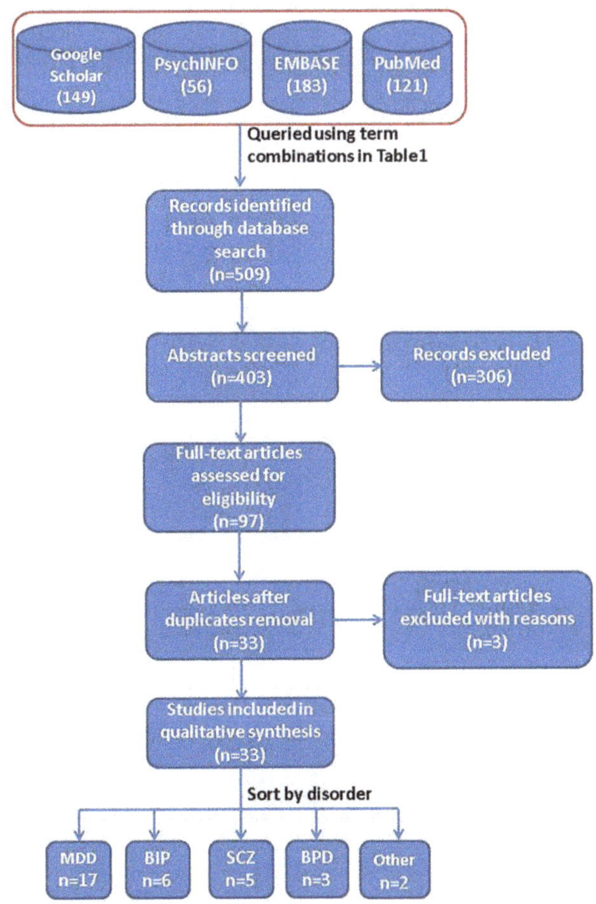

FIGURE 1 | General overview of the methodology. Flow diagram depicting database sources and the steps performed for this systematic review.

TABLE 2 | Main characteristics of articles regarding Major Depressive Disorder and Suicide.

References	*n*	Country	Gender	Age (s.d.)	Brain phenotypes	MRI	Diagnosis	Findings
Gosnell et al. (23)	*n* = 60 (40 patients, 20 controls)	USA	28 F/32 M	MDD suicidal attempt:28.9 (9.98), MDD no suicidal attempt:29.25 (11.1), healthy controls:28.9 (10.0)	Cortical lobes (Frontal, temporal, parietal, occipital), corpus callosum, thalamus, insula, limbic structures, basal ganglia, hippocampus, amygdala.	T1-weighted images on a 3T Siemens Trio MR scanner.	C-SSRS, PHQ, WHOA, DSM-IV	Reduction in right hippocampal volume of the suicidal group compared to healthy controls and frontal and temporal lobe volumes of the suicidal group were diminished compared to the depressed patients.
Colle et al. (24)	*n* = 63 patients	France	~50% F/M	MDD no suicidal attempt: 47.7(12.6), MDD suicidal attempt: 44.2(11.9). Past:47.6(13.4), Acute: 40.2(13.4)	Hippocampal volume.	1.5 or 3-T Philips scanner, SPM5 processing	Hamilton Depression Rating Scale (HDRS) >17, DSM-IVTR.	Depressed patients with a history of suicide attempts had smaller hippocampus than depressed patients without such a history. (TV)
Taylor et al. (25)	*n* = 165 (74 patients, 91 controls)	USA	108 F/57 M	MDD no suicidal: 37.5 (8.9), MDD suicidal: 33.5 (9.1), healthy controls: 29.9 (9.1)	Regional white and gray matter volumes, cortical thickness. Orbitofrontal cortex, cingulate cortex, insula, amygdala, parahippocampus, thalamus and basal ganglia.	Sagittal T1-weighted FreeSurfer processing	DSM-IV, Montgomery–Asberg Depression Rating Scale (MADRS) >15	Depressed group with thoughts of death did exhibit reduced cortical thickness in the left frontal, temporal, parietal regions and the insula but not in regional GMV when compared to the group without thoughts of death.
Peng et al. (26)	*n* = 66 (38 patients, 28 controls)	China	38 F/28 M	MDD suicidal attempt: 27.75(7.21), MDD no suicidal attempt: 31.06 (7.39), healthy controls: 28.61(5.45)	Gray matter volume of the limbic cingulate gyrus, the middle temporal gyrus, the parietal region and the insula.	Philips 3 T, T1-weighted 3D SPM8 processing	Hamilton Depressive Rating Scale (HDRS), DSM-IV, Zung's Self-Rating Depression Scale (SDS).	Patients with a suicide history showed significantly decreased GMV in the right middle temporal gyrus and increased GMV in the right parietal lobe when each group was compared to healthy controls. The suicidal group had a decreased GMV in left limbic cingulate gyrus compared to the non-suicidal group.
Dombrovski et al. (27)	*n* = 52 (33 patients, 19 controls)	USA	30 F/22 M	MDD suicidal attempt: 66.0 (6.4), MDD no suicidal: 67.7 (7.0), healthy controls: 70.5 (7.5)	Basal ganglia gray matter integrity.	T1-weighted images, automated labeling pathway (ALP) processing	SCID/DSM-IV, HDRS-17	Suicide Attempters had lower putamen gray matter voxel counts and lower voxel counts in associative and ventral striatum.

(Continued)

TABLE 2 | Continued

References	*n*	Country	Gender	Age (s.d.)	Brain phenotypes	MRI	Diagnosis	Findings
Wagner et al. (28)	*n* = 60 (30 patients, 30 controls)	Germany	50 F/10 M	MDD high-risk for suicide: 41.0 (12.5), MDD low-Risk for suicide: 34.1 (10.5), healthy controls: 35.1(10.4)	Cortical thickness, dorsolateral prefrontal cortex (DLPFC), ventrolateral prefrontal cortex (VLPFC)	1.5T Siemens scanner, T1-weighted images, FreeSurfer processing	DSM-IV diagnosis, 18 on the 21-item HDRS	Patients with depression and a high risk for suicide had a substantially thinner cortex in the left DLPFC, VLPFC and the anterior cingulate when compared against non-high risk patients.
Cyprien et al. (29)	*n* = 435 (201 patients, 234 controls)	France	222 F/213 M	MDD suicidal attempt: 72.2 (4.3), MDD no suicidal attempt: 71 (3.8), healthy controls: 71 (3.8)	Corpus Callosum volume	T1-weighted imaging, Analyze 9.0 processing	MINI/DSM-IV criteria, Center for Epidemiological Studies-Depression scale (CES-D)	The area of the posterior third of corpus callosum was significantly smaller in suicide attempters than in affective controls and healthy individuals.
Wagner et al. (30)	*n* = 60 (30 patients, 30 controls)	Germany	50 F/10 M	MDD High-risk: 41.0 (12.5), MDD Low-risk: 34.1(10.5), Controls: 35.1 (10.4)	Regional Gray Matter density	Sagittal T1-weighted SPM2 processing	DSM-IV, 18 on the 21-item HDRS	Depressed individuals with higher risk for suicide presented diminished gray matter density in a fronto-striato-limbic network in comparison to healthy controls and in caudate and rostral anterior cingulate cortex when compared to non-high risk patients.
Hwang et al. (31)	*n* = 96 (70 patients, 26 controls)	Taiwan	All Male	MDD suicidal attempt: 79.1(5.6), MDD no suicidal attempt: 79.6 (5.1), healthy controls: 79.5 (4.3)	Regional volumes. GM (insula, posterior cingulate) WM (subcallosal cingulate cortex, floor of lateral ventricles, parahippocampal region, insula, cerebellum).	Siamens 2T T1-weighted imaging, SPM2 processing	17 on the 21-item Hamilton Depression Rating Scale (HDRS), DSM-IV	Suicidal depression was associated with decreased gray matter and white matter volume in the frontal, parietal and temporal lobes, and the insula, lentiform nucleus, midbrain, and cerebellum when compared with non-suicidal individuals.
Pompili et al. (32)	*n* = 99 (all patients)	Italy	57 F/42 M	No suicidal attempt:47.27 (14.54), Suicidal attempt: 45.57 (16.10)	Total White Matter Hyperintensities	T1 & T2-weighted images	DSM-IV-TR diagnosis of major affective disorders (MDD, BIP type I, BIP type II, subst. Abuse), MINI/DSM-IV-TR.	The presence of periventricular white matter hyperintensities was robustly associated with **suicidal behaviors.**
Monkul et al. (33)	*n* = 34 total (17 patients, 17 controls)	USA	All Female	Suicidal: 31.4 (13.9), Non Suicidal: 36.5 (7.5), Healthy controls: 31.3 (8.3)	Regional GM and WM volumes (orbitofrontal cortex, cingulate, amygdala and hippocampus)	1.5T GE Signa Imaging. Signa 5.4.3 software	Structured Clinical Interview for DSM-IV (SCID). (HDRS).	Suicidal depressed patients showed a smaller GMV in the right and left orbitofrontal cortex compared with healthy subjects. Suicidal patients presented larger right amygdala volumes when compared to non-suicidal patients.

(Continued)

TABLE 2 | Continued

References	*n*	Country	Gender	Age (s.d.)	Brain phenotypes	MRI	Diagnosis	Findings
Pompili et al. (32)	$n = 65$ (all patients)	Italy	41 F/24 M	MDD suicidal attempt: 42.17(13.51) MDD no suicidal attempt: 44.61 (13.95)	White Matter Hyperintensities	Axial and coronal T2-weighted Axial and Sagittal T1-weighted	MDD, BIP MINI/DSM-IV diagnosis	The prevalence of white matter hyperintensities was significantly higher in subjects with **past suicide attempts.**
Ehrlich et al. (34)	$n = 102$ (all patients)	USA	68 F/34 M	26.7(5.5)	White matter hyperintensities	T2-weighted	DSM-IV diagnosis.	The prevalence of periventricular white matter hyperintensities was significantly higher in subjects with **past suicide attempts**
Ehrlich et al. (35)	$n = 153$ (all patients)	USA	41 F/112 M	Psychosis: 16.0(3.3), BIP: 14.9 (3.5), Depression: 15.1(2.8)	White matter hyperintensities	T2-weighted	DSM-IV diagnosis	White matter hyperintensities were significantly associated with a higher prevalence of **past suicide attempts**
Ahearn et al. (36)	$n = 40$ (all patients)	USA	34 F/6 M	MDD suicidal attempt: 66.0 (5.8), MDD no suicide attempt: 66.4 (5.7)	Gray matter hyperintensities	1.5 T and T2 weighted imaging	The Hamilton Depression Scale (HDRS)	Unipolar patients with a history of a **suicide attempt** demonstrated significantly more subcortical gray matter hyperintensities compared with patients without such a history
Lee et al. (37)	$n = 38$ (all patients)	South Korea	20 F/18 M	MDD suicidal attempt: 41.95 (10.81), MDD no suicidal attempt: 41.11 (15.15)	Regional gray matter volume differences.	T1-weighted imaging, SPM8 processing	DSM-IV, HDRS	Compared with suicide non-attempters, **suicide attempters** exhibited decreased GM volume in the left angular gyrus and right cerebellum.
Sachs-Ericsson et al. (38)	$n = 246$ (all patients)	USA	190F/55M	MDD suicidal attempt: 66.74 (6.6), MDD no suicidal attempt: 69.8 (7.5)	White matter lesions (WML)	1.5 T imaging MrX processing	MontgomeryeAsberg Depression Rating Scale (MADRS), DSM-IV, MMSE, DIS.	Higher baseline WML in left hemisphere. **Attempt history** predicted growth in WML.

TABLE 3 | Main characteristics of articles regarding Bipolar Disorder and Suicide.

References	*n*	Country	Gender	Age (s.d.)	Brain phenotypes	MRI	Diagnosis	Findings
Johnston et al. (39)	*n* =113 (68 patients, 45 controls)	USA	69 F/44 M	BIP suicidal attempt: 20.5 (3.0), BIP no suicidal attempt: 20.5 (3.0), healthy controls: 20.8 (3.3)	Regional Gray matter volumes	Sagittal, T1-weighted, SPM5 processing	DSM-IV criteria	**Attempters** demonstrated significantly lower GMV than non-attempters in the right orbitofrontal cortex and hippocampus, as well as bilaterally in the cerebellum extending into the vermis.
Lijffijt et al. (40)	*n* = 93 (51 patients, 42 controls)	USA	All Female	BIP suicidal attempt: 36.6 (10.7), BIP no suicidal attempt:41.1 (11.3)	Prefrontal cortex gray matter volume	High resolution 3-D T1-weighted, 1.5-Tesla Intera scanner	DSM-IV(SCID, HDRS, (Young Mania Rating Scale) YMRS.	PFCGM (prefrontal cortex gray matter) volume was lower in patients with than without **attempt history** in those with past psychiatric hospitalization.
Nery-Fernandes et al. (41)	*n* = 62 (40 patients, 22 controls)	Brazilian	41 F/21 M	BIP suicidal: 39.8(11.4), BIP non-suicidal: 42.0(8.6), Healthy controls: 37.7(13.5)	Corpus callosum sub-region area: (rostrum, genu, rostral body, anterior midbody, posterior midbody,isthmus, and splenium).	1.5T Sigma Imaging, ANALYZE AVW processing	DSM-IV axis I (SCID-I), HDRS, YMRS.	No differences were observed for any subregion between Bipolar-Suicidal and Bipolar-Non Suicidal groups. There was a significant reduction in the genu and isthmus areas in bipolar patients compared with HC.
Baldaçara et al. (42)	*n* = 62 (40 patients, 22 controls)	Brazilian	41 F/21 M	BIP suicidal attempt:39.94 (11.12), BIP no suicidal attempt: 41.9 (8.9), Healthy controls:37.72 (13.63)	Cerebellar volume	Sagittal T1, 1.5T Symphony Master/Class Siemens	SCID-I, HDRS, YMRS.	No volumetric differences were found between the BIP subjects with **suicidal attempt** and those without such history.
Matsuo et al. (43)	*n* = 47 (20 patients, 27 controls)	USA	All Female	BIP suicidal: 36.2 (10.1), BIP non suicidal: 44.2 (12.5), Healthy controls: 36.9 (13.8)	Corpus Callosum genu, anterior body, posterior body, isthmus and splenium areas	Philips 1.5 T, Axial 3D T1 weighted	DSM-IV/SCID, HDRS, YMRS.	No significant differences among the three groups on any regional CC areas, although the suicidal BIP patients had the smallest areas.
Duarte et al. (44)	*n* = 59 (39 patients, 20 controls)	Brazillian	34 F/25 M	BIP suicidal attempt: 41.1(12.64), BIP no suicidal attempt: 42.26 (11.70), Healthy controls: 37.40 (10.20)	Whole brain exploratory. Hypothesis driven: OFC (superior lateral, middle lateral, inferior lateral and medial); dorsal lateral PFC (DLPFC) (inferior, middle and superior frontal gyri); ACC; amygdala; hippocampus; insula; and thalamus.	Philips 1.5 T 3D T1 weighted	DSM-IV-TR, MINI-PLUS, HDRS	Attempters showed an increase in GMV in the rostral anterior cingulate cortex, insula and orbitofrontal cortex when compared to non-attempters.

TABLE 4 | Main characteristics of articles regarding Schizophrenia and Suicide.

References	*n*	Country	Gender	Age (s.d.)	Brain phenotypes	MRI	Diagnosis	Findings
Besteher et al. (45)	$n = 87$ (37 patients, 50 controls)	Germany	46 F/41 M	SCZ suicidal attempts: 34.4 (12.1), SCZ no suicidal attempts:28.8 (9.7), Healthy controls:29.5 (7.9).	Cortical thickness (CT)	T1-weighted imaging on 1.5-T Siemens. FreeSurfer processing.	DSM-IV	Suicide attempters had cortical thinning in the bilateral caudal middle frontal gyrus, lateral orbitofrontal and superior frontal gyrus, left pars orbitalis and right caudal ACC, pars opercularis and triangularis when compared with healthy controls.
Giakoumatos (46)	$n = 751$ (489 patients, 262 controls)	USA	387 F/364 M	SCZ no suicidal attempt: 35.9(13.3). SCZ suicidal attempt lethality; High:35.6(11.7), Low:36.9(12.2), Healthy controls:38.1(12.5)	Regional Gray matter volume in temporal, parietal, frontal regions.	High-resolution isotropic T1-weighted imaging, FreeSurfer analysis	DSM-IV-TR/SCID	Attempters had significantly less GMV in bilateral inferior temporal and superior temporal cortices, left superior parietal, thalamus and supramarginal regions, right insula, superior frontal and rostral middle frontal regions when compared to non-attempters.
Spoletini et al. (47)	$n = 100$ (50 patients, 50 controls)	Italy	45 F/55 M	SCZ suicidal attempt: 42.9 (11.3), SCZ no suicidal attempt: 39.8 (11.4), Healthy controls: 40.0 (16.6)	Volumetric data of lateral ventricles, thalamus, hippocampus, amygdala, caudate, putamen, pallidum and accumbens	3D T1-weighted, T2-weighted FSL 4.1 software for processing	DSM-IV-TR, MMSE	An increased volume in the right amygdala was observed in **lifetime suicide attempters** compared non attempter and HC. Increased right amygdala volume was correlated to augmented self-aggression.
Aguilar et al. (48)	$n = 37$ (all patients)	Spain	All Male	SCZ suicidal: 37.12 (10.02), SCZ non Suicidal: 42.65 (10.19)	Gray Matter density	1.5 T, 3D T1-weighted, SPM5 processing	DSM-IV	Reduction in gray matter in the left superior temporal lobe and left orbitofrontal cortex was observed in patients with a **record of suicide attempts** when comparing to non-suicidal patients.
Rüsch et al. (49)	$n = 110$ (55 patients, 55 controls)	Italy	42 F/68 M	SCZ suicidal attempt: 30.3 (6.5), SCZ no suicidal attempt: 37.3 (11.6), Healthy controls: 36.0	Inferior frontal region white matter volumes	T1-weighted 3D SPM2 processing	DSM-IV/SCID-I	Increased bilateral inferior frontal white matter volumes were shown by patients **with a previous suicide attempt** as compared with those patients without such history. Among patients, current self-aggression was positively correlated with white matter volume in the aforementioned regions.

or non-matching controls would receive a score of medium or high risk, respectively. For detailed information on each construct, their interpretation and coding please refer to the **Supplementary Material**.

RESULTS

After applying our quality control and exclusion criteria, we were left with 33 articles (**Figure 2**). Two meta-analysis studies (21, 55), and a study not assessing imaging phenotypes with SB (56) were excluded. Of the selected studies, the majority were related to MDD (17 out of 33) and mainly focused on reporting gray matter volume differences. Characteristics of each individual study are detailed in **Tables 2–5** No single article focusing on NSSI alone was found. Below we summarize the main findings related to specific cortical and subcortical brain regions in MDD, BIP, SCZ, or BPD.

Major Depressive Disorder

MDD affects nearl2y 32 million people worldwide (57). The Diagnostic and Statistical Manual of Mental Disorders 5th edition (DSM-5), describes this psychiatric disorder as characterized by depressed mood and/or diminished interest or pleasure, vegetative symptoms such as disturbed sleep or appetite and persistent thoughts of death, suicidal ideation or previous suicide attempts (58). In fact, up to 50% of all completed suicides annually occur within a depressive episode and MDD patients are 20-fold more likely to die by suicide than healthy individuals (59).

Seventeen studies focused on identifying brain regions associated with SB in patients with MDD (the characteristics of each study are summarized in **Table 2**). Sample size across studies ranged from 34 to 246 individuals aged between 20 and 80 years. Cohorts included participants from the USA, Germany, France, Netherlands and China. With the exception of two studies, all included a combination of both male and female individuals. Most of them compared structural MRI brain phenotypes between depressed suicidal, depressed non-suicidal, and healthy control groups. In addition, the majority of MDD diagnoses were made according to DSM-IV criteria. Phenotypes of interest were mostly gray and white matter regional volumes, but five studies focused on differences in white matter hyperintensities. In this section, we summarize the main findings recovered from these articles, divided into cortical and subcortical phenotypes.

Cortical Regions

We identified four independent studies suggesting a potential link between the **insular cortex** region and suicidal symptoms in MDD. Taylor et al. (25) described reduced cortical thickness in the left insula of MDD patients with death thoughts, compared to MDD patients without death thoughts, but found no significant difference between healthy controls and any of the depressed groups, as reported in two other studies (26, 28). In another study, Hwang et al. (31) found reduced gray matter volumes within the left and right insula of suicidal MDD patients, compared to non-suicidal MDD patients. Taylor et al. (25) argue that the insula may be relevant because it is a component of the salience network and may potentiate the neural response to

TABLE 5 | Main characteristics of articles regarding Borderline Personality Disorder and Suicide.

References	n	Country	Gender	Age (s.d.)	Brain phenotypes	MRI	Diagnosis	Findings
Soloff et al. (50)	$n = 51$ (all patients)	USA	41 F/10 M	BPD High lethality attempers: 36.1 (9.2), BPD Low lethality attempers: 27.4 (5.9)	Regional GM volumes mid-inf. orbital frontal cortex, anterior cingulate cortex, middle-superior temporal cortex, insula, hippocampus, parahippocampus, fusiform gyrus, lingual gyrus and amygdala	1.5T Signa Imaging, Sagittal T1-weighted, (DARTEL) in SPM8 processing	DSMIII-R or DSM-IV (SCID), Diagnostic Interview for Borderlines (DIB).	High lethality attempters had diminished GMV in right midsupperior temporal gyrus, right middle inferior orbitofrontal gyrus, right insular cortex, left fusiform gyrus, left lingual gyrus and right parahippocampal gyrus compared to low lethality attempters.
Soloff et al. (51)	$n = 120$ (68 patients, 52 controls)	USA	76 F/44 M	BPD: 28.3 (7.5), Healthy controls: 25.9 (7.2)	Regional GM concentrations mid-inf. orbitofrontal cortex, mid-sup temporal cortex, anterior cingulate, insula, hippocampus, amygdala, fusiform, lingual and parahippocampal gyri	1.5T Sign, Sagittal T1-weightes imaging, SPM5 processing	DSMIII-R or DSM-IV (SCID), DIB.	BPD attempters had diminished gray matter volumes in the insula, the left hemisphere, the middle superior temporal cortex, the right hemisphere, hippocampus, fusiform gyrus, parahippocampus, anterior cingulate and amigdala when compared to healthy controls.
Goodman et al. (52)	$n = 26$ (13 patients, 13 controls)	USA	20 F/6 M	BPD: 15.8 (1.1), Healthy controls: 16.2 (0.8)	Gray and white matter volume in the prefrontal cortex	T1-weighted MP-RAGE	DSM-IV, DIB, BDI.	Number of suicide attempts was positively associated with smaller overall Brodmann area 24 (ACC) volume.

TABLE 6 | Main characteristics of articles regarding other affective disorders and suicide.

References	n	Country	Gender	Age (s.d.)	Brain phenotypes	MRI	Diagnosis	Findings
Kim et al. (53)	$n = 36$ (all patients)	Korea	23 F/13 M	Panic Disorder suicidal attempt: 33.42 (14.09), Panic Disorder no suicidal attempt: 34.00 (9.38)	Gray Matter and White Matter volumes	3D T1-FSPGR imaging. SPM5 processing	DSM-IV/SCID.	The VBM analysis revealed no significant intergroup difference in the GM and WM volumes.
Thomas et al. (54)	$n = 182$ (61 patients, 121 controls)	USA	93 F/89 M	PTSD: 11.74 (2.4), Healthy Controls: 11.74 (2.7)	Pituitary volumes	T2-weighted images (GE 1.5-Tesla Unit)	DSM-IV	PTSD subjects with a history of suicidal ideation had larger pituitary volumes than healthy controls.

negative stimuli through its connections with the amygdala and the cingulate cortex. Moreover, Hwang et al. (31) add that the insula is preferentially engaged in internally generated emotions and functions as a relay signal station to maintain homeostasis.

The **frontal lobe** was consistently reported as potentially implicated in SB within MDD. Taylor et al. (25) found reduced cortical thickness in the left frontal lobe of MDD patients with death thoughts, compared with non-suicidal MDD patients. Hwang et al. (31) and Gosnell et al. (23) reported significantly decreased volumes in the **right, left and total frontal lobe**, both studies made the observations when comparing suicidal vs. non-suicidal MDD patients. Wagner et al. (30) observed differences in regional gray matter density between MDD patients with high risk for suicide and healthy controls in the **right inferior frontal gyrus**. As mentioned by Gosnell et al. (23), the frontal lobe may inhibit the emotional limbic system, which is probably dysregulated in emotionally unstable individuals and thus could cause the characteristic impulsiveness of SB.

Studies also highlighted differences in the **temporal lobe**; Taylor et al. (25) found reduced cortical thickness in MDD patients with death thoughts, compared with MDD patients without death thoughts. Gosnell et al. (23) observed significantly lower right and total temporal lobe volumes, and Hwang et al. (31) reported reduced gray matter volumes within temporal regions when comparing MDD suicidal patients against non-suicidal MDD patients. Also, Peng et al. (26) reported smaller gray matter volumes in the right middle temporal gyrus of MDD suicidal patients compared to healthy individuals. Both Gosnell et al. (23) and Hwang et al. (31) hypothesize that the temporal cortex may be implicated in emotional dysregulation in suicidal individuals.

Three independent studies associated the **cingulate cortex** with SB in MDD. Wagner et al. (28) observed a cortical thickness reduction in the **anterior cingulate** of MDD patients at high risk for suicide, compared to non-high-risk patients. Moreover, Peng et al. (26) found significantly decreased gray matter volume in the **left limbic cingulate gyrus** of suicidal MDD patients with respect to the non-suicidal depressed group. Finally, Wagner et al. (30) found differences in regional gray matter density between MDD patients at high risk for suicide and healthy controls in the **rostral and dorsal part of the anterior cingulate cortex**, a result later replicated by the same group in 2012 (28). As the cingulate is part of the limbic system, involved in emotional formation and processing, it has been proposed to directly influence the SB of depressed patients (26).

Differences in the **parietal lobe** have also been reported. Taylor et al. (25) described reduced cortical thickness in the **left parietal lobe** in MDD patients with death thoughts, compared to MDD patients without death thoughts. Hwang et al. (31) found reduced gray matter and white matter volumes within parietal regions in suicidal MDD patients compared to non-suicidal MDD patients. On the other hand, Peng et al. (26) observed an increase in gray matter volumes in the **right parietal lobe** in suicidal MDD patients compared to healthy individuals. Peng et al. (26) argue that the parietal lobe is connected to other parietal occipital-temporal areas, which have also been suggested to be altered in MDD patients with suicidal symptoms.

In addition, single studies have implicated **other regions** with suicidal symptoms, but these were not replicated in other studies. For instance, Monkul et al. (33) reported gray matter volume reductions in the **orbitofrontal cortex** of MDD suicidal patients when compared to non-suicidal patients, and Wagner et al. (28) found reduced cortical thickness in the **left dorsolateral and ventrolateral prefrontal cortex** when comparing patients at high suicide risk against non-high-risk patients.

Subcortical Regions

Both Gosnell et al. (23) and Colle et al. (24) found significantly reduced right hippocampal volumes in the suicidal MDD group compared to the healthy controls and non-suicidal MDD patients. This association is consistent with the role of the hippocampus in regulating emotional responses (60) and with findings of hippocampal volumetric decreases as predictors of slower depression recovery (61).

Ahearn et al. (36) reported that MDD patients with a history of a suicide attempt had substantially more subcortical gray matter hyperintensities compared to patients without such a history. Monkul et al. (33) observed larger **right amygdala** volumes in suicidal vs. non-suicidal MDD patients, and Wagner et al. (30) reported a decrease in regional gray matter density between depressed patients at high suicide risk and healthy controls in the **right amygdala–hippocampus formation**. Also, Wagner et al. (30) found differences in regional gray matter density between depressed patients at high risk for suicide and healthy controls in

TABLE 7 | Cortical phenotypes associated with SB across disorders.

Disorder/Area	Frontal	Prefrontal	Orbitofrontal	Parietal	Temporal	Occipital	Limbic (Cingulate)	Insular
MDD Wagner et al. (28)		Reduction DLPFC and VLPFC CT					Reduction anterior CT	
MDD Peng et al. (26)				Increase right GM			Reduction left limbic GM	
MDD Wagner et al. (30)	Reduction GM						Reduction anterior, rostral and dorsal GM	
MDD Taylor et al. (25)	Reduction CT			Reduction left CT	Reduction CT			Reduction left CT
MDD Gosnell et al. (23)	Reduction CV				Reduction CV			
MDD Hwang et al. (31)	Reduction GM, WM			Reduction GM, WM	Reduction GM			Reduction GM
MDD Monkul et al. (33)			Reduction GM					
MDD Duarte et al. (44)			Increase GM				Increase GM	Increase GM
BD Johnston et al. (39)			Reduction GM					
BD Lijffijt et al. (40)		Reduction GM						
BP-P Giakoumatos et al. (46)					Reduction fusiform gyri bilaterian inferior and superior GM			
SCZ Besteher et al. (45)	Reduction CT	Reduction CT	Reduction CT	Reduction left superior CT	Reduction CT	Reduction CT	Reduction right caudal anterior CT	Reduction CT
SCZ Giakoumatos et al. (46)	Reduction GM			Reduction GM	Reduction inferior GM	Reduction right cuneus, pericalcarine GM		Reduction right GM
SCZ Aguilar et al. (48)			Reduction GM		Reduction left superior GM			
SCZ Rusch et al. (49)		Increase WM	Increase WM					
BPD Soloff et al. (51)			Reduction bilateral middle inferior GM		Reduction fusiform gyrus, bilateral middle superior GM	Reduction lingual gyrus GM	Reduction left anterior GM	Reduction right GM
BPD Soloff et al. (50)			Reduction right middle inferior GM		Reduction fusiform gyrus, right middle superior gyrus GM	Reduction left lingual gyrus GM		Reduction right and left GM
BDP Goodman et al. (52)							Reduction CV	

CT, Cortical thickness; CV, Cortical volume; GM, Gray matter volume; WM, White matter volume.

the **caudate nucleus.** Hwang et al. (31) found reduced gray matter volumes within the **lentiform nucleus** when comparing suicidal vs. non-suicidal MDD patients, and reduced gray matter volumes within the cerebellum, an observation later replicated by Lee et al. (37). A cortical volume decrease was reported in single studies in the **corpus callosum** (29) and **putamen** (27) regions.

In the largest neuroimaging study of suicidality in MDD published to date, Rentería et al. (21) conducted a series of

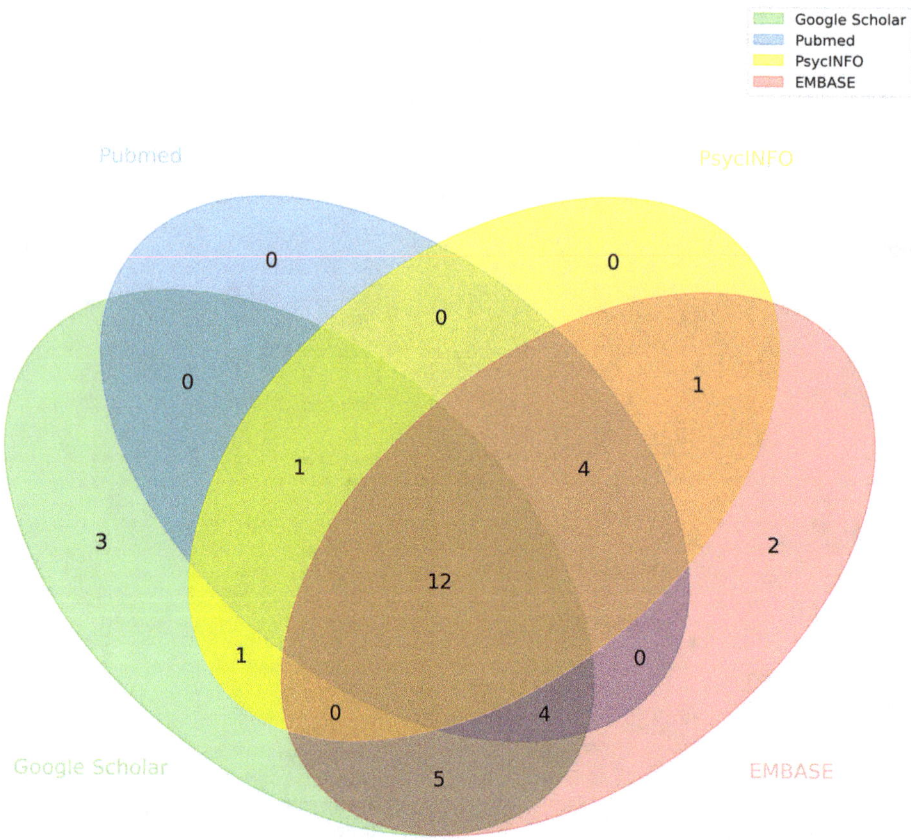

FIGURE 2 | Database source of articles included in this systematic review. Venn diagram illustrating the overlap between studies obtained from different databases.

meta-analyses in 3,097 individuals, including 1,996 healthy controls, 451 MDD patients with suicidal symptoms, and 650 MDD patients without suicidal symptoms. The meta-analyses did not replicate any previously reported associations between subcortical volume and suicidal symptoms (ideation or planning/attempt) in MDD patients. The study reported only a smaller intracranial volume in MDD patients with suicidal symptoms compared with healthy controls, and a study-wide non-significant trend of smaller subcortical volumes and larger ventricular volumes in suicidal patients compared with healthy controls. Importantly, the authors noted that even with those sample sizes the study was underpowered, thus raising the question of statistical power of previous studies with substantially smaller sample sizes (see section Discussion).

White Matter Hyperintensities

Several studies reported on white matter hyperintensities (WMH) and periventricular white matter hyperintensities (PVH) and their association with past suicide attempts (32, 34, 35). Pompili et al. (32) found that lifetime suicidal ideation in the presence of a history of suicide attempt was positively associated with the presence of WMH, and later (62) showed that suicide attempters were more likely to have higher PVH than non-attempters. The same studies reported that suicidal ideation without a history of suicide attempt was not significantly associated with any measure of WMH, PVH, Deep white matter hyperintensities (DWMH), or subcortical gray matter hyperintensities (32, 34), and that DWMH was not significantly associated with suicidality (35, 62). Ehrlich et al. (34) proposed that MDD patients with PVH may be at higher risk of suicide due to the possible disruption of neuroanatomical pathways, as they are associated with ependymal loss and varying degrees of myelination. Although white matter lesions have been linked to aging, they were found to be associated with suicide attempters in an older cohort (38), further supporting the observed correlation with SB.

Bipolar Disorder

The symptoms of BIP include alterations in mood and energy levels and in the person's ability to execute everyday tasks. The characteristic mood episodes go from manic extremely energetic periods to sad, hopeless depressive episodes (63). Suicide rates among BIP patients are 20-fold or higher than in the general population (64). Our literature search identified six scientific articles that investigated neuroanatomical differences in BIP patients with suicidal symptoms. The main characteristics of the studies are summarized in Table 3. Overall, sample sizes ranged from 47 to 113 individuals; participants in 2 studies were exclusively female, whereas 2 other studies had a combination of males and females; national origin of participants was the USA and Brazil. The articles mainly studied regional brain volumes using structural MRI and followed BIP diagnosis criteria in the DSM-IV.

Cortical Regions

Given the relatively few neuroimaging studies analyzing suicidality in BIP patients, most putative brain regions (i.e., cortical and subcortical) have been implicated by only a single study. Johnston et al. (39) showed that BIP patients who attempted suicide had a lower gray matter volume in the **orbitofrontal cortex** than non-attempters. In contrast, Duarte et al. have recently reported an increase in GMV in this region and the **limbic** and **insular** lobes (44). Moreover, Lijffijt et al. (40) reported changes in the **prefrontal cortex** while studying BIP with and without a record of previous psychiatric hospitalization; they also found larger gray matter volume in non-hospitalized patients who had made a suicide attempt relative to patients without history, but lower gray matter volume in BIP suicide attempters compared to those without attempts in the previously-hospitalized group. This last observation could indicate that the severity of the disease (which is correlated with the hospitalization record) could explain the prefrontal cortex differences between BIP suicide attempters and non-attempters.

Subcortical Regions

Contrasting results were found for the cerebellum. Johnston et al. (39) reported significantly lower bilateral gray matter volume in the **cerebellum**, extending into the vermis in the attempter group, compared to non-attempters. On the contrary, Baldaçara et al. (42) had previously reported no total volumetric differences in the **left cerebellum, right cerebellum**, nor the **vermis** between BIP suicide attempters and non-attempters. Importantly, these observations highlight the need for more studies regarding this topic, as more evidence would help clarify this issue.

Johnston et al. (39) reported lower gray matter **hippocampal** volume in BIP suicide attempters compared to non-attempters and healthy controls. Finally, Nery-Fernandes et al. (41) and Matsuo et al. (43) found no significant differences in **total brain**, white matter and gray matter volumes among the BIP suicidal and BIP non-suicidal groups.

Schizophrenia

SCZ is a chronic, severe and disabling psychiatric disorder that is characterized by the presence of hallucinations, delusions, dysfunctional ways of thinking and agitated body movements (65). Up to 40% of premature mortality related to SCZ can be attributed to suicide (66). Various efforts have been undertaken to identify suicide risk factors in the context of this condition (67, 68), but only a few have investigated neuroimaging correlates. We found five articles (summarized in Table 4), with samples sizes ranging from 37 to 751 individuals. All except one included both male and female participants. Psychiatric diagnoses were conducted according to DSM-IV criteria and cross-group comparisons included schizophrenic suicide attempters, non-attempters and healthy controls.

Cortical Regions

Four (of five) independent studies found differences in the **frontal lobe** between suicidal SCZ patients and either non-suicidal individuals or healthy controls (HC). Besteher et al. (45) observed a pronounced cortical thinning in the **right DLPFC** (dorsolateral prefrontal cortex) of suicidal schizophrenic patients compared with non-suicidal patients. Cortical thinning was also observed in the bilateral **caudal middle frontal gyrus**, the lateral **orbitofrontal and superior frontal gyrus**, the left **pars orbitalis**, the left **pars opercularis** and the **triangularis** when comparing healthy subjects with suicidal SCZ patients. A previous study by Giakoumatos et al. (46) had found significantly less gray matter volume in **superior frontal** and **rostral middle frontal regions** in attempters compared to both non-attempers and healthy controls, and Aguilar et al. (48) reported a significant gray matter density reduction in **left orbitofrontal cortex** in patients with a history of attempt, compared with non-suicidal patients. Moreover, Rüsch et al. (49) found significantly increased white matter volumes bilaterally near the **posterior orbital** and the **inferior frontal gyri** in patients with a history of suicide attempt, compared with non-suicidal patients. Also, current self-aggression was positively correlated with white matter volume in the same regions among schizophrenic patients. The link between the **frontal region** and SB of schizophrenic patients was one of the most consistent observations across SCZ studies. Authors hypothesize that since this area is part of a cortical network known to be involved in neural processing, functions such as cognitive control of emotions, impulse control, and inhibition of inappropriate responses its dysregulation could mediate SB (45, 46, 49).

Differences in the **temporal lobe** were reported by three different articles. Besteher et al. (45) reported that SCZ patients with SB showed pronounced cortical thinning in the **right superior** and **middle temporal cortex**, compared to non-suicidal patients. Previously, Giakoumatos et al. (46) had shown that, compared to non-attempters, attempters had significantly less gray matter volumes in the **bilateral inferior temporal** and **superior temporal cortices**, and that both attempters and non-attempters, when compared to HC, had significantly decreased volumes in these regions. In addition, Aguilar et al. (48) encountered a significant gray matter density reduction in the **left superior temporal lobe** in patients who had attempted suicide when comparing with non-suicidal patients. These regions are part of the complex neuronal network that mediates the cognitive control of emotion and impulsivity. Further, as mentioned by Aguilar et al. (48), the left superior temporal lobe is known to be associated with the presence and severity of auditory hallucinations, which could result in emotional dysfunction.

Besteher et al. (45) reported significant cortical thinning in the **right superior** and **middle insular cortex** in suicidal SCZ patients compared to non-suicidal individuals. Moreover, Giakoumatos et al. (46) showed that schizophrenic suicide attempters had significantly lower gray matter volume in the **right insula** compared to both healthy controls and non-attempters. Besteher et al. (45) argue that the **insula** is implicated in delineating the boundary between self and non-self-stimuli, which is impaired in schizophrenic patients in relation to hallucinations, and that this might contribute the presence of suicidal ideation. Finally, Besteher et al. (45) detected significantly lower gray matter volume in the **left superior parietal lobe** in the schizophrenic suicide attempters compared to non-attempters. Similarly, Giakoumatos et al. (46) also reported that attempters had significantly lower gray matter volume in **supramarginal regions**, compared to non-attempters.

Additionally, a number of other brain regions were reported by only one article each. Besteher et al. (45) detected significant cortical thinning in the **right caudal anterior cingulate cortex** when comparing suicidal schizophrenic patients with healthy subjects and in the **temporopolar cortex** relative to non-suicidal patients. Giakoumatos et al. (46) mentioned that among attempters, a history of high lethality attempts in SCZ patients was associated with significantly smaller volumes in the **right cuneus, the left lingual gyrus, the bilateral pericalcarine** and right **lateral occipital area**, compared to low lethality attempters.

Subcortical Regions

In terms of association with subcortical brain regions, Spoletini et al. (47) reported an increased volume in the **right amygdala** in patients with a history of suicidality compared to both patients without a history and HC. Giakoumatos et al. (46) described significantly lower gray matter volume in the **thalamus** of attempters, compared to non-attempters, especially when comparing low lethality attempters against non-attempters and HC. Notably, we identified no consistently SB-associated subcortical region across the five studies related to SCZ included.

Borderline Personality Disorder

BPD is a psychiatric illness characterized by frenetic efforts to avoid real or imagined abandonment, unstable personal relationships that go from idealization to devaluation and persistent suicidal or self-harming behaviors. The prevalence of this condition is estimated between 0.5 and 5.9% in the general population (69). It is a disease for which few genetic studies have been performed (70), and an almost negligible amount of research has been done to determine the brain regions involved in SB and NSSI in this specific disorder. Our methodology found three neuroimaging studies investigating brain structure and suicidality in BPD patients (summarized in **Table 5**). Sample sizes were 26, 51, and 120 individuals from both sexes, aged 13–45 from the USA. BPD diagnoses were determined using the Diagnostic Interview for Borderlines.

Cortical Regions

Most brain phenotypes that exhibited an association with suicidal symptoms were reported in two studies both by Soloff et al. (50, 51), with the exception of diminished gray matter volumes in the **anterior cingulate cortex** (ACC), which was associated with a higher degree of lethality in attempters by only one study (51). Consistently, Goodman et al. found a volumetric reduction in **Brodmann area 24**, which is located in the **ACC** (52). The other brain regions were effectively shared between two studies (50, 51). In 2012, Soloff et al. (51) reported that high lethality BPD attempters had significantly lower **left fusiform gyrus** volume, compared to low lethality BPD attempters. Then, in 2014, they replicated their findings. The fusiform gyrus is primarily associated with facial recognition, and it is hypothesized that a deficit of this function may affect social interactions (50).

Soloff et al. (51) found changes in the **insular cortex**, which had a lower gray matter volume in the right hemisphere of high lethality attempters. In 2014, they also described diminished gray matter volumes in the **right insula** of higher lethality attempters, compared to lower lethality attempters (50). Alterations in the insular cortex may lead patients to misjudge others' intentions and trigger disinhibited responses to perceived rejection; as this region is involved in recognition of one's own internal emotional state, perceived emotions in others, and representation of negative emotional states (50).

These studies also described a significant decrease in gray matter volume in the **left lingual gyrus** and the **right middle superior temporal gyrus** of high lethality attempters, compared to low lethality ones (50, 51). Alterations in these regions may influence social interaction due to their role in facial processing, analysis of others' intentions and reflexive responses to visual social inputs. Lastly, the **right middle inferior orbitofrontal** gyrus and cortex also showed a decrease in gray matter volume in high lethality attempters, compared to low lethality ones. The **orbitofrontal cortex** is associated with executive cognitive functions such as response inhibition, selective attention, conflict resolution, and monitoring and regulating the limbic system. Therefore, damage to this region could result in disinhibition and impulsive and aggressive behavior (50).

Subcortical Regions

A significantly lower gray matter volume in the **left hippocampus** and **parahippocampal gyrus** of BPD high lethality attempters was observed when compared to the low lethality group (50, 51). The parahippocampal gyrus plays a role in memory encoding and retrieval, especially in the familiarity of memory scenes. It also plays a role in identifying sarcasm in verbal communication and participates in complex facial processing. An abnormality in this brain region could impair social functioning and explain SB (50, 51).

Other Disorders

Our methodology identified two further studies assessing neurobiological correlates of SB in other disorders. Their results (**Table 6**) included no significant differences in gray or white matter volumes between suicidal and non-suicidal patients with Panic Disorder (53) and increased pituitary volumes in Posttraumatic stress disorder (PTSD) subjects with a history of suicidal ideation compared to healthy controls (54).

Risk of Bias Assessment

Most instruments for assessing risk of bias in systematic reviews are intended to be used for interventional studies, and a standard instrument for assessing neuroimaging case-control studies is yet to be established. We developed a risk of bias assessment table, partly based on the Cochrane format and in the STROBE checklist, assessing possible design and statistical biases (see **Supplementary Material** and methodology). Our instrument consisted of 15 items assessing potential sources of

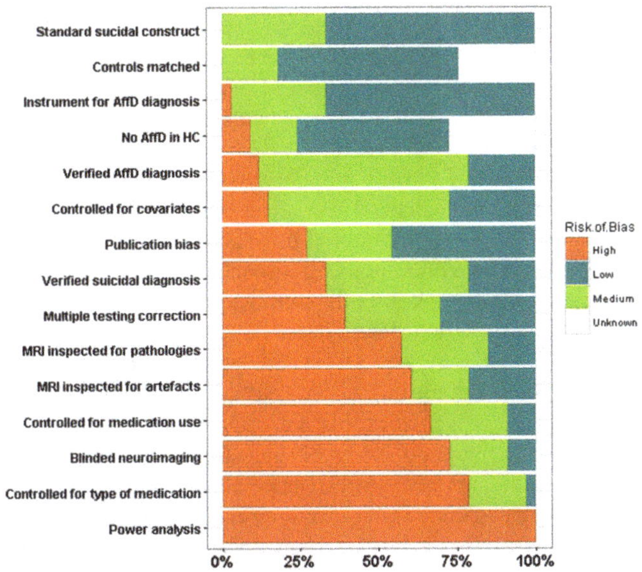

FIGURE 3 | Risk of bias assessment. Stacked bars representing the percentage of literature papers identified at a high, medium, low, or unknown risk of bias for specific possible sources of bias. AffD, affective disorder; MRI, magnetic resonance imaging; HC, healthy controls.

bias. This approach showed an average interrater reliability of ~68%. Notably, we detected no immediate relationship between risk of bias and interrater reliability (**Supplementary Figure 1**). Risk of bias across studies and constructs is reported in the **Supplementary Material**.

A single construct with a high risk of bias across all studies was "***power analysis performed***" (**Figure 3**). The lack of inclusion of this sort of analyses could have serious consequences when interpreting non-significant results [see for e.g., (21)], as a lack of statistical evidence never implies acceptance of a null hypothesis. Other constructs with a high risk of bias across most studies included controlling for medication treatment (e.g., antidepressants) and controlling for the type of medications (**Figure 3**). Effects of medication on cortical phenotypes have been reported (71, 72), so controlling for this covariate is imperative to reduce the risk of bias. Constructs with a medium to high risk of bias across studies were the inclusion of covariates in statistical analyses, correcting for multiple testing and the inspection analysis for MRI artifacts and pathologies. The extent to which the possible sources of bias identified affect each study is not clear. Surprisingly, around 25% of the studies reviewed had either medium or high risk for the construct "***No mental disorder in HC***" suggesting that some studies did not assess mental health in their HC cohorts, or failed to explicitly state it in their publications, reducing their credibility. Finally, We identified that around 60% of the reviewed studies were at medium to high risk for publication bias, reporting only summary statistics and comparisons of statistical significance while not including all other comparisons performed, thus limiting our ability to compare results across studies (**Figure 3**).

DISCUSSION

Here we systematically reviewed the academic literature of neuroimaging studies investigating SB and NSSI in patients with psychiatric disorders. We found 17 articles focusing on MDD, 6 on BIP, 5 on SCZ, 3 on BPD, and single studies focusing on panic disorder and PTSD. Considering the tremendous social and economic costs that result from self-injurious behaviors, and the fact that psychiatric patients are at increased risk, it is evident that more research is needed in this area. In particular, we were unable to identify any neuroimaging studies on NSSI in psychiatric patients. Below, we discuss the most prominent consistencies and inconsistencies within and across disorders.

Major Depressive Disorder

Four studies (32, 34, 35, 62) showed that white matter hyperintensities were significantly associated with a higher prevalence of past suicide attempts. These kind of lesions have also been reportedly associated with aging and dementia (73, 74), and it is unclear whether these hyper-intensities precede or are a consequence of suicidal attempts (75). The fact that these lesions were present even in samples of young adults, where they typically have a lower prevalence (74), suggests that this association might indeed be meaningful. Further, considering that associations between WMH and SB have been observed also in patients with other psychiatric disorders such as BIP, future studies should investigate whether this feature is shared among patients with suicidal symptoms across multiple disorders, and whether hyper-intensities are present in specific brain regions that could indicate which cognitive processes are affected, assuming a causal relationship which has not yet been established.

Gosnell et al. (23) and Colle et al. (24), found significantly reduced right hippocampal volumes in depressed suicidal patients. Although partially agreeing, the 2016 study (23) failed to replicate the total hippocampal volume reduction previously reported by Colle and colleagues. While comparable in several aspects, these studies used different instruments to assess suicidality, which could partially explain the differences reported. A recent ENIGMA-MDD meta-analysis with around 9,000 samples (1,700 cases and 7,200 controls) found hippocampal volume reductions present in MDD patients compared to healthy controls (76). Because of the confounding with the underlying diagnosis, it is currently not possible to establish whether hippocampal volume differences exist between patients with and without suicidality (20).

Three studies (25, 26, 31) detected reduced cortical thickness in frontoparietal regions and the insula in the left hemisphere. The concordance between these studies is surprising given the age differences (around 30, 30 and 65, respectively). However, three other studies (23, 28, 33) failed to replicate these findings. While the sample sizes of the studies ranged from 34 to 160, the number of individuals with *high suicide risk* in all studies was relatively low (between 7 and 27). Also, the study by Taylor et al. (25) only assessed suicidal ideation, or "thoughts of death," whereas Wagner et al. (28) focused on suicide attempt. These and other methodological differences could explain the controversies, but only analyses with harmonized inclusion criteria and well-powered samples can confirm or deny the existence of these alterations.

Bipolar Disorder

Johnston et al. (39) showed that, compared with non-attempters, BIP suicide attempters had significantly lower gray matter volume bilaterally in the cerebellum and vermis. However, Baldaçara et al. (42) had previously found no volumetric differences in any of these regions when comparing attempters with non-attempters. Whilst both studies measured different variables (i.e., gray matter only vs. total volume), these results are not easily conciliated. Both studies reached different conclusions about the association between suicidal attempt and cerebellum phenotypes under BIP disorder. Comprehensive studies, considering both types of volumetric measurement and with larger samples could shed light on this current controversy. Neurobiological alterations could be used as novel suicide risk predictors for bipolar patients, but this would require studies to be replicable. We found no structures consistently associated with SB in BIP cases across the reviewed literature; this could be due to demographic, measurement or diagnosis differences across studies.

Schizophrenia

Three out of the five studies focusing on SCZ detected associations between SB and temporal lobe volume reductions (45, 46, 48). Interestingly, the two other studies (47, 49) studied Italian populations, shared methodological approaches and came from the same groups. Therefore, they are likely to share methodological differences that explain their inconsistency with other reviewed articles. Associations between temporal lobe reductions and SB were also common in other disorders, making this an interesting candidate region. Notably, the temporal lobe is to a great extent associated with epilepsy which is also associated with suicide. An increase in suicide mortality ratio has been reported for epileptic subjects after temporal lobectomy (77), an observation consistent with the aforementioned associations.

Borderline Personality Disorder

When analyzing BPD attempters, Soloff et al. both in 2012 (50) and 2014 (51) observed an association between high lethality attempters and a decrease in gray matter volume in several regions when compared to low lethality attempters. The fact that these studies tried to further stratify SB groups into high lethality and low lethality, is an example of methodological variance that has to be interpreted and harmonized in order to be comparable with results from other studies. Because these studies shared the same diagnostics, imaging, and a similar statistical methodology, and could even have a sample overlap (both recruiting as part of the outpatient program of the Western Psychiatric Institute and Clinic in Pittsburgh), the consistency of their results is not surprising. Nevertheless, we cannot rule out the possibility of some of these consistencies of being artifacts caused by a common bias. Ideally, additional evidence from independent cohorts will be needed to confirm these observations.

Cross-Disorder Regions

Although SB is common in several psychiatric disorders, few efforts have attempted to map its shared neural correlates across different disorders. We hypothesized that there would be some similarities given recent reports of widespread genetic overlap across mental health disorders (22). However, the measurement of several types of cortical phenotypes (e.g., volume, surface, thickness, etc.) and suicidality constructs (e.g., ideation, attempt, severity) in the literature limited our ability to compare studies with different methodological approaches. Below we discuss the brain regions consistently associated with SB across the psychiatric disorders reviewed here.

Cortical phenotypes associated with suicidality were predominantly volume reductions or cortical thinning (**Table 7**). In particular, cortical thickness reduction or lower gray matter volume in the temporal cortex of suicidal patients was reported in MDD, SCZ, and BPD. As discussed above, the temporal lobe has also been associated with increased risk of suicide in epileptic subjects (77). Other cortical areas displaying reductions across disorders are the frontal, limbic, orbitofrontal, and insular lobes. Nonetheless, only reductions in both orbitofrontal and temporal cortex were recurrently reported as associated with suicidality across all four disorders reviewed.

Increases in amygdalar volume were associated with suicidality in MDD (33) and SCZ (47), and a decrease in hippocampal volume was observed in MDD (23, 24), BIP (64), and BPD (50). As previously mentioned, a reduction of this region's volume has been observed in MDD patients compared to HC (76). Furthermore, reductions in the number of synapses, arborisation, dendritic spines, and glial cell numbers have been observed in the hippocampus of depressed patients (78). Whether these changes account for the volumetric difference and are causal or consequential of MDD, as well as its association with suicidal symptoms, still remains debatable. Finally, a cerebellar gray matter reduction was consistently associated with suicidal symptoms in MDD (31) and BIP (39), although a third study in BIP reported no effect (42) (see **Table 8**). Interestingly, we identified no single subcortical brain region associated with suicidality across all four disorders, indicating that better powered (with bigger sample sizes and better-defined groups) studies are needed to detect associations of small effect.

LIMITATIONS

A persistent complication we faced during the elaboration of this review was to establish whether a particular study had analyzed MRI phenotypes different from those reported in their results. In fact, by searching for non-significant or negative results throughout the studies, we detected a publication bias toward the inclusion of positive results. A significant fraction of the studies reported only statistically significant results, without including even as **Supplementary Material**, results for all other regions included in the study and their results (see **Figure 3**). Therefore, our ability to compare studies and identify potential consistencies and inconsistencies was limited by the available information. We encourage the research community to include all the results

TABLE 8 | Subcortical phenotypes associated with SB across disorders.

	Amygdala	Amygdala-hippocampus	Caudate nucleus	Cerebellum	Corpus Callosum	Hippocampus	Lentiform nucleus	Para-hippocampal region	Putamen	Midbrain	Thalamus
MDD Monkul et al. (33)	Increase GM										
MDD Wagner et al. (28)	No difference	Decrease GM	Decrease GM								
MDD Hwang et al. (31)				Decrease GM			Decrease GM			Decrease GM WM	
MDD Cyprien et al. (29)					Decrease CV						
MDD Gosnell et al. (23)	No difference					Decrease CV					
MDD Colle et al. (24)						Decrease CV					
MDD Dombrovski et al. (27)									Decrease GM		
MDD Lee et al. (37)				Decrease GM							
BIP Johnston et al. (39)	No difference			Decrease GM		Decrease GM					
BIP Baldacara et al. (42)				No difference							
SCZ Spoletini et al. (47)	Increase CV										
SCZ Giakoumatos et al. (46)											Decrease GM
BPD Soloff et al. (51)						Decrease left GM		Decrease GM			
BPD Soloff et al. (50)	No difference							Decrease GM			

CT, cortical thickness; CV, cortical volume, GM, gray matter volume; WM, white matter volume.

derived from their analyses, as they might be useful for informing the design of new studies and for conducting meta-analyses, which are scarce in this area (21, 55).

A possible source of bias of the present systematic review is the fact that no mean sample age exclusion criterion was used. Consequently, age-dependent effects may affect the results. We have identified no common regions consistently reported as associated with suicidal symptoms across studies with mean sample age of 60 or greater. Thus, we cannot currently conclude that neural correlates associated with suicidality differ in elderly cohorts. A detailed analysis of possible age effects on SB would be valuable, albeit outside the scope of this review.

Results of several studies reviewed here should be compared with caution, as some of them were conducted in different populations, have samples with differing sex composition (e.g., some including only males while others included only females), and encompass a wide range of ages. Although partly a limitation, as results could be specific to the samples studied, this would increase a bias toward the null, making it harder to identify commonalities across studies reviewed. In spite of this, we have observed some commonalities across studies, which is consistent with recent observations of high genetic correlation between mental health disorders (22). Furthermore, almost all studies assessed suicidal symptoms or suicide risk as part of a standard instrument used for assessing other mental disorders. The convergent and discriminant validity of these different suicide assessment instruments is not clear and makes their comparison difficult. This limiting factor is important, especially considering that a number of current instruments have been reported inadequate for SB risk assessment (13).

Finally, the lack of a standard to assess risk of bias, specifically for neuroimaging case-control studies, motivated us to generate our own. We attempted to follow Cochrane's structure while covering common sources of bias that this kind of studies might have; we partially based our analysis on the STROBE checklist (79). This is an important first step toward reproducible research in neuroimaging studies of suicidality. A key potential source of bias which was not directly addressed by our instrument is the statistical power of the studies taking into account their sample sizes. The median sample size for all studies was 66 including both cases and controls, a value well beyond the estimated sample size of ~2,000 that would be needed to detect relatively low effect sizes at whole brain study-wide significance (21). A meta-analysis of all the selected literature would be a valid approach to achieve a sufficiently powered sample and reliable results, but due to the publication bias mentioned above and the methodological inconsistencies across different studies, this approach was not feasible.

CONCLUSIONS AND PERSPECTIVES

In this review we aimed to collate the results from a variety of structural MRI studies regarding specific cortical and subcortical brain regions implicated in SB and NSSI in patients with a psychiatric disorder. For all the possible combinations of selected keywords (see section Methods) we were only able to recover

50 papers from which just 6 were mainly focused on NSSI or suicidal ideation alone. Unfortunately, after selecting papers that met minimum quality standards and selecting only those that used structural MRI, we were left with 33 papers focusing on SB and no study related to NSSI. Regions most likely associated with suicidality across mental illness include the frontal and temporal cortical regions, as they were consistently reported across the disorders reviewed; as well as the hippocampus, which was implicated by four studies across three disorders.

Notably, we observed that only 11 out of 33 studies included more than 100 individuals in total, and only two meta-analyses have been published so far (21, 55). Meta-analyses and mega-analyses are powerful ways to increase the sample size and achieve better-powered analyses, and we believe the field would greatly benefit from the implementation of these approaches. The majority of the studies we identified were focused mainly on MDD, with fewer studies investigating BIP, SCZ, and BPD. Surprisingly, we found no studies relating SB with eating or anxiety disorders. Research across the variety of psychiatric illnesses might help clarify the question of whether the neural circuits involved in suicidality are shared or unique across distinct mental disorders. Finally, it is critical to standardize the technical and analytical methodologies applied to neuroimaging studies in this area. This would lead to comparable and reproducible research results, which is fundamental to shed light into the underlying mechanisms of SB and NSSI in psychiatric disease. In this regard, the recent establishment of a working group within the Enhancing Neuro-Imaging Genetics through Meta-Analysis (ENIGMA) consortium (80) is of great importance, as it will enable collaborative neuroimaging analyses of unprecedented scale.

AUTHOR CONTRIBUTIONS

CD-B, LG-M, and MR conceived and planned the study. CD-B, LG-M, AC-G, and MR carried out the analysis, drafted, and reviewed the manuscript. All authors provided critical feedback and helped shape the research, analysis, and manuscript.

ACKNOWLEDGMENTS

MR thanks the support of the Australian National Health & Medical Research Council (NHMRC) and the Australian Research Council (ARC), through a NHMRC-ARC Dementia Research Development Fellowship (APP1102821), and through the NHMRC Centre for Research Excellence in Suicide Prevention (CRESP) [GNT1042580]. AC-G is supported by a UQ Research Training Scholarship from The University of Queensland (UQ).

REFERENCES

1. Maciejewski DF, Renteria ME, Abdellaoui A, Medland SE, Few LR, Gordon SD, et al. The association of genetic predisposition to depressive symptoms with non-suicidal and suicidal self-injuries. *Behav Gene.* (2017) 47:3–10. doi: 10.1007/s10519-016-9809-z
2. WHO. *Suicide Data: Wold Health Organization.* (2017) Available online at: http://www.who.int/mental_health/prevention/suicide/suicideprevent/en/
3. Hawton K, Heeringen V. Suicide. *Lancet* (2009) 373:1372–81. doi: 10.1016/S0140-6736(09)60372-X
4. Nock MK, Borges G, Bromet EJ, Alonso J, Angermeyer M, Beautrais A, et al. Cross-national prevalence and risk factors for suicidal ideation, plans and attempts. *Br J Psychiatry* (2008) 192:98–105. doi: 10.1192/bjp.bp.107.040113
5. Briere J, Gil E. Self-mutilation in clinical and general population samples: prevalence, correlates, and functions. *Am J Orthopsychiatry* (1998) 68:609–20. doi: 10.1037/h0080369
6. Klonsky E. Non-suicidal self-injury in United States adults: prevalence, sociodemographics, topography and functions. *Psychol Med.* (2011) 41:1981–6. doi: 10.1017/S0033291710002497
7. Lloyd-Richardson EE, Perrine N, Dierker L, Kelley ML. Characteristics and functions of non-suicidal self-injury in a community sample of adolescents. *Psychol Med.* (2007) 37:1183–92. doi: 10.1017/S003329170700027X
8. Plener PL, Libal G, Keller F, Fegert JM, Muehlenkamp JJ. An international comparison of adolescent non-suicidal self-injury (NSSI) and suicide attempts: Germany and the USA. *Psychol Med.* (2009) 39:1549–58. doi: 10.1017/S0033291708005114
9. Ross S, Heath N. A study of the frequency of self-mutilation in a community sample of adolescents. *J Youth Adolesc.* (2002) 31:67–77. doi: 10.1023/A:1014089117419
10. Zhang H, Chen Z, Jia Z, Gong Q. Dysfunction of neural circuitry in depressive patients with suicidal behaviors: a review of structural and functional neuroimaging studies. *Prog Neuro-Psychopharmacol Biol Psychiatry* (2014) 53:61–6. doi: 10.1016/j.pnpbp.2014.03.002
11. Sher L, Stanley BH. The role of endogenous opioids in the pathophysiology of self-injurious and suicidal behavior. *Arch Suicide Res.* (2008) 12:299–308. doi: 10.1080/13811110802324748
12. Vinod KY, Hungund BL. Role of the endocannabinoid system in depression and suicide. *Trends Pharmacol Sci.* (2006) 27:539–45. doi: 10.1016/j.tips.2006.08.006
13. Harris KM, Syu J-J, Lello OD, Chew YE, Willcox CH, Ho RH. The ABC's of suicide risk assessment: Applying a tripartite approach to individual evaluations. *PLoS ONE* (2015) 10:e0127442. doi: 10.1371/journal.pone.0127442
14. Chapple A, Ziebland S, Hawton K. Taboo and the different death? Perceptions of those bereaved by suicide or other traumatic death. *Sociol Health Illness* (2015) 37:610–25. doi: 10.1111/1467-9566.12224
15. Chesney E, Goodwin GM, Fazel S. Risks of all-cause and suicide mortality in mental disorders: a meta-review. *World Psychiatry* (2014) 13:153–60. doi: 10.1002/wps.20128
16. Bertolote JM, Fleischmann A. Suicide and psychiatric diagnosis: a worldwide perspective. *World Psychiatry* (2002) 1:181.
17. Rihmer Z. Suicide risk in mood disorders. *Curr Opin Psychiatry* (2007) 20:17–22. doi: 10.1097/YCO.0b013e3280106868
18. Rihmer Z, Belsö N, Kiss K. Strategies for suicide prevention. *Curr Opin Psychiatry* (2002) 15:83–7. doi: 10.1097/00001504-200201000-00014
19. Van Heeringen K. Stress-diathesis model of suicidal behavior. In Dwivedi Y editor. *The Neurobiological Basis of Suicide.* Boca Raton: CRC Press (2012). p. 113–124.
20. Maciejewski DF, Creemers HE, Lynskey MT, Madden PA, Heath AC, Statham DJ, et al. Overlapping genetic and environmental influences on nonsuicidal self-injury and suicidal ideation: different outcomes, same etiology? *JAMA Psychiatry* (2014) 71:699–705. doi: 10.1001/jamapsychiatry.2014.89

21. Rentería M, Schmaal L, Hibar DP, Couvy-Duchesne B, Strike LT, Mills NT, et al. Subcortical brain structure and suicidal behaviour in major depressive disorder: a meta-analysis from the ENIGMA-MDD working group. *Translational Psychiatry* (2017) 7:e1116. doi: 10.1038/tp.2017.84
22. Anttila V, Bulik-Sullivan B, Finucane HK, Walters RK, Bras J, Duncan L, et al. Analysis of shared heritability in common disorders of the brain. *Science* (2018) 360:eaap8757. doi: 10.1126/science.aap8757
23. Gosnell SN, Velasquez KM, Molfese DL, Molfese PJ, Madan A, Fowler JC, et al. Prefrontal cortex, temporal cortex, and hippocampus volume are affected in suicidal psychiatric patients. *Psychiatry Res.* (2016) 256:50–6. doi: 10.1016/j.pscychresns.2016.09.005
24. Colle R, Chupin M, Cury C, Vandendrie C, Gressier F, Hardy P, et al. Depressed suicide attempters have smaller hippocampus than depressed patients without suicide attempts. *J Psychiatr Res.* (2015) 61:13–8. doi: 10.1016/j.jpsychires.2014.12.010
25. Taylor WD, Boyd B, McQuoid DR, Kudra K, Saleh A, MacFall JR. Widespread white matter but focal gray matter alterations in depressed individuals with thoughts of death. *Prog Neuro-Psychopharmacol Biol Psychiatry* (2015) 62:22–8. doi: 10.1016/j.pnpbp.2015.05.001
26. Peng H, Wu K, Li J, Qi H, Guo S, Chi M, et al. Increased suicide attempts in young depressed patients with abnormal temporal–parietal–limbic gray matter volume. *J Affect Disord.* (2014) 165:69–73. doi: 10.1016/j.jad.2014.04.046
27. Dombrovski AY, Siegle GJ, Szanto K, Clark L, Reynolds C, Aizenstein H. The temptation of suicide: striatal gray matter, discounting of delayed rewards, and suicide attempts in late-life depression. *Psychol Med.* (2012) 42:1203–15. doi: 10.1017/S0033291711002133
28. Wagner G, Schultz CC, Koch K, Schachtzabel C, Sauer H, Schlösser RG. Prefrontal cortical thickness in depressed patients with high-risk for suicidal behavior. *J Psychiatr Res.* (2012) 46:1449–55. doi: 10.1016/j.jpsychires.2012.07.013
29. Cyprien F, Courtet P, Malafosse A, Maller J, Meslin C, Bonafé A, et al. Suicidal behavior is associated with reduced corpus callosum area. *Biol Psychiatry* (2011) 70:320–6. doi: 10.1016/j.biopsych.2011.02.035
30. Wagner G, Koch K, Schachtzabel C, Schultz CC, Sauer H, Schlösser RG. Structural brain alterations in patients with major depressive disorder and high risk for suicide: evidence for a distinct neurobiological entity? *Neuroimage* (2011) 54:1607–14. doi: 10.1016/j.neuroimage.2010.08.082
31. Hwang J-P, Lee T-W, Tsai S-J, Chen T-J, Yang C-H, Lirng J-F, et al. Cortical and subcortical abnormalities in late-onset depression with history of suicide attempts investigated with MRI and voxel-based morphometry. *J Geriatr Psychiatry Neurol.* (2010) 23:171–84. doi: 10.1177/0891988710363713
32. Pompili M, Ehrlich S, De Pisa E, Mann JJ, Innamorati M, Cittadini A, et al. White matter hyperintensities and their associations with suicidality in patients with major affective disorders. *Eur Arch Psychiatry Clin Neurosci* (2007) 257:494–9. doi: 10.1007/s00406-007-0755-x
33. Monkul E, Hatch JP, Nicoletti MA, Spence S, Brambilla P, Lacerda ALTd, et al. Fronto-limbic brain structures in suicidal and non-suicidal female patients with major depressive disorder. *Molecular Psychiatry* (2007) 12:360. doi: 10.1038/sj.mp.4001919
34. Ehrlich S, Breeze JL, Hesdorffer DC, Noam GG, Hong X, Alban RL, et al. White matter hyperintensities and their association with suicidality in depressed young adults. *J Affect Disord.* (2005) 86:281–7. doi: 10.1016/j.jad.2005.01.007
35. Ehrlich S, Noam GG, Lyoo IK, Kwon BJ, Clark MA, Renshaw PF. White matter hyperintensities and their associations with suicidality in psychiatrically hospitalized children and adolescents. *J Am Acad Child Adolesc Psychiatry* (2004) 43:770–6. doi: 10.1097/01.chi.0000120020.48166.93
36. Ahearn EP, Jamison KR, Steffens DC, Cassidy F, Provenzale JM, Lehman A, et al. MRI correlates of suicide attempt history in unipolar depression. *Biol Psychiatry* (2001) 50:266–70. doi: 10.1016/S0006-3223(01)01098-8
37. Lee YJ, Kim S, Gwak AR, Kim SJ, Kang S-G, Na K-S, et al. Decreased regional gray matter volume in suicide attempters compared to suicide non-attempters with major depressive disorders. *Comprehen Psychiatry* (2016) 67:59–65. doi: 10.1016/j.comppsych.2016.02.013
38. Sachs-Ericsson N, Hames JL, Joiner TE, Corsentino E, Rushing NC, Palmer E, et al. Differences between suicide attempters and nonattempters in depressed older patients: depression severity, white-matter lesions, and cognitive functioning. *Am J Geriatr Psychiatry* (2014) 22:75–85. doi: 10.1016/j.jagp.2013.01.063
39. Johnston JA, Wang F, Liu J, Blond BN, Wallace A, Liu J, et al. Multimodal neuroimaging of frontolimbic structure and function associated with suicide attempts in adolescents and young adults with bipolar disorder. *Am J Psychiatry* (2017) 174:667–75. doi: 10.1176/appi.ajp.2016.15050652
40. Lijffijt M, Rourke E, Swann A, Zunta-Soares G, Soares J. Illness-course modulates suicidality-related prefrontal gray matter reduction in women with bipolar disorder. *Acta Psychiatrica Scand.* (2014) 130:374–87. doi: 10.1111/acps.12314
41. Nery-Fernandes F, Rocha MV, Jackowski A, Ladeia G, Guimarães JL, Quarantini LC, et al. Reduced posterior corpus callosum area in suicidal and non-suicidal patients with bipolar disorder. *J Affect Disord.* (2012) 142:150–5. doi: 10.1016/j.jad.2012.05.001
42. Baldaçara L, Nery-Fernandes F, Rocha M, Quarantini LdC, Rocha G, Guimarães J, et al. Is cerebellar volume related to bipolar disorder? *J Affect Disord.* (2011) 135:305–9. doi: 10.1016/j.jad.2011.06.059
43. Matsuo K, Nielsen N, Nicoletti MA, Hatch JP, Monkul ES, Watanabe Y, et al. Anterior genu corpus callosum and impulsivity in suicidal patients with bipolar disorder. *Neurosci Lett.* (2010) 469:75–80. doi: 10.1016/j.neulet.2009.11.047
44. Duarte DG, Maila de Castro LN, Albuquerque MR, Turecki G, Ding Y, de Souza-Duran FL, et al. Structural brain abnormalities in patients with type I bipolar disorder and suicidal behavior. *Psychiatry Res.* (2017) 265:9–17. doi: 10.1016/j.pscychresns.2017.04.012
45. Besteher B, Wagner G, Koch K, Schachtzabel C, Reichenbach JR, Schlösser R, et al. Pronounced prefronto-temporal cortical thinning in schizophrenia: neuroanatomical correlate of suicidal behavior? *Schizophr Res.* (2016) 176:151–7. doi: 10.1016/j.schres.2016.08.010
46. Giakoumatos CI, Tandon N, Shah J, Mathew IT, Brady RO, Clementz BA, et al. Are structural brain abnormalities associated with suicidal behavior in patients with psychotic disorders? *J Psychiatr Res.* (2013) 47:1389–95. doi: 10.1016/j.jpsychires.2013.06.011
47. Spoletini I, Piras F, Fagioli S, Rubino IA, Martinotti G, Siracusano A, et al. Suicidal attempts and increased right amygdala volume in schizophrenia. *Schizophr Res.* (2011) 125:30–40. doi: 10.1016/j.schres.2010.08.023
48. Aguilar EJ, Garcia-Marti G, Marti-Bonmati L, Lull J, Moratal D, Escarti M, et al. Left orbitofrontal and superior temporal gyrus structural changes associated to suicidal behavior in patients with schizophrenia. *Prog Neuro-Psychopharmacol Biol Psychiatry* (2008) 32:1673–6. doi: 10.1016/j.pnpbp.2008.06.016
49. Rüsch N, Spoletini I, Wilke M, Martinotti G, Bria P, Trequattrini A, et al. Inferior frontal white matter volume and suicidality in schizophrenia. *Psychiatry Res.* (2008) 164:206–14. doi: 10.1016/j.pscychresns.2007.12.011
50. Soloff P, White R, Diwadkar VA. Impulsivity, aggression and brain structure in high and low lethality suicide attempters with borderline personality disorder. *Psychiatry Res.* (2014) 222:131–9. doi: 10.1016/j.pscychresns.2014.02.006
51. Soloff PH, Pruitt P, Sharma M, Radwan J, White R, Diwadkar VA. Structural brain abnormalities and suicidal behavior in borderline personality disorder. *J Psychiatr Res.* (2012) 46:516–25. doi: 10.1016/j.jpsychires.2012.01.003
52. Goodman M, Hazlett EA, Avedon JB, Siever DR, Chu K-W, New AS. Anterior cingulate volume reduction in adolescents with borderline personality disorder and co-morbid major depression. *J Psychiatr Res.* (2011) 45:803–7. doi: 10.1016/j.jpsychires.2010.11.011
53. Kim B, Oh J, Kim M-K, Lee S, Tae WS, Kim CM, et al. White matter alterations are associated with suicide attempt in patients with panic disorder. *J Affect Disord.* (2015) 175:139–46. doi: 10.1016/j.jad.2015.01.001
54. Thomas LA, De Bellis MD. Pituitary volumes in pediatric maltreatment-related posttraumatic stress disorder. *Biol Psychiatry* (2004) 55:752–8. doi: 10.1016/j.biopsych.2003.11.021
55. van Heeringen K, Bijttebier S, Desmyter S, Vervaet M, Baeken C. Is there a neuroanatomical basis of the vulnerability to suicidal behavior? A coordinate-based meta-analysis of structural and functional MRI studies. *Front Hum Neurosci.* (2014) 8:824. doi: 10.3389/fnhum.2014.00824

56. Nanda P, Tandon N, Mathew IT, Padmanabhan JL, Clementz BA, Pearlson GD, et al. Impulsivity across the psychosis spectrum: correlates of cortical volume, suicidal history, and social and global function. *Schizophr Res.* (2016) 170:80–6. doi: 10.1016/j.schres.2015.11.030
57. World Health Organization. *Depression and Other Common Mental Disorders: Global Health Estimates* (2017).
58. AP Association. *Diagnostic and Statistical Manual of Mental Disorders (DSM-5®).* Arlington, VA: American Psychiatric Association (2013). doi: 10.1176/appi.books.9780890425596
59. Otte C, Gold SM, Penninx BW, Pariante CM, Etkin A, Fava M, et al. Major depressive disorder. *Nat Rev Dis Primers* (2016) 2:16065. doi: 10.1038/nrdp.2016.65
60. Phelps EA. Human emotion and memory: interactions of the amygdala and hippocampal complex. *Curr Opin Neurobiol.* (2004) 14:198–202. doi: 10.1016/j.conb.2004.03.015
61. Soriano-Mas C, Hernández-Ribas R, Pujol J, Urretavizcaya M, Deus J, Harrison BJ, et al. Cross-sectional and longitudinal assessment of structural brain alterations in melancholic depression. *Biol Psychiatry* (2011) 69:318–25. doi: 10.1016/j.biopsych.2010.07.029
62. Pompili M, Innamorati M, Mann JJ, Oquendo MA, Lester D, Del Casale A, et al. Periventricular white matter hyperintensities as predictors of suicide attempts in bipolar disorders and unipolar depression. *Prog Neuro-Psychopharmacol Biol Psychiatry* (2008) 32:1501–7. doi: 10.1016/j.pnpbp.2008.05.009
63. Health TNIoM. *Bipolar Disorder 2016* Available online at: https://www.nimh.nih.gov/site-info/citing-nimh-information-and-publications.shtml
64. Tondo L, Isacsson G, Baldessarini RJ. Suicidal behaviour in bipolar disorder. *CNS Drugs* (2003) 17:491–511. doi: 10.2165/00023210-200317070-00003
65. Health TNIoM. *Schizophrenia 2016* Available online at: https://www.nimh.nih.gov/health/topics/schizophrenia/index.shtml
66. Bushe CJ, Taylor M, Haukka J. Mortality in schizophrenia: a measurable clinical endpoint. *J Psychopharmacol.* (2010) 24(4_suppl):17–25. doi: 10.1177/1359786810382468
67. Hor K, Taylor M. Suicide and schizophrenia: a systematic review of rates and risk factors. *J Psychopharmacol.* (2010) 24(4_suppl):81–90. doi: 10.1177/1359786810385490
68. Palmer BA, Pankratz VS, Bostwick JM. The lifetime risk of suicide in schizophrenia: a reexamination. *Arch Gen Psychiatry* (2005) 62:247–53. doi: 10.1001/archpsyc.62.3.247
69. Leichsenring F, Leibing E, Kruse J, New AS, Leweke F. Borderline personality disorder. *Lancet* (2011) 377:74–84. doi: 10.1016/S0140-6736(10)61422-5
70. Bassirnia A, Eveleth MC, Gabbay JM, Hassan YJ, Zhang B, Perez-Rodriguez MM. Past, present, and future of genetic research in borderline personality disorder. *Curr Opin Psychol.* (2018) 21:60–8. doi: 10.1016/j.copsyc.2017.09.002
71. Giakoumatos C, Nanda P, Mathew I, Tandon N, Shah J, Bishop J, et al. Effects of lithium on cortical thickness and hippocampal subfield volumes in psychotic bipolar disorder. *J Psychiatr Res.* (2015) 61:180–7. doi: 10.1016/j.jpsychires.2014.12.008
72. Phillips ML, Travis MJ, Fagiolini A, Kupfer DJ. Medication effects in neuroimaging studies of bipolar disorder. *Am J Psychiatry* (2008) 165:313–20. doi: 10.1176/appi.ajp.2007.07071066
73. Debette S, Markus H. The clinical importance of white matter hyperintensities on brain magnetic resonance imaging: systematic review and meta-analysis. *BMJ* (2010) 341:c3666. doi: 10.1136/bmj.c3666
74. Wardlaw JM, Valdés Hernández MC, Muñoz-Maniega S. What are white matter hyperintensities made of? Relevance to vascular cognitive impairment. *J Am Heart Assoc.* (2015) 4:e001140. doi: 10.1161/JAHA.114.001140
75. Martin PC, Zimmer TJ, Pan LA. Magnetic resonance imaging markers of suicide attempt and suicide risk in adolescents. *CNS Spectrums* (2015) 20:355–8. doi: 10.1017/S1092852915000048
76. Schmaal L, Veltman DJ, van Erp TG, Sämann P, Frodl T, Jahanshad N, et al. Subcortical brain alterations in major depressive disorder: findings from the ENIGMA Major Depressive Disorder working group. *Mol Psychiatry* (2016) 21:806. doi: 10.1038/mp.2015.69
77. Bell GS, Gaitatzis A, Bell CL, Johnson AL, Sander JW. Suicide in people with epilepsy: how great is the risk? *Epilepsia* (2009) 50:1933–42. doi: 10.1111/j.1528-1167.2009.02106.x
78. Serafini G, Hayley S, Pompili M, Dwivedi Y, Brahmachari G, Girardi P, et al. Hippocampal neurogenesis, neurotrophic factors and depression: possible therapeutic targets? *CNS Neurol Disord Drug Targets* (2014) 13:1708–21. doi: 10.2174/1871527313666141130223723
79. Editors PM. Observational studies: getting clear about transparency. *PLoS Med.* (2014) 11:e1001711. doi: 10.1371/journal.pmed.1001711
80. Thompson PM, Stein JL, Medland SE, Hibar DP, Vasquez AA, Renteria ME, et al. The ENIGMA Consortium: large-scale collaborative analyses of neuroimaging and genetic data. *Brain Imaging Behav.* (2014) 8:153–82. doi: 10.1007/s11682-013-9269-5

24

Cue-Induced Brain Activation in Chronic Ketamine-Dependent Subjects, Cigarette Smokers and Healthy Controls: A Task Functional Magnetic Resonance Imaging Study

*Yanhui Liao[1,2,3,4,5], Maritza Johnson[6], Chang Qi[1], Qiuxia Wu[1], An Xie[7], Jianbin Liu[7], Mei Yang[6,8], Maifang Huang[9], Yan Zhang[1], Tieqiao Liu[1], Wei Hao[1] and Jinsong Tang[1,2,3,4,5]**

[1] Department of Psychiatry, The Second Xiangya Hospital, Central South University, Changsha, China, [2] Mental Health Institute, The Second Xiangya Hospital, Central South University, Changsha, China, [3] National Clinical Research Center on Mental Disorders, Changsha, China, [4] National Technology Institute on Mental Disorders, Changsha, China, [5] Hunan Key Laboratory of Psychiatry and Mental Health, Changsha, China, [6] Department of Psychiatry and Biobehavioral Sciences, University of California, Los Angeles, Los Angeles, CA, United States, [7] Department of Radiology, The People's Hospital of Hunan Province, Changsha, China, [8] Department of Addiction Medicine, Shenzhen Mental Health Center, Shenzhen Kangning Hospital, Shenzhen, China, [9] Kangda Voluntary Drug Rehabilitation Center, Changsha, China

***Correspondence:**
Jinsong Tang
tangjinsong@csu.edu.cn

Background: Observations of drug-related cues may induce craving in drug-dependent patients, prompting compulsive drug-seeking behavior. Sexual dysfunction is common in drug users. The aim of the study was to examine regional brain activation to drug (ketamine, cigarette smoking) associated cues and natural (sexual) rewards.

Methods: A sample of 129 [40 ketamine use smokers (KUS), 45 non-ketamine use smokers (NKUS) and 44 non-ketamine use non-smoking healthy controls (HC)] participants underwent functional magnetic resonance imaging (fMRI) while viewing ketamine use related, smoking and sexual films.

Results: We found that KUS showed significant increased activation in anterior cingulate cortex and precuneus in response to ketamine cues. Ketamine users (KUS) showed lower activation in cerebellum and middle temporal cortex compared with non-ketamine users (NKUS and HC) in response to sexual cues. Smokers (KUS and NKUS) showed higher activation in the right precentral frontal cortex in response to smoking cues. Non-ketamine users (NKUS and HC) showed significantly increased activation of cerebellum and middle temporal cortex while viewing sexual cues.

Conclusion: These findings clearly show the engagement of distinct neural circuitry for drug-related stimuli in chronic ketamine users. While smokers (both KUS and NKUS) showed overlapping differences in activation for smoking cues, the former group showed a specific neural response to relevant (i.e., ketamine-related) cues. In particular, the heightened response in anterior cingulate cortex may have important implications for how attentionally salient such cues are in this group. Ketamine users (KUS) showed lower activation in response to sexual cues may partly reflect the neural basis of sexual dysfunction.

Keywords: ketamine users, cigarette smokers, cue, brain activation, functional magnetic resonance imaging

INTRODUCTION

Over the last decade, ketamine has increasingly become a more widely used recreational drug among young people (1, 2). Chronic ketamine use is associated with cognitive changes (2), and our previous studies suggest that these changes are accompanied by marked brain changes that correlate with the magnitude of its use (3, 4).

Drug craving is thought to be a powerful motivational state or a very strong desire that drives the ketamine user to seek ketamine. For example, one subject recruited to our study reported that in the absence of available ketamine she would sniff white powder shaved from a wall. Undoubtedly, craving is clearly an important facet of chronic ketamine use. However, the mechanisms of drug craving in chronic ketamine users are not fully understood. Given that ketamine abuse is a growing problem, which is often accompanied by serious adverse effects such as ketamine-induced ulcerative cystitis, kidney dysfunction, psychosis, depression, cognitive impairment, and neurological changes (2), it becomes exceedingly important to explore and understand how craving drives ketamine or other drug users to use drugs without consideration of negative consequences. One way to address this question is the use of functional magnetic resonance imaging (fMRI) to characterize brain responses to drug-related cues that induce craving (5).

To date, there is a line of evidence indicating that nicotine, alcohol, cocaine, and other drugs of abuse are associated with the activation of some specific brain regions. This fMRI drug-related cue-induced brain activation is often associated with treatment outcomes and relapse (6). For example, in cigarette smokers, fMRI studies indicate smoking-related cue-induced brain activation predominantly in the prefrontal cortex, anterior cingulate cortex, ventral striatum, amygdala, hippocampus, and thalamus (7–13). In addition, smoking cessation selectively reduced responses to smoking cues in the amygdala (14); in heavy drinkers and individuals with alcohol use disorders, a meta-analysis paper demonstrated alcohol cues elicited robust activation in the limbic and prefrontal regions, and showed greater activation in the parietal and temporal regions when compared to controls. Furthermore, cue-elicited ventral striatum activation was most frequently correlated with behavioral measurements and activation in this region often reduced by treatment (15). However, in reviewing the literature, studies using fMRI to examine the effects of cue exposure on different drugs showed mixed findings, making it difficult to identify the reliable patterns of activation in a particular sample or specific drug-related cue exposure paradigm.

In order to characterize ketamine use and cigarette smoking-related cue-induced brain activation, we presented two types of addictive drug cues, ketamine and nicotine, during fMRI to investigate brain activation patterns to ketamine or smoking cues in chronic ketamine users (also smokers), cigarette smokers, and non-ketamine use non-smoking healthy controls (HC).

Based on previous cue-activation studies and behavior studies in illicit and non-illicit substance users, we hypothesized that ketamine use cue-elicited craving of brain activation will be stronger and wider than that of smoking cue-elicited. Also, based on results from our and other previous studies of brain structure changes in prefrontal cortex and anterior cingulate cortex in chronic ketamine users (3, 4, 16) and smoking cue-induced brain-imaging studies (17), we hypothesized that compared with non-ketamine use non-smoking HC, substance use subjects [ketamine use smokers (KUS) and non-ketamine use smokers (NKUS)] would have increased activation in prefrontal cortex and anterior paralimbic structures during ketamine-specific cue and smoking-specific cue presentations.

Loss of sexual interest or pleasure is a common symptom for drug abusers. For example, from a sample of 1,076 substance abusers, 45.2% had been suffering from sexual dysfunctions (18); out of 701 drug abusers, 36.4% reported erectile dysfunction (19); additionally, there is a higher prevalence of sexual dysfunction in female ketamine abusers with cystitis when compared with ketamine abusers without cystitis (20). Thus, we also presented non-addictive but salient cues in the form of sexual stimuli, which are known to induce activation in the hypothalamus, thalamus, amygdala, anterior cingulate gyrus (ACC), insula, fusiform gyrus, precentral gyrus, parietal cortex, and occipital cortex in healthy people (21), and reduce brain responses to sexual stimuli in the anterior cingulate and dorsolateral prefrontal cortex in breast cancer survivors with chemotherapy (22). Evidence shows that chronic illicit drug abusers (including ketamine abusers) commonly demonstrate sexual dysfunction and a previous study showed that cocaine users had smaller activation than the comparison subjects when shown a sex film (23). Given this, we hypothesized that levels of sexual cue-induced brain activation would be lower in chronic ketamine users (KUS) than that in non-ketamine users (NKUS and HC).

MATERIALS AND METHODS

Subjects

One hundred and twenty-nine subjects 129 (40 chronic ketamine and nicotine-dependent subjects/KUS, 45 otherwise healthy nicotine-dependent subjects/NKUS, and 44 non-ketamine use non-smoking HC) were recruited in this study. All subjects were Han Chinese, aged 19–39 with normal or corrected-to-normal vision. Ketamine dependent volunteers were recruited from the Kangda Voluntary Drug Rehabilitation Centers in the Hunan Province and the Department of Addiction Medicine, Hunan Brain Hospital. All ketamine use subjects met the Diagnostic and Statistical Manual of Mental Disorders, fourth edition (DSM-IV) criteria for lifetime ketamine dependence determined from the Structured Clinical Interview (SCID) (24). Ketamine use subjects were excluded if they met criteria for other substance dependence (excluding nicotine dependence; all ketamine dependent subjects smoked at least eight cigarettes for more than 1 year and met DSM-IV criteria for nicotine dependence) at any time. The smokers and non-smokers were screened to ensure that they had no past neurological or psychiatric history. Smokers who had smoked 10 cigarettes per day or more during the previous year and had no period of smoking abstinence longer than 3 months in the past year, and met DSM-IV criteria for nicotine dependence were eligible for this study. All non-smokers in this sample reported no history of smoking behavior in the past. Subjects were excluded if they reported: major medical or psychiatric disorders, current use of psychotropic medications, use of intravenous drugs, pregnancy, and contraindications for MRI. None of the participants reported daily consumption of alcohol, and none reported experiencing social consequences secondary to alcohol use, or any history with difficulty ceasing alcohol intake. Subjects were required to abstain from ketamine for at least 48 h and nicotine for at least 12 h before scanning and from other psychoactive substances for at least 2 weeks. Nicotine patches were provided as needed. A licensed psychiatrist, at MD level, conducted all clinical interviews. The protocol was approved by the university ethics committee (The Second Xiangya Hospital of Central South University Review Board, No. S054, 2008) and the studies were carried out in accordance with the Declaration of Helsinki. Subjects were fully informed about the measurement and MRI scanning procedures in the study. Written informed consent was given and obtained by all subjects.

Ketamine craving and smoking craving were assessed by The Visual Analog Scale for Craving (VASc) (25). The VASc displays a scale from 0 to 10, where 0 represents null craving and 10 represents the most extreme craving.

Stimuli and Design

Three 2-min sexual-related visual films selected from Asian movies of heterosexual activity, which contained hugs, kisses, and sexual acts; three 2-min ketamine-related films made by ketamine user, which visually showed the process of snorting ketamine; and three 2-min smoking-related films made by otherwise healthy smokers, which contained the process of cigarette smoking (Figure S1 in Supplementary Material).

All films intentionally were devoid of other appetitive stimuli (e.g., alcohol, food, tea, caffeine, gaming, etc.). Every film was presented using a Linux laptop computer with in-house stimulus delivery software for 2 min, followed at random by a black screen for 30 s. Additionally, stimulus order was randomized and no stimulus was repeated during the experiments. Together, all films lasted 22 min and 30 s using an Epson (Long Beach, CA, USA) MP 7200 LCD projector onto a screen placed at the feet of the MRI scanner bed and was viewed using a mirror mounted on the head coil.

Imaging Acquisition and Preprocessing

Neuroimaging was conducted using a 3T Siemens Trio MRI scanner. The protocol began with initial structural scans followed by a series of functional runs during which participants completed the ketamine, cigarette, and sexual cues tasks. Structural T1-weighted images were acquired in a sagittal orientation employing a magnetization prepared rapid gradient-echo sequence with the following parameters: slice thickness = 1 mm, gap = 0 mm, repetition time = 2,000 ms, echo time = 2.6 ms, field of view = 256 cm × 256 cm, flip angle = 8°, matrix size = 256 × 256, and slices = 176. Functional MRI data were obtained using a gradient-echo echo-planar imaging (GRE-EPI) sequence with the following parameters: TR/TE = 2,000/30 ms, matrix = 64 × 64, flip angle = 90°, FOV = 220 mm × 220 mm, 32 interleaved axial slices, thickness = 3 mm, slice gap = 1 mm. The first three volumes of each scan were discarded to allow for T1 equilibrium effects.

Imaging analysis was done using SPM5 (Wellcome Trust Centre for Neuroimaging, London, United Kingdom). Images were corrected for the acquisition time delay between different slices and then realigned to the first volume for head-motion correction. Functional images were then normalized according to standard co-registration procedures using the individual's structural scan. Then, all realigned and normalized images were smoothed with an 8 mm × 8 mm × 8 mm full width half maximum Gaussian filter. To remove low-frequency signal drift, a high-pass filter (with cutoff frequency 1/120 Hz) was applied.

Statistical Analysis

Statistical Analysis of MRI data were conducted using SPM5 (Wellcome Trust Centre for Neuroimaging, London, UK). For each subject, fMRI responses were modeled using a canonical hemodynamic response function. The general linear model was used to perform a first level, within-participant analysis on the functional data from each subject individually for the primary contrasts: ketamine minus ketamine baseline, cigarette minus cigarette baseline, and sexual minus sexual baseline. Estimated motion correction parameters were included as additional covariates. Within-group effects were tested using single-sample *t* tests on contrast images for each group separately. Between-group differences were tested using an ANOVA test with variances assumed unequal between groups. Age and sex were included as covariates. Clusters were considered as significant if they reached a combined voxel-extend threshold of an uncorrected voxel level of $p < 0.001$ and cluster extent >10 voxels, as determined based on Monte Carlo simulation with AlphaSim correlation to $p < 0.005$. In order to test the relationship between drug craving scales (VASc) and cue-induced brain activation, ROI based analysis was done according to the fMRI findings.

Demographic and clinical variables analyses were conducted using Statistical Package for Social Sciences (SPSS) version 16. ANOVA test were used for comparison of demographic variables and cognitive tests. Two sample *t* tests were used for comparing the mean smoking variables and drug craving values between ketamine users and smokers.

RESULTS

Participant Characteristics

All subjects were Han Chinese and were characterized typically by upper-middle-income socioeconomic status. The three groups were well-matched in age, gender, handedness, and marriage status. However, levels of education were not quite matched for the three groups. Smoking craving scales in smokers group is stronger than that of ketamine users. Detailed demographic and clinical characteristics for the three groups have been reported previously (26) and are also summarized in **Table 1**.

Functional Brain Activation Analyses of Ketamine Use, Smoking, and Sexual-Related Short Films

Our primary interest was to compare brain activation, elicited in response to different types of addictive substances [i.e., ketamine

TABLE 1 | Demographic and drug use characteristics of patients with ketamine dependence, chronic smokers and HC subjects.

	Ketamine users/smokers (n = 40)	Smokers (n = 45)	Non-smokers (n = 44)	ANOVA, F test	Two sample t test
Demographic variables					
Age, years, mean ± SD	26.8 (4.93)	27.9 (5.60)	26.3 (5.84)	$F = 0.99$ $p = 0.373$	
Range (years)	19–39	19–39	19–38		
Male/female	32/8	37/8 (17.78%)	34/10 (22.7%)		
Subjects' education, years, mean ± SD	11.9 ± 2.8	13.1 ± 2.96	15.0 ± 2.6	$F = 13.22$ $p = 0.000$	
Right/left-handed	39/1	43/2	43/1		
Unmarried/married	25/15	26/19	29/15		
Ketamine use variables					
Age of first use, years, mean ± SD	23.10 ± 5.21	–	–		
Range (years)	14–36	–	–		
Duration, months, mean ± SD	41.7 ± 21.58	–	–		
Range (months)	12–126	–	–		
Times of using ketamine/day	1.85	–	–		
Range (times)	1–4	–	–		
Quantity of using ketamine/time (g)	0.77	–	–		
Range (g)	0.1–2.5	–	–		
Smoking variables					
Age of first smoking, years, mean ± SD	15.5 ± 3.70	18.0 ± 4.25	–		$p = 0.004$
Range (years)	10–30	11–30			
Duration, years, mean ± SD	11.4 ± 4.95	10.2 ± 5.76	–		$p = 0.303$
Range (years)	1.5–21	1.5–21	–		
Smoked cigarette/day, mean ± SD	16.5 ± 7.79	20.3 ± 7.61	–		$p = 0.031$
Range (cigarettes)	8–40	10–40	–		
Drug craving					
Ketamine craving (cm)	6.14 ± 2.81	–	–		
Smoking craving (cm)	5.36 ± 2.28	6.41 ± 1.72	–		$p = 0.016$

TABLE 2 | Regions of brain activation during exposure to ketamine use related films (40 ketamine users VS 45 smokers + 44 non-smokers), smoking (40 ketamine users/also smokers + 45 smokers VS 44 non-smokers), and sexual cue (45smokers + 44 non-smokers VS 40 ketamine users).

Cue	Anatomical region	Cluster size (no. voxel)	Voxel level p uncorrected	Peak T value	Coordinates (mm)			Voxel z value
					x	y	z	
Ketamine use-related cue (K > S + N)	Left anterior cingulate cortex	378	0.000	4.45	−3	39	−6	4.28
	Precuneus	361	0.000	4.19	0	−60	24	4.05
	Cingulate gyrus	77	0.000	3.96	0	−6	30	3.84
	Left inferior parietal cortex	53	0.000	3.76	−42	−69	45	3.66
	Right posterior cingulate	45	0.000	3.76	18	−54	9	3.66
	Left occipital cortex (lingual gyrus)	56	0.000	3.63	−15	−48	0	3.53
	Right parietal cortex (supramarginal gyrus)	53	0.000	3.62	57	−54	27	3.52
Smoking-related cue (K + S > N)	Righ frontal cortex (precentral gyrus)	33	0.000	4.20	51	12	9	4.06
Sexual cue (K < S + N)	Left cerebellum	123	0.000	4.65	−6	−90	−24	4.46
	Middle temporal cortex	80	0.000	4.33	54	−75	18	4.17
Ketamine cue minus smoking cue (K > S)	Left inferior parietal cortex	130	0.000	4.22	−45	−69	48	4.14
	Posterior congulate/precuneus	81	0.000	3.74	6	−51	24	3.68
	Left middle temporal cortex	30	0.000	3.58	−63	−30	−12	3.53

K, ketamine use group (ketamine users were also smokers, n = 40); S, smoking group (n = 45); N, non-smoking group (n = 44).
AlphaSim corrected p < 0.005.

and nicotine in ketamine users and non-ketamine users (smokers, non-smokers)] (see **Table 2** and **Figure 1**). Another interest was to compare substance use and sexual cue-induced brain activation in substance users (ketamine users, smokers) and control subjects. For ketamine use related films and sexual films, there was no significant difference of brain activation between smokers and non-smokers; similarly, for smoking-related films no statistical significance of brain activation between ketamine users (also smokers) and smokers was shown (alphaSim corrected $p < 0.005$). We, therefore, performed between-group comparisons for activity during each condition. In order to remove the effects of gender, we also recalculated the results using male subjects only (see Figure S2 in Supplementary Material).

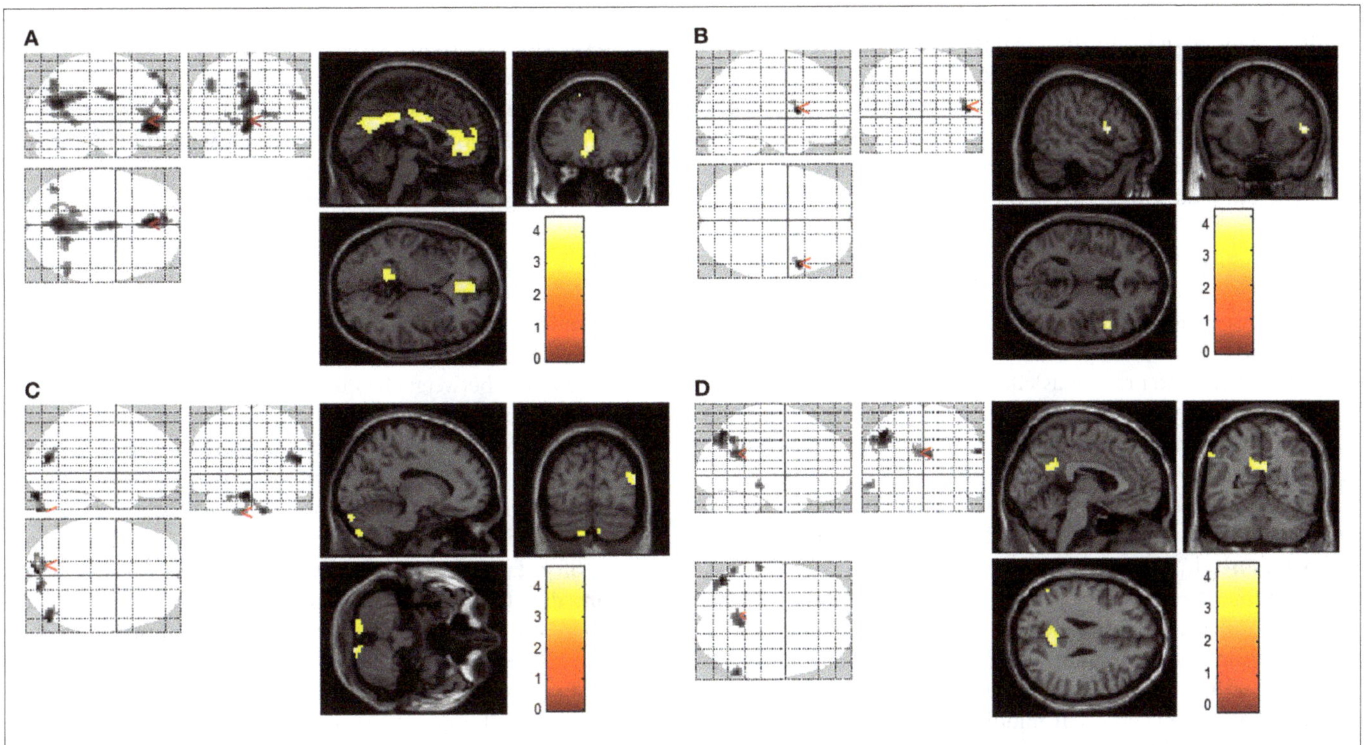

FIGURE 1 | Increased brain regions of activation by different cues. Increased brain regions of activation in chronic ketamine users during exposure to ketamine use-related films when compared with control subjects [smokers and non-smokers **(A)**]; increased brain regions of activation in chronic smokers (chronic ketamine users were also chronic smokers) during exposure to smoking-related films when compared with non-smokers **(B)**; increased brain regions of activation in control subjects (smokers and non-smokers) during exposure to sexual films when compared with chronic ketamine users **(C)**; in respects to ketamime cue minus smoking cue, increased brain regions of activation in chronic ketamine users when compared with chronic smokers **(D)**. AlphaSim corrected $p < 0.005$.

Functional Activation Analyses: Ketamine Craving

In response to ketamine use-related films, we observed greater brain regions of activation in multiple and extensive regions including the left anterior cingulate cortex, precuneus, cingulate gyrus, left inferior parietal cortex, right posterior cingulate, left occipital cortex (lingual gyrus), and right parietal cortex (supramarginal gyrus) in KUS when compared with non-ketamine users (NKUS and HC, see **Table 2** and **Figure 1A**). There were no areas that showed reduced activation for chronic ketamine users. Also, ketamine cue-induced craving showed much more intensive and widespread cortical activation in two regions: anterior cingulate cortex and the precuneus (alphaSim corrected $p < 0.005$) when compared with smoking and sexual cues (see **Table 2** and **Figure 1**). In ROI based association analysis, we found no significant association between ketamine craving scales and ketamine cue-induced brain activation.

Functional Activation Analyses: Smoking Craving

In response to smoking-related films, we only observed greater brain regions of activation in the right frontal cortex (precentral gyrus) in chronic smokers (KUS and NKUS) when compared with non-smokers (HC) (see **Table 2** and **Figure 1B**). In ROI-based association analysis, we found no significant association between smoking craving scales and smoking cue-induced brain activation.

Functional Activation Analyses: Sexual Cues

For sexual films, increased brain regions of activation in the left cerebellum and middle temporal cortex were observed in non-ketamine users (NKUS and HC) when compared with chronic ketamine users (KUS) (see **Table 2** and **Figure 1C**). In other words, KUS showed reduced activation in those two regions.

Functional Activation Analyses: Ketamine Minus Smoking Cues

In order to explore the unique and relatively strong brain activation of ketamine cues, the following analyses has been applied: ketamine cue versus another substance (i.e., smoking/nicotine) cue for KUS compared to the same contrast for NKUS. In respect to ketamine minus smoking cues, we only observed greater brain regions of activation in the left inferior parietal cortex, posterior congulate/precuneus, and left middle temporal cortex in KUS when compared with NKUS (see **Table 2** and **Figure 1D**).

DISCUSSION

To the best of our knowledge, this is the first study using fMRI to examine the brain regional activation associated with ketamine use, cigarette smoking, and sexual visual cues in a sample of KUS (with ketamine and nicotine dependence, KUS), NKUS (only with nicotine dependence, NKUS) and non-ketamine use non-smoking HC. The present study found that KUS showed significant increased activation mainly in the anterior cingulate cortex and precuneus in response to ketamine cues. Smokers (KUS and NKUS) showed higher activation in the right precentral frontal cortex in response to smoking cues. None-ketamine users (NKUS and HC) showed significant increased activation of cerebellum and middle temporal cortex while viewing sexual cues.

As for *ketamine cues*, this study revealed a wide distribution of brain regions that showed significant greater activation in the ketamine users (KUS) as the ketamine cues were being viewed. Besides those two mainly activated regions (i.e., the anterior cingulate cortex and precuneus), the cingulate gyrus, left inferior parietal cortex, right posterior cingulate, left occipital cortex (lingual gyrus), and right parietal cortex (supramarginal gyrus) were also activated during ketamine craving in KUS when compared with non-ketamine users (NKUS and HC). When compared with smoking, ketamine cue-induced craving was more intensive and widespread, which is consistent with our hypothesis that ketamine use cue-elicited craving of brain activation will be stronger and wider than that of smoking cue-elicited craving. For ketamine minus smoking cues, we observed only greater brain regions of activation (in the left inferior parietal cortex, posterior congulate/precuneus, and left middle temporal cortex) in KUS when compared with NKUS. Higher levels of sensation seeking and novelty-seeking in several classes of addiction (such as heroin and ketamine) in comparison with others (such as alcohol and tobacco) (27) may partly explain why stronger activation occurred during ketamine cues. It is plausible to conclude, however, that the widespread and strong regional (mostly in the limbic system) activations induced by ketamine use in the present study reflect the unique circuitry of ketamine users. A further understanding of these uniquely large responses (i.e., PPI or DCM connectivity analysis) may cast new light on the concept of ketamine dependency and how chronic ketamine use affects normal brain systems for desire, leading to its dependence.

Activation of the anterior cingulate cortex has been reported in cigarette smoking (12, 28) and other substances, such as cocaine (23, 29) and alcohol (30) induced craving. Additionally, this activation is seen in non-substance abuse such as internet gaming (31) induced craving, and has been thought to play a role in drug-seeking behavior (32), cognitive and emotional process (33). The current study further supports an important role for the anterior cingulate cortex in craving—one of the key factors resulting in relapse.

The precuneus, a medial prefrontal-mid-parietal neural network with the association of cortical and subcortical structures, is linked with visual-processing, attention, as well as integrates the related memory and complexity of behavioral specializations (34). While viewing ketamine cues, our study showed activation of the precuneus in KUS compared with NKUS and HC. This finding is also consistent with the previously documented cue-induced craving research in alcohol dependent subjects (35) and internet addictions (31, 36), which suggests a role of the precuneus in cue-induced craving.

In response to *cigarette smoking cues*, this study observed greater activation only in the right precentral frontal cortex in smokers (both KUS and NKUS) when compared with non-smokers (HC). Smoking induced brain activation was found in reward-related brain areas (frontal cortex) in the processing of other smoking-related stimuli (8, 37, 38). However, previous similar studies reported extended regional activation (7–11, 39). The severity of nicotine dependence (i.e., heavily dependent smokers' craving was more stable than moderately dependent smokers) (40), and even menstrual cycle phase (41) may have resulted in mixed findings. Unfortunately, in the present study, we did not assess both factors. Besides a different design, participants and stimuli are possible factors for mixed findings. Furthermore, our study did not show any differences of smoking cue-induced brain activation between chronic KUS and NKUS.

For *sexual cues*, NKUS and HC showed significant increased activation of cerebellum and middle temporal cortex while viewing sexual cues when compared with KUS, which means chronic ketamine users showed hypo-activation in those two regions. These results may partly reflect the neural basis for the reduced ability of ketamine-dependent subjects to experience sexual pleasure due to their sexual dysfunction. Cocaine users also revealed decreased brain activation induced by watching sexual films (23), and treatment-seeking male cocaine patients showed "unseen" sexual cues elicited strong limbic activations (42). The hypo-activation by natural stimuli (sexual cues) in drug users may suggest its role in drug dependence, treatment, and relapse.

Limitation

An earlier fMRI study with cocaine users (23) reported that brain response to cocaine cues was stronger than that to sexual cues. From this point of view, we should attempt to directly compare the magnitude of the brain activation associated with cues for a natural (sexual) reward and drug (ketamine or nicotine) reward. However, history of ketamine use, smoking, and sexual experience are uncontrolled variables in the present study. It is difficult to equate the cues on a critical dimension, i.e., their relevance for the individuals' unique learning history, even when the cue types are otherwise approximately equated on visual characteristics (brightness, hue, shape, orientation, complexity, etc.). Thus, we did not directly compare the brain response to them. Further preclinical fMRI research could offer a novel alternative for establishing and directly comparing brain activation to cue categories for natural and drug rewards. In addition, although the study showed no differences of brain activation during smoking cues between KUS and NKUS, we need to admit that only ketamine users' abstinence from ketamine use and smoking has been controlled, while smokers' abstinence from smoking was based only on their self-reported answer.

CONCLUSION

In conclusion, KUS showed intense and widespread cortical activation in anterior cingulate cortex and precuneus when they were viewing ketamine cues. Smokers (KUS and NKUS) showed higher activation in right precentral frontal cortex when compared with non-smokers. In contrast with smoking cues, ketamine cues induced much stronger and widespread brain activation. Based on the common symptom of sexual dysfunction, ketamine users (KUS) showed lower activation in cerebellum and middle temporal cortex compared with non-ketamine users (NKUS and HC) in response to sexual cues, which may partly reflect the neural basis of sexual dysfunction. These findings show clearly the engagement of distinct neural circuitry for drug-related stimuli in chronic ketamine users. While smokers (both KUS and NKUS) showed overlapping differences in activation for smoking cues, the former group showed a specific neural response to relevant (i.e., ketamine-related) cues. In particular, the heightened response in anterior cingulate cortex may have important implications for how attentionally salient such cues are in this group.

Clinical Implications

Cue-induced drug craving is often cited as a major determinant in drug relapse. Identifying patterns of whole-brain activation associated with cue categories for natural and drug rewards may have clinical implications; for example, helping optimize therapeutic interventions that block craving and attenuate compulsive drug-seeking behavior. Encouragingly, this implicates that cue exposure treatment [Cue Exposure Therapy (43)], with multiple methodological innovations for addiction may be a speculative used therapy in clinical settings.

AUTHOR CONTRIBUTIONS

All of the authors contributed to the study conception and design, interpretation of findings, and manuscript preparation and revision. YL originated the study and drafted the manuscript. JT conducted the statistical analyses and revised the manuscript. WH advised on the statistical analysis, interpretation of findings, and reviewed drafts of the manuscript.

FUNDING

The study was supported by the National Natural Science Foundation of China (Grant No. 81371480 to JT, 81671325 to YL, and 81371465 and 81671324 to TL). The authors would like to acknowledge all the participants. The grant had no role in study design, data collection and analysis, decision to publish, or preparation of the manuscript. The lead author would like to acknowledge Dr. Paul C. Fletcher for providing invaluable analytical and editorial assistance. The authors thank the subjects who participated in this study.

REFERENCES

1. Jia Z, Liu Z, Chu P, McGoogan JM, Cong M, Shi J, et al. Tracking the evolution of drug abuse in China, 2003–10: a retrospective, self-controlled study. *Addiction* (2015) 110(Suppl 1):4–10. doi:10.1111/add.12769
2. Morgan CJ, Curran HV. Ketamine use: a review. *Addiction* (2012) 107(1):27–38. doi:10.1111/j.1360-0443.2011.03576.x
3. Liao Y, Tang J, Ma M, Wu Z, Yang M, Wang X, et al. Frontal white matter abnormalities following chronic ketamine use: a diffusion tensor imaging study. *Brain* (2010) 133(Pt 7):2115–22. doi:10.1093/brain/awq131
4. Liao Y, Tang J, Corlett PR, Wang X, Yang M, Chen H, et al. Reduced dorsal prefrontal gray matter after chronic ketamine use. *Biol Psychiatry* (2011) 69(1):42–8. doi:10.1016/j.biopsych.2010.08.030
5. Wilson SJ, Sayette MA. Neuroimaging craving: urge intensity matters. *Addiction* (2015) 110(2):195–203. doi:10.1111/add.12676
6. Courtney KE, Schacht JP, Hutchison K, Roche DJ, Ray LA. Neural substrates of cue reactivity: association with treatment outcomes and relapse. *Addict Biol* (2016) 21(1):3–22. doi:10.1111/adb.12314
7. David SP, Munafo MR, Johansen-Berg H, Mackillop J, Sweet LH, Cohen RA, et al. Effects of acute nicotine abstinence on cue-elicited ventral striatum/nucleus accumbens activation in female cigarette smokers: a functional magnetic resonance imaging study. *Brain Imaging Behav* (2007) 1(3–4):43–57. doi:10.1007/s11682-007-9004-1
8. Franklin TR, Wang Z, Wang J, Sciortino N, Harper D, Li Y, et al. Limbic activation to cigarette smoking cues independent of nicotine withdrawal: a perfusion fMRI study. *Neuropsychopharmacology* (2007) 32(11):2301–9. doi:10.1038/sj.npp.1301371
9. Lee JH, Lim Y, Wiederhold BK, Graham SJ. A functional magnetic resonance imaging (FMRI) study of cue-induced smoking craving in virtual environments. *Appl Psychophysiol Biofeedback* (2005) 30(3):195–204. doi:10.1007/s10484-005-6377-z
10. McClernon FJ, Hiott FB, Huettel SA, Rose JE. Abstinence-induced changes in self-report craving correlate with event-related FMRI responses to smoking cues. *Neuropsychopharmacology* (2005) 30(10):1940–7. doi:10.1038/sj.npp.1300780
11. Rubinstein ML, Luks TL, Moscicki AB, Dryden W, Rait MA, Simpson GV. Smoking-related cue-induced brain activation in adolescent light smokers. *J Adolesc Health* (2011) 48(1):7–12. doi:10.1016/j.jadohealth.2010.09.016
12. Bourque J, Mendrek A, Dinh-Williams L, Potvin S. Neural circuitry of impulsivity in a cigarette craving paradigm. *Front Psychiatry* (2013) 4:67. doi:10.3389/fpsyt.2013.00067
13. Moran-Santa Maria MM, Hartwell KJ, Hanlon CA, Canterberry M, Lematty T, Owens M, et al. Right anterior insula connectivity is important for cue-induced craving in nicotine-dependent smokers. *Addict Biol* (2015) 20:407–14. doi:10.1111/adb.12124
14. McClernon FJ, Hiott FB, Liu J, Salley AN, Behm FM, Rose JE. Selectively reduced responses to smoking cues in amygdala following extinction-based smoking cessation: results of a preliminary functional magnetic resonance imaging study. *Addict Biol* (2007) 12(3–4):503–12. doi:10.1111/j.1369-1600.2007.00075.x
15. Schacht JP, Anton RF, Myrick H. Functional neuroimaging studies of alcohol cue reactivity: a quantitative meta-analysis and systematic review. *Addict Biol* (2013) 18(1):121–33. doi:10.1111/j.1369-1600.2012.00464.x
16. Roberts RE, Curran HV, Friston KJ, Morgan CJ. Abnormalities in white matter microstructure associated with chronic ketamine use. *Neuropsychopharmacology* (2014) 39(2):329. doi:10.1038/npp.2013.195
17. Engelmann JM, Versace F, Robinson JD, Minnix JA, Lam CY, Cui Y, et al. Neural substrates of smoking cue reactivity: a meta-analysis of fMRI studies. *Neuroimage* (2012) 60(1):252–62. doi:10.1016/j.neuroimage.2011.12.024
18. Hossain KJ, Nandi AK, Karim MR, Haque MM, Kamal MM. Pattern of mental illness on substance abusers. *Mymensingh Med J* (2012) 21(2):251–8.
19. Bang-Ping J. Sexual dysfunction in men who abuse illicit drugs: a preliminary report. *J Sex Med* (2009) 6(4):1072–80. doi:10.1111/j.1743-6109.2007.00707.x
20. Jang MY, Long CY, Chuang SM, Huang CH, Lin HY, Wu WJ, et al. Sexual dysfunction in women with ketamine cystitis: a case-control study. *BJU Int* (2012) 110(3):427–31. doi:10.1111/j.1464-410X.2011.10780.x
21. Kuhn S, Gallinat J. A quantitative meta-analysis on cue-induced male sexual arousal. *J Sex Med* (2011) 8(8):2269–75. doi:10.1111/j.1743-6109.2011.02322.x
22. Versace F, Engelmann JM, Jackson EF, Slapin A, Cortese KM, Bevers TB, et al. Brain responses to erotic and other emotional stimuli in breast cancer survivors with and without distress about low sexual desire: a preliminary fMRI study. *Brain Imaging Behav* (2013) 7(4):533–42. doi:10.1007/s11682-013-9252-1
23. Garavan H, Pankiewicz J, Bloom A, Cho JK, Sperry L, Ross TJ, et al. Cue-induced cocaine craving: neuroanatomical specificity for drug users and drug stimuli. *Am J Psychiatry* (2000) 157(11):1789–98. doi:10.1176/appi.ajp.157.11.1789

24. Spitzer RL, Williams JBW, Gibbon M, First MB. The Structured Clinical Interview for DSM-III-R (SCID). I History, rationale, and description. *Arch Gen Psychiatry* (1992) 49(8):624–9. doi:10.1001/archpsyc.1992.01820080032005
25. Mottola CA. Measurement strategies: the visual analogue scale. *Decubitus* (1993) 6(5):56–8.
26. Liao Y, Tang J, Liu J, Xie A, Yang M, Johnson M, et al. Decreased thalamocortical connectivity in chronic ketamine users. *PLoS One* (2016) 11(12):e0167381. doi:10.1371/journal.pone.0167381
27. Le BO, Basiaux P, Streel E, Tecco J, Hanak C, Hansenne M, et al. Personality profile and drug of choice; a multivariate analysis using Cloninger's TCI on heroin addicts, alcoholics, and a random population group. *Drug Alcohol Depend* (2004) 73(2):175–82. doi:10.1016/j.drugalcdep.2003.10.006
28. Zhao LY, Tian J, Wang W, Qin W, Shi J, Li Q, et al. The role of dorsal anterior cingulate cortex in the regulation of craving by reappraisal in smokers. *PLoS One* (2012) 7(8):e43598. doi:10.1371/journal.pone.0043598
29. Maas LC, Lukas SE, Kaufman MJ, Weiss RD, Daniels SL, Rogers VW, et al. Functional magnetic resonance imaging of human brain activation during cue-induced cocaine craving. *Am J Psychiatry* (1998) 155(1):124–6. doi:10.1176/ajp.155.1.124
30. Grusser SM, Wrase J, Klein S, Hermann D, Smolka MN, Ruf M, et al. Cue-induced activation of the striatum and medial prefrontal cortex is associated with subsequent relapse in abstinent alcoholics. *Psychopharmacology (Berl)* (2004) 175(3):296–302. doi:10.1007/s00213-004-1828-4
31. Ko CH, Liu GC, Yen JY, Chen CY, Yen CF, Chen CS. Brain correlates of craving for online gaming under cue exposure in subjects with Internet gaming addiction and in remitted subjects. *Addict Biol* (2013) 18(3):559–69. doi:10.1111/j.1369-1600.2011.00405.x
32. Volkow ND, Wang GJ, Fowler JS, Tomasi D, Telang F. Addiction: beyond dopamine reward circuitry. *Proc Natl Acad Sci U S A* (2011) 108(37):15037–42. doi:10.1073/pnas.1010654108
33. Bush G, Luu P, Posner MI. Cognitive and emotional influences in anterior cingulate cortex. *Trends Cogn Sci* (2000) 4(6):215–22. doi:10.1016/S1364-6613(00)01483-2
34. Cavanna AE, Trimble MR. The precuneus: a review of its functional anatomy and behavioural correlates. *Brain* (2006) 129(Pt 3):564–83. doi:10.1093/brain/awl004
35. Liu J, Calhoun VD, Chen J, Claus ED, Hutchison KE. Effect of homozygous deletions at 22q13.1 on alcohol dependence severity and cue-elicited BOLD response in the precuneus. *Addict Biol* (2013) 18(3):548–58. doi:10.1111/j.1369-1600.2011.00393.x
36. DU W, Liu J, Gao X, Li L, Li W, Li X, et al. [Functional magnetic resonance imaging of brain of college students with internet addiction]. *Zhong Nan Da Xue Xue Bao Yi Xue Ban* (2011) 36(8):744–9. doi:10.3969/j.issn.1672-7347.2011.08.008
37. Hayashi T, Ko JH, Strafella AP, Dagher A. Dorsolateral prefrontal and orbitofrontal cortex interactions during self-control of cigarette craving. *Proc Natl Acad Sci U S A* (2013) 110(11):4422–7. doi:10.1073/pnas.1212185110
38. Brody AL, Mandelkern MA, Olmstead RE, Jou J, Tiongson E, Allen V, et al. Neural substrates of resisting craving during cigarette cue exposure. *Biol Psychiatry* (2007) 62(6):642–51. doi:10.1016/j.biopsych.2006.10.026
39. Ray LA, Courtney KE, Ghahremani DG, Miotto K, Brody A, London ED. Varenicline, naltrexone, and their combination for heavy-drinking smokers: preliminary neuroimaging findings. *Am J Drug Alcohol Abuse* (2015) 41(1):35–44. doi:10.3109/00952990.2014.927881
40. Vollstadt-Klein S, Kobiella A, Buhler M, Graf C, Fehr C, Mann K, et al. Severity of dependence modulates smokers' neuronal cue reactivity and cigarette craving elicited by tobacco advertisement. *Addict Biol* (2011) 16(1):166–75. doi:10.1111/j.1369-1600.2010.00207.x
41. Wetherill RR, Jagannathan K, Hager N, Maron M, Franklin TR. Influence of menstrual cycle phase on resting-state functional connectivity in naturally cycling, cigarette-dependent women. *Biol Sex Differ* (2016) 7(1):1. doi:10.1186/s13293-016-0078-6
42. Childress AR, Ehrman RN, Wang Z, Li Y, Sciortino N, Hakun J, et al. Prelude to passion: limbic activation by "unseen" drug and sexual cues. *PLoS One* (2008) 3(1):e1506. doi:10.1371/journal.pone.0001506
43. Martin T, LaRowe SD, Malcolm R. Progress in cue exposure therapy for the treatment of addictive disorders. *Open Addic J* (2010) 3:92–101. doi:10.2174/1874941001003020092

Permissions

All chapters in this book were first published by Frontiers; hereby published with permission under the Creative Commons Attribution License or equivalent. Every chapter published in this book has been scrutinized by our experts. Their significance has been extensively debated. The topics covered herein carry significant findings which will fuel the growth of the discipline. They may even be implemented as practical applications or may be referred to as a beginning point for another development.

The contributors of this book come from diverse backgrounds, making this book a truly international effort. This book will bring forth new frontiers with its revolutionizing research information and detailed analysis of the nascent developments around the world.

We would like to thank all the contributing authors for lending their expertise to make the book truly unique. They have played a crucial role in the development of this book. Without their invaluable contributions this book wouldn't have been possible. They have made vital efforts to compile up to date information on the varied aspects of this subject to make this book a valuable addition to the collection of many professionals and students.

This book was conceptualized with the vision of imparting up-to-date information and advanced data in this field. To ensure the same, a matchless editorial board was set up. Every individual on the board went through rigorous rounds of assessment to prove their worth. After which they invested a large part of their time researching and compiling the most relevant data for our readers.

The editorial board has been involved in producing this book since its inception. They have spent rigorous hours researching and exploring the diverse topics which have resulted in the successful publishing of this book. They have passed on their knowledge of decades through this book. To expedite this challenging task, the publisher supported the team at every step. A small team of assistant editors was also appointed to further simplify the editing procedure and attain best results for the readers.

Apart from the editorial board, the designing team has also invested a significant amount of their time in understanding the subject and creating the most relevant covers. They scrutinized every image to scout for the most suitable representation of the subject and create an appropriate cover for the book.

The publishing team has been an ardent support to the editorial, designing and production team. Their endless efforts to recruit the best for this project, has resulted in the accomplishment of this book. They are a veteran in the field of academics and their pool of knowledge is as vast as their experience in printing. Their expertise and guidance has proved useful at every step. Their uncompromising quality standards have made this book an exceptional effort. Their encouragement from time to time has been an inspiration for everyone.

The publisher and the editorial board hope that this book will prove to be a valuable piece of knowledge for researchers, students, practitioners and scholars across the globe.

List of Contributors

Yuqun Zhang, Rongrong Bian, Wenhao Jiang, Yingying Yin, Yingying Yue, Zhenghua Hou and Yonggui Yuan
Department of Psychosomatics and Psychiatry, ZhongDa Hospital, School of Medicine, Southeast University, Nanjing, China
Institute of Psychosomatics, School of Medicine, Southeast University, Nanjing, China

Yuan Yang
Department of Respiration, Zhong Da Hospital, Southeast University, Nanjing, China

Ze Wang
Center for Cognition and Brain Disorders and the Affiliated Hospital, Hangzhou Normal University, Hangzhou, China

Ranran Li, Jin Zhao, Ying Wang, Renrong Wu, Jingping Zhao and Wenbin Guo
Department of Psychiatry, Second Xiangya Hospital of Central South University, Changsha, China

Feng Liu
Department of Radiology, Tianjin Medical University General Hospital, Tianjin, China

Qinji Su and Zhikun Zhang
Mental Health Center of the First Affiliated Hospital, Guangxi Medical University, Nanning, China

Xiao Li, Huaqing Meng, Yixiao Fu, Lian Du, Haitang Qiu, Tian Qiu and Qinghua Luo
Department of Psychiatry, The First Affiliated Hospital of Chongqing Medical University, Chongqing, China

Qibin Chen
Department of Anesthesiology, The First Affiliated Hospital of Chongqing Medical University, Chongqing, China

Zhiwei Zhang
Department of Radiology, The First Affiliated Hospital of Chongqing Medical University, Chongqing, China

Yi Yin, Shishun Fu, Kelei Hua, Yunfan Wu and Guihua Jiang
Guangdong Second Provincial General Hospital, Third School of Clinical Medicine, Southern Medical University, Guangzhou, China

Qianying Tang and Wei Qu
Department of Psychology, Affiliated Southwest Hospital, Army Medical University, Chongqing, China

Meng Li, Xiaofen Ma, Jianhao Yan, Tianyue Wang and Wenfeng Zhan
Department of Medical Imaging, Guangdong Second Provincial General Hospital, Guangzhou, China

Chao Li
Guangdong Second Provincial General Hospital, Third School of Clinical Medicine, Southern Medical University, Guangzhou, China

Zhiwei Zuo, Shuhua Ran, Yao Wang, Chang Li, Qi Han and Haitao Li
Department of Radiology, Affiliated Southwest Hospital, Army Medical University, Chongqing, China

Simeng Gu
School of Psychology, Jiangsu University Medical Center, Zhenjiang, China
School of Psychology, Institute of Emotional Studies, Nanjing University of Chinese Medicine, Nanjing, China

Liyuan Jing and Yang Li
School of Psychology, Institute of Emotional Studies, Nanjing University of Chinese Medicine, Nanjing, China

Jason H. Huang
Department of Neurosurgery, Baylor Scott & White Health, Temple, TX, United States

Fushun Wang
School of Psychology, Institute of Emotional Studies, Nanjing University of Chinese Medicine, Nanjing, China
Department of Surgery, Texas A&M University, Temple, TX, United States

Shuang Liu and Jian Xu
Department of Rheumatology and Immunology, First Affiliated Hospital of Kunming Medical University, Kunming, China
Yunnan Key Laboratory of Laboratory Medicine, Kunming, China

Yuqi Cheng
Yunnan Key Laboratory of Laboratory Medicine, Kunming, China
Department of Psychiatry, First Affiliated Hospital of Kunming Medical University, Kunming, China

Zhongqi Xie, Aiyun Lai, Zhaoping Lv and Yueyin Zhao
Department of Rheumatology and Immunology, First Affiliated Hospital of Kunming Medical University, Kunming, China

Xiufeng Xu
Department of Psychiatry, First Affiliated Hospital of Kunming Medical University, Kunming, China

Chunrong Luo and Hongjun Yu
Magnetic Resonance Imaging Center, The First Hospital of Kunming, Kunming, China

Baoci Shan
Key Laboratory of Nuclear Analysis, Institute of High Energy Physics, Chinese Academy of Sciences, Beijing, China

Lin Xu
Key Laboratory of Animal Models and Human Disease Mechanisms, Kunming Institute of Zoology, Chinese Academy of Sciences, Kunming, China

Yishul Wei, Jennifer R. Ramautar and Bart H. W. te Lindert
Department of Sleep and Cognition, Netherlands Institute for Neuroscience (NIN), An Institute of the Royal Netherlands Academy of Arts and Sciences, Amsterdam, Netherlands

Michele A. Colombo
Department of Sleep and Cognition, Netherlands Institute for Neuroscience (NIN), An Institute of the Royal Netherlands Academy of Arts and Sciences, Amsterdam, Netherlands
Bernstein Center Freiburg and Faculty of Biology, University of Freiburg, Freiburg, Germany
Centre for Chronobiology, Psychiatric Hospital of the University of Basel (UPK), Basel, Switzerland

Eus J. W. Van Someren
Department of Sleep and Cognition, Netherlands Institute for Neuroscience (NIN), An Institute of the Royal Netherlands Academy of Arts and Sciences, Amsterdam, Netherlands
Department of Psychiatry, Amsterdam UMC, Vrije Universiteit Amsterdam, Amsterdam, Netherlands
Department of Integrative Neurophysiology, Center for Neurogenomics and Cognitive Research (CNCR), Amsterdam Neuroscience, Vrije Universiteit Amsterdam, Amsterdam, Netherlands

Xiaofen Ma, Guihua Jiang, Shishun Fu, Jin Fang, Yunfan Wu, Mengchen Liu and Tianyue Wang
Department of Medical Imaging, Guangdong Second Provincial General Hospital, Guangzhou, China

Guang Xu
Department of Neurology, Guangdong Second Provincial General Hospital, Guangzhou, China

Lei He, Lidan Fan, Yining Li, Jun Liu and Ru Yang
Department of Radiology, The Second Xiangya Hospital, Central South University, Changsha, China

Ping Li
Department of Radiology, The First Hospital of Hunan University of Chinese Medicine, Changsha, China

Jun Zhang
Hunan Judicial Police Academy, Changsha, China

Shucai Huang and Yuanyuan Dai
Department of Psychiatry, The Fourth People's Hospital of Wuhu, Wuhu, China

Zhixue Zhang, Lidan Fan and Jun Liu
Department of Medical Imaging, The Second Xiangya Hospital, Central South University, Changsha, China

Changcun Zhang
Pingtang Isolated Compulsory Drug Rehabilitation Center in Hunan Province, Changsha, China

Cheng Yang, Wei Hao and Hongxian Chen
Department of Psychiatry, The Second Xiangya Hospital, Central South University, Changsha, China
Hunan Key Laboratory of Psychiatry and Mental Health, Chinese National Clinical Research Center on Mental Disorders (Xiangya), Chinese National Technology Institute on Mental Disorders, Mental Health Institute of the Second Xiangya Hospital, Central South University, Changsha, China

Qiuxia Wu
Department of Psychiatry, The Second Xiangya Hospital, Central South University, Changsha, China
Mental Health Institute, The Second Xiangya Hospital, Central South University, Changsha, China
Chinese National Clinical Research Center on Mental Disorders, Second Xiangya Hospital, Central South University, Changsha, China
National Clinical Research Center on Mental Disorders, Changsha, China
National Technology Institute on Mental Disorders, Changsha, China
Hunan Key Laboratory of Psychiatry and Mental Health, Changsha, China
Department of Psychological Sciences, Texas Tech University, Lubbock, TX, United States

Zhixue Zhang
Department of Radiology, The Second Xiangya Hospital, Central South University, Changsha, China
Department of Radiology, The First Hospital of Hunan University of Chinese Medicine, Changsha, China

Chang Qi, Jiang Long, Yanhui Liao, Xuyi Wang, Wei Hao, Tieqiao Liu and Jinsong Tang
Department of Psychiatry, The Second Xiangya Hospital, Central South University, Changsha, China
Mental Health Institute, The Second Xiangya Hospital, Central South University, Changsha, China
Chinese National Clinical Research Center on Mental Disorders, Second Xiangya Hospital, Central South University, Changsha, China
National Clinical Research Center on Mental Disorders, Changsha, China
National Technology Institute on Mental Disorders, Changsha, China
Hunan Key Laboratory of Psychiatry and Mental Health, Changsha, China

An Xie and Jianbin Liu
Department of Radiology, Hunan Provincial People's Hospital, Changsha, China

Yiyuan Tang
Department of Psychological Sciences, Texas Tech University, Lubbock, TX, United States

Baozhu Yang
Department of Psychiatry, Yale University School of Medicine, New Haven, CT, United States

Huixia Zhou
Center on Ageing Psychology, CAS Key Laboratory of Mental Health, Institute of Psychology, Beijing, China
Department of Psychology, University of Chinese Academy of Sciences, Beijing, China

Bibing Dai
Center on Ageing Psychology, CAS Key Laboratory of Mental Health, Institute of Psychology, Beijing, China
Institute of Psychology, Tianjin Medical University, Tianjin, China

Juan Li
Center on Ageing Psychology, CAS Key Laboratory of Mental Health, Institute of Psychology, Beijing, China
Department of Psychology, University of Chinese Academy of Sciences, Beijing, China
Magnetic Resonance Imaging Research Center, Institute of Psychology, Chinese Academy of Sciences, Beijing, China
State Key Laboratory of Brain and Cognitive Science, Institute of Biophysics, Chinese Academy of Sciences, Beijing, China

Sonja Rossi
Clinic for Hearing-, Speech- and Voice Disorders, Medical University of Innsbruck, Innsbruck, Austria

Wenhan Yang, Ru Yang, Jing Luo, Lei He and Jun Liu
Department of Radiology, Second Xiangya Hospital of Central South University, Changsha, China

Jun Zhang
Hunan Judicial Police Vocational College, Changsha, China

Feng Wu, Lingtao Kong and Yue Zhu
Department of Psychiatry, The First Affiliated Hospital of China Medical University, Shenyang, China

Qian Zhou
Department of Psychiatry, The First Affiliated Hospital of China Medical University, Shenyang, China
Shanghai Mental Health Center, Shanghai, China

Xiaowei Jiang
Department of Radiology, The First Affiliated Hospital of China Medical University, Shenyang, China
Brain Function Research Section, The First Affiliated Hospital of China Medical University, Shenyang, China

Miao Chang and Ke Xu
Department of Radiology, The First Affiliated Hospital of China Medical University, Shenyang, China

Yifang Zhou
Department of Gerontology, The First Affiliated Hospital of China Medical University, Shenyang, China

Yang Cao
Shenyang Mental Health Center, Shenyang, China

Fei Wang
Department of Psychiatry, The First Affiliated Hospital of China Medical University, Shenyang, China
Department of Radiology, The First Affiliated Hospital of China Medical University, Shenyang, China

Yanqing Tang
Department of Psychiatry, The First Affiliated Hospital of China Medical University, Shenyang, China
Department of Gerontology, The First Affiliated Hospital of China Medical University, Shenyang, China

Jiashu Yao
Department of Psychiatry, Sir Run Run Shaw Hospital, Hangzhou, China

Danmei Lv
School of Medcine, Zhejiang University, Hangzhou, China

Wei Chen
Department of Psychiatry, Sir Run Run Shaw Hospital, Hangzhou, China

Xiaomei Luo, Guanmao Chen, Shaojuan Qiu, Feng Chen, Zhangzhang Qi, Li Huang and Ying Wang
Medical Imaging Center, First Affiliated Hospital of Jinan University, Guangzhou, China
Institute of Molecular and Functional Imaging, Jinan University, Guangzhou, China

JiaYing Gong
Institute of Molecular and Functional Imaging, Jinan University, Guangzhou, China
The Sixth Affiliated Hospital of Sun Yat-sen University, Guangzhou, China

Lianping Zhao
Medical Imaging Center, First Affiliated Hospital of Jinan University, Guangzhou, China
Department of Radiology, Gansu Provincial Hospital, Lanzhou, China

Yishul Wei
Department of Sleep and Cognition, Netherlands Institute for Neuroscience, An Institute of the Royal Netherlands Academy of Arts and Sciences, Amsterdam, Netherlands

Tessa F. Blanken
Department of Sleep and Cognition, Netherlands Institute for Neuroscience, An Institute of the Royal Netherlands Academy of Arts and Sciences, Amsterdam, Netherlands
Department of Integrative Neurophysiology, Center for Neurogenomics and Cognitive Research, Amsterdam Neuroscience, Vrije Universiteit Amsterdam, Amsterdam, Netherlands

Eus J. W. Van Someren
Department of Sleep and Cognition, Netherlands Institute for Neuroscience, An Institute of the Royal Netherlands Academy of Arts and Sciences, Amsterdam, Netherlands
Department of Integrative Neurophysiology, Center for Neurogenomics and Cognitive Research, Amsterdam Neuroscience, Vrije Universiteit Amsterdam, Amsterdam, Netherlands
Department of Psychiatry, Amsterdam UMC, Vrije Universiteit Amsterdam, Amsterdam, Netherlands

Chun-Hong Liu
Beijing Hospital of Traditional Chinese Medicine, Beijing Institute of Traditional Chinese Medicine, Capital Medical University, Beijing, China
Beijing Key Laboratory of Mental Disorders, Department of Radiology, Beijing Anding Hospital, Capital Medical University, Beijing, China

Yanbin Jia, Shuming Zhong and Shunkai Lai
Department of Psychiatry, First Affiliated Hospital of Jinan University, Guangzhou, China

Jing Guo and Cun-Zhi Liu
Acupuncture and Moxibustion Department, Beijing Hospital of Traditional Chinese Medicine, Capital Medical University, Beijing, China

Shun-Li Lu, Li-Rong Tang and Chuan-Yue Wang
Beijing Key Laboratory of Mental Disorders, Department of Radiology, Beijing Anding Hospital, Capital Medical University, Beijing, China

Jin Fan
Department of Psychiatry, Icahn School of Medicine at Mount Sinai, New York, NY, United States

Lihong Wang
Department of Psychiatry, University of Connecticut Health Center, Farmington, CT, United States

Qing-Quan Liu
Beijing Hospital of Traditional Chinese Medicine, Beijing Institute of Traditional Chinese Medicine, Capital Medical University, Beijing, China

Xia-an Bi, Qian Xu, Qi Sun and Zhigang Wang
College of Information Science and Engineering, Hunan Normal University, Changsha, China

Xianhao Luo
College of Mathematics and Statistics, Hunan Normal University, Changsha, China

Ningzhi Gou, Zhening Liu, Yunzhi Pan, Xudong Chen, Haojuan Tao, Guowei Wu, Xuan Ouyang, Zheng Wang and Zhimin Xue
Mental Health Institute, Second Xiangya Hospital, Central South University, Changsha, China
Key Laboratory of Psychiatry and Mental Health of Hunan Province, The China National Clinical Research Center for Mental Health Disorders, National Technology Institute of Psychiatry, Changsha, China

Lena Palaniyappan
Departments of Psychiatry and Medical Biophysics & Robarts and Lawson Research Institutes, University of Western Ontario, London, ON, Canada

Mingding Li
Zhejiang University School of Medicine, Zhejiang University, Hangzhou, China

Taotao Dou
Department of Neurosurgery, The First affiliated Hospital of Xinjiang Medical University, Urumqi, China

Weidan Pu
Medical Psychological Center, Second Xiangya Hospital, Central South University, Changsha, China
Medical Psychological Institute of Central South University, Changsha, China

Carmen Domínguez-Baleón and Luis F. Gutiérrez-Mondragón
Licenciatura en Ciencias Genómicas, Centro de Ciencias Genómicas, Universidad Nacional Autónoma de México, Cuernavaca, Mexico

Adrián I.Campos-González and Miguel E. Rentería
Department of Genetics & Computational Biology, QIMR Berghofer Medical Research Institute, Brisbane, QLD, Australia
Faculty of Medicine, The University of Queensland, Herston, QLD, Australia

Yanhui Liao and Jinsong Tang
Department of Psychiatry, The Second Xiangya Hospital, Central South University, Changsha, China
Mental Health Institute, The Second Xiangya Hospital, Central South University, Changsha, China
National Clinical Research Center on Mental Disorders, Changsha, China
National Technology Institute on Mental Disorders, Changsha, China

Maritza Johnson
Department of Psychiatry and Biobehavioral Sciences, University of California, Los Angeles, Los Angeles, CA, United States

Chang Qi, Qiuxia Wu, Yan Zhang, Tieqiao Liu and Wei Hao
Department of Psychiatry, The Second Xiangya Hospital, Central South University, Changsha, China

An Xie and Jianbin Liu
Department of Radiology, The People's Hospital of Hunan Province, Changsha, China

Mei Yang
Department of Psychiatry and Biobehavioral Sciences, University of California, Los Angeles, Los Angeles, CA, United States
Department of Addiction Medicine, Shenzhen Mental Health Center, Shenzhen Kangning Hospital, Shenzhen, China

Maifang Huang
Kangda Voluntary Drug Rehabilitation Center, Changsha, China

Index

M

N

O

P

R

S

T

V

W

Printed in the USA
CPSIA information can be obtained
at www.ICGtesting.com
LVHW080736221023
761596LV00011B/2152